DIAGNOSTIC
ULTRASOUND
APPLIED TO
OBSTETRICS AND
GYNECOLOGY

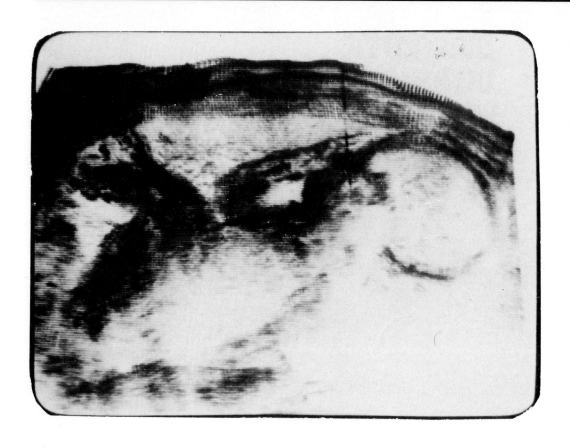

EDITED BY
RUDY E. SABBAGHA, M.D.

ASSOCIATE PROFESSOR OF OBSTETRICS AND GYNECOLOGY
DIRECTOR, DIAGNOSTIC ULTRASOUND CENTER
NORTHWESTERN UNIVERSITY MEDICAL SCHOOL
PRENTICE WOMEN'S HOSPITAL AND MATERNITY CENTER

WITH 29 CONTRIBUTING AUTHORS

DIAGNOSTIC ULTRASOUND

APPLIED TO OBSTETRICS AND GYNECOLOGY

HARPER & ROW, PUBLISHERS

HAGERSTOWN

CAMBRIDGE
NEW YORK
PHILADELPHIA
SAN FRANCISCO

LONDON
MEXICO CITY
SÃO PAULO
SYDNEY

1817

THIS BOOK IS DEDICATED TO
MY MENTOR T. TERRY HAYASHI, AND
TO MY FAMILY
FOR THEIR SUPPORT AND UNDERSTANDING.

ISBN 0-06-142310-6

Library of Congress Catalog Card Number 79-27666

3   5   6   4   2

Library of Congress Cataloging in Publication Data

Main entry under title:

Diagnostic ultrasound applied to obstetrics and
   gynecology.

   Includes index.
   1. Ultrasound in obstetrics.   2. Generative
organs, Female—Diseases—Diagnosis.   3. Diagnosis,
Ultrasonic. I. Sabbagha, Rudy E.
[DNLM: 1. Ultrasonics—Diagnostic use.
2. Pregnancy complications—Diagnosis.   3. Genital
diseases, Female—Diagnosis.   4. Obstetrics.
WP141   D536]
RG527.5.U48D48   618   79-27666

CONTENTS

CONTRIBUTORS

Usama Abdulla, M.B., Ch.B., MRCOG

Chapter 3
Senior Lecturer
Department of Obstetrics and Gynecology
University of Liverpool
Royal Liverpool Hospital
Prescot Street
Liverpool, England   L78XP

Alex A. Bezjian, M.D.

Chapters 20, 21
Associate Professor
Departments of Obstetrics and Gynecology,
   and Radiology
University of Miami Professional Art Center
1150 N.W. 14th Street
Miami, Florida   33136

James D. Bowie, M.D.

Chapter 22
Associate Professor of Radiology
Director, Division of Ultrasound
Duke University Medical Center
Durham, North Carolina 27710

Donn J. Brascho, M.D., FACR

Chapter 23
Professor and Vice-Chairman
Department of Radiation Oncology
University of Alabama
619 South 19th Street
Birmingham, Alabama   35233

Alan V. Cadkin, M.D.

Chapters 14, 21
Director of Ultrasound Section
Attending Physician
Department of Diagnostic Radiology
Michael Reese Hospital and Medical Center
University of Chicago
Pritzker School of Medicine
2929 South Ellis
Chicago, Illinois   60616

Ernest N. Carlsen, M.D., Ph.D.

Chapter 2
Director of Diagnostic Ultrasound
Loma Linda University School of Medicine
1899 Commere Center West
Suite 302
San Bernardino, California   92408

Allan G. Charles, M.D.

Chapter 17
Attending Physician and Clinical Professor
Department of Obstetrics and Gynecology
Michael Reese Hospital and Medical Center
30 N. Michigan Avenue, Suite 607
Chicago, Illinois   60616

Richard Depp, M.D.

Chapter 11
Director, Division of Obstetrics
Department of Obstetrics and Gynecology
Northwestern University Medical School
Prentice Women's Hospital and Maternity Center
333 East Superior Street
Chicago, Illinois   60611

Daniel I. Edelstone, M.D.

Chapter 16
Assistant Professor
Department of Obstetrics and Gynecology
University of Pittsburgh
Magee Women's Hospital
Forbes and Halket Street
Pittsburgh, Pennsylvania   15213

Sherman Elias, M.D.

Chapter 15
Co-Director, Clinical Genetics Services
Assistant Professor of Obstetrics and Gynecology
Department of Obstetrics and Gynecology
Northwestern University Medical School
Prentice Women's Hospital and Maternity Center
333 East Superior Street, Room 1102
Chicago, Illinois   60611

Harold E. Fox, M.D.

Chapter 18
Associate Professor of Clinical Obstetrics and
  Gynecology
College of Physicians and Surgeons of Columbia
  University
Medical Director, Western and Upper Manhattan
  Perinatal Network
Columbia Presbyterian Medical Center
630 W. 168th Street
New York, New York   10032

William J. Garrett, M.D., Ph.D., F.R.C.O.G

Chapter 4
Director
Department of Diagnostic Ultrasound
Royal Hospital for Women
Oxford Street
Paddington, Sydney, Australia

Y.B. Gordon, M.D., MRCOG, FCOG (SA)

Chapter 13
Senior Lecturer
Department of Obstetrics and Gynecology
Royal Free Hospital School of Medicine
University of London
Academic Department of Obstetrics and Gynecology
Royal Free Hospital, Pond Street
London   NW3 2QG

Charles R. Griffith, M.S., F.A.C.R.

Chapter 1
Adjunct Associate Professor
Radiological Science
Chicago Medical School
Chicago, Illinois

J.G. Grudzinskas, MRCOG

Chapter 13
WHO Research Fellow
Royal Free Hospital School of Medicine
University of London
Academic Department of Obstetrics and Gynecology
Royal Free Hospital, Pond Street
London   NW3 2QG

John C. Hobbins, M.D.

Chapter 12
Associate Professor of Obstetrics and
  Gynecology, and Diagnostic Radiology
Yale University School of Medicine
Department of Obstetrics and Gynecology
333 Cedar
New Haven, Connecticut   06510

Charles W. Hohler, M.D.

Chapter 25
Assistant Professor of Obstetrics and Gynecology
University of Southern California
Los Angeles County Women's Hospital
Los Angeles, California 90033

Michael John Hughey, M.D.

Chapters 5, 7
Assistant Attending Physician
Department of Obstetrics and Gynecology
Northwestern University Medical School
Evanston Hospital
2650 Ridge
Evanston, Illinois   60201

Elizabeth Kelly-Fry, ScM, EdD

Chapter 24
Associate Professor
Indiana University Hospital
Ultrasound Research Laboratory, Room A-32
1100 West Michigan Street
Indianapolis, Indiana   46202

Ingrid Kipper, R.T.

Chapter 6
Senior Medical Sonographer
Department of Diagnostic Ultrasound, Room 170
Northwestern University Medical School
Prentice Women's Hospital and Maternity Center
333 East Superior Street
Chicago, Illinois   60611

Frank A. Manning, M.D.

Chapter 28
Head, Division of Maternal-Fetal Medicine
University of Manitoba
Manitoba, Winnipeg, Canada

Sheridan N. Meyers, M.D.

Chapter 27
Assistant Professor of Medicine
Director of Cardiac Catheterization
  Laboratory
Department of Medicine
Northwestern University Medical School
Chicago, Illinois   60611

Martin N. Motew, M.D., F.A.C.O.G.

Chapter 17
Attending Physician
Assistant Clinical Professor
Department of Obstetrics and Gynecology
Michael Reese Hospital
30 N. Michigan Avenue, Suite 607
Chicago, Illinois   60611

Harvey L. Neiman, M.D.

Chapter 26
Associate Professor of Radiology
Chief, Angiography and Sectional Imaging
Department of Radiology
Northwestern Memorial Hospital
Wesley Pavilion
250 East Superior Street
Chicago, Illinois 60611

Lawrence D. Platt, M.D.

Chapter 28
Assistant Professor
Division of Maternal-Fetal Medicine
Department of Obstetrics and Gynecology
Los Angeles County/USC Medical Center
Los Angeles, California   90033

Rudy E. Sabbagha, M.D., F.A.C.O.G.

Chapters 6, 9 (with Tamura), 8, 10, 19, 14 (with Cadkin),
*   21 (with Bezjian and Cadkin)*
Associate Professor of Obstetrics and
    Gynecology
Director, Diagnostic Ultrasound Center
Northwestern University Medical School
Prentice Women's Hospital and Maternity Center
333 East Superior Street
Chicago, Illinois   60611

Joe Leigh Simpson, M.D.

Chapter 15
Head, Section of Human Genetics
Department of Obstetrics and Gynecology
Northwestern University Medical School
Prentice Women's Hospital and Maternity Center
333 East Superior Street
Chicago, Illinois   60611

James V. Talano, M.D.

Chapter 27
Associate Professor of Medicine
Department of Medicine
Northwestern University Medical School
Chicago, Illinois   60611

Ralph K. Tamura, M.D.

Chapter 9
Fellow, Maternal and Fetal Medicine
Department of Obstetrics and Gynecology
Northwestern University Medical School
Prentice Women's Hospital and Maternity Center
333 East Superior Street
Chicago, Illinois   60611

PREFACE

In the past decade impressive technological advances have led to the development of refined sonar equipment with capabilities extending to gray-scale and real-time imaging. During the same time the usefulness of ultrasound as a diagnostic tool in a wide variety of clinical situations has been extensively researched. As a result, the medical literature dealing with ultrasound is, at present, enormous.

This book was conceived with the intent of including all of the applications of sonography to the field of obstetrics and gynecology, in one volume. The first two chapters, however, deal with basic physics and ultrasound instrumentation. Echograms of fetal organs are then shown to illustrate the resolution of modern sonar equipment.

Subsequently, the ultrasonic methods used to define gestational age and fetal growth are analyzed in depth. For example, some of the issues discussed pertain to the reasons for discrepancies apparent in charts used to relate fetal biparietal diameter to the length of gestation—the use of a standard chart to assess fetal development is stressed. In addition, a coherent plan of identifying the growth patterns of symmetric and asymmetric intrauterine-growth-retarded fetuses is presented, and the methodology leading to antenatal recognition of fetuses at high risk for macrosomia is described.

Recent observations relating fetal biophysical characteristics (such as breathing, movement, and tone) to fetal well-being suggest that pregnancies can also be evaluated by the assessment of fetal dynamic functions using real-time imaging—these areas are adequately covered.

The usefulness of ultrasound in helping physicians manage urgent and difficult obstetrical problems is addressed separately. Further, a comparison of the value of a variety of antenatal tests used to evaluate fetal status is made.

The ultrasonic characteristics of abnormal pregnancies including hydatidiform mole are presented in detail. Similarly, the entity of placenta previa is completely described. A rationale is also formulated for using ultrasound to localize the placenta and the fetus prior to amniocentesis and intrauterine transfusion. The diagnosis of fetal congenital anomalies by sonography and the use of ultrasound to differentiate between true- and false-positive elevations of α-fetoprotein are allotted a separate chapter.

The ultrasound diagnosis of pelvic masses, including the differentiation between ovarian and uterine tumors associated with pregnancy, is outlined in Chapters 20 through 22. The application of sonography to the specialized field of gynecologic oncology is presented in Chapter 23.

Three chapters are devoted to cover the state of the art in echography of the breast, heart, abdomen, neck and extremities, because the specialist in obstetrics and gynecology should be in a position to know how ultrasound is used for the diagnosis of abnormalities outside the pelvis.

Finally, the extent to which pregnancies are examined by real-time imaging within the confines of the private offices of obstetricians and gynecologists is examined.

As I look at the whole manuscript, I cannot but feel a deep sense of gratitude to all the contributors for the time they spent in the preparation of their respective chapters. I am also very grateful to David Hampton, M.S. for the many hours he devoted to the statistical analysis of a large segment of the data presented in many areas of the book. Additionally, my appreciation goes to Scott and Kathryn Sisson and to Cindy Tinnes for their splendid contributions to the artwork displayed in the book. Finally, I am indebted to my administrative assistant Colleen Nelson and to the publishers for their relentless attention to detail.

Rudy E. Sabbagha, M.D.

1

Basic physics

CHARLES R. GRIFFITH

Sound, like x-ray, is a phenomenon for the transfer of energy. Unlike x-rays, however, which can travel through a vacuum, sound must have matter through which to pass. Sound waves are actually vibrations, and the matter present vibrates to transmit the sound waves and produce sound.

This vibration represents one of the most important physical factors related to sound—frequency. **Frequency** is the number of vibrations of the material per unit of time. The unit of frequency is the hertz (Hz). One hertz is equal to one vibration (cycle) per second. The characteristic frequency of a given material causes air particles to vibrate and carry energy to the receptive ear, and this results in hearing.

The normal human hearing range is from 20 to 20,000 (20K) hertz (Hz). Frequencies well above human hearing range, in the order of 1–20 million (20M) Hz, are used for diagnostic ultrasound studies (Fig. 1–1). Different frequencies are required, depending on certain anatomic characteristics.

The ringing of a bell provides a good example of the basic characteristics of sound. The bell represents the transducer, or the producer of the sound. When a bell is struck with a hammer, an impulse is created within the bell. This impulse results in the bell's vibration. Based on its design, the bell vibrates with a given frequency or pitch. Differently designed bells produce different frequencies. Characteristic frequencies cause characteristic sounds to be produced.

Since various ultrasound procedures depend on certain anatomic characteristics' requiring different frequencies to be used, different transducers must be available for different procedures. Transducer characteristics are discussed later.

CHARACTERISTICS OF THE SOUND WAVES

Sound travels through material by causing it to vibrate. As was already discussed, sound has a frequency characteristic of the material used to generate the sound. The movement of each particle of matter as it vibrates back and forth is the amplitude of the sound strength and is referred to as the **sound pressure.**

As Figure 1–2 illustrates, the sound from the transducer compresses the material adjacent to the transducer. This material then expands, owing to its elasticity, and compresses adjacent material. This process continues as sound moves through the material. Thus, sound moves through material in a series of compressions and expansions. The frequency of these compressions and expansions is determined by the transducer. The pressure applied to the material is determined by the strength of the transducer pulse. For example, if the bell mentioned before is hit with a light hammer blow (pulse), it rings with a given frequency (pitch) but is not very loud. If the bell is struck with a heavy hammer, it

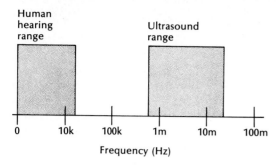

FIG. 1-1. Frequency associated with human hearing and that used in diagnostic ultrasound.

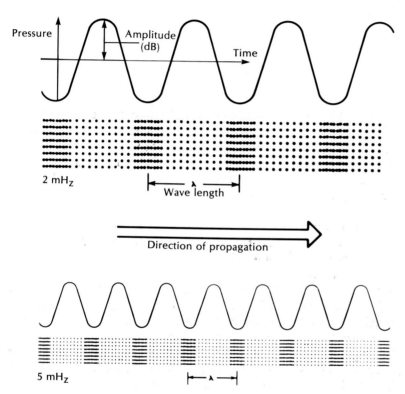

FIG. 1-2. Sound transmission by compression and expansion of the medium through which it travels.

again rings with the given frequency but much louder. The loudness illustrates the pressure and is determined by the force of the hammer blow.

Again referring to Figure 1–2, we plot the pressure of the sound as it travels through matter. We see that a typical sine curve function is created, similar to the characteristic curve of x-rays.

The height of the curve above the base line is the pressure or amplitude of the sound beam. Sound beam amplitude of echo (A_2) is measured in decibels (dB). Incident initial amplitude is (A_1).

$$dB = 20 \log \frac{A_1}{A_2}$$

The length of one complete cycle as shown is referred to as one wavelength and represented by the symbol λ.

The velocity of the sound wave through matter depends on the material itself and not the sound. We find that there is a relationship between frequency (μ), velocity (c), and the wavelength (λ). This relationship is expressed in the equation: $c = \lambda \cdot \mu$. Table 1–1 lists the velocity of sound in various anatomic materials.

It should be remembered that the equipment bases its depth indication on the average sound velocity in soft tissue of 1540 m/sec. The differences in depth indications for sound traveling through other tissue types will be a little in error, but this error is very small and usually may be disregarded.

TRANSDUCERS

The transducer, our bell in the previous example, is the [unit that physically produces the sound pulse.] As such, it is an important component of the total system. The frequency of the sound is characteristic of the transducer used; therefore, several transducers should be available to supply different frequencies for different functions.

The heart of the transducer is a piezoelectric crystal. These crystals have a very interesting property that makes them vital to the production of sound. When a potential of 300–700 volts is applied across the crystal, it expands slightly. After the potential is turned off, the crystal returns to normal size. When the polarity of the potential is reversed, the crystal contracts slightly. (Fig. 1–3) The expansion and contraction creates a pressure wave when in physical contact with the skin. This is an ultrasound beam created by the crystal, and it travels into tissue. When a reflection, or echo, returns and strikes the crystal with a slight pressure, a small voltage is created at the electrodes.

Thus, the function of the piezoelectric crystal is to create the ultrasound beam by an applied potential and also to create a potential when an echo returns to the crystal. The greater the amplitude of the echo, the greater the pressure on

TABLE 1-1. VELOCITY OF SOUND IN VARIOUS ANATOMIC MATERIALS

Tissue	Velocity (m/sec)
Blood	1570
Fat	1450
Brain	1541
Liver	1549
Kidney	1561
Muscle	1585
Lens of eye	1620
Skull, bone	4080
Lung (air)	331

the crystal, and more voltage is generated by the crystal, which represents the amplitude of the returning echo.

The characteristic frequency of the crystal is determined primarily by the thickness of the crystal. When a given crystal is excited by an electrical impulse, it rings owing to internal resonance, again similar to a bell's being struck by a hammer.

As shown in Figure 1–4, the piezoelectric crystal is encased with an acoustic backing that permits the absorption of the sound emitted in the opposite direction. The package shown in the drawing is the transducer.

CHARACTERISTICS OF THE SOUND BEAM

The sound beam emitted from the face of the transducer is affected by two factors, namely, the diameter of the piezoelectric crystal and the wavelength of the sound beam. The beam of sound emitted from the transducer is divided into two definite areas of interest: the near zone (Fresnal Zone); and the far zone (Fraunhofer Zone).

FIG. 1–3. Piezoelectric phenomenon of crystals used in ultrasound.

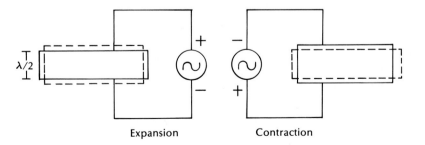

Expansion   Contraction

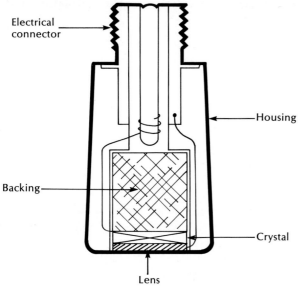

Electrical connector

Housing

Backing

Crystal

Lens

FIG. 1–4. Typical ultrasound transducer.

The typical compression wave emitted from the face of the crystal is composed of many waves emitted from the many parts of the crystal surface, as if the crystals themselves were made up of many small individual crystals. These many waves due to reinforcement caused by in-phase, coincident compressions create a common wave front. This common wave front tends to move in a cylindrical path approximately the diameter of the crystal and constitutes the near zone (Fresnal Zone). The depth of the cylindrical near zone is determined by the equation:

$$D = \frac{R^2}{\lambda}.$$

D = Near zone depth (cm)
R = Radius of transducer (cm)
λ = Wavelength (cm)

In Table 1–2 it is evident that, with a fixed radius, the higher the frequency (smaller wavelength), the greater the near zone depth. Similarly, with a fixed frequency, the greater the radius, the greater the near zone depth.

At the point where the near zone ends and the far zone begins, the sound beam starts to spread. The spread of the beam in the far zone (Fraunhofer Zone) is found by using the equation:

$$\sin \theta = \frac{0.61\lambda}{R}$$

θ = Angle of spread, degrees
λ = Wavelength (cm)
R = Radius of transducer (cm)

In Table 1–3 it is seen, on the basis of this equation and with a fixed transducer radius, that the higher the frequency (smaller wavelength), the lesser the beam spread. Also, at a fixed frequency, as the radius increases, the spread of the beam decreases.

Consequently, the crystal diameter and the

TABLE 1-2. FRESNAL ZONE DEPTH $D = \frac{R^2}{\lambda}$

As a function of frequency (transducer diameter constant at 1 cm)

Frequency (MHz)	Wavelength (cm)	Zone Depth (cm)
0.5	0.30	0.83
1.0	0.15	1.67
2.0	0.075	3.33
4.0	0.0325	7.80
8.0	0.0163	15.33

As a function of transducer diameter (frequency constant at 1.5MHz)

Diameter (cm)		Zone Depth (cm)
0.5		0.6
1.0		2.5
2.0		10.0
4.0		40.0

Table 1-3. ANGLE OF SPREAD OF ULTRASONIC BEAMS IN WATER
Relationship: Sin $\Theta = \dfrac{.61\lambda}{R}$

As a function of frequency (transducer diameter = 1 cm)

Frequency (MHz)	Spread angle (degrees)
0.5	21.5
1.0	10.5
2.0	5.2
4.0	2.3
8.0	1.1

As a function of transducer diameter (frequency = 1.5 MHz)

Diameter (cm)	Spread angle (deg)
0.5	14.1
1.0	7.0
2.0	3.5
4.0	1.7

frequency of the sound are the two main variables that must be understood so that the proper transducer is used for the part of the body to be examined.

INTERACTION OF THE SOUND BEAM IN THE BODY

The transducer and some of the sound beam properties being understood, now consider how the sound beam travels through tissue and interacts with specific tissues. As sound travels through a medium, it loses sound intensity or is attenuated. Attenuation may occur owing to the absorption of the sound in the material and also to the scattering of the sound, again a direct result of the material.

The attenuation can be expressed by the equation:

$$I_x = I_o e^{-2ax}$$

I_o = Initial sound intensity (watts/cm^2)
I_x = Intensity at depth × (watts/cm^2)
e = Base of natural logs
x = Depth in tissue (cm)
a = Amplitude absorption coefficient

Interestingly, in this equation the absorption coefficient (a) of a given material increases as the frequency of the sound increases. As the equation illustrates, the total depth possible is inversely related to the frequency. Consequently,

for a deep penetration, a lower frequency must be used, and for a very small depth, a high frequency should be used.

Loss of intensity by absorption is the most important aspect of attenuation and should be given special consideration. The absorption loss resulting from sound energy's moving through tissue is given by the following equation:

$$S = \frac{20 \log \dfrac{A_o}{A_x}}{x}$$

S = Absorption (dB/cm)
A_o = Amplitude at zero depth (dB)
A_x = Amplitude at depth x (dB)
x = Depth in tissue (cm)

According to the equation, sound absorption in tissue is approximately 1 dB loss/cm/MHz (see Table 1–4).

TABLE 1-4. ATTENUATION OF ULTRASOUND BEAMS IN BIOLOGIC MATERIALS

Tissue	Mean db cm^{-1} MHz^{-1}
Blood	0.18
Fat	0.63
Brain	0.85
Liver	0.94
Kidney	1.00
Muscle	1.30
Lens of eye	2.00
Skull, bone	20
Lung (air)	41

ACOUSTIC IMPEDANCE

Acoustic impedance is probably the most important factor in this discussion of ultrasound.

Acoustic impedance is one of the factors that determines the amount of sound energy reflected from, or transmitted through, different body materials. Acoustic impedance (z) is determined by the density (p) of the material and the velocity (c) of the sound through the material.

$$Z = pc$$

Table 1–5 lists the acoustic impedance of some of the common biological materials of the body.

**TABLE 1–5. ACOUSTIC IMPEDANCES OF
BIOLOGICAL MATERIALS**

Material	Characteristic impedance $(\text{gm cm}^{-2}\text{sec}^{-1}) \times 10^{-3}$
Water	1.48
Fat	1.38
Brain	1.58
Blood	1.61
Kidney	1.62
Human tissue	1.63
Spleen	1.64
Liver	1.65
Muscle	1.70
Lens of eye	1.84
Bone, skull	7.80

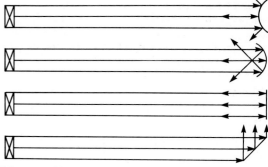

FIG. 1–5. The reflectivity (echo) produced by different boundary surfaces.

Sound traveling through material continues until it comes to another material of a different impedance. Two adjacent materials of different acoustic impedance establish an acoustic boundary. Depending on the impedance of each material, a reflection occurs.

When the incident sound beam is perpendicular to this acoustic boundary or interface, an echo results based on the following equation:

$$R = \left[\frac{Z_2 - Z_1}{Z_2 + Z_1} \right]^2 \times 100$$

R = Percent of sound beam reflected
Z_1 = Acoustic impedance of one material
Z_2 = Acoustic impedance of second material

Also at each interface, a certain percentage of the beam is transmitted across the acoustic boundary. The percentage transmission also depends on the acoustic impedance of the material on each side of the boundary. The following equation gives the amount of sound transmitted through the boundary:

$$T = \frac{4Z_2 \cdot Z_1}{[Z_2 + Z_1]^2} \times 100$$

T = Percent of sound beam transmitted

The total reflected and transmitted at a boundary must equal 100%: $R + T = 100$.

In these calculations it is assumed that the beam is perpendicular to the acoustic boundary. In actual practice on the human body, however, this is sometimes difficult. One must, therefore, appreciate the fact that a boundary not perpendicular to the beam axis will reflect a greater per-centage than this equation indicates. Also, the reflected beam is not directed back to the transducer but follows the laws of optics, which state that the angle of reflection is equal to the angle of incidence. Figure 1–5 shows how the sound beam is reflected from various surfaces in the body. The technologist operating the transducer must appreciate this and realize that the transducer must always be perpendicular to the acoustic boundary before a signal (echo) can be detected and recorded.

RESOLUTION

The importance of transducer characteristics and the interaction of sound with tissue is better understood when we discuss the system's resolution capabilities.

Resolution is the capability of a system to demonstrate two points of information (acoustic boundary) that lie parallel to the beam (axial resolution) or that lie perpendicular to the beam (lateral resolution). The closer these two points can be resolved, the better the resolution of the system. Resolution is expressed in millimeters (mm). If a system has the capabilities to resolve 5 mm, two boundaries 5 mm apart are detected as two echoes in the image. If the two boundaries are closer than 5 mm, only one echo results.

AXIAL RESOLUTION

Axial resolution is the resolution along the path of the sound beam. Axial resolution, then, is the capability of a system to see boundaries directly behind each other. It is mainly determined by the time duration of each pulse. The sound beam is not continuous but is a series of pulses less than 5% of the time, the transducer actually listening for returning echoes more than 95% of the time. Each pulse is about 1 microsecond (one millionth of a second) in duration. If the sound pulse is on for 1 μsec and the sound is traveling at 1540 m/sec in tissue, then: 1 μsec × 1540 meter/sec = 1.54 mm, this representing the length of the sound pulse.

An analysis of this reveals that the axial resolution can be no better than one-half the pulse length (Fig. 1–6). Therefore, for this situation with a 1 μsec pulse, the best resolution possible would be 1.54 mm/2 = 0.77 mm.

Another basic rule is that axial resolution cannot be better than one wavelength. Knowing the frequency of the transducer and using sound velocity of 1540m/sec, one can use the equation $\lambda = \mu/c$ to determine wavelength.

Example: A 3.5-MHz transducer will produce a 0.44-mm wavelength.

Therefore, as frequency increases, resolution also increases. This is a theoretical increase because there are other limiting factors on resolution, such as the recording and display monitors. Often the transducer may be capable of a given resolution, but the oscilloscope or the TV moni-

FIG. 1–6. Axial resolution determined by the effect of pulse length. If the lines A and B are separated by a distance greater than one-half the pulse length (L), both the echoes from A and B will be seen separately with no overlap. The second drawing shows lines A and B separated by less than half the pulse length and the echoes from A and B overlap and appear as one echo.

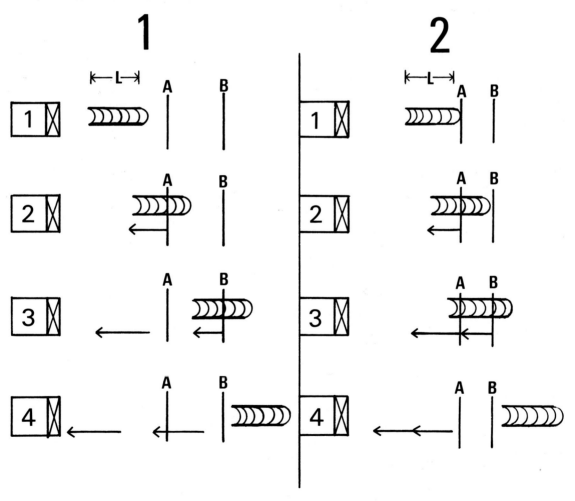

tor cannot display it. When contemplating the purchase of new equipment, be certain of the displayed resolution, as well as of the resolution of the transducer.

LATERAL RESOLUTION

Lateral resolution refers to the ability of the system to resolve two acoustic boundaries that lie perpendicular to the axis of the sound beam. Lateral resolution is limited to the beam width at a given depth. Two acoustic boundaries closer together than the width of the sound beam produce only a single echo, whereas if the two boundaries are farther apart than the beam width, then both boundaries produce echoes and can be visualized. Figure 1–7 demonstrates this principle.

Beam width is affected by several factors discussed earlier in this chapter. Recall that sound can be focused and therefore plastic lenses can be used in conjunction with the piezoelectric crystal to give the smallest beam width at the focal point of the lens used.

Obviously, lateral resolution is not as good as axial resolution, and it is, therefore, the limiting factor of the total transducer resolution.

IMAGE DISPLAY MODES

As has been discussed up to this point, an ultrasound beam directed into the body, on the basis of all the parameters discussed, results in an echo at an acoustic interface and, if the geometry is correct, returns to the transducer and produces a small electrical pulse. This small electrical signal is amplified and passed on to an oscilloscope or some other device for visual display.

Instrumentation for producing the sound and for displaying the visual pulse is discussed in Chapter 2. To complete the basic discussion in this chapter, however, a brief description of the several modes of echo display follows.

Image display modes can be limited to four basic modes: A-mode, B-mode, M-mode, and B-scan.

A-MODE DISPLAY (AMPLITUDE MODULATION)

After being amplified, the returning echoes are displayed on an oscilloscope screen. An oscilloscope is a device that displays the amplitude of an electrical signal on the vertical axis while the moving base-time line sweeps across the screen. The speed of sweep of the base-time line (hori-

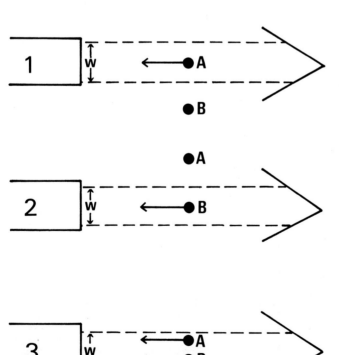

FIG. 1–7. Lateral resolution is determined by beam width. If points A and B are separated by a distance greater than the beam width, two echoes are seen on the monitor. If the distance between A and B is less than the beam width, then only a single echo is recorded.

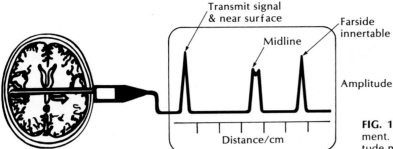

FIG. 1-8. Pulse echo, midline measurement. A-mode display based on amplitude modulation of the returning echoes.

zontal axis) is calibrated to correspond to the speed of sound in tissue (1540 m/sec). Therefore, the position of the displayed echo along the base-time line indicates the position of the acoustic boundary within the body.

The height of the echo signal on the vertical axis is directly proportional to the amplitude of the returning echo—hence, the name A-mode (amplitude modulation). The greater the amplitude of the echo, the higher the signal presented on the oscilloscope. Figure 1-8 demonstrates A-mode.

A-mode is useful for making measurements along a single line of sight of the transducer and for assessing the consistency of tissue along that line. Both the transducer and the reflecting surfaces are stationary.

B-MODE DISPLAY (BRIGHTNESS [INTENSITY] MODULATION)

In B-mode display, echoes appear as dots along the invisible time-base. B-mode is practically the same as A-mode, except the pulses are shown as dots instead of spikes (Fig. 1-9).

M-MODE DISPLAY (INTENSITY MODULATION)

M-mode (intensity modulation) is known as time-motion presentation. Echoes are displayed as dots along the horizontal time-base line, and their strength is indicated by the brightness rather than by amplitude. The display sweeps across the screen in a direction perpendicular to the time-base to add the dimension of time and thus chart the motion of the individual echoes. This mode is useful in tracking moving structures such as the heart, components of the heart,

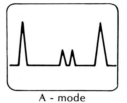

A - mode

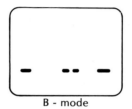

B - mode

echo motion

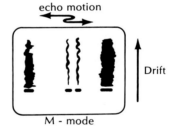

Drift

M - mode

Drifting the invisible baseline up the screen gives graphic presentation of moving echoes

FIG. 1-9. A-mode, B-mode, and M-mode display of the returning echoes.

and the great vessels. In M-mode the transducer position remains stationary. The echo-producing surface is moving (Fig. 1-9).

B-SCAN

B-scan combines a B-mode type of display on an axial moving time-base line. B-scan is produced by using the B-mode type of display and

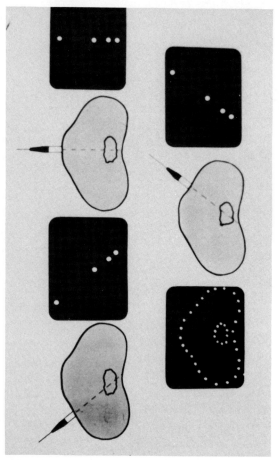

sweeping the transducer across the area of interest, producing a tomographic effect. In B-scan, an exact electronic positioning procedure must be used to maintain the invisible time-base line of the monitor to be in the exact same position as the transducer, or sound beam axis.

This procedure is extremely useful in producing outlines of organs and mass, and also the consistency and density variations within (Fig. 1–10).

The foregoing discussion of physics is basic. It is intended to give the reader some of the fundamentals of ultrasound so that the material presented in this book will be better understood.

It is highly recommended that both the physician and the technologist read more extensively on the physics of ultrasound. Such reading will aid each in a better understanding of the procedures involved and the principles of this rapidly expanding new means of diagnosis.

FIG. 1–10. B-scan display using B-mode plus an axial moving time-base line synchronized with the transducer position.

2

Ultrasound instrumentation

ERNEST N. CARLSEN

Ultrasound instrumentation has proliferated during the recent past. Several types of apparatus have been introduced for diagnostic purposes. General approaches to two-dimensional ultrasound imaging are discussed, but no attempt is made to judge the various claims made by manufacturers regarding the performance characteristics of the instruments.

If any judgment is applied it relates to issues such as simplicity of operation, reproducibility, clarity of anatomy, and economic impact.

The discussion presents the technology and application of ultrasound instrumentation not only for the large imaging laboratories but also for the office practice.

GENERAL INSTRUMENTATION PRINCIPLES

The basic ultrasound instrument consists of components that can generally be compartmentalized. The minimum requirements of the instrument are a transmitter, transducer, receiver, and display (oscilloscope) (Fig. 2-1). To provide a two-dimensional image, the instrument requires a sensing mechanism to determine location and direction of the sound beam (Fig. 2–2). A brief description of all the components that contribute to the resolution of the image is presented. There is virtually no difference in concept of the components, whether they are for

static imaging or real-time imaging ultrasound instrumentation.

THE TRANSMITTER

The transmitter provides the electrical impulse that strikes the piezoelectric crystal of the transducer to provide the packet of sound transmitted into the tissue. The magnitude, time period, and shape of the voltage are carefully matched to the transducer. Axial resolution is determined in part by the pulsing circuitry and the characteristics of the transducer.

THE RECEIVER

The main purpose of the receiver is to amplify the echo information. The sound wave returning to the transducer is changed to an electrical charge by the piezoelectric crystal. From these very small electrical signals the amplifier multiplies the signals to a size that can be then processed. The amplification of the receiver, including the time gain compensation amplification, must be in the range of 100–120 db of noise-free amplifcation for modern grey-scale systems. This is to provide good display of the soft-echo information from deep within the body. Continued improvement in amplifier design has led to amplifiers that not only are quiet but also have good frequency response. This means that the amplifier must have the ability to

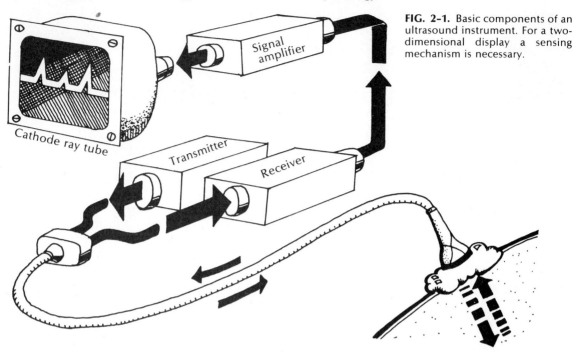

FIG. 2-1. Basic components of an ultrasound instrument. For a two-dimensional display a sensing mechanism is necessary.

amplify large- and small-echo information accurately as well as to process information from different frequency transducers. The receiver electronics also relate to the axial resolution of the system.

SIGNAL PROCESSING

The purpose of grey-scale ultrasound imaging is to provide an image in which the pattern, distribution, and amplitude of the internal echoes can be assessed easily. A term that can be applied to this is contrast resolution. Typically the data obtained from the tissues range from 80 to 100 db. Since most systems can display only 10–20 db of information, a logarithmic compression curve is applied to the data to provide contrast resolution and meaningful information to the diagnostician.

STORAGE GRAY-SCALE IMAGING

The backbone of two-dimensional ultrasound instrumentation has been the contact grey-scale instrument. Its proliferation was due to the quality of its image reproducibility and its relative

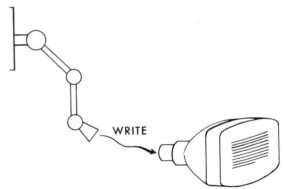

FIG. 2-2. Articulated contact arm of a B-scan system translates the location and direction of the sound beam for presentation on the video screen.

simplicity of operation compared with previous instrumentation. The heart of the display system is a scan converter. This may be an analog system or a digital system.

ANALOG SCAN CONVERTERS

The analog unit has the ability to store approximately 32 levels of grey-scale information in a matrix of approximately 1000 × 1000. The construction of the scan converter tube is similar to that of an oscilloscope tube in which the electrons from the cathode ray gun are directed at the target by beam deflection plates. The functions of the scan converter are to receive spatial data, record and display the data, and provide amplitude information. The data may be added to or erased. Silicon crystals are used as the storage medium. The data are generally displayed in a television format.

In the evaluation of the analog scan converter the following two major limitations were noted early in its use: background nonuniformity and overwrite. These have been greatly reduced in the present systems and are a major limitation to the storage and processing of the information. The longevity of the analog system remains undetermined.

DIGITAL SCAN CONVERTERS AND MEMORIES

More recently digital memories have been introduced to ultrasound. The size of the matrix and depth of the memory (shades of gray) are currently controlled by economics. The price of acceptable memory size is still mildly prohibitive but is becoming less every year. Their use has been the same as that of the analog systems—the recording and displaying of spatial and amplitude data. To date, no computer enhancement techniques have been developed to make the data more easy to perceive.

The data from tissues are apparently not in a simple relationship but in a complex measure. Tissue interrogation by the ultrasound beam provides the returning echo information in regard to the changes in tissue density and/or elasticity. These are not absolute terms, but they provide a local reference between information points that is much more easily perceived by the human eye than by computers. Specialized programs for making the data more perceptible may make the computer more than just an intelligent operator.

Presently, good gray-scale imaging, whether static or real time, depends on instrumentation that has wide band amplifiers and good signal-to-noise ratios. This provides for adequate amplification of the sound wave from deep within the body.

We analyze the future from the points of view that the instrumentation must be developed to provide reproducibility and yet remain simple to operate, and the anatomy presented should be more easily recognized, and if possible, tissure signatures should be employed in the diagnosis.

TRENDS IN ULTRASOUND INSTRUMENTATION FOR OBSTETRIC-GYNECOLOGIC USE

TRANSDUCERS

Future improvements in diagnostic ultrasound will certainly continue to center around the transducer design, as well as the electronics of the system. Two improvements in transducer design can be expected. One is the improvement in sensitivity, and the other is the development of narrower beam profile. (Improved sensitivity generally means improvement in our ability to evaluate the signal from the far field.) Generally more sensitivity also means the ability to use higher frequency transducers to provide imaging to the same depth as older instrumentation. With higher frequency the axial resolution is improved, but more importantly, lateral resolution is improved. (The higher frequency is less diverging and more tightly focused, which results in better lateral resolution.) A general adage that holds true is "For better resolution use transducers that are focused in the zone of interest and use the highest frequency that will penetrate to the desired depth."

REAL-TIME ULTRASOUND

Real-time ultrasound is a slight misnomer. It is very rapid scanning in which the speed of sound limits line density, frame rate, and field of view. Each pulse of sound must still pass into the tissues and the echoes return before a new pulse can be started. For each given area to be viewed, therefore, one can calculate the maximum number of lines for any given frame rate when the depth of the image is known.

Several means have been developed for increasing the line rate of the display. One method of increasing the visual acceptability of the

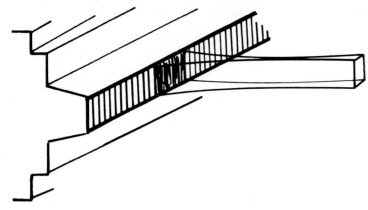

FIG. 2-3. Linear-array system. The line density is improved by pulsing a group of small crystals together and then moving down one element of the array with each pulse.

image is to interlace the line of the image informations contained in two or more frames. Another method is to interpolate information digitally to fill in the space between the true lines of data. These methods are currently under development and in some instances appear to improve the apparent resolution of the system.

TYPES OF REAL-TIME INSTRUMENTATION

Real-time ultrasound instrumentation can be classified in several ways. One method is to classify by the method of obtaining two-dimensional images.

LINEAR ARRAYS

The general concept of a sequenced linear array is that each of the transducer elements is pulsed separately in a sequential manner. The image is formed by B-mode presentation of each individual line. By the appropriate rapid switching the image is continuously updated to provide a dynamic display.

To correct the problem of beam divergence, the crystals have to be large to produce an adequate aperture that decreases the line density of the resulting image, though this creates poor line density.

To improve the line density of the image, the crystals can be reduced in size and then pulsed in a group, sequentially moving down one element of the array with each pulsing (Fig. 2–3). Even-

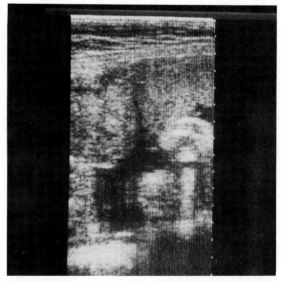

FIG. 2-4. Image illustrating a linear-array image. A view through the fundus demonstrating the location of the placenta.

odd grouping of elements has further increased the line density. This feature, along with focusing of the beam, has been introduced with linear arrays.

To date, all these features have been tested clinically and have improved the image quality of the linear arrays. In addition digital memories have added the capability of stop framing, which is very useful in diagnosis. Anatomy can be clarified in a still frame, and this reduces the number of poor photographs taken (Fig. 2–4).

In considering the linear array in the abdomen the major problems are encountered because of ribs and gas. Ribs tend to create poor contact and/or obscure detail by shadowing. In obstetrics the only real limitation involves viewing the lower uterine segment in late pregnancy.

For gynecologic uses, gas in the abdomen causes total loss of information beyond the gas; consequently, limited views of the anatomy are often produced. The array can, however, be used to massage the gas away from an area of interest, and in many instances adequate acoustic windows can be attained. This, along with a full bladder, provides the best approach to the problem.

The true value of the linear array is certainly in its lower cost and mobility. With high-frequency transducers adequate resolution for good diagnosis may well be achieved. The high-frequency array is valuable in superficial organs and vessels such as the breast and femoral-iliac vessels.

SECTOR SCANNERS

Sector scanners produce an image that is generally listed in degrees of a sector and depth. The displays vary from 30° to 120° sectors with depths between 5 and 20 cm. The same problems explained about line density and frame rate exist in sector scanners except that they vary with depth and scan angle. The information lines radiate out from a point at the transducer (Fig. 2–5).

The advantages of sector scanners are related to ease of access to structures where it is difficult to find a good acoustic window, such as around ribs or through gas. Because the transducer is very maneuverable, it provides freedom of movement for locating often very small acoustical windows. The sector can then be adjusted to look beneath the superficial obstructions. The disadvantages of these scanners are in the aperture size of the transducers and the general lack of focus variability in all planes. The field of view at the surface is also very small and often

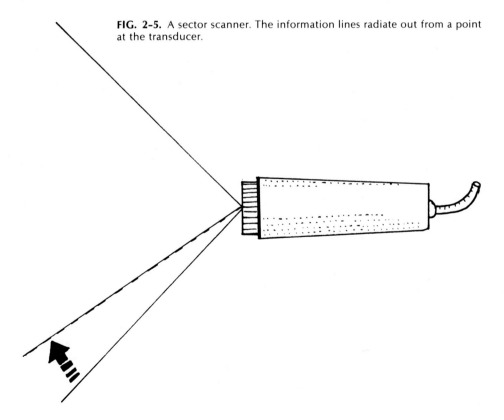

FIG. 2-5. A sector scanner. The information lines radiate out from a point at the transducer.

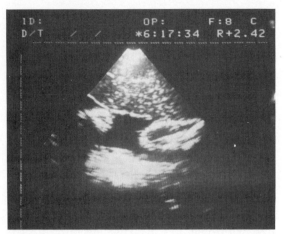

FIG. 2–6. Image illustrating a sector array image. The anterior placenta can be identified, though the anterior field of view is limited.

obscured by the main bang of the transducer (Fig. 2–6). Generally it provides a more difficult image to interpret during the third trimester. The bladder provides an adequate standoff window for early pregnancy and gynecologic diagnosis.

Two general groups of sector scanners have been developed, mechanical and electronic.

Mechanical Sectors. In general, mechanical sector scanners combine mechanical motion of a conventional transducer. One technique spins a wheel with multiple transducers, appropriately addressing the proper transducer through the prescribed sector. The most popular mechanical sector scanning technique is accomplished by oscillating a single transducer (Fig. 2–7).

Electronic Phased Array. The beam can be swept through an arc electronically. This type of technique is called phased array. The phased-array transducer is a series of elements placed in a single row or in several rows. The beam can not only be steered but also focused. In fact the focusing can be dynamic on receive, tracking the source of the echo with the best received focus for the given aperture. (Aperture size determines the focus and thus the lateral resolution.)

The advantages of the phased array over the mechanical sector scanner lie in the facts that it has no moving parts and the focal zones are adjustable. These advantages are, however, outweighed by the complexity of the electronic structures (generally one pulser and receiver for each transducer element), which makes these instruments more expensive. In general these systems have wider angles of view (approximately 90° sectors) for the same apertures at the skin level. Mechanical sectors can also produce 90° sector scans but generally require a large window at the skin level for the same acoustic aperture. Disadvantages of the electronic scanners relate to image degradation caused by diffraction gratings and side pulses. The basic effect is an increase in the noise within the image. Generally another disadvantage is the plane thickness. The phased-array resolution at right angles to the scan plane is less than that of the single-element mechanical sector.

FIG. 2–7. Mechanical sector scanner consists of a single-element transducer that is mechanically moved rapidly through an arc. Basic components are transducer, mechanical drive, and electrical motor.

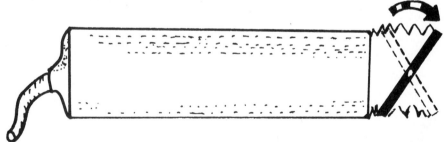

WATER PATH REAL-TIME SCANNERS

Another variation to real time that was first introduced in the late 1960s is a parabolic-mirror-equipped, multiple-transducer rotational scanner. The system employs a water path and soft membrane to form the coupling with the skin. The system provides a linear image that can be seen with the sector scanner. Image quality in this system lacks lateral resolution and in many respects would be greatly improved with larger aperture transducers that are focused. The soft membrane of this water path system makes it amenable to irregular skin surfaces.

COAXIAL ANNULAR ARRAY

A system that provides high resolution and real time is a coaxial annular array–water path system in which the beam steering is mechanical. So that the reverberation echo from the water path does not interfere with the images of interest, the water path must be as long as the depth of the image being displayed. One approach has

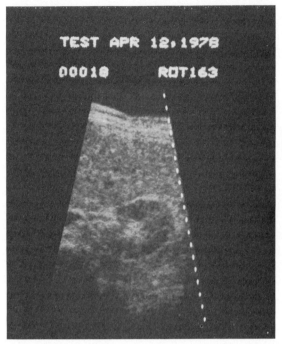

FIG. 2-9. Image from a real-time water path scanner demonstrating liver and right kidney.

been to use a mirror system in which the transducer is stationary and the mirror moves through an arc creating a sector (Fig. 2–8). This type of head is more compact, requires less volume of water, and is, therefore, lighter and more easily maneuvered.

The large coaxial phased array provides excellent resolution in both azimuth planes (Fig. 2–9).

AUTOMATED SCANNERS

Automated scanners include the real-time scanners, which, in turn, include linear arrays, sector scanners and water path scanners.

Another group of automated scanners are multiple-transducer water path scanners in which the multiple transducers are synchronously swept. The beams from each transducer cross the area of interest. This overlapping sector motion permits detection of specular reflectors within the body that are not in the plane of a single transducer. The image produced is an integrated image.

FIG. 2-8. Annular phased-array water path system. The sound beam is focused by the annular array and swept through a sector by a mechanically moving mirror system.

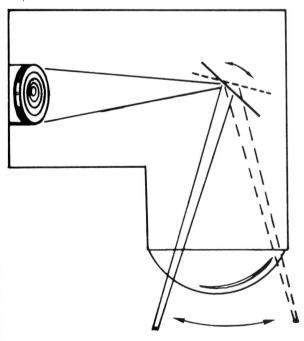

Automated scanners reduce technique and improve reproducibility. The main advantage of multiple-transducer instruments is a large field of view. Additionally a high degree of precision in calibration of the mechanical mechanisms is maintained. To date, such systems are high-priced instruments with good throughput capabilities and are used on a very limited basis.

SUMMARY

Ultrasound instrumentation has undergone vast improvements over the past few years and will continue to do so. The most significant improvements have come through the use of gray-scale imaging and real-time scanning. Future improvements will relate to ease of use and clarity of anatomic details.

3

Biologic effects of ultrasound

USAMA ABDULLA*

"I may, therefore, say that no science advances except doubt be first shown upon what is taught or written upon it."

Dr. Benjamin Ridge (91)

Ultrasound has become one of the most popular diagnostic tools in medicine. As a noninvasive technique, both its popularity and range of clinical application have steadily increased over the last 20 years. Now it is being successfully used in almost every branch of medicine. There is no doubt that in recent years diagnostic ultrasound has influenced the practice of modern obstetrics and gynecology (30–32). It is now widely used in early pregnancy (1, 2, 92), as well as in all other stages of pregnancy, to monitor fetal growth and development (21). It is also used, in its Doppler form, for fetal heart detection, antenatal fetal heart monitoring, and fetal heart monitoring in labor.

In any invesigative technique it is important to establish that it causes no harmful effects, especially when used in pregnancy, where delicate targets are involved. These targets include not only the developing tissues and organs of the fetus but also the maternal and fetal gonads, where harmful effects may be delayed and may not, therefore, be discovered for many generations. In medicine the ideal diagnostic technique should be not only safe but also accurate and without discomfort to the patient. In considering these principles, diagnostic ultrasound scores very well, for to date there have been no reported harmful effects to the patients or their offspring; it has proved itself a reliable technique whereby almost instantaneous results can be obtained; and, lastly but equally importantly, it can be used easily on patients and with no discomfort, even to those who are ill.

Although the possibility of harmful effects from the use of diagnositc ultrasound has been the concern of both clinician and workers in this field, they have, nevertheless, continued to use it in the honest belief that it is "safe" and that its advantages are overwhelmingly greater than possible disadvantages. Furthermore, there is no doubt that diagnostic ultrasound will continue to be used so long as no recognizable harm comes to light.

We must not, however, forget the tragic lesson learned from the incautious use of diagnostic x-rays earlier in this century. It was not until many years later that the damaging effects of ionizing radiation were discovered, and by that time damage had already been inflicted on a signifi-

* I should like to thank Dr. Stanley Walker, Cytogenetic Unit, University of Liverpool, and Dr. Malcolm Brown, Bio-Engineering and Medical Physics Unit, Liverpool Area Health Authority (Teaching), for their valuable help and advice. I am also grateful for the secretarial assistance of Mrs. D. Williams.

cant number of children born to mothers who had been x-rayed during the various stages of pregnancy. Diagnostic ultrasound has, similarly, become widely used before adequate knowledge of its safety parameters and full understanding of its interactions with the human body have been obtained. It would, therefore, be most advisable to continue using ultrasound with caution until we have the complete answer to its interactions with the developing human cells, tissues, and organs and to its safety limits.

Perhaps at this stage we ought to draw a distinction between the two types of ultrasound, the gentle diagnostic ultrasound and the ferocious power ultrasound. Whereas the former, with its low energy levels, has proved itself an important diagnostic tool, the latter, with its high intensity levels, is capable of destroying living cells and organisms. Power ultrasound is mostly known for its use in industry, where, for example, it can clean or drill metals. Power ultrasound can also be used in medicine as a therapeutic tool, where, for example, physiotherapists use it because of its selective and deep heating capabilities (72). Also, at much higher energy levels, power ultrasound can be used to destroy tissue deliberately, as in the treatment of Meniere's disease (99).

Although there are recognizable differences between diagnostic and power ultrasound, one still wonders whether diagnostic ultrasound is free from any deleterious effects. This chapter may help to clarify aspects regarding the safety of diagnostic ultrasound and perhaps answer some of the queries relating to the possibility of its damaging effects.

First there is an outline of the physical aspects of ultrasound and the mechanisms of its interaction. The rest of the chapter then deals with the various biologic effects.

PHYSICAL ASPECTS

Ultrasound can be defined as mechanical vibratory waves that are transmitted through media at frequencies above those heard by the human ear. These waves travel at different velocities through different media. In the human

being, the velocity of ultrasound through most soft tissue is approximately 1500 m/sec (83). Sound waves travel in a number of ways, but ultrasound in soft tissue propagates as longtitudinal (compression) waves.

The frequencies commonly employed in diagnostic ultrasound equipment are 1–10 megahertz (MHz), while those for therapeutic equipment are 0.75–3 MHz (83). An important feature of ultrasound is that it can be projected in a narrow beam, and in the body it behaves very like a beam of light passing through layers of transparent but different media, reflections and refractions occurring at each interface.

Diagnostic apparatus falls into two categories, Doppler equipment (continuous wave) for detection of movement within the body and pulsed equipment for imaging. Pulsed ultrasound usually has a pulse repetition frequency between 100 and 3000/sec and a pulse length of about 1 μsec.

The intensity of ultrasound is the energy that passes each second through a specified cross-sectional area, usually quoted in watts per square centimeter (W/cm^2). The intensity varies along and across the ultrasound beam, owing to the characteristics of the transducer mechanism and the properties of the transmission media (tissue).

For continuous-wave apparatus the transmitted intensity is usually between 1 and 5 W/cm^2 for therapeutic instruments, and between 0.5 and 30 mW/cm^2 for obstetric Doppler instruments. For pulsed apparatus the time-averaged intensity is similar, typically 1–20 mW/cm^2; however the energy is transmitted in very short pulses that individually may have peak intensities from 1–100 W/cm^2 (58). Real-time scanners, now becoming popular in obstetrics, can be expected to have characteristics similar to those of conventional pulsed scanners.

Ultrasound intensity can be measured directly in vitro by using a radiation pressure balance (69). It can also be measured indirectly by other methods such as detecting temperature rise in sound-absorbing materials (119), by tiny microphones (hydrophones) (57), and by reflection methods (52). Some of these methods can be applied in vivo (8, 41, 52).

As with a beam of light, the intensity of ultrasound diminishes with distance from the source owing to divergence of the beam and to absorption. This situation is modified when the beam is specially focused or when there are "standing waves."

In assessing the biologic hazards the relevant factors to be considered include ultrasonic intensity, ultrasonic frequency, pulse duration, repetition frequency, and the total time of exposure. The relevant intensity here is, of course, that measured, not at the transducer, but at the target.

BIOPHYSICAL MECHANISMS

The biophysical mechanisms of ultrasonic action are not fully understood, particularly in relation to diagnostic intensity levels. The effects of ultrasound on various biological entities may be due to one or a combination of any of the following:

1. Heating effects
2. Cavitational effects
3. Mechanical effects

Hill (56) described three mechanisms of action as thermal effects, cavitation, and "direct" mechanisms. When Dunn and Fry (36) published their experimental results on focal lesions in the mammalian central nervous system following exposure to ultrasound, they also described three mechanisms of action and referred to them as heat, cavitation, and mechanical factors.

In general, heating and cavitation are associated only with high average intensities not found in diagnostic equipment. Mechanical or direct effects that may affect cell function may also, however, occur at the relatively low average intensity levels. The complex effects caused by short pulsed waveforms with high peak but low average intensity are particularly difficult to assess.

HEATING EFFECTS

The absorption of ultrasound wave energy results in heat production. Although we do not fully understand the mechanisms leading to sound absorption in complex media, a number of relevant factors are known. We know, for instance, that ultrasound absorption varies with viscosity and sound frequency. In most media the absorption increases with frequency (45, 70). Because ultrasound is strongly absorbed by bone, it results in local rise of temperature at the insonatee bone surface. For this reason therapeutic intensities are employed in physiotherapy to heat joint capsules and sinovial membranes (72). Such treatments are usually of short duration. Longer exposure periods may result in deep periosteal pain or even periosteal damage (73).

Diagnostic equipment operating at low intensity is very unlikely to cause heat production even when there are standing waves or adventitious localized focusing. On the other hand, equipment delivering high average intensity can lead to heat production and possible tissue damage. In the human being, heating to above 50° C causes irreversible tissue damage. Experimental animal work suggests that tissue necrosis after ultrasonic exposure can be largely attributed to this effect.

Temperature rise can be directly measured by the use of implanted microthermocouples (88). The actual rise depends on ultrasound intensity, duration of exposure, and the absorption coefficient of the tissue. Another important factor is the heat dissipation, which is dependant on blood circulation and tissue vascularity.

CAVITATION EFFECTS

The tensile strength of liquids may be overcome when they are subjected to large local variations of pressure, resulting in cavities within the liquid. Moreover, liquids contain microgas bubbles that are usually stabilized against dissolution but may expand under suitable stress, for example, when they are in the path of high-intensity ultrasound. In an ultrasound field the microgas bubbles may grow by a process of "rectified diffusion," wherein there is alternating but unbalanced diffusion of gases. Mammalian soft tissues are quasi-liquids that exhibit cavitation in strong ultrasonic fields.

There are two types of cavitation, stable and unstable. Stable cavitation, also known as resonant cavitation, occurs when microgas bubbles grow to a certain size and then resonate at the ultrasonic frequency. Their amplitude of oscillation is very much greater than that of particles in liquid in the absence of such resonant microbubbles (56). Tissues in the vicinity of cavitation bubbles are subjected to enormous stresses that may break macromolecules and even cell membranes. Because stable cavitation bubbles take time to develop, they are, therefore, more usually produced by continuous-wave ultrasound or long pulses.

Unstable (collapse) or transient cavitation is more violent. An ultrasonic wave subjects the tissue to laternating cycles of high and low pressure. At high intensities the low pressure may produce vapor-filled cavities. The subsequent high pressure allows collapses of the cavities with subsequent release of energy in the form of strong shock waves that in turn may disrupt and damage the tissues (63). The shock waves are associated with enormous pressures and temperatures, causing chemical as well as physical changes. Free radicals that have longer term effects are said to be released into solution. The estimated pressure attained during the shock wave from a collapsing cavity 10^{-3} mm in diameter in incompressible surrounds can be 1000 atm (102). Other cavities can then be opened by the shock wave, resulting in a chain reaction called "interaction cavitation" (106).

Diagnostic ultrasound is unlikely to cause unstable cavitation, for the threshold level in water is approximately 300 W/cm^2 at 1 MHz (61) and is said to be even higher in soft tissues. Unstable cavitation in liquids can be detected without difficulty. There are, however, many difficulties with regard to methods of assessing stable cavitation, especially in tissues.

MECHANICAL EFFECTS

An ultrasonic wave is propagated by the vibration of particles in the medium through which it travels. These vibrations, which are present at all ultrasonic intensities, cause a range of mechanical or "direct" effects on living tissue particles that are not satisfactorily defined or understood. The mechanical effects may result from the particle acceleration, pressure vibrations, radiation pressure, or shearing forces that occur. A secondary effect is streaming, by which radiation pressure causes movement of particles away from the transducer.

Hawley et al (53) describe a direct mechanical effect disrupting macromolecules in the absence of cavitation. They reported on DNA degradation with use of an ultrasonic intensity of 30 W/cm^2 at 1 MHz. The implications of such a possibility can be far reaching when the hazardous effects of ultrasound are considered.

The transport properties of cell membranes can also be affected both reversibly and irreversibly. Such changes may occur instantaneously with the onset of insonation and may produce sublethal changes that, though not killing the cells, may alter their structure and function (22) in important ways. Recent electron microscopic studies show damage to cell membrane and intracellular components (39, 60).

The function of spinal cord cells was shown by Dunn (35) to be totally arrested after insonation of mice with 1 MHz ultrasound at 50–300 W/cm^2, and this caused immediate paralysis. Cavitational and thermal effects were avoided by operating at high pressure and low temperature. Dunn suggested that, since the functional effect was present some 10–15 minutes before the appearance of any histologic lesion, such action was at a submicroscopic level intimately associated with physiologic function.

Chemical changes may also occur that may be attributable to the agitation of the particles or to streaming. Woodcock (121), using 3 MHz ultrasound, reported the in vitro acceleration of sucrose hydrolysis at intensities of about 3 W/cm^2 and attributed this chemical change to the "direct" effect of ultrasound.

Williams (120) suggested local intravascular microstreaming as the cause of platelet adhesion or fusion to normal endothelial surface after insonating mice blood vessels in vivo. He showed, by electron microscopy, evidence of platelet membrane rupture in spite of intact endothelial surface of the insonated blood vessels.

BIOLOGIC INTERACTIONS

Undoubtedly, our present-day knowledge of the various interactions of ultrasound with human or animal organs, tissues, cells, or subcellular components is still limited, in spite of ample and varied literature on the biologic effects of ultrasound (35, 56, 63, 104, 118). We are still in the early stages of understanding the many mechanisms of such interactions, which often may have multiple effects. The majority of the early reports on the biologic effects of ultrasound are of limited value, for they contained insufficient data with regard to the different experimental conditions, the varied ultrasonic parameters, and dosimetry.

To assess adequately the many safety aspects of diagnositc ultrasound, we need to gain both deep and extensive understanding of how ultrasound interacts with the complex biologic systems of the body as it is transmitted through these systems.

There is no doubt that meaningful data can be acquired in future safety studies if workers in this field endeavor, whenever possible, to measure and assess human or animal ultrasound dosages, especially since such measurement techniques are now being developed (8, 40, 52).

I now discuss and evaluate the reported studies on the biologic effects of ultrasound under one or more of the following main groups:

1. Cell (genetic) studies
2. Animal studies
3. Human studies
4. Delayed effects

CELL (GENETIC) STUDIES

The various genetic experiments on cells are subdivided into cytogenetic experiments and other mutation experiments.

CYTOGENETIC EXPERIMENTS

The search for chromosomal changes in tissue cultures has proved most valuable in assessing the harmful effects of electromagnetic radiation. It was Bender who, in 1957, published the first quantitative study on x-ray-induced chromosome aberrations in human tissue cultures (13). Since then various cultures have been widely used to study the extent of chromosomal damage after exposure to x-irradiation (9). It is not, therefore, surprising that possible cellular or chromosomal damage from diagnostic ultrasound has always been in the forefront of clinicians' minds. Such cautious thoughts were equally shared by the various workers in the field of medical ultrasound. It was, however, the publication of Macintosh and Davey from South Africa in 1970 that finally set the cat among the pigeons (80). The findings of their preliminary communication on chromosomal aberrations following the use of an ultrasonic fetal heart detector was an alarm signal for all those concerned with medical ultrasonics. It even alarmed some pregnant patients at that time who came to hear about this report. I clearly remember the barrage of telephone calls to the ultrasonic department of the Queen Mother's Hospital in Glasgow from frightened patients seeking reassurance or even canceling their next ultrasonic appointments.

The publication of Macintosh and Davey has impelled a large number of clinicians, physicists, and engineers from different parts of the world to set up experiments for detecting possible chromosomal damage following insonation (I prefer the use of the word *insonation* or *sonication* to *irradiation* when denoting exposure to ultrasound). There were some similarities in the experiments, but on the whole they varied in duration of exposure, ultrasonic frequency, and intensity levels. The intensities used ranged from low diagnostic to very high average power levels, some of which reached a few thousand times higher than average diagnostic levels.

The cytogenetic studies are included under in vitro or in vivo experiments after a brief discussion on some of the cytogenetic aspects.

CYTOGENETIC ASPECTS

In tissue cultures the cell cycle is conventionally divided into pre-DNA synthesis phase (G_1), DNA synthesis phase (S), post-DNA synthesis phase (G_2), and mitosis (M). This cell cycle in cultured human lymphocytes usually takes some 15–22 hours to be completed. The approximate duration of each phase is outlined in Figure 3–1, the G_1 phase being the most variable and sometimes quite prolonged. In in vitro lymphocyte cell cultures there is usually an approximate 24-hour delay before the cycle starts when lympho-

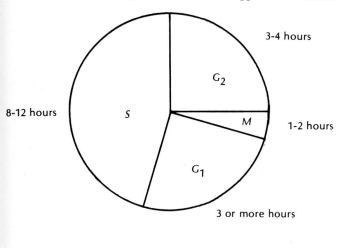

G_1 = presynthesis gap

S = DNA synthesis phase

G_2 = postsynthesis gap

$\left.\begin{array}{}\\ \\ \\ \\ \end{array}\right\}$ Interphase

M = mitosis

FIG. 3-1. The phases and duration of the human lymphocyte cell cycle, in vitro culture.

cytes that are in G_1 phase are stimulated by phytohemagglutinin that is contained in the culture medium to proceed to phases S and G_2 and then the first mitosis. This first mitosis occurs at approximately 46–48 hours after initiation of the culture.

Routine cytogenetic cultures are usually harvested at approximately 72 hours, when the second and probably a few third waves of mitosis

FIG. 3-2. More frequent chromosome aberrations.

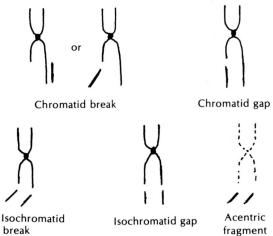

Chromatid break   Chromatid gap

Isochromatid   Isochromatid gap   Acentric
break   fragment

have occurred. In these routine cultures spontaneous chromosomal aberrations (including gaps) up to 5% are acceptable (26). However, the effect of possible damaging agents, for example, x-rays or ultrasound, on chromosomes (Figs. 3–2 and 3–3) is best assessed after the first wave of mitosis. For this reason we (3), as well as some other workers, have harvested the cell cultures after 48 hours. If such cytogenetic assessment is carried out on cells after a longer period of culture, some of the cells will have completed more than their first division and the number of chromatid aberrations may be exaggerated, whereas the number of unstable and more complex aberrations, like dicentric chromosomes, may be lost after the first mitosis (112).

In cell studies, the type of chromosomal damage depends on the phase of the cell cycle during which cells have been exposed to harmful agents. If cells are exposed during G_1 phase and part of S phase, the whole chromosome will be affected (isochromatid damage), whereas if cells are exposed during most of S and G_2 phases, only part of the chromosome may be affected (chromatid damage).

In other studies where cells such as those obtained from liquor amnii (mainly fibroblastic) are cultured, the cells require 2 to 4 weeks in culture and would have been through many division cycles since exposure to ultrasound, and hence, cells with chromosomal damage may be lost.

In recent years much experimental work has been performed to evaluate the possibility of chromosomal damage from exposure of cells to ultrasound. Either the cells studied were insonated while in tissue cultures or the patients were insonated first and then cells obtained from such patients were subsequently cultured. These studies are now respectively discussed under in vitro and in vivo experiments.

In Vitro Chromosome Experiments. The value of Macintosh and Davey's contribution in 1970 was that it instigated many research workers from various centers to publish the results of their experiments, which otherwise would not have found their way into medical literature. Their findings of chromosomal damage following the exposure of human blood cultures to continuous-wave ultrasound at diagnostic levels (30 mW/cm²) prompted us to report an entirely different experience with similar experiments (18), which were done in 1966 and were briefly referred to by Donald in 1969 (31). In these experiments we exposed human lymphocyte cultures to both pulse and continuous-wave diagnostic ultrasound but were unable to detect chromosomal damage in these cultures when compared with uninsonated cultures.

Other workers have reported the lack of chromosomal damage in human lymphocyte cultures when exposed to diagnostic ultrasound, whether in continuous-wave form (14, 17, 19, 71, 93) or in both pulsed and continuous-wave forms (4, 18, 115). In some of these experiments (4, 18, 115) high average intensities in the therapeutic range or even higher have also been used. Some experiments, primarily designed to use high-intensity ultrasound whether in pulse or continuous-wave form, have also failed to demonstrate chromosomal damage in human cell cultures (25, 71, 84, 94).

Hill et al exposed Chinese hamster cells to 1 MHz high-intensity pulsed ultrasound employing peak intensities of 150–200 W/cm² and extended the pulse duration to 50 μsec without finding significant difference in chromosomal aberrations between the insonated cells and the controls (59). Bleaney et al (16), also using the hamster, have exposed suspensions of its lung cells to high-intensity ultrasound and have demonstrated no direct effect of ultrasound on cell reproductive integrity.

Loch et al (75), using both diagnostic and therepeutic ultrasound intensities, showed that diagnostic ultrasound did not interfere with cell growth and proliferation. They found that in the therapeutic range there was some cell damage and loss of ability to proliferate. However, the cells they used in the tissue culture were human amniotic fibroblasts and cervical cancer cells (see discussion relating to amniotic fluid cell cultures under in vivo experiments section).

Coakley et al (24), using high-intensity ultrasound, reported chromosomal damage similar to that reported by Macintosh and Davey in 1970, but on changing the technique of insonation the damage was no longer observed. They suggested that the similarity of chromosome damage

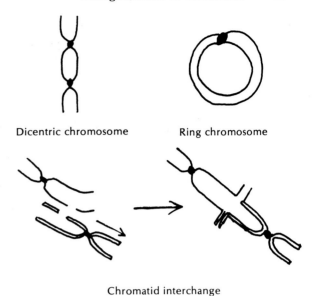

Dicentric chromosome   Ring chromosome

Chromatid interchange

FIG. 3-3. Less frequent chromosome aberrations.

found by Macintosh and Davey and themselves may be due to the release of "toxins" from the polythene bags containing the blood cultures, especially when the high number of chromatid aberrations were still present when the cells were harvested after 72 hours. However, Buckton and Baker, in an attempt to conform the observations of Macintosh and Davey found no increase in chromosome aberrations over the controls when they used glass containers (19). Macintosh (78) suggested that the incidental focusing effect he noticed with his transducer in using Schlieren photographs may explain the discrepancy between his and Davey's preliminary report and the negative reports by other workers.

Macintosh and Davey published in 1972 their second joint paper (81) in which they studied the effect of varying the intensity of 2 MHz continuous-wave ultrasound on chromosomal damage in human blood cultures. When they varied the intensity from 0–80 mW/cm², they reported a relationship between intensity of ultrasound and chromosomal aberrations induced, with a threshold at an ultrasound intensity of 8.2 mW/cm² below which they did not detect chromosomal damage under the experimental conditions they described. They also suggested a further threshold at ultrasound intensity of 18.4 mW/cm² above which more serious aberrations such as dicentric chromosomes may be seen. In an addendum to their paper they suggested another explanation for their high rate of chromosomal damage based on the formation of resonant microbubbles as well as on differences in scoring techniques. However, Coakley et al (25) subjected human blood cultures to ultrasound of sufficiently high intensity to expose some of the cells to cavitation, but they were unable to show increased chromosomal damage in cells surviving cavitation as compared with the controls.

In 1975 Macintosh and colleagues in Cardiff repeated the Capetown experiments using not only the same instrument and culture media but also the same blood donor and were unable to reproduce the high chromosomal aberration rate (79). In view of these results they felt that the chromosomal aberrations originally found in the experiments from South Africa were produced by an artifact that they could not identify, but at the same time they felt that these aberrations were not related to the exposure of cultures to ultrasound.

In vitro DNA Experiments. The effects of ultrasound at the subcellular level on macromolecules like deoxyribonucleic acid (DNA) have been reported in a number of in vitro experiments. It is well known that power ultrasound can cause degradation of mammalian DNA (23, 53). Galperin-Lemaitre et al (49) have reported on the damage to purified calf-thymus DNA when exposed to ultrasound at therapeutic levels of 1.5 W/cm^2, as well as at levels of 200 mW/cm^2. They found no damage when the same in vitro DNA solution was exposed to ultrasound at 20 mW/cm^2. More recently Prasad (90) observed up to 14% reduction in DNA synthesis after exposing hela cells to pulsed ultrasound at an intensity of 4 mW/cm^2. It must, however, be pointed out that DNA is rather unstable in solution, and such results cannot, therefore, lead to a conclusion concerning the in vivo implications. In addition, Thacker (109) points out that DNA degradation arises from hydrodynamic shear forces set up around oscillating or collapsing gas bubbles in insonated liquids and that, to generate comparable fluid forces in tissue, a higher intensity would be required than what degrades DNA in solution; moreover, where these forces are sufficient to

disrupt DNA in chromosomes, it is likely that damage to other cellular structures will be expensive enough to cause cell disruption and death.

In vivo Chromosome Experiments. Another report describing an increased frequency of chromosomal damage in cells after exposure to diagnostic ultrasound also appeared in 1970, but this was an in vivo study. In this study Serr et al (96) observed the effect of diagnostic continuous-wave ultrasound on fetal cells obtained by amniocentesis after exposing the mothers to ultrasound for 10 hours. They reported on the possibility of ultrasound-induced change, for they found an increased rate of chromosomal breakages and aberrations in the exposed amniotic fetal cells as compared with the controls. Any study done in search of possible chromosomal damage from ultrasound using long-term fibroblast culture is both inappropriate and unacceptable, for cells examined after long periods of culture may show an increase in chromatid aberrations that have been produced by replication of chromosome aberrations, or cells carrying more complex and unstable chromosomal abnormalities are eliminated with each cell cycle (112, 116). Dewhurst (29), also rejecting the suggestion of Serr et al, stated that they did not employ standard genetic terminology, that they gave no details of cytogenetic technique, and that the polyploidy phenomenon they alleged to be due to the effect of ultrasound is not infrequently reported in routine amniotic fluid fibroblast cultures without exposure to ultrasound (66, 85).

Boyd et al (18) studied the effect of both continuous-wave and pulsed diagnostic ultrasound on chromosomes in blood cultures from infants whose mothers have been exposed to ultrasound at various stages of pregnancy. There was no evidence of damage due to ultrasound on the chromosomes of these newborn infants when compared with the same number of matched controls.

In another in vivo experiment Abdulla and co-workers (3) studied the effect of both continuous-wave and pulsed diagnostic ultrasound on maternal and fetal chromosomes in patients admitted for termination of pregnancy by hysterotomy. A total of 35 patients were exposed to

1 hour of pulsed ultrasound and 10 hours of continuous-wave ultrasound some 16–24 hours before hysterotomy. There was no increase in the number of chromosome aberrations in blood cultures from insonated mothers and fetuses when compared with 11 control mothers and their fetuses.

Lucas et al (76) reported on the effect of continuous-wave fetal heart monitoring on chromosomes of 24 newborn infants whose mothers had been insonated in labor for up to 9½ hours. They found no increased chromosomal breakage when these infants were compared with controls born to mothers on whom ultrasound was not used during pregnancy or labor. No x-rays were used in pregnancy in either the insonated or the control group. Watt and Stewart (116) in a similar experiment cultured white blood cells from cords of 10 newborn infants and from their mothers after 2–10 hours of exposure to a fetal heart monitor in labor but found no chromosomal damage when comparing the results with those in the controls. In another similar negative experiment lkeuchi et al (64) assessed the effect of 40 mW/cm^2 continuous-wave ultrasound on chromosomes of embryonic fibroblast cultures where the cells were obtained from 97 fetuses who were aborted immediately after exposure to ultrasound. When they compared these fetuses with 103 controls, there was no significant difference in the rate of chromosomal aberration between the two groups. Galperin-Lemaitre et al (48) studied the in vivo effect of power ultrasound on marrow cell chromosomes, exposing the femoral and humoral areas of golden hamsters to 1 and 1.5 W/cm^2 continuous-wave ultrasound for 2 and 5 minutes. Because the bone marrow cells divide naturally and continuously, they harvested the cells 1 hour and 24 hours after insonation. In comparing the insonated marrow cells with the controls, they found no significant increase in chromosome aberrations.

OTHER MUTATION EXPERIMENTS

An important assessment of the hazards of any agent is to study the possibility of its mutagenic effects. Thacker (108) used four different yeast genetic systems to study the effect of ultrasound in inducing mutation or changing the distribu-

tion of genetic material within a population of cells (recombination). He found no increase in the mutation of recombination frequency when the yeast cells were insonated with intensity levels similar to diagnostic, therapeutic, or even very high (cavitational) levels. He found some genetic changes only under conditions due to heating and free radical formation. The overall evidence from his genetic experiments was that no hazard was likely from ultrasound at diagnostic intensity levels but that there was a small chance of genetic hazard from therapeutic levels. At the same time he pointed out the difficulties in extrapolation and the need for genetic studies using multicellular organisms. Such experiments are discussed under the genetic section of Animal Studies.

ANIMAL STUDIES

There was practically no animal experimentation before diagnostic ultrasound was introduced into clinical practice. The absence of any recognizable damage site or pattern, together with limited understanding of the biologic interaction mechanisms, created difficulties in setting up appropriate animal toxicity experiments. Such experiments either showed no detectable physical effect, or when an effect was observed, damage persisted or there was an ultimate recovery. In these experiments the animals were exposed to intensity levels similar to those used in current ultrasonic diagnosis or much higher levels. The various reports on any observed damage or change in animals after exposure to ultrasound are now discussed under the following:

A. Structural changes
B. Functional changes
C. Behavioral changes
D. Developmental changes
E. Genetic changes

STRUCTURAL CHANGES

The early toxicity experiments were designed to study possible structural damage in animal tissues or organs. No such damage was detected when Donald et al (33) studied the effect of pulsed diagnostic ultrasound on the brains of kittens. Smyth (100), in a more elaborate experiment, also using low-average-intensity pulsed ultrasound, studied mice and rats after exposing them for 20 minutes a day for 5 consecutive days. He was unable to detect any effect of ultrasound on brain tissue when comparing insonated rats with controls. He also insonated the liver, cardiac, and gonadal areas of mice and compared them with controls but was unable to demonstrate any histologic change in the liver, the cardiac area, or the gonads. The local irritation of the costochondral area that he noticed was attributed to the effect of the harness restraint used. He also studied the blood and some enzyme values but showed no differences between the insonated and control groups. Abramowski et al (5) exposed the brains of 154 rabbit fetuses to low-intensity continuous-wave ultrasound for up to 8 hours but found no evidence of histologic damage in any of them.

The literature contains many studies wherein varying levels of power ultrasound were used to illustrate damage in different animal tissues. Such studies included the assessment of damage in nerve tissue (10, 34, 44, 47, 74, 88, 97, 101, 106), liver tissue (12, 27, 103, 105), as well as other tissues, including muscle and blood (11, 42, 55, 111, 113). Although heating seems to be the mechanism of damage in most of these experiments, mechanical forces and stable cavitation have also been implicated. In recent experiments attempts have been made to establish threshold levels for intensity, frequency, and duration of exposure (36, 44, 106). These studies are invaluable in elucidating some of the interaction mechanisms. Certainly there is a need for more experimental work to be done using wider frequency range and variable intensity, pulse repetition, and pulse duration.

BEHAVIORAL CHANGES

Almost no experimental work has been done to detect alterations in animal behavior after exposure to ultrasound. Smyth (100) trained rats for a conditioned-escape response and then insonated them, using low-intensity pulsed ultrasound, for periods of 52–120 min after initially giving them a light anesthetic. He then tested the rats on Days 1, 2, and 7 after insonation and found no difference between the conditioned-escape response of these rats when compared with the control group.

FUNCTIONAL CHANGES

Reversible and irreversible functional changes have been reported in many animal experiments. Dyson et al (40) used relatively low-intensity continuous-wave ultrasound and found complete but reversible arrest of blood flow in chick embryos. In a later report Dyson et al (39) concluded that the minimum intensity required for stasis in vessels of chick embryo was 0.5 W/cm^2 when continuous-wave ultrasound was used. They concluded that the threshold intensity varied with the type, size, and orientation of the vessel, as well as with the heart rate of the chick embryo. Assessing a different functional end point, Hrazdira and Konečný (61) insonated the thyroid gland of 38 rabbits using therapeutic ultrasound intensities (up to 2 W/cm^2) and found a decrease in radioiodine uptake.

High-intensity ultrasound has been used to produce paraplegia. Fry et al (44, 46) used pulsed ultrasound to produce spinal paralysis in the frog. Dunn (34) produced irreversible paraplegia as well as brain focal lesions when using pulsed ultrasound. Taylor and Pond (106) insonated the spinal cord of adult rats and used pulsed ultrasound at low MHz frequencies and extended pulse duration amounting to a few thousand times more than that used in ultrasonic diagnosis.

Using low-intensity pulsed ultrasound, Dyson et al (38) observed stimulation of growth of injured rabbit ear. In 1976 Dyson et al (37) reported on the effect of ultrasound in stimulating healing of varicose ulcers.

DEVELOPMENT CHANGES

The majority of this type of experimental work was done on mice and rats with conflicting results. The biologic end points included the assessment of litter size, fetal viability, and congenital malformations.

Woodward et al (122), experimenting on mice, could detect no increase in the abnormality rate despite using varied peak intensities (20

W/cm^2 up to 490^2), pulse duration and exposure time. Garrison et al (51) found no significant effect on fetal viability when using high-average-intensity ultrasound on pregnant rats. Warwick et al (114) also found no significant effect on the litter size or the rate of abnormality when they exposed 297 pregnant mice to high-average-intensity pulsed ultrasound. A similar conclusion was reached by Mannor et al (82) after exposing pregnant mice to variable intensities of continuous-wave ultrasound.

Andres (6) employed standard diagnostic equipment to insonate frog spawn at different developmental stages (during the first 11 days), but when the tadpoles hatched, no gross structural defects were detected nor was there increased developmental abnormality rate. Smyth (100) also used low-intensity ultrasound but found no congenital abnormalities in 348 offspring born to mice that he insonated for 5 days during the premating period, for 10 days during the mating period, and, with the exception of the last 2 days, throughout pregnancy.

There are also experiments suggesting development changes caused by ultrasound. Weinland (117), using low-intensity continuous-wave ultrasound, subjected pregnant hamsters during various pregnancy stages; as a result there were either no living embryos, or among those that survived, several were growth retarded. Shoji et al (98) found significant effect on late fetal death in one of the two mice strains exposed to continuous-wave ultrasound at low levels. Curto (28), using continuous ultrasound on pregnant mice, found a significant decrease in the neonatal survival of the offspring at intensities of 125 mW/cm^2. O'Brien (86) also used continuous ultrasound on pregnant mice and found a significant decrease in fetal weight at intensitites of 0.5–5.5 W/cm^2.

Although it is difficult to draw a conclusion from these developmental experiments, the results should be carefully considered.

GENETIC CHANGES

Animal experiments designed to assess genetic hazards after exposure to ultrasound are quite important in the study of ultrasonic safety.

Although the early genetic experiments dem-onstrated definite genetic changes, the ultrasound intensities used were well above those employed for diagnostic purposes. Pourhadi et al (89) exposed testes of rabbits to ultrasound at intensities of 2.5–4 W/cm^2. They reported histologic damage, as well as mitotic abnormalities of spermatocytes and spermatogonia. Severely affected spermatocytes and spermatids have also been reported by Andrianov (7) when he exposed rats to ultrasonic intensities of 0.2–2 W/cm^2. Okauchi reported similar experience on insonated mice testes (87). He argued that, since animal gonads are sensitive to heat, the heating effect of high-intensity ultrasound is the most likely cause of the observed damage. Similarly, heating may be responsible for the reported damage in the other two reports.

The fruit fly Drosophila has been used to study the possibility of postinsonation mutation. Lethal mutations have been reported by Bushnell and Wallace (20) and Kato (65). In both these reports high ultrasound intensities have been employed that would have led to considerable internal heating, which can be mutagenic to the Drosophila (107). However, Fritz-Niggli and Boni (43) observed no increase in the frequency of lethal mutation in the Drosophila after exposure to ultrasonic intensities of 0.3–1.8 W/cm^2. More recently Thacker and Baker (110) also used the Drosophila to study the possibility of genetic hazard after exposure to ultrasound. They employed intensities of 0.05–2 W/cm^2 but found no significant increase in the rate of recessive lethal mutation. They concluded that there was little risk of genetic damage to multicellular organisms following exposure to ultrasound at currently employed diagnostic frequencies and intensities.

In another series of well-designed experiments Lyon and Simpson (77) insonated mice to study the possibility of genetic effects. They employed both continuous-wave and pulsed ultrasound. The intensity of the continuous-wave source was 1.6 W/cm^2. The pulsed ultrasound employed two types of pulse durations, 1 msec and 30 μsec with average intensities of 0.9–1.6 W/cm^2 and peak intensities of 6.4–45 W/cm^2. They aimed at intensities higher than those used in medical diagnosis but lower than those causing cavitation. They argued that, since their experiments were designed to cover various stages of spermatogenesis and maturation of oocyte, it was unlikely that damage at a specific stage could have been missed. They concluded from their experimental studies that diagnostic ultrasound as used antenatally was unlikely to cause genetic hazards to the fetus or its mother.

HUMAN STUDIES

There is no doubt that the final assessment of the safety of any diagnostic tool used in medicine is incomplete without relying on satisfactory evidence from human studies. A small number of such studies have been carried out in an attempt to detect the possibility of deleterious effects following the use of diagnostic ultrasound. Bishop (15) in 1966 used a Doppler instrument on 600 obstetric patients and detected no clinical side effects. He found no harmful effects when assessing 255 of their infants at postnatal examination. Kohorn et al (67) in 1967 found no change in the electroencephalographic (EEG) pattern before and after exposing 20 infants to pulsed ultrasound for 5 minutes. In the same year Garg and Taylor (50), also using pulsed ultrasound, reported similar EEG responses when they insonated 6 terminal cancer patients for 1 hour. They also studied brain histology and tissue enzymes but found no abnormal changes.

In three epidemiologic studies there has been no evidence to incriminate diagnostic ultrasound. Using a diagnostic Doppler instrument on pregnant patients, Bernstine (14) examined their 720 infants and found 4 of them with anomalies, amounting to 0.55%. He indicated that comparable statistics of congenital anomalies for the same period of time was 1.3% in noninsonated cases. The results of the largest of these studies meant laudable evidence for the safety of diagnostic ultrasound. Hellman et al (54), in a joint survey from three different centers in New York, Glasgow, and Lund, studied a total of 3297 women who were examined at various stages of pregnancy. The examinations, mainly using pulsed ultrasound, were undertaken for a number of reasons, such as diagnosis of early pregnancy, placental localization, and growth and development studies. They analyzed 1114 patients who apparently had normal pregnancies and for whom the following information was obtained:

1. Previous abnormal children
2. Weeks of gestation at first examination
3. Total number of ultrasound examinations
4. Reason for ultrasound examination
5. Pregnancy outcome
6. Number of infant malformations
7. Detection of normality or abnormality at first ultrasonic visit

The analyzed data from the 1114 patients in the normal group showed a fetal abnormality rate of 2.7%, whereas the rate in all 3297 patients was 3.7%, excluding abortions, which amounted to 10.1% of cases scanned before 20 weeks' pregnancy. These authors indicated that they cannot validly compare these results with the incidence of abnormality in the general population, for their patients were selected to be scanned for specific indications and not chosen at random. Nevertheless, the incidence of their fetal abnormality compares favorably with that of 4.8% in a large survey of 63,236 single births in the United States of America. They concluded, therefore, that neither the gestation period at the first ultrasound examination nor the number of examinations seemed to increase the risk of fetal abnormality. Koryani et al (68) performed a smaller but similar study and again reported the absence of increased congenital fetal abnormality where patients had antenatal ultrasonic examinations.

Although there is uncertainty regarding the possibility or the nature of damage from ultrasonic examination in pregnancy, especially in the early stages, observations and studies so far indicate the improbability of discovering gross fetal defects. Nevertheless, one should consider the possibility of damage to specialized organs of the developing embryo, such as its sensory organs, which might ultimately affect certain functions in the child, for example, hearing. There is, therefore, a growing demand for a large clinical trial that should be both prospective and controlled so that the possibility of hazards from diagnostic ultrasound in pregnancy can be accurately assessed. The various ultrasonic parameters should be carefully recorded, as well as the length of each ultrasonic examination during the various stages of pregnancy. The mother and the newborn should be carefully assessed in the postnatal period. The child can then have long-term pediatric follow-up so that its progress and development can be critically assessed.

DELAYED EFFECTS

The possibility of long-term or delayed hazards from any modality or agent used in clinical practice must always be considered, especially when all the safety aspects of such an agent are not fully recognized. In using the example of ionizing irradiation in pregnancy, the possibility of delayed effects is now well recognized, for there is increased risk of leukemia in children whose mothers have been x-rayed during pregnancy. The answers to the possibility of delayed effects from ultrasound can be obtained only through continual assessment of every available hazard information that may relate to the earlier use of ultrasound. Such valuable data may be obtained only through analyzing data from many large clinical trials.

CONCLUSION

The evidence from animal experiments indicates that diagnostic ultrasonography, as used at present, most probably has a wide margin of safety. Moreover, so far there has been no clinical evidence to suggest any harmful effects from diagnostic ultrasound. Although this is rather encouraging, it must be remembered that the absence of demonstrable ultrasonic hazards in the human being does not exclude the possibility of either immediate unrecognized or delayed effects. This is particularly so when, as yet, we do not fully understand the various mechanisms of interaction, nor have we established adequate safety limits. It must, therefore, be emphasized that, though the development of new ultrasonic equipments and new ultrasonic systems should continue, it would be most advisable to decrease, or at least not to exceed, the present average and peak intensity levels, pulse repetition frequency, and length of pulses. Changes in these ultrasonic parameters may otherwise be readily incorporated to improve resolution and diagnostic capabilities. Ultrasonic examination time should also be kept to the minimum required to obtain adequate information, especially when patients are scanned in early pregnancy. It is hoped that, while the necessary information is obtained, it may be possible to reduce the intensity levels, the scanning time, or both.

Whereas further research into the mechanisms of interaction must continue with an endeavor to devise more sensitive biologic tests, care must be taken in extrapolating the results to man when one attempts to define threshold levels and safety limits. Evidence for ultrasonic safety in the human being may require the setting up of epidemiologic studies, but above all there is a need for a well-controlled prospective study wherein children born to insonated and uninsonated mothers should have intensive developmental, behavioral, and functional assessment for a number of years.

REFERENCES

1. ABDULLA U: Sonar in very early pregnancy. In Böck J, Ossoinig K (eds): Ultrasonographia Medica. Vienna, Wiener Medizinischen Akademie, 1971, p 185

2. ABDULLA U: Early diagnosis and follow up of twin-pregnancy using a two-dimensional ultrasonic scanner. Acta Genet Med Gemellol (Roma) 25: 317, 1976

3. ABDULLA U, CAMPBELL S, DEWHURST J et al: Effect of diagnostic ultrasound on maternal and fetal chromosomes. Lancet 2: 829, 1971

4. ABDULLA U, TALBERT D, LUCAS M et al: Effect of ultrasound on chromosomes of lymphocyte cultures. Br Med J 3: 797, 1972

5. ABRAMOWSKI PK, STRUM KW, JUNG H et al: Der Einfluss der Ultraschall-Langzeitapplikation auf das fetale Gehirn. Z Gerburtshlife Perinatol 176: 286, 1972

6. ANDREW DS: Ultrasonography in pregnancy—an enquiry into its safety. Br J Radiol 37:185, 1964

7. ANDRIANOV VM: Submicroscopic studies of the cells of the spermatogenic epithelium after exposure of white rats to ultrasound. Fiziolog Zh 12:404, 1966

8. BANG J: The intensity of ultrasound in the uterus during examination for diagnostic purposes. Acta Pathol Microbiol Scand [A] 80:341, 1972

9. BARTALOS M, BARAMKI TA: Medical Cytogenetics, The Effect of Ionizing Radiation on Chromosomes. Baltimore, Williams & Wilkins, 1967

10. BASAURI L, LELE PP: A simple method for the production of trackless focal lesions with focussed ultrasound: statistical evaluation of the effects of irradiation on central nervous system of the cat. J Physiol (Lond) 160:513, 1962

11. BAUM G: The effect of ultrasonic radiation upon the eye and occular adnexa. Am J Opthalmol 42:696, 1956

12. BELL E: Action of ultrasound on adult and embryonic organ systems. Am J Phys Med 37:184, 1958

13. BENDER MA: X-ray induced chromosome aberrations in normal diploid human tissue cultures. Science 126:974, 1957

14. BERNSTINE R: Safety studies with ultrasonic Doppler technic—a clinical follow-up of patients and tissue culture study. Obstet Gynecol 34:707, 1969

15. BISHOP EH: Obstetric uses of the ultrasonic motion sensor. Am J Obstet Gynecol 96:863, 1966

16. BLEANEY BI, BLACKBURN P, KIRKLEY J: Resistance of CHLF hamster cells to ultrasonic radiation of 1.5 MHz frequency. Br J Radiol 45:354, 1972

17. BOBROW M, BLACKWELL N, UNRAU AE et al: Absence of any observed effect of ultrasonic irradiation on human chromosomes. J Obstet Gynaecol Br Commonw 78:730, 1971

18. BOYD E, ABDULLA U, DONALD I et al: Chromosome breakage and ultrasound. Br Med J 2:501, 1971

19. BUCKTON KE, BAKER NV: An investigation into possible chromosome damaging effects of ultrasound on human blood cells. Br J Radiol 45:340, 1972

20. BUSHNELL RJ, WALLACE RH: Induction of sex-linked mutations in Drosophila with ultrasonic treatment. Anat Rec 101:690, 1948

21. CAMPBELL S, NEWMAN GB: Growth of the fetal biparietal diameter during normal pregnancy. J Obstet Gynaecol Br Commonw 78:513, 1971

22. CHAPMAN IV: The effect of ultrasound on potassium content of rat thymocytes in vitro. Br J Radiol 47:411, 1974

23. COAKLEY WT, DUNN F: Degradation of DNA high intensity focussed ultrasonic fields at 1 MHz. J Acoust Soc Am 50:1539, 1971

24. COAKLEY WT, HUGHES DE, SLADE JS et al: Chromosome aberrations after exposure to ultrasound. Br Med J 1:109, 1971

25. COAKLEY WT, SLADE JS, BRAEMAN TM: Examination of lymphocytes for chromosome aberrations after ultrasonic irradiation. Br J Radiol 45:328, 1972

26. COURT BROWN W, BUCKTON KE, JACOBS PA et al: Chromosome studies on adults. Eugen Lab Mem 42, New York, Cambridge University Press, 1966

27. CURTIS JC: Action of intense ultrasound on the intact mouse liver. In Kelly E (ed): Ultrasonic Energy. Urbana, University of Illinois Press, 1965, p 85

28. CURTO KA: Early postpartum mortality following ultrasound radiation. In White D, Barnes R (eds): Ultrasound in Medicine. New York, Plenum Press, 1976, p 535

29. DEWHURST CJ: The safety of ultrasound. Proc R Soc Med 64:966, 1971

30. DONALD I: Ultrasonics in obstetrics. Br Med Bull 24:71, 1968

31. DONALD I: On launching a new diagnostic science. Am J Obstet Gynecol 103:609, 1969

32. DONALD I: New problems in sonar diagnosis. Am J Obstet Gynecol 118:299, 1974

33. DONALD I, MACVICAR J, BROWN TG: Investigation of abnormal masses by pulsed ultrasound. Lancet 1:1188, 1958

34. DUNN F: Temperature and amplitude dependence of acoustic absorption in tissue. Am J Phys Med 34:1545, 1962

35. DUNN F: Interaction of ultrasound and tissue. In Böck J, Ossoinig K (eds): Ultrasonographia Medica. Vienna, Wiener Medizinischen Akademie, 1971, p 451

36. DUNN F, FRY FJ: Ultrasonic threshold dosages for the central mammalian nervous system. IEEE Trans Bio Eng 18:253, 1971

37. DYSON M, FRANKS C, SUCKLING J: Stimulation of healing of varicose ulcers by ultrasound. Ultrasonics 14:232, 1976

38. DYSON M, POND JB, JOSEPH J et al: Stimulation of tissue regeneration by pulsed plane wave ultrasound. IEEE Trans Sonics Ultrasonics SU 17:133, 1970

39. DYSON M, POND JB, WOODWARD B et al: The production of blood cell stasis and endothelial damage in the blood vessels of chick embryos treated with ultrasound in a stationary wave field. Ultrasound Med Biol 1:133, 1974

40. DYSON M, WOODWARD B, POND JB: Flow of red blood cells stopped by ultrasound. Nature 232:572, 1971

41. ETIENNE J, FILIPCZYNSKI L, FIREK A et al: Intensity determination of ultrasonic focussed beams used in ultrasonography in the case of gravid uterus. Ultrasound Med Biol 2:119, 1976

42. FISHMAN SS: Biological effects of ultrasound: in-vivo and in-vitro hemolysis. Proc West Pharmacol Soc 11:147, 1968

43. FRITZ-NIGGLI H, BONI A: Biological experiments on Drosophila melanogaster with supersonic vibrations. Science 112:120, 1950

44. FRY FJ, KOSSOFF G, EGGLETON RC et al: Threshold ultrasonic dosages for histological changes in the mammalian brain. J Acoust Soc Am 48:1413, 1970

45. FRY WJ, DUNN F: Ultrasound: analysis and experimental methods in biological research. In Nastuck WL (ed): Physical Techniques in Biological Research. London, Academic Press, 1962, p 261

46. FRY WJ, TUCKER D, FRY FJ et al: Physical factors involved in ultrasonically induced changes in living systems. II. Amplitude duration relations and the effect of hydrostatic pressure for nerve tissue. J Acoust Soc Am 23:364, 1951

47. FRY WJ, WULFF VJ, TUCKER D et al: Physical factors involved in ultrasonically induced changes in living systems. I. Identification of non-temperature effects. J Acoust Soc Am 22:867, 1950

48. GALPERIN-LEMAITRE H, GUSTOT P, LEVI S: Ultrasound and marrow-cell chromosomes. Lancet 2:505, 1973

49. GALPERIN-LEMAITRE H, KIRSCH-VOLDERS M, LEVI S: Ultrasound and mammalian DNA. Lancet 2:662, 1975

50. GARG AG, TAYLOR AR: An investigation into the effects of pulsed ultrasound on the brain. Ultrasonics 5:208, 1967

51. GARRISON BM, BO WJ, KRUEGER WA et al: The influence of ovarian sonication on fetal development in the rat. J Clin Ultrasound 1:316, 1973

52. HALL AJ: An investigation into certain aspects of the safety of diagnostic ultrasound. MSc thesis, University of Glasgow, 1974

53. HAWLEY SA, MACLEOD RM, DUNN F: Degradation of DNA by intense non-cavitating ultrasound. J Acoust Soc Am 35:1285, 1963

54. HELLMAN LM, DUFFUS GM, DONALD I et al: Safety of diagnostic ultrasound in obstetrics. Lancet 1:1133, 1970

55. HERRICK JF: Temperatures produced in tissues by ultrasound: experimental study using various technics. J Acoust Soc Am 25:12, 1953

56. HILL CR: The possibility of hazard in medical and industrial applications of ultrasound. Br J Radiol 41:561, 1968

57. HILL CR: Calibration of ultrasonic beams for biomedical applications. Phys Med Biol 15:241, 1970

58. HILL CR: Acoustic intensity measurements on ultrasonic diagnostic devices. In Böck J, Ossoinig K (eds): Ultrasonographia Medica. Vienna, Wiener Medizinischen Akademie, 1971, p 21

59. HILL CR, JOSHI GP, REVELL SH: A search for chromosome damage following exposure of Chinese hamster cells to high intensity, pulsed ultrasound. Br J Radiol 45:333, 1972

60. HRAZDIRA I: Changes in cell ultrastructure under direct and indirect action of ultrasound. In Böck J, Ossoinig K (eds): Ultrasonographia Medica. Vienna, Wiener Medizinischen Akademie, 1971, p 457

61. HRAZDIRA I, KONEČNÝ M: Functional and morphological changes in the thyroid gland after ultrasonic irradiation. Am J Phys Med 45:238, 1966

62. HUETER TF, BOLT RH: Sonics. New York, John Wiley & Sons, 1955

63. HUGHES DE, NYBORG WL: Cell disruption by ultrasound. Science 138:108, 1962

64. IKEUCHI T, SASKI M, OSHIMURA M et al: Ultrasound and embryonic chromosomes. Br Med J 1:112, 1973

65. KATO M: Inductivity of recessive lethal mutations in Drosophila melanogaster by ultrasonic vibration. Osaka Med School Bull: 12:108, 1966

66. KOHN G, ROBINSON A: Tetraploidy in cells cultured from amniotic fluid. Lancet 11:778, 1970

67. KOHORN EI, PRITCHARD JW, HOBBINS JC: The safety of clinical ultrasonic examination. Obstet Gynecol 29:272, 1967

68. KORYANI G, FALUS M, SOBEL M et al: Follow-up examination of children exposed to ultrasound in utero. Acta Paediatr Acad Sci Hung 13:231, 1972

69. KOSSOFF G: Balance technique for the measurement of very low ultrasonic outputs. J Acoust Soc Am 38:880, 1965

70. KOSSOFF G, ROBINSON DE, GARRETT WJ: Acoustic properties of materials. Sydney, CAL Report 31, 1965

71. KUNZE-MÜHL E, GOLOB E: Chromosomenanalysen nach Ultraschalleinwirkung. Hum Genet 14:237, 1972

72. LEHMANN JF, DE LATEUR BJ, SILVERMAN DR: Selective heating effects of ultrasound in human beings. Arch Phys Med Rehabil 46:331, 1966

73. LEHMANN JF, KRUSEN FH: Therapeutic applications of ultrasound in physical medicine. Am J Phys Med 37:173, 1958

74. LELE PP: Effects of focussed ultrasonic radiation on peripheral nerve with observations on local heating. Exp Neurol 8:47, 1963

75. LOCH EG, FISCHER AB, KUWERT E: Effect of diagnostic and therapeutic intensities of ultrasonics on normal and malignant human cells in vitro. Am J Obstet Gynecol 110:457, 1971

76. LUCAS M, MULLARKEY M, ABDULLA U: Study of chromosomes in the newborn after ultrasonic fetal heart monitoring in Labour. Br Med J 3:795, 1972

77. LYON MF, SIMPSON GM: An investigation into the possible genetic hazards of ultrasound. Br J Radiol 47:712, 1974

78. MACINTOSH IJC: Chromosome breakage and ultrasound. Br Med J 3:703, 1971

79. MACINTOSH IJC, BROWN RC, COAKLEY WT: Ultrasound and 'in vitro' chromosome aberrations. Br J Radiol 48:230, 1975

80. MACINTOSH IJC, DAVEY DA: Chromosome aberrations induced by an ultrasonic fetal pulse detector. Br Med J 4:92, 1970

81. MACINTOSH IJC, DAVEY DA: Relationship between intensity of ultrasound and induction of chromosome aberrations. Br J Radiol 45:320, 1972

82. MANNOR SM, SERR DM, TAMARI I: The safety of ultrasound in fetal monitoring. Am J Obstet Gynecol 113:653, 1972

83. Manual on Non-Ionizing Radiation Protection: Ultrasound Radiation. To be published by the World Health Organization, Regional Office for Europe. (in press, 1979/80)

84. MERMUT S, KATYAMA KP, DEL CASTILLO R et al: The effect of ultrasound on human chromosomes in vitro. Obstet Gynecol 41:4, 1973

85. MILUNSKY A, LITTLEFIELD JW, ATKINS L: Tetraploidy in amniotic fluid cells. Lancet 2:979, 1970

86. O'BRIEN WD: Ultrasonically induced fetal weight reduction in mice. In White D (ed): Ultrasound in Medicine 2. New York, Plenum Press, 1976, p 531

87. OKAUCHI K: Effects of heating of testes on spermatogenesis in mice. In Animal Breeding Abstracts. Bulletin of the Faculty of Agriculture, University of Miyazaki 15:186, 1968

88. POND JB: The role of heat in the production of ultrasonic focal lesions. J Acoust Soc Am 47:1607, 1970

89. POURHADI R, BONHOMME CH, TURCHINI JP: Action des ultrasons sur la spermatogenese (Souris). Etude histologique. Arch Anat Microsc Morphol Exp 54:847, 1965

90. PRASAD N: Ultrasound and mammalian DNA. Lancet 1:1181, 1976

91. RIDGE B: Principles of Organic Life. London, Robert Hardwicke, 1875, p 17

92. ROBINSON HP: Sonar measurement of fetal crown-rump length of pregnancy as a means of assessing maturity in first trimester. Br Med J 4:28, 1973

93. ROTT HD, HUBER HJ, SOLDER R et al: Chromosomenuntersuchungen nach Einwirkung von Ultraschall auf Menschliche Lymphozyten in vitro. Elektromedica 1:14, 1972

94. ROTT HD, SOLDER R, VAN ZYL J: Zur Wirkung von Ultraschall auf menschliche Chromosomen in vitro. Geburtshilfe Frauenheilkd 32:662, 1972

95. SCHEIDT PC: Letter: questions: safety of ultrasound. Paediatrics 57:162, 1976

96. SERR DM, PADEH B, ZAKUT H et al: Studies on the effects of ultrasonic waves on the fetus. In Huntingford PJ, Beard RW, Hytten FE et al (eds): Perinatal Medicine. Basel, Karger, 1970, p 302

97. SHEALEY CN, HENNEMAN E: Quantitative neuro-anatomic studies implemented by ultrasonic lesions. Arch Neurol 6:374, 1962

98. SHOJI R, MURAKAMI U, SHIMIZU T: Influence of low-intensity ultrasonic irradiation on prenatal development of two inbred mouse strains. Teratology 12:227, 1975

99. SLEEMAN RM: The treatment of Meniére's disease with ultrasound. NZ Med J 64:446, 1965

100. SMYTH MG: Animal toxicity studies with ultrasound at diagnostic power levels. In Grossman CC, Holmes JH, Joyner C et al (eds): Diagnostic Ultrasound. New York, Plenum Press, 1966, p 296

101. TAKAGI SF, HIGASHINO S, SHILKURYA T et al: The actions of ultrasound on the myelinated nerve, the spinal cord and the brain. Jpn J Physiol 10:183, 1960

102. TALBERT DG, CAMPBELL S: Physical aspects of diagnostic ultrasound. Br J Hosp Med 8:501, 1972

103. TAYLOR KJW, CONNOLLY CC: Differing hepatic lesions caused by the same dose of ultrasound. J Pathol 98:291, 1969

104. TAYLOR KJW, DYSON M: Possible hazards of diagnostic ultrasound. Br J Hosp Med 8:571, 1972

105. TAYLOR KJW, POND JB: The effects of ultrasound of varying frequencies on rat liver. J Pathol 100:287, 1970

106. TAYLOR KJW, POND JB: A study of the production of haemorrhagic injury and paraplegia in rat spinal cord by pulsed ultrasound of low megahertz frequencies in the context of the safety for clinical usage. Br J Radiol 45:343, 1972

107. THACKER J: The possibility of genetic hazard from ultrasonic radiation. Curr Top Radiat Res Q 8:235, 1973

108. THACKER J: An assessment of ultrasonic radiation hazard using yeast genetic systems. Br J Radiol 47:130, 1974

109. THACKER J: Ultrasound and mammalian DNA. Lancet 2:770, 1975

110. THACKER J, BAKER NV: The use of Drosophila to estimate the possibility of genetic hazard from ultrasound irradiations. Br J Radiol 49:367, 1976

111. TORCHIA RT, PURNELL W, SOKOLLU A: Cataract production by ultrasound. Am J Ophthalmol 64:305, 1967

112. United Nations Scientific Committee Report on the Effect of Atomic Radiation. New York, United Nations, 1969

113. VALTONEN EJ: A histological method for measuring the influence of ultrasonic energy on living tissue under experimental conditions. Acta Rheum Scand 14:35, 1968

114. WARWICK R, POND JB, WOODWARD B et al: Hazards of diagnostic ultrasonography—study with mice. IEEE Trans Sonics Ultrasonics SU 17:158, 1970

115. WATTS PL, HALL AJ, FLEMING JEE: Ultrasound and chromosome damage. Br J Radiol 45:335, 1972

116. WATTS PL, STEWART CR: The effect of fetal heart monitoring by ultrasound on maternal and fetal chromosomes. J Obstet Gynaecol Br Commonw 79:715, 1972

117. WEINLAND LS: Production of abnormal hamster embryos with ultrasound. Penn Acad Sci 37:48, 1963

118. WELLS PNT: Physical Principles of Ultrasonic Diagnosis. London, Academic Press, 1969, p 222

119. WELLS PNT, BULLEN MA, FOLLETT DH et al: The dosimetry of small ultrasound beams. Ultrasonics 1:106, 1963

120. WILLIAMS AR: Intravascular mural thrombi produced by acoustic microstreaming. Ultrasound Med Biol 3:191, 1977

121. WOODCOCK J: The action of non-cavitating ultrasound on the hydrolysis of sucrose solution. London, British Acoustical Society Meeting, 1967

122. WOODWARD B, POND JB, WARWICK R: How safe is diagnostic sonar? Br J Radiol 43:719, 1970

4

Fetal organ imaging

WILLIAM J. GARRETT

There is a great gulf between the rough fetal outlines of Donald's pioneering paper published 20 years ago (2) and the high-quality gray-scale pictures obtained today. The technologic advances of those years have developed systems by which fetal soft-tissue anatomy can be studied in detail and the state of health of the various tissues can be qualitatively assessed. The next few years will see the development of quantitative tissue characterization studies by computerized analysis of the physical factors involved when sound passes through tissues or is reflected or scattered by them.

With bistable equipment an echo had to be of a certain amplitude to light the persistence screen, and when it did so, the spot was fully illuminated. In compound scanning, if the transducer "looked" at one point from eight different angles, eight small echoes were generated, but if each of these echoes was not sufficiently large to light the screen, nothing was recorded and the information was lost. By contrast, one echo four times the intensity of one of these hypothetical small echoes might be strong enough to light the screen even though its intensity was only half the sum of the smaller ones. The bistable system was good at displaying interfaces with significant mismatch of acoustic impedance such as boundaries between organs and at displaying noise and other odd echoes giving a snow storm appearance to many echograms. The system gave virtually no information about the tissue content of

an organ, though this could be obtained in a rough way by switching to A-mode.

Despite the limitations of bistable echograms, much anatomic detail of the fetus was identified (1, 15, 21). The fetal spine, kidney, bladder, and heart were seen, and measurements of the heart and bladder were obtained (14, 23). With the original UI Water Delay Echoscope designed by Kossoff (17), fine structures such as the aorta, interventricular cardiac septum, and ductus venosus were recorded (15), but in 1969 with the introduction of gray scale also by Kossoff, a new era began. His system was simple enough (17, 19). A standard cathode ray oscilloscope was used in place of the persistence screen. The gain was adjusted so that the background that should be black on the echogram was just not black but was the darkest shade of gray possible. Under these circumstances, every echo above background noise level no matter how small produced a spot of light on the screen. By opening the shutter of the Polaroid camera just before scanning began and by closing it at the completion of the scan, the film stored the multitude of small echoes and no information was lost. The borders of organs were still present, but now the parenchyma of the fetal organs and the placental tissue began to appear with an appearance related to their histology. These tissues scatter much of the incident ultrasound, but among this scattered ultrasound a few small echoes are returned to the transducer to be accurately re-

35

corded. This is the essence of gray scale. It is not just getting a picture with a grayish blur but rather the faithful record of every echo no matter how small.

The open-shutter method is suitable for both contact and water delay machines. With a hand-held transducer the open-shutter technique calls for considerable skill in scanning, and there may be a lot of difference in the results achieved by different operators. Such difficulties are dispelled in a water delay system where mechanically driven transducers are employed. The smooth mechanical oscillation of the transducers produces a perfectly smooth scanning motion with excellent gray scale on the film with both simple and compound scanning.

With the advent of scan converters, gray-scale pictures have been obtained more easily, and the scan converter has given great impetus to ultrasound as a diagnostic modality. The scan converter gray scale is, however, obtained at a price in that the picture quality is degraded by the television lines and lacks the fine detail of echograms obtained by the open-shutter system. In my department the four B-mode echoscopes designed by the Ultrasonics Institute under the direction of Kossoff have scan converters on them, but these have been used only to indicate to the sonographer the plane of section being examined. The echograms are taken from a separate oscilloscope by the open-shutter method.

Since 1962 we have used a water delay system wherein the patient presses her abdomen against the polythene membrane of a water bath in which a single transducer is immersed. The transducer oscillates four times as it moves in an arc around the patient so getting eight "looks" at the patient. The system has required approximately 16 sec to obtain each echogram, and with a repetition rate of 500/sec this has meant that much irrelevant information has been received. The transducer has produced eight pulses between one discernibly different position of the transducer and the next so that seven times the information required has been generated. Such unnecessary repetition is avoided in the UI Octoson (18), where eight 3-MHz transducers mounted on an arm and immersed in a water bath "look" up from below into the patient (Fig. 4–1). The transducers oscillate synchronously every 2½ sec through an angle of 50° to produce each echogram. The transducers are energized in order one after another at 650 μsec intervals. By the time the transmit pulses have energized all eight transducers and the cycle is ready to begin again, the transducers as a whole have moved through an angle of 0.1°, which is the next discernibly different position. No line of sight of any transducer is repeated, so that no unnecessary information is obtained. The position of the arm on which the transducers are mounted is controlled from a console. The arm

FIG. 4–1. The principle of operation of the Octoson. The eight transducers "looking" up from below move simultaneously through an angle of 50° as each echogram is obtained. The water surface is covered with a polythene membrane.

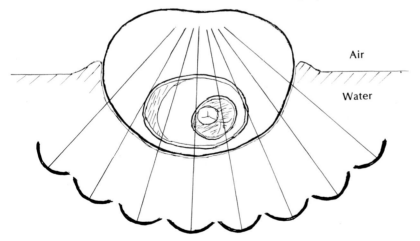

Air

Water

may be raised or lowered to put the focus in the area of greatest interest. Transverse-section echograms are obtained with the transducer arm lying transversely across the machine. The position of this transverse plane can be moved cranially or caudally by 1-, 2-, 5-, 10- or 20-mm steps, either one section at a time or in an automatic mode whereby sections are taken serially every 2½ sec at planes the selected distance apart. This scanning time is shortened if fewer than eight transducers are used and the scanning angle is reduced. With one transducer and a narrow angle quasi-real time is possible.

Longitudinal sections are obtained by rotating the arm through 90°, and the single-step or automatic mode is available to take sections appropriate distances apart as required. For in-

clined planes, the arm may be tilted, and for some special examinations the plane may be rotated about a point. Both simple and compound scanning modes are available, and any combination of the eight transducers can be used.

For examining the fetus and placenta, the patient lies prone on the padded examination top of the instrument (Fig. 4–2). The central section is not unlike a water bed in that it has a polythene cover to the water tank in which the transducers are immersed. Oil is the coupling medium, and good coupling to the flanks is achieved by raising the water level, which causes the polythene membrane to rise and wrap itself around the patient's abdomen. To the patient, the procedure is both comfortable and brief, the examination usually taking about 10 min. The

FIG. 4–2. An obstetric patient being examined on the UI Octoson.

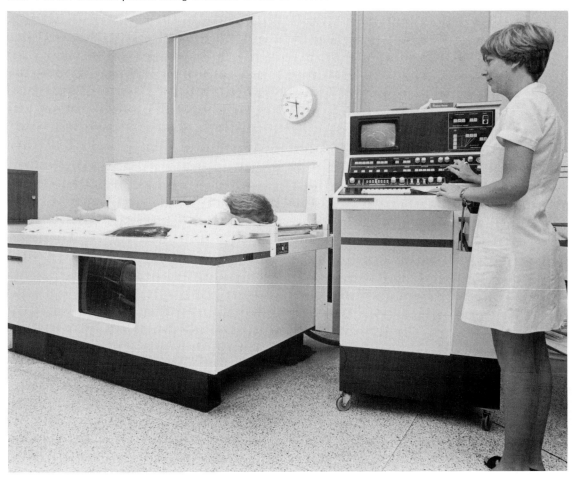

full set of transverse and longitudinal echograms is obtained in about 30 sec each way. The rest of the time is taken in the administrative details of the procedure.

THE FETAL HEAD AND SPINE

The flexed fetal head is easily seen as a circle in transverse-section echograms, and its transverse diameters or cross-sectional area may be measured. Where the head is extended, the cranial vault appears more oval in transverse section, and with a considerable degree of extension, the bony orbits and eyes may be identified (Fig. 4–3). It is usually difficult to see the eyes with the head flexed, for the plane of section commonly passes through all the facial bones, which return such strong echoes that identifying the landmarks of the face is difficult.

Within the cranial vault the falx is identified from the early second trimester, and on either side of it a parallel line is recorded corresponding to the lateral wall of the bodies of the lateral ventricles. In neonates, ventricular size is measured by estimating the lateral ventricular ratio, which is calculated by dividing the width of the body of the lateral ventricle by half the internal biparietal diameter of the skull. The normal range for the lateral ventricular ratio (LVR) in neonates and young children is 0.26–0.36 (10, 11). Although no figures are available for the LVR in fetuses, it would be reasonable to accept these figures for the last 4 weeks of pregnancy until the normal fetal range is established. In identifying the lateral ventricles in the fetus, care should be taken not to mistake the echo from the sulcus over the insula for the echo from the lateral wall of the lateral ventricle or to confuse the brain stem and basal nuclei with the lateral ventricles. Myelinated nerve tissue generates few echoes, and though myelination is incomplete in the fetus, the brain stem may on occasions look like lateral ventricles in coronal section.

In the ultrasonic examination of the fetal head and spine, the main variations to seek are hydrocephaly, microcephaly, anencephaly, and meningomyeloceles. There may be previous or family history of these conditions; if so, amniocentesis will be performed in the earlier weeks. Hydrocephaly is first suspected by finding the head larger than it should be for the stated period of amenorrhea or larger than the size the fetal trunk would suggest should be the case. Where the underlying cause is severe stenosis or blockage of the aqueduct, the increased head size is present from the earliest weeks. The head may grow at a regular rate and the hydrocephaly may not be immediately obvious on clinical examination. An example is recorded where the head was 5 weeks' size bigger than it should be, and yet the head grew at the normal rate (15). More commonly the stenosis is such that it makes its mark only in the later weeks of pregnancy. Either the stenosed aqueduct, which has previously coped with the flow of cerebrospinal fluid, fails and the lateral ventricles expand rapidly or the production of cerebrospinal fluid increases considerably with a similar result (Fig. 4–4).

Finding a large fetal head is not enough to diagnose hydrocephaly unless the enlargement is gross. Gross cases are obvious, and while early diagnosis is helpful, it is not usual for the obstetrician to interfere until cephalopelvic disproportion is present. Craniotomy or some related drainage operation is undertaken in labor to reduce the size of the head and relieve the obstruction to delivery. Happily the fetus does not survive and a mistake in the diagnosis is unlikely to occur.

In cases of hydrocephaly of mild or moderate degree, increased head size may or may not be present. The lateral ventricles will be dilated, and good gray scale allows them to be identified and measured (5). The obstetrician is then alerted and the difficult decision between delivery by Caesarean section or by the vaginal route must be made. Large ventricles in themselves do not necessarily indicate significant brain damage. Cortical thickness is a better parameter, and this can be judged from good-quality gray-scale echograms where the cerebral tissue is clearly differentiated from the cerebrospinal fluid within the ventricles.

Anencephaly is easily identified in late pregnancy by the absence of the calvarium. In bi-

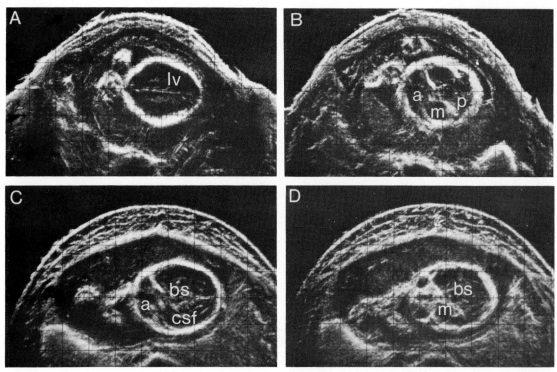

FIG. 4-3. Normal fetal heads. **A.** transverse section at the level of the bodies of the lateral ventricles LVR 0.36. **B.** section 3 cm lower than A, showing cranial fossae. **C.** an extended head with section through anterior fossa and brain stem. The symmetrical collections of CSF under the parietal bones are not infrequently seen in fetuses and infants. In young babies they are to be distinguished from subdural hematomas. **D.** section 2 cm lower than C, showing orbits middle fossa and brain stem (a, anterior fossa; bs, brain stem; csf, cerebrospinal fluid; f, falx; lv, lateral wall of lateral ventricle; m, middle fossa; p, posterior fossa).

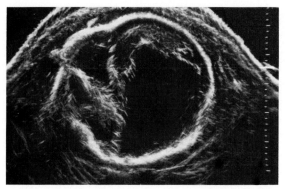

FIG. 4-4. Hydrocephaly, showing the brain tissue distorted by grossly enlarged ventricles.

stable days it was not unknown to mistake the fetal trunk for a head, but today there is no excuse for such confusion, for viscera of the thorax and abdomen are visible landmarks. Anencephaly is commonly associated with polyhydramnios, and indeed this is the usual reason why ultrasonic examination is sought. Polyhydramnios is not, however, a constant sign, and extreme oligohydramnios may occur (5). In twin pregnancy with one anencephalic fetus, the polyhydramnios affects only one sac (4) (Fig. 4–5).

If we are to make a significant contribution to the diagnosis of anencephaly, the diagnosis must be made early when termination of pregnancy can be undertaken before the patient has felt fetal movements (3). Amniocentesis for alpha fetoprotein is done at the 15th to 16th weeks of amenorrhea; at that time anencephaly can be directly confirmed in the B-mode examination. Fetal movement may be a problem with an active headless little fetus in a relatively large pool of amniotic fluid. With UI Octoson, when the angle of sweep of the transducers is narrowed from 50° to 30° to cover the length of the fetus only and the central four transducers are used instead of the full rank of eight, the examination time for each echogram is reduced to 0.6 sec. The ill effects of fetal movement are thus significantly reduced. Another approach is to use a freeze-frame system on a real-time scanner, but there the poorer resolution is a considerable difficulty when one is looking for the absence of a

FIG. 4–5. Anencephaly in one of twins. Note that the polyhydramnios is restricted to the amniotic sac of the abnormal fetus. (c, cord; H1, T1, head and trunk normal fetus; H2, T2, head and trunk anencephalic fetus.)

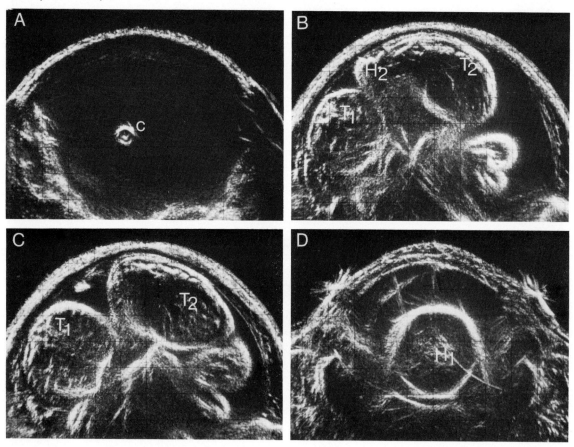

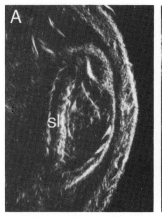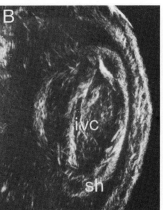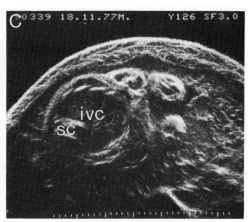

FIG. 4–6. Normal spine, showing the difficulty in diagnosing spina bifida. **A, B.** longitudinal sections 2 cm apart. **C.** transverse section (ivc, inferior vena cava; s, spine; sc, spinal canal; sh, shoulder).

very small cranial vault. It is easy to say a head is present and to state its size, but to be certain of the absence of part of it may be problematic.

Microcephaly is generally diagnosed on size alone. Warkeny (22), in his authoritative work on congenital abnormalities, states that it is diagnosed where the size of the head is more than three times the standard deviation below the norm. We have found microcephaly difficult to diagnose in fat patients. The fetus generally presents as a vertex, and the tiny head lies low in the pelvis (5), but its measurement is possible.

Spina bifida may be a very real problem for ultrasonic diagnosis. With a fetus immersed in amniotic fluid, the intrauterine pressure may equal the pressure of the cerebrospinal fluid in the dilated neural tube, so that the surface contour of the myelocele may be flat and be at the level of the normal skin if that had been present. Where a membrane covers the defect, alpha fetoprotein is usually detected by amniocentesis in the early weeks, but where the membrane is unduly thick or the defect is covered by skin, this biochemical test may prove negative. The classic lumbosacral cystic mass seen in the nursery is not necessarily present at birth and may develop following delivery when the intrauterine pressure is replaced by the very much lower air pressure. The fetus with such a flat myelocele may press its back against the uterine wall to defy diagnosis in transverse-section echograms by the best high-resolution echoscopes.

With longitudinal-section echograms the plane of section may be adjusted to correspond to the axis of the spine, but the spinal canal, being gently curved, is not generally seen in its entirety in any one plane. The plane of section may falsely give the impression of a spindle-shaped enlargement that can be falsely interpreted as a major neural tube deformity. If the plane is misjudged, the inferior vena cava may be confused with the spinal canal (Fig. 4–6). With good resolution individual vertebrae can be seen at 11½ weeks (7).

THE FETAL THORAX

The fetal thorax is usually best seen in transverse-section echograms. The heart is identified as a circular structure a little to the left of the midline, and its size and position are noted. The chambers of the heart can be identified (Fig. 4–7), even though the heart may have contracted 2–40 times during the examination. Occasional lucky-shot echograms show clearly intracardiac structures such as the mitral valve (15), but this is not to be relied on for diagnosis.

Congenital anomalies of the fetal heart are difficult to diagnose, and only those with an unusual rhythm are likely to be detected with real-time equipment. Fetal heart failure produces the classic signs of ascites and generalized edema, which is particularly marked over the scapula region, around the chest, and in the scalp (Fig. 4–8). Occasionally a pleural effusion

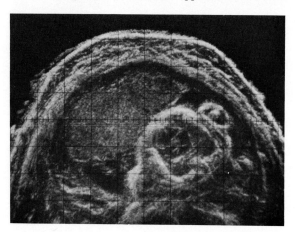

FIG. 4-7. Normal fetal heart and lungs. Note the septa within the heart, the echo-free chambers, and the gray pattern of the lung tissue.

FIG. 4-8. Hydrops fetalis from rhesus isoimmunization. **A.** head. **B.** upper chest and massive edema of shoulders. **C.** the very small heart. **D.** ascites and edema of the abdominal wall (a, ascites; e, edema; h, heart; sh, shoulder; t, thorax).

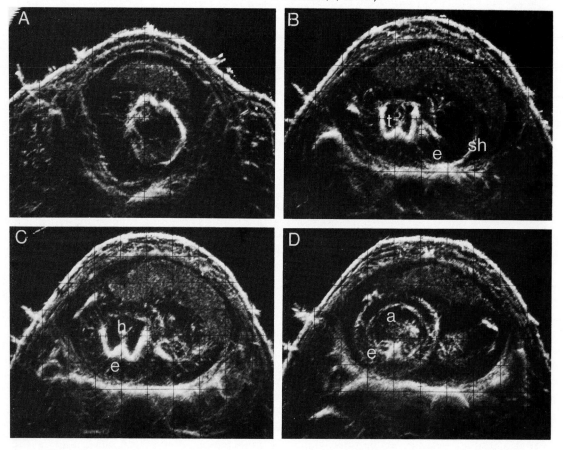

is seen. The earliest sign of heart failure in post-natal life may be an increase in heart size, but in the fetus this is not usual. The ratio of the transverse diameter of the fetal heart to the transverse diameter of the chest at the same level is 0.52 (SD-0.05). The transverse diameter of the left ventricle is greater than that of the right ventricle by a factor of 1.2, and the angle the interventricular septum makes with the sagittal plane is very variable and in normal cases has been measured at 0–57° (mean 32°) (14).

Fetal cardiac failure is always secondary to some other condition. It is commonly associated with fetal anemia of one variety or another or with interference to the circulation. The interference may be due to direct obstruction to the outflow tracts at the base of the heart by a lung tumor or cyst or by blockage of the inflow, as with transfusion syndrome in twins or massive placental infarction (Fig. 4–9 and 4–10). A more detailed list of the causes of hydrops is included under the differential diagnosis of fetal ascites.

A case of hamartoma of the fetal lung with congestive cardiac failure has been described (12). The diagnostic signs were massive edema, ascites, and displacement of the heart to the left by a solid, ill-defined mass (Fig. 4–11). A similar picture is seen with a pulmonary cyst (Fig. 4–12) where the cyst presses on the great vessels on the base of the heart. The cyst has a firm outline and is apparently under some pressure, which distinguishes it from diaphragmatic hernia, where the dilated stomach forms a cystic structure above the level of the heart (9). The stomach being soft and deformable, it molds itself to the surrounding structures and does not interfere with the circulation.

Dextrocardia may be seen in echograms of the fetus (8), but its diagnosis is likely to be missed, for there is no sign other than the reversed geometry. Because of the variations in fetal presentation and position, the diagnosis of fetal situs inversus may not be immediately obvious.

With pulmonary atresia, the fetal chest is smaller than usual and polyhydramnios is present. In the example shown (Fig. 4–13), the head corresponds in size with the usual measurements for 29 weeks' amenorrhea, the abdomen corresponds in size with the usual measurements at 27 weeks, and the fetal chest is very much smaller than this. The lecithin-sphingomyelin ratio never reached mature levels. At birth no respiratory effort occurred.

FETAL ABDOMEN

In transverse sections, the landmarks in the fetal abdomen are the spine, the fetal kidneys, and the ductus venosus, which can always be identified. The fetal stomach, urinary bladder, gall bladder, and, less commonly, loops of colon are seen when their lumens are distended with fluid. It is sometimes difficult to distinguish the inferior surface of the normal fetal liver from the collapsed bowel.

The stomach is commonly seen in transverse sections in the upper left quadrant of the fetal abdomen as a circular cystic structure surrounded on all sides by echo-producing "gray" tissue. It is usually at or slightly above the level of the ductus venosus, which is the continuation of the umbilical vein in its intraabdominal course to the inferior vena cava.

The fetal stomach does not normally measure more than 25 mm in transverse diameter and may be seen distended beyond this size in atresia of the small bowel (8). In small bowel obstruction other echo-free, liquid-filled, dilated loops of bowel are recorded that in jejunal and duodenal atresia may be restricted to the upper part of the abdomen. Bowel obstruction is commonly associated with polyhydramnios. Dilated loops of bowel are to be distinguished from mesenteric cysts (20); where the stomach is not significantly dilated, there is no polyhydramnios, and the cysts, unlike the fetal bladder, do not empty periodically.

In meconium ileus the dilated bowel returns echoes from within its lumen corresponding to the abnormal meconium, and these are distinguished from the normal bowel pattern by being at a lower level than usual (Fig. 4–14).

The ductus venosus is a regularly seen landmark that presents as two parallel lines corresponding to its walls as it runs from the umbilicus toward the inferior vena cava. With the UI Octoson, the blood flow within the ductus can be measured. The transverse-plane section through the ductus is first put on the screen by compound

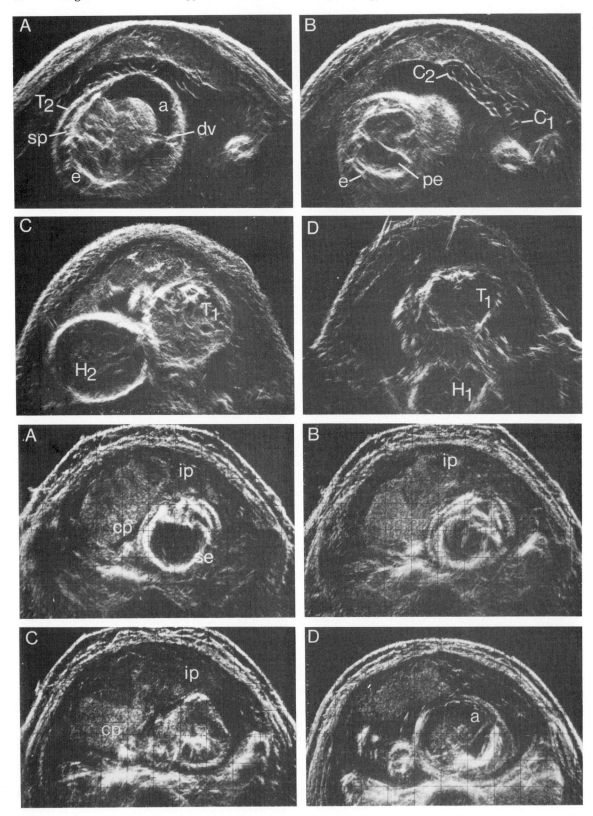

◀ **FIG. 4-9.** Transfusion syndrome in twins (a, ascites; C1 and C2, cords of first and second fetuses; dv, ductus venosus; f, edema; H1, H2 and T1, T2, heads and trunks of first and second fetuses; pe, pleural effusion).

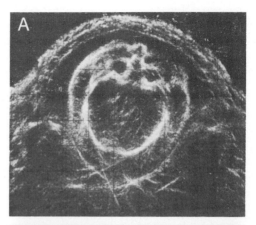

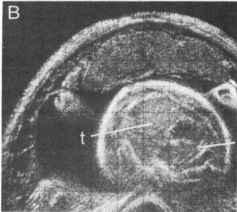

scanning. With one transducer, a line of sight is laid down so that the angle between this line of sight and the ductus can be measured. The transducer selected is the one that will make this angle conveniently small. By special adjustment the equipment is switched to record Doppler changes in frequency associated with blood flow within the vessel and by calculation; the cosine of the angle and the width of the ductus being known, the flow is assessed (16). In a short series this has been calculated as 100 ml/min/kg of fetus in the third trimester.

Where there is a defect in the abdominal wall such as with exompahlos, the bowel extrudes into the herniation and there may be some free fluid distending the sac (Fig. 4–15). The sac is variable in size. It may be quite small or so large that it may at first sight be confused with the amniotic sac. Reference to the whole series of sections instead of reliance on one or two planes makes the diagnosis obvious.

In prune belly syndrome there is a lack of musculature in the anterior abdominal wall; this occurs most commonly between the pubic symphysis and umbilicus. The peritoneum and skin are separated only by a layer of areolar or thin fibrous tissue so that a diffuse ventral hernia develops (Fig. 4–17b). Where there is concurrent severe oligohydramnios, care should be taken in diagnosing prune belly syndrome from echograms. Under these conditions, a normal fetal abdomen may assume an unusual shape, and with the plane of section not absolutely transverse in relation to the fetus, a very similar picture may be obtained.

Ascites is the commonest cause of abdominal distension in the fetus. This may be part of the syndrome of congestive cardiac failure secondary to a very severe anemia (Fig. 4–16) or circu-

FIG. 4-11. Case of hamartoma of the lung displacing the heart to the left and causing congestive cardiac failure. **A.** head, showing massive edema of the face and scalp. **B.** transverse section through the heart. Note the characteristic ground glass appearance of the placenta in heart failure (t, tumor; h, heart).

◀ **FIG. 4-10.** Massive placental infarction leading to congestive cardiac failure. **A.** transverse section through the head. **B, C, D.** 1, 3, and 9 cm respectively above A. (a, ascites; cp, congested placenta; ip, infarcted placenta; se, scalp edema.)

latory obstruction or may be associated with an intraabdominal condition. Where the ascites is associated with a renal abnormality, there is commonly oligohydramnios. In contrast to adults, liver disease is an unusual cause of ascites in the fetus but is not unknown and has been seen with calcification of the liver (20). In male fetuses with open inguinal canals, unilateral or bilateral hydrocele may be noted. A list for the differential diagnosis of ascites can thus be given.

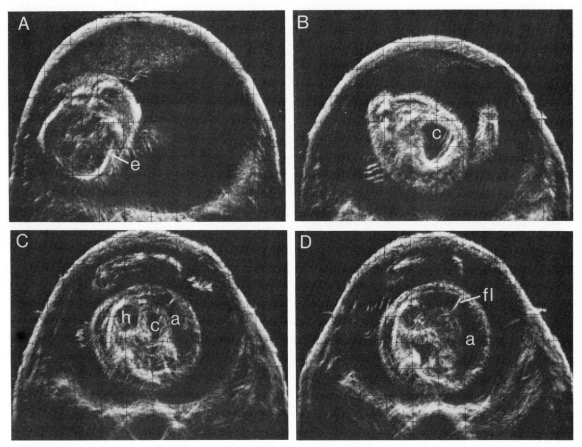

FIG. 4–12. Fetal lung cyst with polyhydramnios and cardiac failure. **A.** scalp edema. **B.** lung cyst pressing on base of heart. **C.** displaced heart. **D.** ascites (a, ascites; c, cyst; fl, falciform ligament; h, heart).

CAUSES OF FETAL ASCITES

Anemia causes
   Rh isoimmunization
   ABO incompatibility
   Leukemia
   Congenital hemolytic anemia
Circulatory causes
   Transfusion syndrome in twins
   Lung tumor
   Lung cyst
   Congenital heart disease
   Massive placental infarction
Abdominal causes
   Multicystic kidney
Other causes
   Absent kidney
   Liver disease
   Exomphalos
   Toxoplasmosis
   Idiopathic

The kidneys are well seen in both transverse section and longitudinal echograms, and their size and position are noted. The normal renal parenchyma returns very low-level echoes and not infrequently seems to be echo free. The collecting system produces a characteristic high-level echo in the center of the kidney. In normal cases the lumen of the renal pelvis cannot be resolved. In one patient who subsequently developed a nephroblastoma, the kidney failed to show a collecting system in the middle of the kidney during fetal life, and it is tempting to postulate that it was pushed to one side at an early stage, even though there was no enlargement of the kidney. The commonest fetal renal abnormality is multicystic or polycystic kidney (6), which may or not be associated with ascites or oligohydramnios.

Obstructive lesions to the collecting system occur at various levels. Blockage at the pel-

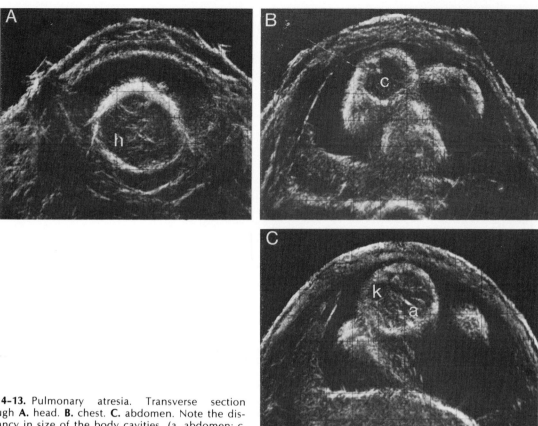

FIG. 4–13. Pulmonary atresia. Transverse section through **A.** head. **B.** chest. **C.** abdomen. Note the discrepancy in size of the body cavities. (a, abdomen; c, chest; h, head; k, kidney.)

FIG. 4–14. Meconium ileus and volvulus. **A.** transverse section at the level of the kidneys. A dilated loop of bowel returns echoes from its lumen. **B.** longitudinal section showing loops of bowel (b, bowel; k, kidney; s, spine).

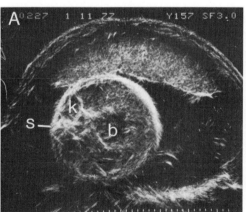

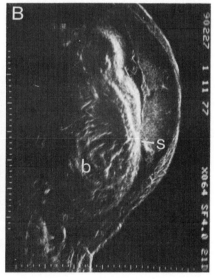

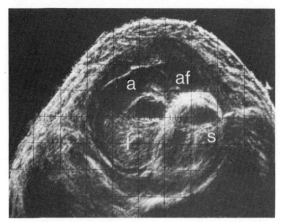

FIG. 4–15. Large exomphalos (a, ascites; af, amniotic fluid; l, liver; s, spine).

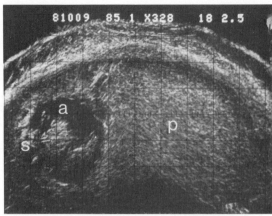

FIG. 4–16. Fetal leukemia, showing ascites, grossly congested placenta, and absent amniotic fluid, the reason for which is obscure (a, ascites; s, spine; p, placenta).

viureteric junction causes unilateral hydronephrosis. Blockage at the ureterovesical orifice, which may be bilateral, produces hydronephrosis or hydroureter, or both. Bilateral hydroureter can be quite gross and yet need not be accompanied by significant hydronephrosis (Fig. 4–17). Urethral blockage may be absolute with either a valve or atresia (13) (Fig. 4–18) or partial and lead to bilateral hydronephrosis. Urethral stenosis is sometimes associated with ureteric stenosis, and the latter may be the more significant lesion (13). The fetal urine production has been estimated at 9.6 ml/hour at 30 weeks' amenorrhea, and this rate increases to 27.3 ml/hour at 40 weeks (23). There does not appear to be a diurnal variation in fetal urinary output or a variation due to sex of the fetus. In light of these figures it is not surprising to find rapid increase in the size of the fetal bladder with megacystis; a fetal bladder containing 3 liters of urine was recorded at the 34th week (13).

THE LIMBS

Ultrasound will demonstrate gross abnormalities of the limbs, but owing to the limitations of two-dimensional sections and the angles at which flexed limbs dispose themselves, such

diagnoses are unduly difficult. The signs of achondroplasia and osteogensis imperfecta are generally identified when echograms are reviewed after the clinical diagnosis is made. Where the possibility of a disease of bone is present, radiologic examination is to be preferred.

PRACTICAL APPLICATIONS

The prenatal diagnosis of a congenital abnormality that inevitably proves fatal is always a disappointment, but it is a disappointment that may be tempered with kindliness and good sense. The obstetrician can prepare the patient and her husband for losing the child so that a psychologic scar is not added to the obstetric loss. In appropriate cases, labor may be induced prematurely and risks related to the fetus are not taken. Morphine may replace demerol in labor.

When the abnormality is such that survival is a possibility, risks to the fetus are then minimized. The fetus with exomphalos, gut atresia, or diaphragmatic hernia is delivered at the hospital with full pediatric surgical facilities. The defect is repaired within a few hours of birth and before fluid balance problems have begun to complicate the picture.

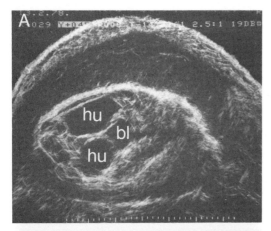

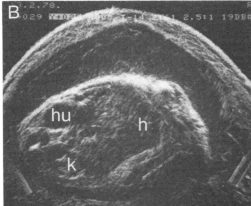

FIG. 4–17. Bilateral hydroureter, small polycystic kidney, and prune belly syndrome. **A.** massive dilatation of both ureters and normal size bladder. **B.** section 2 cm higher through small polycystic kidney and showing broad anterior herniation due to prune belly (bl, bladder; h, herniation; hu, hydroureter; k, kidney).

In rhesus isoimmunization, the timing of intrauterine transfusion can be assisted by detecting the earliest moment when edema and ascites appear. These can come on very quickly, and the patient must be examined every second day if major degrees of hydrops are to be avoided. Following intrauterine transfusion, the rate of absorbtion of the induced hemoperitoneum can be monitored.

FIG. 4–18. Urethral blockage with megacystis. **A.** the head pushed to one side by the massive bladder at 17 weeks' amenorrhea. **B.** section 2 cm lower. Note absence of amniotic fluid (b, bladder; s, spine.)

Accurate prenatal diagnosis of congenital abnormalities makes possible the introduction of prenatal surgery. If needles can be placed in the fetal peritoneal cavity with ease, they can be placed in other cystic structures to relieve pressure or obstruction. A lung cyst pressing on the vessels at the base of the heart could be collapsed. A megacystis could be drained; by using a self-retaining catheter, as was previously used for intrauterine transfusions, it should be possible to puncture the bladder and leave the free end of the catheter in the amniotic sac. An intrauterine suprapubic cystostomy would thus be established and the obstructive problem could be sorted out after delivery.

The earlier diagnosis of transfusion syndrome presents a problem of management. When one fetus is healthy and the other is in failure, can the failure be treated with drugs? If not, could the affected fetus be converted into a fetus papyraceous by putting an endoscopic clip on the cord

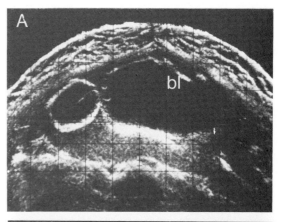

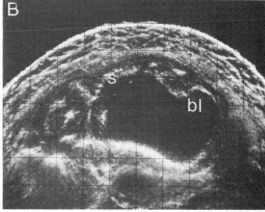

or by some other method? Such a suggestion may seem both heroic and theoretic, but it may not be so unreasonable given special circumstances.

The new information on fetal anatomy provided by high-grade ultrasonic echoscopes solves many problems that have worried obstetricians in the past, but like all technical advances, the new information available poses problems not previously thought possible to challenge the clinician in the practice of the art.

REFERENCES

1. CAMPBELL S: The antenatal detection of fetal abnormality by ultrasonic diagnosis. Amsterdam, Exerpta Medica, Int Congr Ser No. 310, 1973, pp 240–247

2. DONALD I, MACVICAR J, BROWN TG: Investigation of abdominal masses by pulsed ultrasound. Lancet 1:1188, 1958

3. FIELD B, MITCHELL G, GARRETT W, KERR C: Prenatal diagnosis and selective abortion for anencephaly and spina bifida. Med J Aust 1:608–610, 1974

4. FISHER CC, GARRETT WJ, KOSSOFF G: Anencephaly in one of twins diagnosed by ultrasonic echography. Aust NZ J Obstet Gynaecol 15:108–110, 1975

5. GARRETT WJ, FISHER CC, KOSSOFF G: Hydrocephaly, microcephaly and anencephaly diagnosed in pregnancy by ultrasonic echography. Med J Aust 2:587–589, 1975

6. GARRETT WJ, GRUNWALD G, ROBINSON DE: Prenatal diagnosis of fetal polycystic kidney of ultrasound. Aust NZ J Obstet Gynaecol 10:7–9, 1970

7. GARRETT WJ, KOSSOFF G: An obstetric test for resolution by ultrasonic echoscopes. Ultrasonics 13:217–218, 1975

8. GARRETT WJ, KOSSOFF G: Selection of patients by ultrasonic echography for fetal and immediate neonatal surgery. Aust Paediatr J 12:313–318, 1976

9. GARRETT WJ, KOSSOFF G: Gray scale examination of the fetus. In Sanders RC, James AE (eds): Ultrasonography in Obstetrics and Gynecology. New York, Appleton-Century-Crofts, 1977, pp 175–179

10. GARRETT WJ, KOSSOFF G, CARPENTER DA, RADOVANOVICH G: The Octoson in use. In White DN, Barnes R (eds): Ultrasound in Medicine, Vol 2. New York, Plenum, 1976, pp 341–349

11. GARRETT WJ, KOSSOFF G, JONES RFC: Ultrasonic cross-sectional visualization of hydrocephalus in infants. Neuroradiology 8:279–288, 1975

12. GARRETT WJ, KOSSOFF G, LAWRENCE R: Gray scale echography in the diagnosis of hydrops due to fetal lung tumor. J Clin Ultrasound 3:45–50, 1975

13. GARRETT WJ, KOSSOFF G, OSBORN RA: The diagnosis of fetal hydronephrosis, megaureter and urethral obstruction by ultrasonic echography. Br J Obstet Gynaecol 82:115–120, 1975

14. GARRETT WJ, ROBINSON DE: Fetal heart size measured in vivo by ultrasound. Pediatrics 46:25–27, 1970

15. GARRETT WJ, ROBINSON DE: Ultrasound in Clinical Obstetrics. Springfield, IL, Thomas, 1970

16. GILL RW: Quantative blood flow measurement in deep lying vessels using pulsed doppler with the Octoson. In White DN (ed): Ultrasound in Medicine, 4:341–348, 1978

17. KOSSOFF G: Developments in ultrasonic echoscopy. 9th International Conference on Medical Biol Engineering, 1971, p 58

18. KOSSOFF G, CARPENTER DA, RADOVANOVICH G, ROBINSON DE, GARRETT WJ: Octoson: a new rapid multitransducer general purposes water-coupling echoscope. Amsterdam, Exerpta Medica, Int Congr Ser No. 363, 1975, pp 90–95

19. KOSSOFF G, GARRETT WJ, CARPENTER DA, JELLINS J, DADD MJ: Principles and classification of soft tissues by grey scale echography. Ultrasound Med Biol 2:89–105, 1976

20. KOSSOFF G, GARRETT WJ, RADOVANOVICH G: Grey scale echography in obstetrics and gynaecology. Aust Radiol 18:62–111, 1974

21. ROBINSON DE, GARRETT WJ, KOSSOFF G: Fetal anatomy displayed by ultrasound. Invest Radiol 3:442–449, 1968

22. WARKENY J: Congenital Malformations. Chicago, Year Book Medical, 1971

23. WLADIMIROFF JW, CAMPBELL S: Fetal urine-production rates in normal and complicated pregnancy. Lancet 1:151–154, 1974

5

The ultrasound scan

MICHAEL JOHN HUGHEY

ROLE OF HUMAN RELATIONS

No review of ultrasonic scanning technique is complete without at least a passing comment on the role of human relations, the art rather than the science of diagnostic ultrasound. Whereas technical expertise in ultrasound scanning is a desirable goal, ultrasonographers should not lose their sense of perspective of the role of diagnostic ultrasound in medicine. This role exists solely for the benefit of patients, aiding their physicians in diagnosing and treating disease, or ensuring safe passage through potentially dangerous life experiences, such as childbirth. Patients undergoing ultrasound scanning should be treated with courtesy, respect, and a kindness in word and action that conveys to the patient the sympathetic feelings of the operator. Condescension, belligerence, or a cold, unfeeling attitude is inappropriate in any patient-care setting and is not tolerable in diagnostic ultrasound, where patient cooperation is vital if beneficial service is to be given.

Ultrasonographers should maintain humility, paying careful attention to the limitations of their skills and of the science. Great disservice has been done in the past by well-intentioned but ill-informed sonographers whose ability to "read" their own suppositions into the eight confusing shades of gray of an image was limited only by the depths of their imaginations. Enthusiasm for the science of diagnostic ultrasound should be tempered by an immediate under-standing of the limits of the equipment. It is not always possible to distinguish between a uterine leiomyoma and a solid ovarian tumor. It is not always possible to distinguish between a low-lying placenta and a placenta previa. Pelvic masses are not always identified by ultrasound examination, and bowel configurations can sometimes resemble a pelvic mass, misleading even the most astute sonographer.

Overly timid interpretations of ultrasound images are also to be discouraged. The words "may be," "apparent," "possibly could represent," and other such words and phrases are used too frequently. Every time such a word is used, the value of the ultrasound scan to the patient and her physician is proportionately diminished. Such inexact reporting can delay needed intervention or precipitate unnecessary intervention. Sonographers should interpret their findings simply and with precision, indicating areas of doubt where they exist and expressing to the managing physician the confidence limits of the predictions whenever possible. The sonographer must neither overread nor underread the images produced.

The sonographer must also guard against intervening between the patient and the referring physician. Ultrasonic evaluation, while often important or critical to a diagnostic evaluation, cannot be the sole determinant of clinical management. The sonographer does not have the same depth of knowledge of the patient possessed by the referring physician. Because of this limitation, questions regarding management must be directed to the referring physician. Such referral can be easily done, without apology or embarrassment.

Ultrasonographers should not avoid patient contact. It is not only appropriate but also desirable that sonographers ask questions of their patients, such as "When was your last normal menstrual period?" or "When did you last feel the baby move?" Such questions provide additional clinical information that greatly enhances the value of an ultrasonic evaluation. When the operator is skilled in the performance of bimanual pelvic examinations, such an examination can be particularly helpful in evaluating a pelvic mass. In short, the role of the ultrasonographer in patient care is that of a consultant who should apply all of his or her clinical skills and acumen to aid the referring physician in caring for the patient.

There is no question that the best interpretation of ultrasound findings will be given by the individual performing the examination. There are fine details, appearing with slight changes in gain or plane, that are not captured on film and will be appreciated only by the operator. An "ultrasonographer" who sits in the office waiting for a technician to bring in some 30 photographic images of a patient will be forever mired in mediocrity, never developing the full potential of ultrasound science or its skills. Whereas many routine scans can be performed by technicians, the ultrasonographer should perform those scans that are most difficult and challenging.

A question frequently arising is how much information the ultrasonographer should give to the patient upon completing the examination. The answer is variable, depending on the circumstances. Consider a woman referred for examination because both she and her obstetrician suspect her fetus has expired. Upon examination with real-time imaging, the fetus is obviously moving, kicking, demonstrating fetal breathing motions, and the fetal heart is seen to be beating vigorously. It would be cruelly inhuman to withhold this information from such a patient, letting her anxiously await hearing from her physician. Under such circumstances, it is perfectly appropriate for the ultrasonographer to convey to the patient the news that the fetus appears alive and normal to the extent that ultrasound evaluation can determine (1). Consider a second example, that of a woman referred for evaluation of a pelvic mass. Ultrasound imaging shows a cystic mass in the pouch of Douglas. The patient asks, "Do I need surgery?" The sonographer should not attempt to answer this question, because the answer is not entirely dependent on ultrasonic findings. The referring physician needs to consider the ultrasound report along with other diagnostic modalities, combine them with knowledge of the patient and best clinical judgment, and then arrive at a diagnosis and plan of management (4). The ultrasonographer, lacking knowledge of these other diagnostic modalities, clinical judgment, and knowledge of the patient, should not attempt to answer the question but should politely explain that the patient's physician is the one best qualified to answer her questions.

Pregnant patients undergoing ultrasound scanning should have a thorough explanation of the ultrasound procedures as they are occurring (1). The patient should be reassured that the examination is painless and (to the best of our knowledge) harmless to both mother and fetus and will give valuable information to the woman's physician. An explanation of what the mother is seeing can be helpful in reducing her anxiety, increasing her cooperation, and aiding in mother–infant bonding. For these reasons I often have the husband accompany the patient during the scanning procedure, a reflection of my belief that the benefits to the family in reducing anxiety and promoting family involvement far outweigh the minor inconvenience of having an extra person in the scanning area. In hospitals where family-oriented obstetrics is practiced, having the fathers accompany their wives during ultrasound scanning has been enthusiastically received by the patients.

The atmosphere of the scanning area should be relaxing, to reduce patient anxiety and promote cooperation. Sonographers should remember that their patients are often frightened by the size and appearance of diagnostic ultrasound equipment and must be reassured that the examination will not hurt and is harmless. Even with these reassurances, every effort should be made

to humanize the examination. Soft, soothing music played at an appropriate sound level is helpful in creating a relaxed, nonthreatening atmosphere. Human touches, such as paintings, pictures, wall coverings, or other such items help reduce the sterile atmosphere of an institution. Softening the lighting from the standard overhead institutional fluorescent lamps is also helpful. Patients should be greeted by their names, and their names should be used often during the examination. Whereas children should be addressed by their first names, adults should be addressed by their formal names, "Mr. Jones," "Miss Smith," or "Mrs. Adams." Older patients in particular resent the use of their first name by individuals considerably their junior. Patients should be treated with dignity and respect, and care taken not to offend their sensitivities.

The operators of diagnostic ultrasound equipment need the human relations skills necessary to maintain a light conversation while performing examinations. The sonographer should demonstrate to the patient that he or she is interested in the patient as a human being, not just as a patient with a pelvic mass. "Small talk" or a brief discussion about the weather, the post office, cooking, or other extraneous matters helps relax the patient and add warmth to the examination atmosphere.

Sonographers need to be attentive to the special needs of a patient. Many scanning areas are unseasonably cold, and the application of mineral oil or scanning jelly to the abdomen can further increase the patient's discomfort. Having extra blankets available for such circumstances is thoughtful and always appreciated. Some patients cannot lie flat on their backs for any length of time without discomfort. Rather than demonstrate anger that the patient cannot fully cooperate with the scan, the sonographer should show sympathy and choose appropriate rest periods wherein the patient may move freely to a comfortable position before resuming the scanning procedure. Pregnant women often experience supine hypotension (sudden onset of faintness, dizziness, nausea, ringing in the ears, numbing of the extremities) when lying flat. The sonographer must remain attentive to pregnant patients so that detection of such hypotension

occurs early, allowing immediate treatment by turning the patient to her left side. Some patients cannot lie flat for an examination; in this case, ultrasound technique must be altered, the scanning being performed with the patient sitting, prone, or in lateral decubitus position. The technique should be matched to the patient's clinical situation.

Most ultrasound scans are not emergencies, and if the patient feels ill on a particular day, it is appropriate to cancel the scan for that day and reschedule the patient for a later time when she will feel better. Some scans require the patient to have a full bladder. This can create an uncomfortable situation for the patient, and the sonographer should try to perform scans in this patient with speed and adeptness. When finished, the sonographer should allow the patient the opportunity to empty her bladder immediately and not leave her waiting on the examining table while the forms are filled out and the next patient is summoned. In each of these cases, a knowledge of the needs of the patient and a sensitivity to those needs are necessary if the best patient care is to be delivered.

SCANNING TECHNIQUES

CONVENTIONAL SCANNING OF THE ABDOMEN

During conventional scanning a patient is placed in the supine position, arms at her side, with her head supported by a small pillow. The room is darkened to a level permitting optimal visualization of the imaging screen by the operator and enough light to permit ordinary movement in the room with an unimpeded view of the instruments. The patient's abdomen is exposed, from the costal margin to the pubic symphysis, and a generous layer of contact medium is applied. The contact medium provides a necessary linkage between the scanning transducer and the abdomen (sound travels poorly through air). Specially designed scanning jelly may be used and has the advantage of water solubility so that it does not stain clothing. Mineral oil may be used for this purpose but requires special handling to avoid damage to the patient's clothing. If the contact medium should dry during the ex-

amination, additional medium is added as necessary to provide for excellent sonic contact.

For certain scans a full bladder is necessary. Ultrasound energy travels poorly through air (such as is found in the large and small bowel) or bone but quite well through fluid; consequently the bladder is used to aid in sonically identifying structures within the pelvis. In this way the full bladder acts as a "window" through which the uterus, tubes, and ovaries may be seen. To fill the bladder, a patient should drink 3–4 glasses of water or juice (28–32 oz) approximately 45 min to an hour before the examination is to begin. Some patients require longer periods of time for bladder filling. If the bladder fills too rapidly, the patient is allowed to empty her bladder halfway, a task accomplished with only minor difficulty.

On occasion an intravenous solution of 5% dextrose in water may be given to fill the bladder. When time is of great importance and other methods cannot be reasonably applied, a catheter may be inserted in the bladder and approximately 250–300 cc of sterile saline slowly infused. Whenever this procedure is performed, all routine precautions should be taken to provide asepsis and prevent infection.

After 12–14 weeks' gestation a full bladder is not generally necessary, since the amniotic fluid acts as the transmitting medium and the enlarged uterus pushes the bowel away from the anterior abdominal wall.

In diagnosing placenta previa, it is important for the bladder to be partially filled, not only to provide better visualization of internal structures, but also to provide a landmark by which the margins of the placenta may be judged. Usually there is little difficulty in identifying with precision the position of the placenta. The diagnostic challenge is to determine the proportion of placental tissue extending to the lower uterine segment and approaching the cervical internal os (Chapter 16). The presence of a partially full bladder helps to identify the internal os and the lower uterine segment. Note, however, that a full bladder also distorts the shape of the lower uterine area and may give the false impression of placenta previa. Because of this ambiguity, in cases of suspected placenta previa,

the lower uterus should be imaged with the bladder filled and also with it empty.

Machine warm-up time must be allowed before accurate scanning and imaging are possible. Warm-up times vary from machine to machine, and this information can be found in the service manual.

The transducer is placed on the patient's abdomen and a preliminary midline image obtained and properly centered. For a supine midline scan, custom places the patient's feet on the right of the screen and the patient's head to the left. (Transverse scans place the patient's left side on the right side of the image, as though the cut section of abdomen were being viewed from the perspective of the feet.)

The TGC control (time/gain compensation) is adjusted to ensure even imaging at all depths of tissue (Fig. 5–1). The TGC control is necessary because of the inherent properties of sound energy within tissue. As the sound waves traverse tissues, a certain amount of energy is lost, absorbed, or scattered. The amplitude (loudness) of echoes returning from deep tissues is not as great as echoes returning from nearby tissues. To avoid this problem of uneven imaging, the equipment automatically amplifies the returning signals at variable rates, depending on the distance from the transducer (determined as a function of time, thus the terminology of time/gain compensation). Most conventional ultrasound machines have an adjustable TGC control to allow the operator to finely tune the instrument to give even reproduction throughout the depths of the particular tissue being scanned (Figure 5–1).

Near-signal suppression is also an adjustment that should be made. Because of the uneven interface of the transducer with the skin and because of acoustic reverberation, a considerable amount of artifactual noise is generated at the skin surface and extends into the image of the abdomen. In most cases clarity of images within a centimeter or two of the transducer is unimportant, and therefore variable suppression is offered on most conventional machines to squelch the accoustic noise at the surface of the abdomen.

Once the TGC and near-field suppression

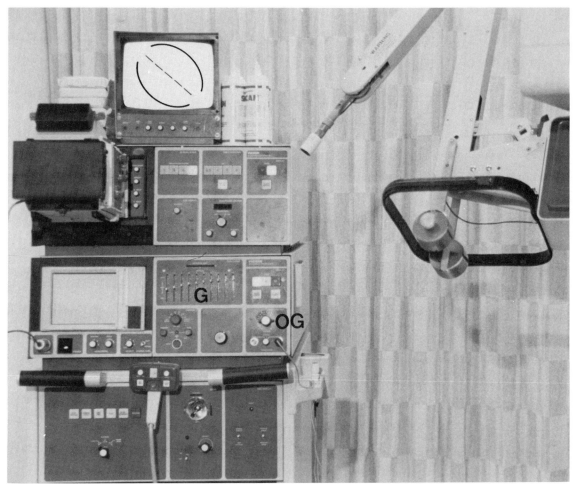

FIG. 5–1. G, Time-Gain-Control (TGC) knobs (seen above letter G). The TGC curve is such that posterior gain is higher than anterior gain; OG, Overall gain knob used to increase TGC proportionally for gray-scale imaging. Note transducer in transverse position (to account for angle of pelvic inclination) and directed perpendicular to falx cerebri of the fetal head. The latter is seen in occiput oblique position on the TV monitor.

controls are properly adjusted, the overall gain must be regulated to give the best image. The bladder and amniotic fluid should appear echo free, the uterus assuming a faintly speckled appearance on B-scan or a fine gray shade on gray scale. Convention dictates that a distinction should be made between cystic (bladder) and solid (uterus) components within the abdomen.

Regardless of the method of photographing the images created during standard imaging, the camera should be inspected to see that the correct and customary speed, f-stop, and focus adjustments are made and that film is in the camera.

Several methods of scanning are possible with conventional equipment. Arc-scanning involves maintaining the transducer perpendicular to the contour of the skin while the operator moves the transducer through the plane of examination. In radial scanning, the transducer remains at the same point on the skin, but the angle of incidence is rocked back and forth, creating a wedge-shaped image with the transducer at the apex (5). A third system, compound-sector scanning, combines the two methods (5). Each of these systems has application in different areas of the body and in different clinical conditions. The basic priniciple of all these methods is that the most accurate imaging occurs when sound energy is reflected perpendicularly off an interface.

After the initial midline image is created and photographed, the scanning arm is shifted laterally 0.5–1.0 cm, and a second sagittal section is obtained. Additional sagittal sections are photographed until the entire abdomen has been sonically sliced into slabs from one side of the abdomen to the other. The transducer arm is then rotated 90° and transverse sections are obtained and photographed in the same fashion, beginning at the symphysis pubis and extending at 0.5–1.0 cm intervals to the costal margin. From 30 to 40 photographs will be produced that sequentially view the entire abdomen from two separate points of perspective. Where certain areas of special interest are concerned, additional imaging is necessary. When pelvic masses are being evaluated, it is necessary to make use of the full bladder to better define such pelvic masses. Oblique views through the bladder using sector scanning may occasionally be helpful in delineating these structures.

When one is attempting to obtain a fetal biparietal diameter (BPD), considerable maneuvering is necessary if the results are to even vaguely reproduce the true BPD. From the first midline scan, the position of the fetus is usually apparent. In the most common situation, with a cephalic presentation, the fetal head is inclined slightly toward the floor of the scanning room, rather than parallel to it (Fig. 5–2). This angle of lateral flexion is measured and the transducer arm rotated 90° to perform a transverse scan (Fig. 5–2). The transducer is angled to the same extent as the angle of lateral cephalic flexion, so that the beam of sonic energy strikes the fetal head at right angles to the falx cerebri, the midline of the fetal head. Correct angling of the transducer arm will be confirmed by the image of symmetrically opposed fetal skull tables with a loud (bright) midline echo. If the skull images are oval, then the transducer needs to be simply moved a few millimeters or centimeters cephalad and caudad, creating images at a number of

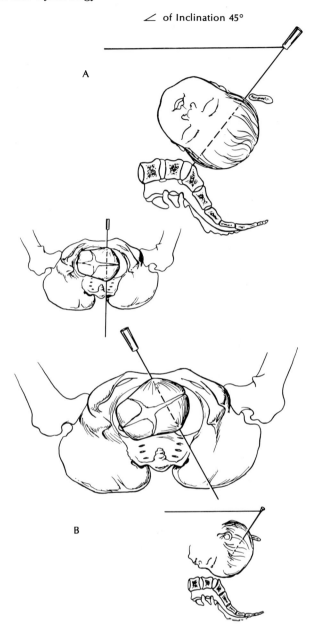

FIG. 5–2. A. If fetal head is in occiput–transverse position, the ultrasonic transducer is adjusted only to account for "lateral flexion" of the fetal head as the latter accommodates to the angle of maternal pelvic inclination (approximately 45°). In this way the sound beam will be perpendicular to the falx cerebri and an accurate biparietal diameter measurement can be obtained. **B.** If the occiput of the fetal head is rotated anteriorly or posteriorly, the ultrasonic transducer is adjusted to account for angle of lateral flexion (as in A), and angle of occipital rotation (as in B). In this way the sound beam will be perpendicular to the falx cerebri and an accurate biparietal diameter measurement can be obtained.

different planes to capture the widest transverse diameter of the fetal head. If the skull image is not oval, then the fetal head is flexed and a slight adjustment of the transducer arm away from the direct transverse scan to a more oblique approach is necessary.

On occasion, rather than lie in an occiput transverse position (with the fetus looking toward a maternal hip), the fetus will lie in a more direct occiput anterior or posterior position (the fetus looking down at the floor or up at the ceiling). When this occurs, an accurate BPD cannot be obtained. Trendelenburg position may be used to encourage a fetal head to disengage from the pelvis and assume the occiput-transverse position. Gentle stimulation of the fetus by abdominal manipulation may also cause the fetus to move out of this inaccessible position. If these attempts fail, an approximate BPD should be obtained and reported as such. The patient should return at another time for another scan.

The method described here for obtaining a BPD with conventional scanning is admittedly not as accurate as might be obtained with nonpersistent image scanning or with real-time ultrasonography. Fetal motion is a complicating factor and the confidence limits of predictions based on BPDs obtained in this manner should be widened accordingly.

To obtain a BPD from a breech or transverse-lie fetus, the same principles are involved, ensuring that the transducer beam approaches the midline of the fetal head at the perpendicular. Again, the widest transverse diameter is used to predict fetal age.

NONPERSISTENT IMAGE SCANNING

Conventional scanning with the B-scan or gray-scale modalities leads ultimately to an image displayed on a storage oscilloscope. This frozen image may be enhanced by additional scanning in the same plane. However, such a system has some inherent liabilities: the stored image may lack detail, particularly if any movement on the part of the object being scanned occurs. In addition, capturing the correct plane featuring anatomic landmarks is difficult and time consuming.

These major drawbacks are avoided to a large extent by nonpersistent image scanning or NPIS (5). With NPIS the image created on the oscilloscope screen fades immediately unless scanning is continued. Images are stored, not on the screen, but rather in the mind of the sonographer, and because of continuous updating of information, any motion of the object scanned is visualized. NPIS permits the operator to select the best plane featuring a particular anatomic finding.

NPIS has particular application to the field of fetal cephalometry, where fetal motion is a constant problem and slight changes in scanning angle or level of approach have profound consequences in gestational age prediction. To apply NPIS to fetal cephalometry, the pregnant patient is scanned in routine fashion, the operator determing fetal position, angle of lateral cephalic flexion, and degree of anteroposterior cephalic flexion (ie, occipital rotation, Fig. 5–2). The transducer arm is then moved cephalad and caudad while the operator watches the nonstorage oscilloscope. The image of the fetal head will grow in diameter until the widest BPD is obtained, at which point the diameter image will grow smaller. By moving the image plane slowly back and forth across the true BPD, the widest diameter is easily visualized by the operator. When this widest BPD is obtained, the oscilloscope is switched back to storage, and in a single scanning motion the fetal head image is captured. It is this BPD that is most accurate, giving the greatest reproducibility (5).

NPIS may also be used to advantage in scanning of pelvic masses, where fine distinctions between acoustic properties of different tissues may be more fully appreciated than on a storage oscilloscope. Gray-scale imaging also helps with these distinctions, once the correct plane is identified by NPIS.

REAL-TIME IMAGING

The introduction of real-time ultrasonic imaging has added a new dimension, time, to conventional two-dimensional imaging modes. Because of its continuous and automatic updating of the ultrasonic image, it allows for extremely rapid scanning. Further, because the transducer is not attached to any scanning arm (Chapter 6), the operator is able to make fine adjustments in the angle of incidence through three different planes simultaneously. In this way the most accurate and reproducible measurements of moving objects, such as of a fetal head can be obtained (3). With real-time ultrasound, fetal viability can be confirmed as early as 7 weeks' gestation by visualization of fetal heart motion and "end-over-end tumbling" of the early fetus. Later in pregnancy, fetal heart activity, fetal breathing motions, and the filling and emptying of the fetal bladder are clearly visible (2, 3). The speed of these examinations is impressive. For routine obstetric purposes, the information that would require a skilled technician 20–45 minutes to obtain with 30–40 photographs using conventional scanning methods can be obtained in 30–40 sec by use of one or two photographs with real-time imaging equipment. The economic implications of this technologic advance are important and may realistically allow for routine scanning of all pregnant patients on a cost-effective basis.

In the linear array real-time system (Chapter 2) the transducer is not attached to a scanning arm but is held by the operator and swept across the abdomen or held motionless while the image is automatically and continuously updated (Chapters 2 and 6).

For most obstetric scans, the real-time imaging transducer is used to identify fetal position, number of fetuses, position of the placenta, and the biparietal diameter—determinations that are quickly performed with the scanner. After observing the midline image with the real-time scanner and visualizing the location of the fetal head and angle of lateral flexion, the operator rotates the transducer 90° to the transverse position and makes small corrections in angle, tilt, and position of the scanning plane. These motions are continued until the widest fetal BPD is visualized by the operator, creating an image of symmetrically opposed skull tables, oval in shape, with a midline echo perpendicular to the direction of sonic energy.

Whereas real-time imaging has been very helpful in most obstetric scanning areas, some technical limitations have yet to be solved. Lateral resolution with real-time imaging units is not of the same quality as in most conventional scanning units. For many purposes this limitation is not critical, but for fine delineation of detail of a fixed object within the pelvis, conventional scanning techniques appear to give superior results. With further technologic advancement this liability of real-time imaging may be overcome.

REFERENCES

1. American Hospital Association: A Patient's Bill of Rights. Adopted 1973
2. CAMPBELL S, WLADMIROFF JW, DEWHURST DJ: The antenatal measurement of fetal urine production. J Obstet Gynecol 80:680, 1973
3. FOX HE, HOHLER CW: Fetal evaluation by real-time imaging. Clin Obstet Gynecol 20:339, 1977
4. HOGSHEAD HP: The art of delivering bad news. Chicago Med 79:1069, 1976
5. SABBAGHA RE, TURNER JH: Methodology of B-scan sonar cephalometry with electronic calipers and correlation with fetal birth weight. Obstet Gynecol 40:74, 1972

6

The first-trimester pregnancy

RUDY E. SABBAGHA, INGRID KIPPER

Ultrasonic imaging of the pregnant uterus has been recently enhanced by two developments. The first is the capability of magnifying fetal echoes, and the second is the introduction and widespread use of real-time diagnostic ultrasound (Chapter 5). Despite these advances ultrasonic evaluation of pregnancy in the first trimester is still not performed on a routine basis. The reasons, although complex, are realted in part to cost-effectiveness and availability of both equipment and personnel. The indications, at present, for the sonographic study of a gravida in the first 12 weeks of gestation are listed in Table 6–1.

This chapter deals with the assessment of early pregnancy by ultrasonic measurement of fetal crown–rump length (CRL) and gestational sac. Further, the methods of establishing fetal viability prior to 12 weeks' gestation are presented.

SONAR FETAL CRL—METHODOLOGY AND REPRODUCIBILITY

In the first trimester of pregnancy the technique for sonar measurement of the CRL involves localizing the fetal axis or lie by obtaining parallel longitudinal scans across the gestational sac. The ultrasound transducer is then moved to the plane joining the fetal poles and an echogram of the longest fetal axis or sonar CRL is produced (9).

This methodology, described by Robinson, is feasible and practical only when nonpersistent image scanning (NPIS) is used, Chapter 5. Even then, fetal motion in early pregnancy is sometimes excessive and the procedure is prolonged.

Fortunately, the recent use of real-time sonography has alleviated the difficulty in obtaining sonar CRL measurements by conventional scanning. In this exciting modality of imaging, fetal motion is visualized as it occurs (Chapter 5). Additionally, the transducer in real-time echography is freely mobile (it is not attached to a scanning arm) and can be quickly directed to capture the correct plane featuring the fetal CRL, Figure 6–1. Photographs of the crown–rump length in three fetuses of varying gestational ages are shown in Figures 6–2 to 6–4.

The margin of error of CRL measurements using NPIS is $\pm$ 1.2 mm (2 SD) (11) and is similar to the reproducibility of sonar BPDs derived either by NPIS or by real-time imaging (Chapter 7).

FETAL CRL VERSUS GESTATIONAL AGE

In the management of high-risk pregnancies it is important to establish gestational age not only in women with suspect dates (1, 3) but also in those with known dates (Chapter 8). In the latter situation the menstrual history is sometimes inaccurate (12), and confirmation of the duration of pregnancy can be reliably achieved by measurement of fetal CRL.

TABLE 6–1. INDICATIONS FOR SONOGRAPHIC STUDY OF GRAVIDAS IN THE FIRST TRIMESTER OF PREGNANCY

Indications	Applicable to	Ultrasound examination
To confirm menstrual dates	Maternal Rh sensitization, diabetes mellitus, hypertension, and repeat C-sections	C-R length
To establish gestational age	Unknown or suspect dates, inconclusive pelvic exam (as in women for pregnancy termination)	C-R length
First trimester vaginal bleeding	Normal pregnancy, ectopic pregnancy, poor obstetric history, missed abortion, blighted ovum, hydatidiform mole	C-R length Fetal motion Serial sonography for fetal growth
"Large for dates"	Possible ovarian tumors or uterine myomas, multiple gestation	C-R length Ultrasound evaluation of adnexa and uterus
"Small for dates"	Poor obstetric history, oligomenorrhea, suspect dates, previous use of oral contraceptive	C-R length Fetal motion Serial fetal growth

FIG. 6–1. Note real-time transducer in oblique position across abdomen. Transducer is freely mobile and not attached to a scanning arm.

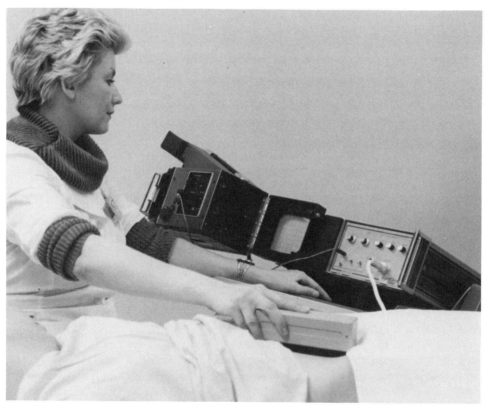

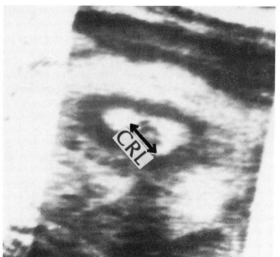

FIG. 6–2. CRL, crown–rump length. Fetal CRL 1 cm corresponding to a gestational age of 7 weeks.

FIG. 6–3. CRL, crown–rump length. Fetal CRL is 2.8 cm corresponding to a gestational age of 9½ weeks.

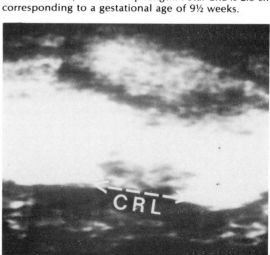

FIG. 6–4. CRL, crown–rump length. Fetal CRL is 6.5 cm corresponding to a gestational age of 13 weeks.

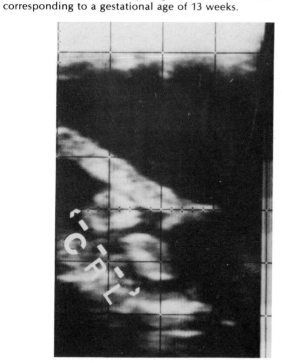

Crown-rump length (mm)

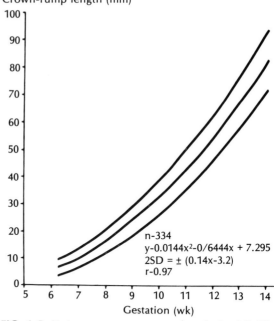

n-334
$y-0.0144x^2-0/6444x + 7.295$
$2SD = \pm (0.14x-3.2)$
r-0.97

Gestation (wk)

FIG. 6–5. Note mean crown–rump length (and 2 SD limits) corresponding to gestational weeks.

Robinson and Fleming drived the mean CRL and its 95% confidence limits from a population of women with reliable menstrual dates (9, 11), Figure 6–5. They showed that fetal age estimates in the first trimester of pregnancy vary from ± 4.7 to ± 2.7 days in 95% of gravidas, depending on whether one or three CRL measurements are obtained respectively.

FETAL CRL VERSUS SONAR EDD

Drumm et al scanned 40 pregnant women in whom ovulation dates were established by basal body temperature records, and found a close correlation between CRL measurements and fetal age (5). Additionally, Drumm showed that the onset of spontaneous labor could be accurately predicted by using fetal CRL values to estimate the expected date of delivery (EDD) (4). Specifically, in his report approximately 95% of pregnant women delivered within ± 12 days of the sonar (CRL) EDD.

The results of the study by Drumm suggest that in his series the incidence of preterm and postterm deliveries is only 5%—a figure smaller than the normal biologic frequency (10–16%) noted in the general population of gravidas. For example, in Yerushalmy's report (14), based on evaluation of a very large number of pregnancies, approximately 10 and 6% of women went into spontaneous labor before 38 and after 42 weeks' gestation, respectively, Figure 6–6.

It should be emphasized that accurate definition of gestational age should not imply that a greater number of women will go into spontaneous labor at or close to the 40th week of pregnancy. Many pregnant women assume that they will deliver within ± 1–5 days of the sonar EDD (derived from a fetal CRL measurement). Such misconceptions can be easily corrected if personnel in ultrasound laboratories take a few minutes to explain to gravidas the difference between a sonar EDD and spontaneous delivery.

FETAL CRL VERSUS REAL-TIME IMAGING

The authors have gained wide experience in obtaining fetal CRL measurements by real-time imaging and find that the correlation with gestational age in accordance with the data in Table 6–2 is satisfactory (11). We feel, however, that, in defining the length of pregnancy, it is simpler to obtain fetal CRL after 8 weeks' gestation because during this interval it is possible to display the fetal head and trunk clearly on the screen,

FIG. 6–6. Onset of spontaneous delivery in about 400,000 women. Approximately 84% of women deliver ± 2 weeks of the 40th week or EDD. (Yerushalmy J: Clin Obstet Gynecol 13:107, 1970)

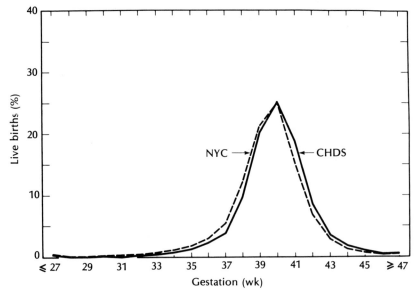

TABLE 6-2. CORRELATION OF CRL* WITH GESTATIONAL AGE

Menstrual maturity (weeks + days)	Corrected "regressional analysis" (cm), mean values	Menstrual Maturity (weeks + days)	Corrected "regressional analysis" (cm), mean values
6 + 2	0.55	10 + 2	3.32
6 + 3	0.61	10 + 3	3.46
6 + 4	0.68	10 + 4	3.60
6 + 5	0.75	10 + 5	3.74
6 + 6	0.81	10 + 6	3.89
7 + 0	0.89	11 + 0	4.04
7 + 1	0.96	11 + 1	4.19
7 + 2	1.04	11 + 2	4.35
7 + 3	1.12	11 + 3	4.51
7 + 4	1.20	11 + 4	4.67
7 + 5	1.29	11 + 5	4.83
7 + 6	1.38	11 + 6	5.00
8 + 0	1.47	12 + 0	5.17
8 + 1	1.57	12 + 1	5.34
8 + 2	1.66	12 + 2	5.52
8 + 3	1.76	12 + 3	5.70
8 + 4	1.87	12 + 4	5.88
8 + 5	1.97	12 + 5	6.06
8 + 6	2.08	12 + 6	6.25
9 + 0	2.19	13 + 0	6.43
9 + 1	2.31	13 + 1	6.63
9 + 2	2.42	13 + 2	6.82
9 + 3	2.54	13 + 3	7.02
9 + 4	2.67	13 + 4	7.22
9 + 5	2.79	13 + 5	7.42
9 + 6	2.92	13 + 6	7.63
10 + 0	3.05	14 + 0	7.83
10 + 1	3.18		

* The mean crown–rump length (CRL) values are shown. The 2 SD limits of gestational age are ± 4.7 days (Robinson HP, Fleming JEE: Br J Obstet Gynecol 82:702, 1975)

Figure 6–4. As a result, the sonographer can be certain that a particular echogram does in fact represent the true CRL, and definition of fetal age is more likely to be accurate.

GUIDELINES FOR USING CRL MEASUREMENTS

Assessment of gestational age by fetal CRL is particularly useful in managing pregnant women sensitized by Rh disease, because the variation in the length of pregnancy corresponding to a specific CRL value is smaller than that noted in relation to a single biparietal diameter (BPD) measurement.

Once the duration of pregnancy is defined by fetal CRL, the first sonar BPD should be obtained between 31 and 33 weeks' gestation and used to assess whether in a given pregnancy cephalic growth falls into a large, average, or small bracket (Chapter 10).

A third ultrasound examination is then performed at approximately 36 weeks' gestation and should consist of a BPD measurement and a circumference of the trunk obtained at the area of the fetal liver showing the ductus venosus (Chapters 9, 10).

The third sonar examination is significant in that it allows the obstetrician to relate fetal growth in relation to its potential and to delineate symmetric from asymmetric intrauterine growth retardation as described in Chapter 10.

GESTATIONAL SAC DIMENSIONS

The normal intrauterine pregnancy is first visualized by 5–6 weeks' gestation (menstrual dates) and appears as a ring or circular structure

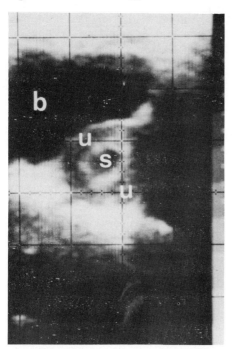

FIG. 6-7. Note: b, bladder; u, uterus; s, fluid compartment within gestational sac. Transverse scan shows gestational sac at 6 weeks after the first day of the last menstrual period. No fetus is seen yet.

FIG. 6-8. Note: b, bladder; u, uterus; s, gestational sac. Longitudinal scan of same patient in Figure 6-7. Note change in appearance of gestational sac between this sac, longitudinal, and the transverse scan in Figure 6-7.

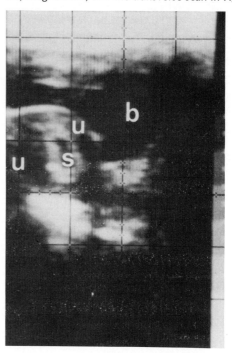

TABLE 6-3. FETAL DIMENSIONS ACCORDING TO GRAY-SCALE ULTRASOUND MEASUREMENTS IN 24 PATIENTS

Menstrual Weeks	Gestational Sac (mm)	"Crown-rump" (mm.)	Head* (mm.)	Trunk (mm.)
3				
4				
5	10			
6	20			
7	30	10		
8	45	17	10	
9	60	25	12	
10	70	32	14	
11		40	17	
12		55	?1	18
13		65	25	21
14		80	29	24
15		100	33	28

* Head represents shortest fetal dimension from 8–11 weeks and BPD from 12 weeks (Chilcote Ws, Asokan S: Clin Obstet Gynecol 20:253, 1977).

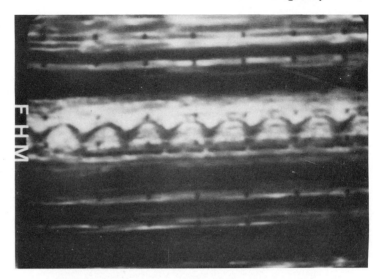

FIG. 6–9. FMH, fetal heart motion as seen on time–motion (TM) study.

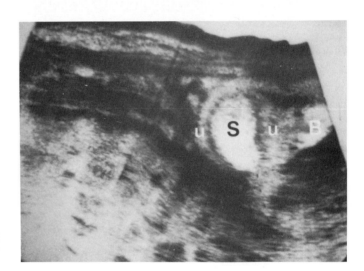

FIG. 6–10. U, uterus; B, bladder; S, cavity within gestational sac. Note absence of fetal echoes, diagnostic of blighted ovum.

within the uterus. This echo pattern of early pregnancy is universally referred to as a gestational sac, Figure 6–7. The presence of a gestational sac in the uterus not only confirms pregnancy but also indirectly rules out ectopic gestation (in the majority of cases). By the 8th week fetal echoes are seen rather distinctly within the sac (Fig. 6–2), and fetal CRL can be obtained as discussed elsewhere.

Some investigators have attempted to relate spontaneous abortion in early pregnancy to a low uterine implantation site, but a cause-and-effect relationship has not been established, Chapter 14; others have tried to relate fetal age to the diameter, cross section, or volume of gestational sacs (6–8, 10, 13). The latter approach is time consuming and has not been clinically useful. The reasons are as follows: first, the 95% confidence limits of fetal age estimates corresponding to a specific gestational sac dimension are approximately ± 12 days, whereas in relation to a fetal CRL the range is only ± 1–5 days. Second, the shape of the gestational sac varies not only in different pregnancies but also in the same pregnancy depending on bladder volume and plane of scanning, that is, longitudinal versus transverse, Figure 6–8.

The mean gestational sac, CRL, and BPD

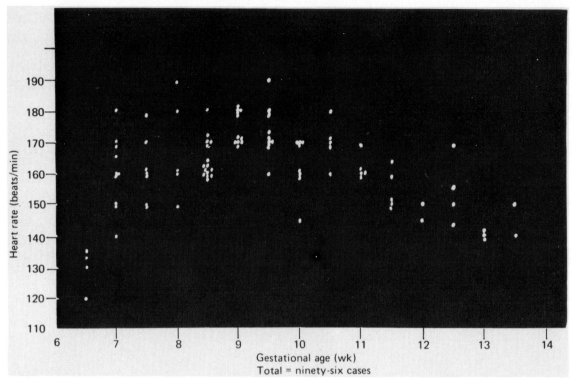

FIG. 6-11. Heart rate in first trimester of pregnancy recorded by ultrasound imaging. Note peak at about 9 weeks' gestation. (Chilcote WS, Asokan S: Clin Obstet Gynecol 20:253, 1977)

measurements obtained from a small series of gravidas (with known dates) in the first trimester of pregnancy are shown in Table 6-3. These values may be useful only in providing a basis for comparison of these different dimensions in early gestation (2).

FETAL VIABILITY

Objective confirmation of fetal life in the first trimester of pregnancy is mandatory for the proper management of pregnant women who relate a poor obstetric history or who present with vaginal bleeding. In these women fetal life can be established by approximately the 7th week of gestation, particularly if real-time imaging is used. In the latter modality fetal motion, including heart motion, is visualized directly and can be seen by both sonographer and patient. Nonetheless, documentation of fetal heart motion is necessary and can be achieved by recording the scan either on video-tape or directly on a polaroid photograph, Figure 6-9. The absence of a fetus by 7-8 weeks of pregnancy is consistent with the diagnosis of a blighted ovum, Figure 6-10.

Note that some investigators have reported a difference in the mean fetal heart rate between 7 and 14 weeks' gestation (2), Figure 6-11. This observation may be of clinical value at some future date as we learn more about the characteristics of fetuses in early pregnancy.

REFERENCES

1. CAMPBELL S: The assessment of fetal development by diagnostic ultrasound. Clin Perinatol 1:2, 507, 1974
2. CHILCOTE WS, ASOKAN S: Evaluation of first trimester pregnancy by ultrasound. Clin Obstet Gynecol 20:253, 1977
3. DEWHURST CJ, BEAZLEY JM, CAMPBELL S: Assessment of the fetal maturity and dysmaturity. Am J Obstet Gynecol 113:147, 1972
4. DRUMM JE: The prediction of delivery date by ultrasonic measurement of fetal crown-rump length. Br J Obstet Gynaecol 84:1, 1977

5. DRUMM JE, CLINCH J, MACKENZIE G: The ultrasonic measurement of fetal crown-rump length as a method of assessing gestational age. Br J Obstet Gynaecol 83:417, 1976

6. HELLMAN LM, KOBAYASHI M, FILLISTI L, LAVENHAR M: Growth and development of the human fetus prior to the twentieth week of gestation. Am J Obstet Gynecol 103:789, 1969

7. JOUPILA P: Ultrasound in the diagnosis of early pregnancy and its complications, a comparative study of A, B, and Doppler methods. Acta Obstet Gynecol Scand [Supp] 50 (15):3, 1971

8. KOHORN EI, KAUFMAN M: Sonar in the first trimester of pregnancy. J Obstet Gynecol 44:473, 1974

9. ROBINSON HP: Sonar measurement of the fetal crown-rump length as a means of assessing maturity in the first trimester of pregnancy. Br Med J 4:28, 1973

10. ROBINSON HP: Gestation sac volumes as determined by sonar in the first trimester of pregnancy. Br J Obstet Gynaecol 82:100, 1975

11. ROBINSON HP, FLEMING JEE: A critical evaluation of sonar crown-rump length measurements. Br J Obstet Gynaecol 82:702, 1975

12. SABBAGHA RE: Ultrasound in managing the high-risk pregnancy. In Spellacy WN (ed): Management of the High-Risk Pregnancy. Baltimore, University Park Press, 1976

13. TROOSTWIJK A: Echoscopie in de Jonge Zwangerschap. M.D. Thesis, Free University of Amsterdam

14. YERUSHALMY J: Relation of birth weight, gestational age, and rate of intrauterine growth to perinatal mortality. Clin Obstet Gynecol 13:107, 1970

7

Fetal cephalometry

MICHAEL JOHN HUGHEY

DETERMINATION OF BIPARIETAL DIAMETER

Although the fetal biparietal diameter (BPD) can be measured with any one of several ultrasonographic modes, differences exist among the modes. A knowledge of these differences is required to avoid errors. The usefulness of fetal cephalometry is directly related to its accuracy, which in turn is related to the skill of the operator and the operator's strict attention to detail. In some areas ultrasound technology has gained an undeserved reputation for inaccuracy that would not have occurred if local sonographers had exercised greater diligence in the pursuit of precision and shown more attentiveness to the subtleties of diagnostic ultrasound technique.

DIFFERENT IMAGING MODES

Several imaging modes may be used to perform fetal cephalometry. Although the original A-scan mode is now obsolete when used alone, it is still used in some areas in combination with B-scan imaging (combined B–A scan) (2); in this method B-scan imaging is used to obtain the correct cephalic plane for BPD determinations. A second oscilloscope is used to project the equivalent A-scan image for the fetal BPD, and measurements of the fetal BPD are taken from that image. The most reproducible measurement from an A-scan image obtained in this fashion is from the same point of the leading edges of the near and far skull echo complexes. These points are believed to correspond to the fluid/scalp interface of the near and the dura/bone interface of the far tables. Some sonographers use peak-to-peak measurements with some success, but such measurements have not been shown to have the same high degree of reproducibility of the leading edge measurements.

B-scan imaging is commonly used to obtain the fetal BPD (Fig. 7–1). Using this imaging mode, the gain (amplitude applied to the returned signal) is reduced to the point at which a clear image of the fetal skull is seen, with the thinnest possible skull tables. Measurements are taken from the leading edge of the near table (fluid/scalp interface) to the leading edge of the far table (dura /skull interface). In this way the measurements are comparable to those obtained by the combined B–A scan method (14) and are reproducible (3, 8, 11, 13).

The development of gray-scale imaging added greater definition of tissue characteristics and greater complexity of interpretation. With this mode, ultrasonic imaging has the capability of reflecting each of the fetal head layers in a recognizable pattern (Fig. 7–2). Although gray-scale imaging clearly depicts the different layers, it does not reproduce those layers *exactly* as they exist in nature, because of the inherent properties of sound energy.

Willocks (17) found the average scalp of the term fetus to measure 1.2 mm and the average

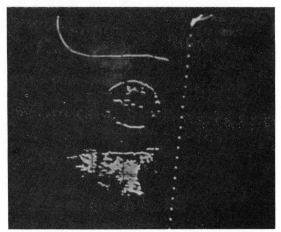

FIG. 7-1. B-scan image showing biparietal diameter. Note small width of skull tables. The distance between the outer and inner aspects of the fetal head is measured in comparison to 1-cm markers (shown adjacent to fetal head).

skull thickness to be 1.3 mm. Consider a term fetus with such scalp and bone thicknesses and a brain width of 90 mm (true, anatomic BPD = 1.2 + 1.3 + 90 + 1.3 + 1.2mm = 95 mm). These measurements will not be faithfully reproduced by any diagnostic ultrasound mode, because of differences in the speed of sound in the different tissues. Processing of the returned echoes involves careful measurement of the time interval

FIG. 7-2. Gray-scale image showing fetal biparietal diameter. For best reproducibility, width of skull tables should not exceed 3–5 mm (see text). (Hughey M, Sabbagha RE: Am J Obstet Gynecol [in press])

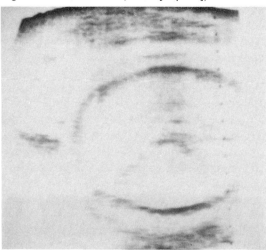

(t) between echoes. By assuming the speed of sound (v) in the object being scanned, the distance between echoes (d) is estimated and reproduced graphically, according to the relationship:

$$v = d/t \text{ or } vt = d$$

Ultrasound equipment in North America is calibrated to an assumed speed of sound of 1540 meters per second (m/sec), a figure generally accepted as representing the *average* speed of sound. It is known, however, that the speed of sound in bone is much faster than 1540 m/sec, some estimates running as high as 4080 m/sec. Similarly, the speed of sound in brain tissue is less than 1540 m/sec and has been recorded at 1515 m/sec (10).

These figures being used and applied to the example of the term fetus just described, the fetal skull that in reality measures 1.3 mm will be portrayed on the ultrasound screen as only 0.49 mm in thickness (1540/4080 × 1.3). The fetal brain that, in reality, measures 90 mm in width will be portrayed as measuring 91.49 mm (1540/1515 × 90). The sum total of these differences will be the image of a fetus with a sonographic BPD of 94.87 mm rather than 95.0 mm (1.2 + 0.49 + 91.49 + 0.49 + 1.2 = 94.87). The difference between the sonic image BPD and the true anatomic BPD is not significant, only because the apparent narrowing of the skull bones is balanced by an apparent widening of the brain. Clinically, it is important to recognize that, though the BPD measurement portrayed on the ultrasound screen is quite accurate, its component parts are distorted, the brain being 1½% larger and the skull bones 60% smaller than real life.

A second important consideration in gray-scale imaging is the role of "gain" in determining fetal BPD. Hughey and Sabbagha (8) demonstrated that altering the gain led to significant changes in BPD measurements regardless of which diameter was measured, outer edge to outer edge (O–O), outer edge of near table to inner edge of far table (O–I), middle of near to middle of far (M–M), or inner side of both tables (I–I) (Fig. 7–3). The O–I diameter was the least affected by changes in gain, and when medium gain was used (skull tables 3–5 mm thick) with

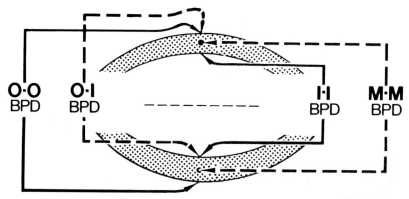

FIG. 7–3. Different cephalic points used to measure the biparietal diameter. BPD, biparietal diameter; O-O, BPD measured from outer points of cephalic contour; O-I, BPD measured from outer to inner aspect of cephalic contour (i.e., leading edge); M-M, BPD measured from midpoints of cephalic contour; I-I, BPD measured from inner aspect of cephalic contour. (Hughey M, Sabbagha RE: Am J Obstet Gynecol [in press])

O–I measurements, the results were very reproducible (2 SD = ± 0.8 mm), Table 7–1.

Measurements of other than the O–I diameter can be used with gray-scale images, but none of them are as reproducibly accurate as the O–I (3, 8, 11, 13). In theory, the M–M diameter should measure the same as the O–I diameter. In practice, unless the two skull table images are precisely the same thickness (a goal always sought but difficult to attain), a small difference will exist between them. The I–I diameter varies widely according to the gain applied, and this measurement should not be used to determine the fetal BPD. The O–O diameter offers one advantage: it more closely approximates the true anatomic BPD (useful for obstetric considerations). Unfortunately, the O–O BPD suffers

from significant variations in thickness of skull tables, depending on the gain applied to the image. The true anatomic BPD in term fetuses can be very accurately approximated by adding 4 mm to the medium-gain, gray-scale, O–I diameter (8), obviating the need for a separate measurement of true anatomic BPD.

Real-time imaging has added a new dimension, time, to standard gray-scale imaging modes (Fig. 7–4). Two separate anlyses of real-time imaging modes have demonstrated that no important differences in BPD measurements exist between real-time and gray-scale imaging and they may be used interchangeably (8). The only points of distinction between these two modes are greater reproducibility of BPD measurements with real-time imaging (unless some form

TABLE 7-1. ERROR* IN BPD MEASUREMENTS DERIVED BY DIFFERENT SCANNING MODALITIES

Investigator	Scanning techniques	Width of skull tables	BPD measurement error in mm (2SD)
Campbell (3)	B–A scan & NPIS	—	<1.0
Davison et al (6)	B–A scan & NPIS	—	±2.42
Davison et al (6)	B–A scan & NPIS	—	±4.06
Poll (11)	B–A scan & NPIS	—	±1.6
Sabbagha et al (13)	B–scan & NPIS	—	±1.0
Sabbagha et al (13)	Gray-scale & NPIS	—	±1.6
Sabbagha et al (13)	Gray-scale & stored imaging	—	±2.8
Cooperberg (5)	Real-time	—	±1.54
Hughey & Sabbagha (8)	Real-time	3–5 mm	±0.8

* Errors noted represent ±2SD.

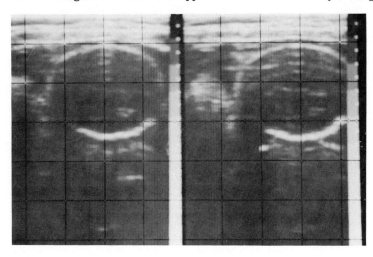

FIG. 7-4. Real-time image showing fetal biparietal diameter. For best reproducibility, width of skull tables should not exceed 3–5 mm (see text). (Hughey M, Sabbagha RE: Am J Obstet Gynecol [in press])

of nonpersistent image scanning is used) and the short time with which BPDs can be obtained with real-time equipment.

FINDING THE BPD PLANE

Regardless of the mode used to identify the BPD, due regard must be given to the plane selected for the measurement of the BPD. Most sonographers have demonstrated that the widest fetal BPD has the greatest reproducibility if the following criteria are met: skull tables are symmetrically opposed and of equal thickness creating an oval shape, and a midline echo perpendicular to the line of travel of the sonic energy is seen (8). Other sonographers choose a plane containing the BPD with a fixed relationship to an identifiable fetal landmark, such as 1.0 cm below the falx. The use of such arbitrary planes is not encouraged, for several reasons. The overwhelming majority of published series on fetal BPDs were taken with the widest fetal BPD, not an arbitrarily defined plane. Secondly, none of the arbitrary planes bears any relationship to the true anatomic BPD, which the obstetrician may require in certain clinical situations. The reporting of a BPD that, in reality, may underestimate the true anatomic BPD by as much as a centimeter or more may eventually lead to an obstetric catastrophe, as, for example, in the assessment of feasibility of vaginal delivery in a breech presentation (Ch. 12). Under

these circumstances both the sonographic (O–I BPD) and the true anatomic BPD (O–O BPD) should be included in the report.

STANDARD IMAGING AND NONPERSISTENT IMAGE SCANNING (NPIS)

When standard imaging is employed with either a B-scan or gray-scale unit, the operator sonically slices the maternal abdomen into approximately 1-cm slabs horizontally and vertically, taking a photograph of each slab. The 30-odd photographs are then evaluated and the one image that shows the best fetal head diameter is selected for measuring the BPD. The only advantage to this approach is that the technique is easily performed by an inexperienced technician. However, there are several disadvantages: 1) this approach ignores the lateral flexion of the fetal head, leading to images that approach the fetal head obliquely rather than perpendicular, and leading to gross inaccuracies; 2) this approach fails to provide for the occurrence of the widest BPD *between* rather than at the 1-cm divisions; 3) this approach ignores the fact that the fetuses are frequently moving. Because of this motion the standard scanning technique may fail even to approximate the fetal BPD. Each of these disadvantages can be overcome through the use of some form of NPIS. Functionally, NPIS involves the continuous updating of the sonic image to accommodate fetal motion while small changes in the scanning plane are made to capture the widest BPD (Ch. 5). Real-time ultrasonography performs this function automatically and continuously, and it is this characteristic of real-time imaging that leads to the greatest reproducibility of fetal BPD images. Where real-time imaging is available, it should be used to give the most accurate BPDs. Where it is not available, NPIS may give very accurate results. Least desirable and least accurate is the conventional form of imaging. Where conventional imaging is the only mode available, confidence limits of predictions based on these relatively inaccurate measurements must be altered accordingly.

PREDICTION OF GESTATIONAL AGE FROM BPD

An accurate fetal BPD having been obtained, care must be exercised in selecting an appropriate gestational age chart. Most of the available charts are unsatsifactory. The reasons are several. First, in the majority of the charts derived by early B-mode equipment electronic calipers were rarely used. Rather, BPDs were measured in relation to a horizontal grid overlying a nonflat oscilloscope face. Thus, because of parallax, BPD values were artificially reduced—the reduction being greater in large BPDs. For example, an actual O–I BPD of 9.4 cm would be reduced by a minimum of 5.0 mm to 8.9 cm. Upon discovery of this phenomenon flat-faced oscilloscope tubes were used and BPDs were derived in relation to 1-cm markers displayed along the axis of the BPD.

Secondly, many charts were not carefully derived (ie, use of NPIS in a large numbers of patients, each with a totally reliable menstrual history, in whom predicted gestational age was confirmed by physical examination of each newborn), and they should not, therefore, be used.

Even when care is used in selecting a gestational age chart, important differences (related to the velocity of ultrasound used) arise between the charts. Table 7–2 shows the differences that occur in the published gestational age charts from four investigators, each of whom obtained their data with care and due regard for the caveats listed earlier. To understand fully why these differences arise, the methodology of each of these investigators should be examined.

In 1971 Campbell and Newman (4) reported the results of ultrasonic cephalometry of 574 patients (1029 measurements). In each case the last menstrual period (LMP) was reliably known, labor occurred within 1 week of the EDC, pregnancies were single and uncomplicated, and the babies were above the 5th percentile of weight for 40 weeks' gestation. To obtain the BPD, they located the largest transverse fetal head diameter with a B-scan image and then measured that diameter with an A-scan image (combined B–A scan). Electronic calipers, calibrated to an assumed speed of sound in tissue of 1600 m/sec, were placed on the leading edges of the proximal and distal skull echo complexes. The distance between the caliper dots was taken to represent the fetal BPD. Campbell and Newman used an assumed speed of sound of 1600 m/sec rather than 1540 m/sec to compensate for their observation that a leading-edge B-scan BPD underestimates the true anatomic BPD by failing to measure the width of the distal skull and scalp. By artificially inflating their leading-edge BPDs by a factor of 1600/1540, they found experimentally that the true anatomic BPD was closely approximated.

TABLE 7-2. GESTATIONAL AGE AND BIPARIETAL DIAMETER*

Investigator	Weeks	18	20	22	24	26	28	30	32	34	36	38	40
Campbell and Newman (4)		44	50	57	64	70	76	81	86	90	93	96	98
Levi and Smets (9)		41	48	54	59	66	71	77	81	85	89	92	94
Varma (16)		—	50	55	61	67	72	78	82	87	91	94	95
Sabbagha et al (12)		43	47	53	59	66	72	78	83	87	90	93	95

* BPD in mm, gestational age in weeks from last normal menses.

TABLE 7-3. GESTATIONAL AGE AND BIPARIETAL DIAMETER* AFTER STANDARDIZATION†

Investigator	Weeks	18	20	22	24	26	28	30	32	34	36	38	40
Campbell and Newman (4)		42	48	55	62	67	73	78	83	87	90	93	94
Levi and Smets (9)		42	48	54	60	66	73	78	82	86	89	92	95
Varma (16)		—	50	55	61	67	73	79	83	88	92	95	96
Sabbagha et al (12)		43	47	53	59	66	72	78	83	87	90	93	95

* BPD in mm, gestational age in weeks from last normal menses.
† Original measurements corrected to an assumed speed of sound in tissue of 1540 m/sec.

TABLE 7-4. COMPOSITE MEAN OF 7059 FETAL SONOGRAPHIC BPDs FROM 14 TO 40 WEEKS' GESTATION AT DIFFERENT ASSUMED SPEEDS OF SOUND IN TISSUE

Weeks	Speed of sound (m/sec)		
	1540*	1529*	1600†
14	2.8	2.8	2.9
15	3.2	3.2	3.3
16	3.6	3.6	3.7
17	3.9	3.9	4.1
18	4.2	4.2	4.4
19	4.5	4.5	4.7
20	4.8	4.8	5.0
21	5.1	5.1	5.3
22	5.4	5.4	5.6
23	5.8	5.8	6.0
24	6.1	6.1	6.3
25	6.4	6.4	6.6
26	6.7	6.7	7.0
27	7.0	6.9	7.3
28	7.2	7.1	7.5
29	7.5	7.4	7.8
30	7.8	7.7	8.1
31	8.0	7.9	8.3
32	8.2	8.1	8.5
33	8.5	8.4	8.8
34	8.7	8.6	9.0
35	8.8	8.7	9.1
36	9.0	8.9	9.4
37	9.2	9.1	9.6
38	9.3	9.2	9.7
39	9.4	9.3	9.8
40	9.5	9.4	9.9

* BPDs given in centimeters from leading edge of the near-skull table to the leading edge of the far-skull table, i.e., from outer to inner aspects of fetal head (0–I BPDs).
† BPDs given in centimeters from outer to outer aspects of fetal head (0–0 BPD).

Thus, 1600 m/sec was chosen as the most desirable assumed speed of sound in tissue for cephalometric purposes.

In 1973 Levi and Smets (9) reported their results from examining 1011 normal patients (3032 examinations). They used the combined B–A scan method of Campbell and Newman (4) but employed electronic calipers calibrated to an assumed speed of sound in tissue of 1529 m/sec instead of 1600 m/sec.

Varma (16) reported the results of serial cephalometry in 100 normal pregnancies with birthweights above the 10th percentile (1966 measurements). She used the combined B–A scan method of Campbell and Newman (4) and equipment calibrated to 1540 m/sec.

Sabbagha et al (12) reported in 1976 the results of serial cephalometry of 198 normal pregnancies (600 measurements). They decreased the B-scan gain producing the thinnest possible skull tables, and to minimize parallax used electronic calipers (1540 m/sec) to measure the distance from the leading edge to the trailing edge of the second echo complex. However, since the width of the second echo complex was invariably less than 1 mm (Fig. 7–1), their data are statistically comparable to the leading-edge data derived by other investigators (14).

At first glance large differences appear in the gestational age charts developed by these investigators. Table 7–2 shows the mean or 50th percentile data from each of these published charts, and Table 7–3 shows the same data after standardization to compensate for differences in the assumed speed of sound. The data of Campbell and Newman were reduced by a factor of 1540/1600; those of Levi and Smets were increased by a factor of 1540/1529. The differences that existed in the charts are largely corrected by this standardization, most of the measurements falling within 1 mm of the mean after standardization.

Sabbagha and Hughey (14) have statistically analyzed these data and found that, from 16 to 40 weeks' gestation, the mean BPD values from these studies are not significantly different from the composite mean gestational age chart, constructed from each of the studies and representing 7059 measurements of 1883 pregnant women (Table 7–4).

The finding that there are no significant differences in BPD measurements from these studies, despite the fact that they were derived by different investigators, from different populations, at different centers in the United States and Europe, is important. Sabbagha, Barton, and Barton (12) analyzed the BPD variations between two different populations and reached the same conclusion, that there are no important BPD differences between populations, Figure 7–5. Because of this finding sonographers need not develop gestational age charts for their particular region (an enormously time-consuming and costly effort if it is to be done well) but may use any of the established charts that have been carefully derived, such as any of the ones listed here. The composite mean chart, an amalgamation of each of the four carefully constructed BPD charts, may also be used with confidence, when the calibrated assumed speed of sound is matched with the appropriate chart. The composite mean chart is useful if single BPD measurements are obtained. However, if serial cephalometry is employed, assessment of gestational age is enhanced by using a GASA (15) chart in lieu of the composite mean chart, as detailed in Chapter 8. It should be emphasized that the composite mean BPD chart represents data derived from gravidas living in geographic areas relatively close to sea level and may not apply to determine gestational age in pregnant women residing at very high altitude (5000–6000 ft above sea level) (14).

Gestational age is always expressed in weeks following the onset of the last normal menstrual period. This obstetric terminology is universally accepted, and thus an average duration of pregnancy is 40 weeks. A few sonographers have, in the past, attempted to express gestational age in terms of the presumed time of conception, with the mistaken impression of improving accuracy. Instead, the practice has led only to confusion. The standard, accepted terminology for obstetric purposes gives gestational age in weeks following the last normal menstrual period, or 40 weeks for a term pregnancy.

A fetal BPD having been matched with the corresponding gestational age, due regard must be given to the confidence limits of that prediction. Like many biologic systems, gestational ages are distributed around a given BPD in a bell-shaped curve. Although the mean gestational age for a given BPD may be 34 weeks, the limitations of the technique confine the accuracy of that prediction to plus or minus several weeks. Table 7–5 shows the observed variation in gestational age predictions (90% and 95% confidence limits) when some form of NPIS is used (12). If a BPD is derived by a less accurate method (without some form of NPIS), the confidence limits are wider. Thus, the practice of reporting a precise gestational age in relation to a third-trimester BPD is dangerous and should be eschewed. For example, a BPD reported as 8.2 representing 32.3 weeks' gestation (1) conveys to the obstetrician a false sense of predictive accuracy, implying that 32.3 weeks can be distinguished in some way from 32.4 or 32.2 weeks. In fact the normal variation from a single third-trimester BPD is about ± 3 weeks, and the

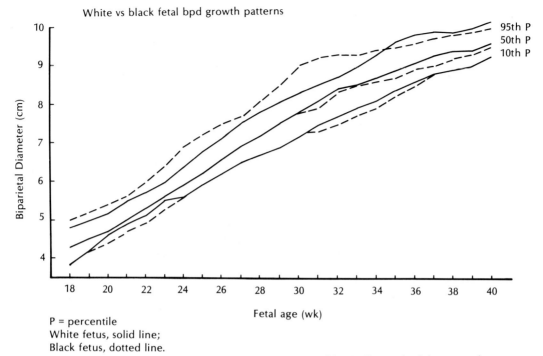

White vs black fetal bpd growth patterns

P = percentile
White fetus, solid line;
Black fetus, dotted line.

FIG. 7–5. The mean BPDs for white and black fetuses, measured by similar methodology, are almost identical. P, percentile; white fetus shown by solid line; black fetus shown by dotted line. (Sabbagha RE, Barton FB, Barton BA: Am J Obstet Gynecol 126:479, 1976)

sonographer does a disservice to the obstetrician when he attributes greater accuracy to the prediction than truly exists. Whenever a gestational age prediction based on cephalometric data is given, the obstetrician must also be informed of the confidence limits of such a prediction (see Ch. 8).

Each of the four carefully derived gestational age charts listed in Tables 7–2 and 7–3 was formulated with use of B-scan or B–A scan data. Since most centers in this country are now em-

TABLE 7–5. OBSERVED VARIATION IN GESTATIONAL AGE PREDICTED BY BPDs OBTAINED DURING THE SECOND AND THIRD TRIMESTERS OF PREGNANCY (11a, 12)

Week of pregnancy BPD is obtained	Variation in gestational age by days
16*	±7
17–26†	±10–11
27–28*	±14
29–40*	±21

  * The reported variation in gestational age is applicable to 90% of fetuses (10).

  † The reported variation in gestational age is applicable to 95% of fetuses (11a).

ploying gray-scale or real-time imaging modes, the question of interchangeability of these modes arises. Hughey and Sabbagha (8) and Cooperberg et al (5) have demonstrated that O–I gray-scale or real-time BPDs taken at medium gain are interchangeable with O–I (leading-edge) B-scan BPDs. This finding is fortuitous in that it demonstrates that new charts for gray-scale or real-time imaging are not required. These investigators also found, however, that, when other measurements (such as O–O, M–M, or I–I) at other than medium gain were used, differences in measurements arose that were sufficiently different to disallow the use of existing B-scan charts.

From these data, Sabbagha and Hughey (14) proposed standardization of BPD measurements, based on the most accurate and reproducible methodology currently available. They proposed that all cephalometric measurements be made from the leading edge of the near-skull echo complex to the leading edge of the far-skull echo complex with medium gain applied (skull tables 3–5 mm thick) with either gray-scale or real-time imaging modes, which would corre-

TABLE 7-6. CORRELATION OF FETAL BPD AND BIRTH WEIGHT*

Author	Date	Mode	95% weight margin (g)
Brown	1971	A-scan	±638
Stocker et al	1974	B-real time	±652
Campbell	1974	B–A-scan	±812
Johnson and Tosach	1954	Fundal height	±454 in 80%
Lind	1970	Clinical guess at 3300 g	±454 in 70%

* Modified from Sabbagha RE: Clin Obstet Gynecol 20:297, 1977

spond to the commonly accepted practice throughout the world of measuring the leading-edge diameters from B-scan images. Similar or identical charts could then be used in all centers and communication between centers improved. Obstetricians requiring the true anatomic BPD in term fetuses presenting as breech need only add 4.0 mm to the sonographic BPD to account for the additional skull and scalp not measured by O–I determinations.

OTHER USES OF FETAL CEPHALOMETRY

ESTIMATION OF FETAL WEIGHT

Although the use of ultrasonic measurements to estimate fetal weight is described later (Ch. 10), it is worthwhile to note that fetal cephalometry has been used alone to estimate fetal weight (Table 7–6). These reports demonstrate that the 95% confidence limits of fetal weight estimation are so wide that cephalometry alone offers no improvement over simple clinical estimates. Some success has been found in predicting fetal weights ≥ 2500 g in 97%–100% of fetuses with BPDs greater than a certain fixed diameter. Unfortunately, that diameter varies in different studies from 8.7 to 9.4 cm, probably because of methodologic differences mainly related to parallax. Investigators are beginning to accept a BPD close to 9.4 cm to represent attainment of a minimum weight of 2500 g.

EVALUATION OF FETAL GROWTH

Serial fetal cephalometry has important applications in the field of high-risk obstetrics to evaluate fetal growth in a potentially hostile environment. This application is more thoroughly described in Chapters 8 through 11.

DIAGNOSIS OF HYDROCEPHALY

Fetal cephalometry can accurately predict hydrocephalus. Classically a BPD of more than 10.7 or 11 cm has denoted hydrocephaly. This classical understanding has not been substantiated clinically, because it is not uncommon for a fetus suffering from scalp edema or diabetic macrosomia to display head sizes of at least that magnitude. At all stages of pregnancy the fetal head should approximate the fetal trunk. Before the diagnosis of fetal hydrocephalus can be made, the fetal BPD must be shown to substantially exceed the thoracic diameter or abdominal circumference (Chapter 19). In addition an evaluation of the size of cerebral ventricles should be attempted, see Chapter 19.

DIAGNOSIS OF ANENCEPHALY

The absence of a fetal head is usually readily apparent particularly when real-time or NPIS imaging is used. Patients with a history of open neural tube defects are at significantly greater risk for the development of anencephaly and should undergo ultrasound scanning in early pregnancy to allow for termination if that should be desired. Similarly, patients with polyhydramnios are at greater than average risk for the presence of anencephaly, and these patients should undergo ultrasonic scanning. When the diagnosis is not clear from ultrasound evaluation alone, radiographic studies may prove useful.

INTRAUTERINE FETAL DEMISE

Certain cephalometric findings are frequently seen in patients with intrauterine fetal death (IUFD). Serial scans showing a persistant decline in head size is one such finding. Clear distortion of the fetal skull or overriding skull bones has also been seen in patients with IUFD. The classical "halo" sign must be interpreted with caution. Scalp edema creating the "halo" sign may occur 24–28 hours after fetal demise. Other conditions can mimic this sign, and other methods of determining IUFD should be used. Certainly, the absence of a visible fetal heart beat by real-time imaging is the most reliable method with an accuracy close to 100% (7).

REFERENCES

1. BROWN RE: Ultrasonography: Basic Principles and Clinical Applications. St. Louis, Warren H. Green, 1975

2. CAMPBELL S: An improved method of fetal cephalometry by ultrasound. J Obstet Gynaecol Br Commonw 75:568, 1968

3. CAMPBELL S: Ultrasonic fetal cephalometry during the second trimester of pregnancy. J Obstet Gynaecol Br Commonw 77:12, 1970

4. CAMPBELL S, NEWMAN GB: Growth of the fetal biparietal diameter during normal pregnancy. J Obstet Gynaecol Br Commonw 78:513, 1971

5. COOPERBERG PL, CHOW T, KITE V, AUSTIN S: Biparietal diameter: a comparison of real-time and conventional B-scan techniques. J Clin Ultrasound 4:421, 1976

6. DAVISON JN, LIND T, FARR V, WHITTINGHAM TA: The limitations of ultrasonic fetal cephalometry. J Obstet Gynaecol Br Commonw 80:769, 1973

7. HOBBINS JC, WINSBERG F: Ultrasonography in Obstet-rics and Gynecology. Baltimore, Williams & Wilkins, 1977

8. HUGHEY M, SABBAGHA RE: Cephalometry by real-time imaging: a critical evaluation. Am J Obstet Gynecol, 131:825, 1978

9. LEVI S, SMETS P: Intrauterine fetal growth studied by ultrasonic biparietal measurements. Acta Obstet Gynecol Scand 52:193, 1973

10. LUDWIG GD: The velocity of sound through tissues and the acoustical impedence of tissues. J Accoust Soc Am 22:862, 1950

11. POLL V: Precision of ultrasonic fetal cephalometry. Br J Obstet Gynaecol 83:217, 1976

11a. SABBAGHA RE, TURNER JH, ROCKETTE H, MAZER J, ORGILL J: Sonar BPD and fetal age: definition of the relationship. Obstet Gynecol 43:7, 1973

12. SABBAGHA RE, BARTON FB, BARTON BA: Sonar biparietal diameter. I. Analysis of percentile growth differences in two normal populations using same methodology. Am J Obstet Gynecol 126:479, 1976

13. SABBAGHA RE, CHILCOTE WS, MARTIN AO, GRASSE D: Reproducibility of ultrasonic cephalometry using B-scan and gray-scale imaging. Ultrasound Med Biol 3A:663, 1977

14. SABBAGHA RE, HUGHEY M: Standardization of sonar cephalometry and gestational age. Obstet Gynecol 52:402, 1978

15. SABBAGHA RE, HUGHEY M, DEPP R: Growth adjusted sonographic age: a simplified method. Obstet Gynecol 51:383, 1978

16. VARMA TR: Prediction of delivery date by ultrasound cephalometry. J Obstet Gynaecol Br Commonw 80:316, 1973

17. WILLOCKS J, DONALD I, DUGGAN TC, DAY N: Fetal cephalometry by Ultrasound. J Obstet Gynaecol Br Commonw 71:11, 1964

8

Biparietal diameter and gestational age

RUDY E. SABBAGHA

The differentiation between normal and altered fetal growth is dependent on accurate knowledge of gestational age because the length of pregnancy expressed in weeks or days forms the X-coordinate of graphs depicting fetal cephalic growth and weight, Figure 8–1. Similarly, many laboratory tests pertaining to fetal well-being cannot be interpreted unless fetal age is defined. For example, the significance of a given maternal estriol value as an index of a failing feto-placental unit (24) rests on whether a fetus is premature or small for gestational age (SGA), Figure 8–2. The same logic is applicable to biochemical determinations of human placental lactogen (HPL) during pregnancy (23).

In addition the placement of a fetus affected by Rh-disease in any of Liley's three zones delineating the severity of red blood cell hemolysis depends on correct dating of the pregnancy, Figure 8–3. Finally, the concentration of alpha-fetoprotein in amniotic fluid or maternal serum used to predict neural tube defects is related to gestational age, Figure 8–4.

HOW GESTATIONAL AGE IS DEFINED

Until recently the length of pregnancy has been mainly defined by the menstrual history, i.e., from the first day of the last menstrual period (LMP), because the errors in assessment of gestational age incurred by using certain clinical or laboratory parameters are unacceptable. For example, the distance between symphysis pubis and uterine fundus varies considerably depending on maternal height, amniotic fluid volume (1), and presence of uterine or ovarian tumors (15). Likewise, the proportion of "fat cells" or the concentration of creatinine in amniotic fluid are indices of fetal age applicable only to pregnancies close to term (13). Furthermore, fetograms obtained to demonstrate the appearance of distal femoral epiphyses lack sensitivity and specificity (7).

Reliance on the menstrual history for defining fetal age is not always effective, because 20%–40% of women cannot relate the last menstrual period accurately (5, 8). Some reasons for this inaccuracy are listed here:

1. History of oligomenorrhea
2. History of metrorrhagia
3. Irregular bleeding with IUD
4. Implantation bleeding
5. Pregnancy following use of oral contraceptive or IUD removal
6. Pregnancy during interval of postpartum amenorrhea

Even if the LMP is known, confirmation of gestational age, by a simple and objective method,

Percentile chart—sonar BPD at intervals of one week.

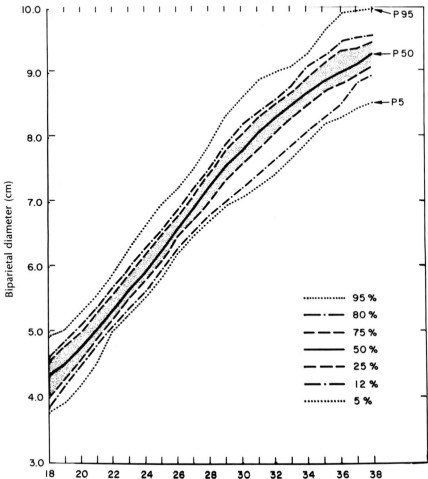

FIG. 8-1. Gestational age as X-coordinate of graph depicting normal growth of the bi-parietal diameter (BPD); maximum separation of large versus small BPDs between 30–33 weeks' gestation. (Sabbagha RE, Barton FB, Barton BA: Am J Obstet Gynecol 126:479, 1976)

at least in high-risk pregnancies, is highly desirable because: 1) in approximately 15% of women, the given date of the LMP is inaccurate (15); and 2) in elective repeat cesarean sections, approximately 8% of neonates are inadvertently delivered prematurely (2).

The objective definition of fetal age in relation to measurements of the fetal CRL is detailed in Chapter 6. In the remaining part of this chapter the relation between sonar BPD and fetal age is outlined.

SONAR BPD VERSUS FETAL AGE

Campbell was the first investigator to link fetal BPD to gestational age. In his study he obtained sonar BPD measurements at each gestational week from a large number of normal gravidas in whom: 1) LMP was known and 2) delivery occurred spontaneously within ±1 week of the menstrual EDD. Using these data he defined the mean BPD values corresponding to each week in gestation. Subsequently he showed that in

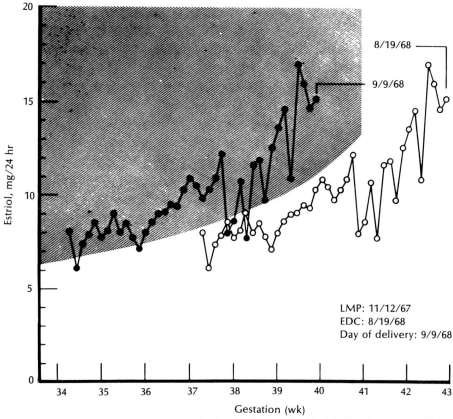

FIG. 8–2. Gray area represents normal estriol levels. Correct EDC is 9-9-68 rather than 8-19-68. Estriol levels fall below 2 SD if wrong dates are used. (Merkatz I, Solomon S: Clin Obstet Gynecol 13:665, 1970)

84% of gravidas with uncertain dates delivery occurred within ±9 days of the sonar EDD, if the latter is derived from BPDs obtained in the second trimester of pregnancy (4). Varma in a similar study confirmed Campbell's report (25). These results imply that the BPD is a reliable index of gestational age, particularly since 84% of gravidas are normally expected to deliver within ±2 weeks of the menstrual EDD (26).

Sabbagha et al (18, 22) then defined the confidence limits of fetal age in relation to second and third trimester BPDs, Figure 8–5 and Table 8–1. They showed that: 1) prior to 26 weeks' gestation a single BPD can be used to predict gestational age within a range of ±7–11 days (with 95% confidence); 2) after 26 weeks' gestation BPDs vary markedly around these mean values and are inaccurate indices of fetal age;

and 3) serial cephalometry leads to a better definition of gestational age by application of the principle of growth-adjusted sonographic age (GASA).

SERIAL CEPHALOMETRY VERSUS GROWTH-ADJUSTED SONOGRAPHIC AGE (GASA)

Serial cephalometry in monkey and human fetuses have clarified two important fetal cephalic growth phenomena (17, 21).

NORMAL VARIATION IN FETAL BPDS

Starting from approximately the 20th week of pregnancy, BPDs in fetuses of the same gesta-

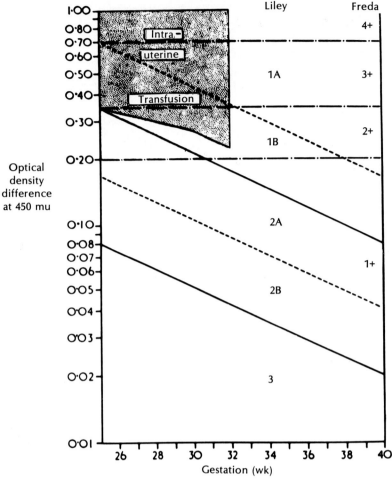

FIG. 8–3. Liley's three zones. (Queenan JT: Clin Obstet Gynecol 14:505, 1971)

tional age show a normal biologic variation and can be separated into three divisions: 1) large (BPDs ≥ 75th percentile); 2) average (BPDs varying from the 25th to the 75th percentiles); and 3) small (BPDs ≤ 25th percentile). Thus, as shown in Figure 8–6, a single BPD measurement can be applicable to three fetuses of different gestational ages. The first is a young fetus with a large BPD, the second is of average cephalic size and age, and the third is more advanced in gestational age but has a small BPD.

In correlating a given BPD value to the duration of pregnancy, sonographers make no differentiation between fetuses with large or small cephalic sizes. Thus, by assigning a second tri-

mester fetus with a relatively large BPD a mean gestational age, corresponding to that of a fetus with average cephalic size, pregnancy duration is overestimated by 7–11 days (depending on whether the BPD is at the 75th or 95th percentile), Table 8–2. In other words, gestational age is always incorrectly advanced in the young fetus with a large BPD, Figure 8–6. Similarly, by assigning a second trimester fetus with a small BPD a mean gestational age corresponding to that of a fetus with average cephalic size, pregnancy duration is underestimated by 7–11 days (depending on whether BPD is at the 25th or 5th percentiles), Table 8–2. In other words, gestational age is always incorrectly underestimated

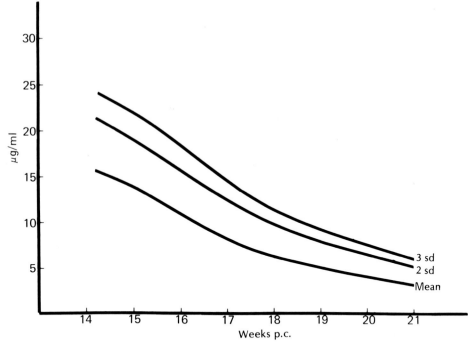

FIG. 8–4. Amniotic fluid alpha-fetoprotein levels are related to gestational age. (Cowchock FS: Clin Obstet Gynecol 19:871, 1976)

in the older fetus with a small BPD, Figure 8–6.

Because of these biologic differences in BPD size the variation in fetal age corresponding to a single BPD obtained prior to 26 weeks' gestation is ±10–11 days (2 SD). The magnitude of error in defining the length of pregnancy during the third trimester by assigning the mean gestational age to a fetus with a large or small BPD is even greater, namely: ±3 weeks, Figure 8–7.

By using serial cephalometry, assessment of gestational age can be enhanced. The reason is related to characteristic patterns of BPD growth.

BPD GROWTH PATTERNS

The following observations regarding the BPD growth pattern have been noted (17): first, at least 90% of fetuses with large, average, or small BPDs tend to maintain their relative cephalic rank with advancing gestation. Second, the maximum biologic variation in the length of BPDs occurs by 30 weeks' gestation, Figure 8–1.

These growth phenomena make it possible to place each fetus into a large, average, or small cephalic bracket if two BPD readings are obtained at approximately the 21st and 31st weeks of pregnancy. The second BPD is used to adjust the error in gestational age incurred by the first BPD. Thus, if the second BPD measurement falls on or above the 75th percentile (large BPD), gestational age is adjusted to make the fetus 7–11 days younger, ie, a growth-adjusted sonar age (GASA) is used. Similarly, if the second BPD falls on or below the 25th percentile (small BPD), a GASA is assigned to advance fetal age by 7–11 days.

By using a GASA, estimates of gestational age based on second trimester BPDs are enhanced yielding smaller 95% confidence limits of approximately ±1–3 days (17).

In a small minority of fetuses with severe intrauterine growth retardation (IUGR) the BPD may fall from an average to a lower percentile rank between 21–31 weeks' gestation, ie, during the time BPDs should be obtained for a GASA. In these fetuses the length of pregnancy may be

Percentiles of growth

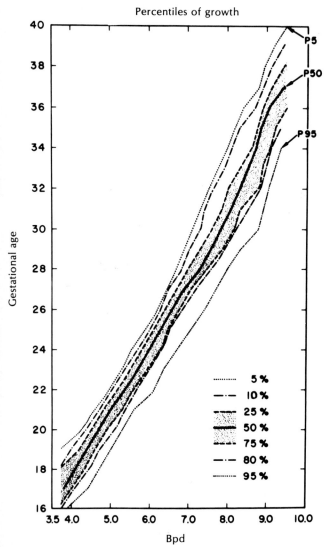

FIG. 8-5. The 95% confidence limits of gestational age in relation to single BPD measurements.

TABLE 8-1. OBSERVED VARIATION IN GESTATIONAL AGE PREDICTIONS BY BPDs OBTAINED DURING THE SECOND AND THIRD TRIMESTERS OF PREGNANCY

Week of pregnancy BPD is obtained	Variation in gestational age by days
16	±7*
17–26	±10–11†
27–28	±14*
29–40	±21*

* The reported variation in gestational age is applicable to 90% of fetuses (Sabbagha RE, Barton FB, Barton BA: Am J Obstet Gynecol 126:479, 1976)

† The reported variation in gestational age is applicable to 95% of fetuses (Sabbagha RE, Turner JH, Rockette H, Mazer J, Orgill J: Obstet Gynecol 43:7, 1974)

Similarly, about 5% of fetuses may accelerate BPD growth from a lower to an upper percentile rank during the interval that BPDs are measured to obtain a GASA. This pattern may sometimes exist in normal gravidas, and possibly in some pregnancies associated with maternal diabetes mellitus. Again, in these fetuses the length of pregnancy may be incorrectly underestimated by approximately 1 week if a GASA is used, a relatively acceptable error.

HOW TO ASSIGN FETUSES A GASA

A simple GASA chart that lends itself to routine clinical use is presented, Table 8–3. This chart clearly indicates that the first BPD should be obtained prior to 26 weeks' gestation because then the variation in fetal age is ±11 days. The second BPD should be measured at least 6 weeks later and between 30–33 weeks' gestation. The latter interval is important for three reasons. First, BPDs show a maximal spread then, Figure 8–1. Second, IUGR usually occurs after 32 weeks of pregnancy (9). Third, preliminary data show that FDMs (fetuses of diabetic mothers) who show an increase in BPD do so after 32–33 weeks' gestation.

The assignment of a GASA in five fetuses with different BPD growth patterns is illustrated in Table 8–4.

incorrectly overestimated by approximately 1 week if a GASA is used. Nonetheless, this error is small in relation to the wide range in fetal age estimates defined by a single BPD value: namely ±11 days. In addition such fetuses, with severe IUGR, continue to show a drop in the BPD to lower percentile levels with advancing gestation—and this growth pattern should alert the astute physician to the diagnosis of severe IUGR.

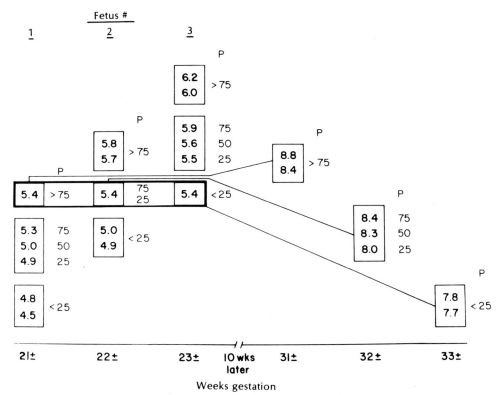

FIG. 8-6. Fetal growth patterns from biparietal diameter (BPD) of 5.4 cm. A BPD of 5.4 cm represents any of three fetuses of differing fetal ages as shown. A second BPD reading obtained 10 weeks later will identify the fetus as large, average, or small and lead to a closer assessment of fetal age. +, 1–3 days; −, 1–3 days; P, percentile. (Sabbagha RE, Barton BA, Barton FB et al: Am J Obstet Gynecol 126:485, 1976; Sabbagha RE, Hughey M, Depp R: Obstet Gynecol 51:383, 1978)

VALIDITY OF THE GASA CHART (TABLE 8-3)

At present, a number of charts are used to estimate the mean gestational age corresponding to a given BPD value. Most of these charts have been derived by B-scan or B–A scan methods, and the BPDs reported represent the distance between the outer and inner aspects of the fetal head—O-I BPDs (see Ch. 7).

The need for all these charts has recently been questioned (19) (Ch. 7) because: 1) BPD measurements derived by the early modalities of scanning are statistically comparable to BPDs obtained by gray-scale or real-time imaging—if medium gain is used (11) (ie, skull tables produced are 3–5 mm wide); 2) the differences in the mean BPD values derived from four large fetal populations (studied at altitudes close to sea level) are not significantly different from zero (19) see Chapter 7.

The GASA chart, Table 8–3, is derived from a group of fetuses constituting one of the four populations in whom the BPDs are statistically comparable (19). The advantages of using the GASA chart are the following:

1. It is simple and lends itself to routine use for assigning a GASA in busy ultrasound departments.
2. It clearly separates BPDs into those obtained before and after 26 weeks' gestation in accordance with the accuracy of the BPD as an estimator of fetal age.
3. It shows the range in BPD measurements during the third trimester for fetuses with large, average, and small cephalic sizes.

TABLE 8-2. FETAL AGE PERCENTILE VALUES FOR BPD's FROM 3.5 to 9.5 CM

	Fetal age percentiles (wk)*						
BPD	5	10	25	50	75	80	95
3.5	17+	17	16+	16	16−	16−	15+
3.6	18	17+	17	16+	16	16	15+
3.7	19	18		17−	16	16	16
3.8	19	18+	18+	17	16+	16+	16
3.9	19+	19	18+	17+	17−	17−	16
4.0	19+	19	19−	18−	17	17−	16
4.1	19+	19	19−	18	17+	17+	16
4.2	20−	19+	19	18+	17+	17+	16+
4.3	20	20−	19+	19−	18−	18−	17−
4.4	20+	20	20−	19	18+	18	17
4.5	21−	20+	20	19+	19−	18	17+
4.6	21	21−	20+	20−	19	18+	18−
4.7	21+	21	21−	20	19+	19	18
4.8	21+	21	21	20+	20−	19+	18+
4.9	22−	21+	21+	21	20	19+	19−
5.0	22	22	22−	21	20+	20−	19
5.1	22+	22	22−	21+	20+	20	19+
5.2	23−	22+	22	22−	21−	20+	20−
5.3	23	23−	22+	22−	21	21−	20
5.4	24−	23+	23−	22	21+	21+	20+
5.5	24	24−	23	22+	22−	21+	21−
5.6	24	24−	23+	23−	22	22−	21
5.7	24+	24	24−	23	22+	22+	21+
5.8	25−	24+	24	23+	23−	23−	21+
5.9	25	25−	24+	24−	23	23−	22−
6.0	25+	25	25−	24	23	23	22−
6.1	26−	25+	25	24+	23+	23+	22
6.2	26	26−	25+	25−	24−	23+	22+
6.3	26+	26	26−	25	24	24	23−
6.4	27−	26+	26	25+	24+	24+	23+
6.5	27+	27	26+	26−	25	25	24−
6.6	28−	27+	27−	26	25+	25+	24−
6.7	28	28−	27	26+	26−	26−	24
6.8	28+	28	27+	27−	26	26−	24+
6.9	29	28+	28−	27	26+	26+	25−
7.0	29+	29−	28	27+	27−	26+	25−
7.1	30	30−	28+	28−	27	27−	25+
7.2	31−	30−	29−	28−	27+	27	25+
7.3	31	30	29	28	28−	27+	26−
7.4	32−	31	29+	28+	28−	27+	26
7.5	32	32−	30−	29−	28+	28−	26+
7.6	33−	32	30	29	28+	28	27−
7.7	33	32	30+	30−	29−	28+	27
7.8	33	32+	31−	30	29−	29−	27+
7.9	33+	33	31+	30+	29	29	28−
8.0	34	33+	32	31−	29+	29+	28
8.1	34+	34	32+	31	30−	30−	28+
8.2	35	35−	33−	31+	30	30	29−
8.3	36−	35	33	32	31	30+	29
8.4	36	36−	33+	32+	31	31−	29
8.5	36+	36−	34−	33	31+	31	29+
8.6	36+	36−	34	33+	31+	31	29+
8.7	37−	36	35−	34	32−	31+	30−
8.8	37	36+	35+	34+	32	32−	30
8.9	38−	37	36	35+	33	32+	31
9.0	38+	37+	37−	36−	33+	33	32−
9.1	39−	38	37	36+	34	34	32+
9.2	39	39−	37+	36+	35	35	33
9.3	39+	39−	38−	37−	35	35	34−
9.4	40−	39	38	37	36−	35	34+
9.5	40	39+	38+	37+	36	35	35−

* + = 1 to 3 days; − = 1 to 3 days. (Sabbagha RE, Barton BA, Barton FB et al: Am J Obstet Gynecol 126:485, 1976)

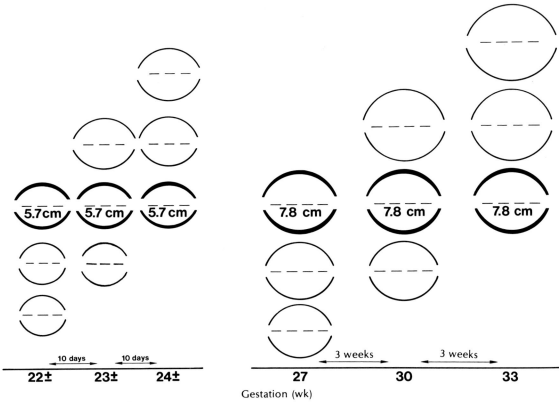

FIG. 8-7. 5.7 cm, length of BPD prior to 26 weeks' gestation; 7.8 cm, length of BPD after 26 weeks' gestation; +, 1–3 days; −, 1–3 days. Variation in gestational age corresponding to a single second trimester BPD is ± 10–11 days (2 SD). But variation in gestational age corresponding to a single third trimester BPD is ± 3 weeks (2 SD). (Sabbagha RE, Barton BA, Barton FB et al: Am J Obstet Gynecol 126:485, 1976)

4. It is derived from precise intervals of gestation as shown in Figure 8–8. Thus, it is applicable to pregnant women, regardless of when they are scanned in relation to their last menstrual period.

5. Its use leads to the placement of fetal BPDs in specific percentile growth brackets by 31–33 weeks' gestation, Table 8–3 and 8–4. This is significant because the growth potential of each fetus and the risk for growth retardation can then be defined (Ch. 10).

HOW TO REPORT SONAR ESTIMATES OF GESTATIONAL AGE

In the assessment of gestational age from sonar BPDs, a clear distinction has to be made between single BPDs obtained before or after 26 weeks' gestation and serial BPD measurements.

SINGLE BPD MEASUREMENTS

A single BPD obtained prior to 26 weeks' gestation predicts fetal age within ±11 days (95% confidence limits). Such BPDs are particularly useful in dating gravidas prior to amniocentesis used for detection of biochemical or cytogenetic fetal abnormalities (Ch. 15). If the BPD measurement is not repeated by 30–33 weeks' gestation, the distinction between young fetuses with large BPDs (as in infants of diabetic mothers) and older fetuses with small BPDs (as in IUGR) cannot be made. As a result, assessment of fetal age and appreciation of the dynamics of fetal growth in high-risk pregnancies are not possible.

TABLE 8-3 CHART FOR ASSIGNING FETUSES A GROWTH-ADJUSTED SONOGRAPHIC AGE (GASA)

	First sonar* (BPD as fetal age percentile)		Second sonar (BPD percentile range)			
BPD	Range large fetus vs small fetus (wk)	Average fetus (age accepted temporarily)	Fetal age (wk)	Average fetus (× 25 to 75)	Large fetus (75 to 95)	Small fetus (5 to 25)
2.8	± 1	14				
3.2	± 1	15				
3.5	± 1	16	29	7.4–7.7	7.8–8.3	6.8–7.3
3.6	± 1.6	16+	29+	7.5–7.8	7.9–8.4	6.9–7.4
3.7	± 1.6	17−	30−	7.6–7.8	7.9–8.5	7.0–7.5
3.8	± 1.6	17	30	7.7–7.9	8.0–8.6	7.1–7.6
3.9	± 1.6	17+	30+	7.8–8.0	8.1–8.7	7.2–7.7
4.0	± 1.6	18+	31−	7.8–8.0	8.1–8.7	7.2–7.7
4.1	± 1.6	18	31	7.9–8.1	8.2–8.8	7.3–7.8
4.2	± 1.6	18+	31+	8.0–8.2	8.3–8.9	7.4–7.9
4.3	± 1.6	19−	32−	8.0–8.2	8.3–8.9	7.4–7.9
4.4	± 1.6	19	32	8.1–8.3	8.4–9.0	7.5–8.0
4.5	± 1.6	19+	32+	8.2–8.4	8.5–9.0	7.6–8.1
4.6	± 1.6	20−	33−	8.3–8.4	8.5–9.1	7.6–8.2
4.7	± 1.6	20	33	8.4–8.5	8.6–9.1	7.7–8.3
4.8	± 1.6	20+	33+	8.5–8.6	8.7–9.2	7.8–8.4
4.9	± 1.6	21−	34−	8.5–8.7	8.8–9.2	7.8–8.4
5.0	± 1.6	21	34	8.6–8.8	8.9–9.3	7.9–8.5
5.1	± 1.6	21+	34+	8.7–8.9	9.0–9.4	8.0–8.6
5.2	± 1.6	22−	35−	8.7–8.9	9.0–9.5	8.1–8.6
5.3	± 1.6	22−	35	8.8–9.0	9.1–9.6	8.2–8.7
5.4	± 1.6	22	35+	8.9–9.0	9.2–9.6	8.2–8.8
5.5	± 1.6	22+	36−	8.9–9.1	9.3–9.6	8.2–8.8
5.6	± 1.6	23−	36	9.0–9.2	9.3–9.7	8.3–8.9
5.7	± 1.6	23	37	9.1–9.3	9.4–9.8	8.4–9.0
5.8	± 1.6	23+	38	9.2–9.4	9.5–9.9	8.5–9.1
5.9	± 1.6	24−	39	9.3–9.5	9.6–10.0	8.7–9.2
6.0	± 1.6	24	40	9.5–9.6	9.7–10.1	8.9–9.4
6.1	± 1.6	24+				
6.2	± 1.6	25−				
6.3	± 1.6	25				
6.4	± 1.6	25+				
6.5	± 1.6	26−				
6.6	± 1.6	26				
7.5	± 3	29−				
8.5	± 3	33				
9.5	± 3	37+				

BPD = biparietal diameter, measured from outer to inner aspects of fetal head; + = plus 1–3 days; − = minus 1–3 days.

* First sonar is done prior to 26 weeks because of small variation in fetal age of ± 11 days. Second sonar: 1) must be done between 30–33 weeks because of maximal variation in fetal BPD size in this interval and prior to onset of IUGR in most cases; 2) must be done at least 6 weeks after first BPD. The second sonar BPD places a fetus in a large or average or small growth bracket and a growth-adjusted sonographic age (GASA) is used—see text and Table 8-4. (Sabbagha RE, Hughey M, Depp R: Obstet Gynecol 51:383, 1978)

The accuracy in prediction of gestational age from a single BPD obtained after 26 weeks of pregnancy is ±3 weeks, Figure 8–7. Nonetheless, as shown in Table 8–5, because approximately 2/3 of fetuses in the third trimester have BPDs of average length, gestational age may be reported to fall within a range of 2–4 weeks. For example, a BPD of 8.4 cm is shown to correspond to a fetal age of 31–35 weeks. This means that in 2/3 of normal gravidas the length of gestation in a fetus who attains a BPD of 8.4 cm will not be less than 31 weeks or more than 35 weeks. When Table 8–5 is used, it is mandatory to report to the obstetrician that the range in fetal age is applicable only to 2/3 of pregnancies. In this way he is clearly reminded that fetuses

TABLE 8-4. ASSIGNMENT OF A GASA IN FIVE FETUSES WITH DIFFERENT BPD GROWTH PATTERNS

First sonar 18 to 26 weeks*			Second sonar 30 to 33 weeks						
Date	BPD (cm)	Average fetal age accepted temporarily (wk)	Date§	Internal between scans (wk)	Age of average fetus (wk)	BPD Expected for fetus of average size	BPD obtained	GASA‡	BPD percentile for GASA
8–12	4.2	18+	11–11	13	31+	8.0–8.2	8.2 (Same as expected)	31+. No change	25th–75th
1–10	5.8	23+	3–10	9–	32–	8.1–8.2	8.5 (Larger than expected)	31–. 1 week younger	75th–95th
2–15	5.1	21+	5–10	12	33+	8.5–8.6	9.1 (Much larger than expected)	32. Approximately 10 days younger	□95th
4–10	6.0	24	5–30	7+	31+	8.0–8.2	7.5 (Much smaller than expected)	33. Fetus is very small	□ 5th

BPD = biparietal diameter: + = plus 1–3 days: − = minus 1–3 days.

* First sonar is done prior to 26 weeks because of small variation in fetal age of ± 11 days.

† Second sonar: 1) must be done between 30–33 weeks because of maximal variation in fetal BPD size in this interval and prior to onset IUGR in most cases, and 2) must be done at least 6 weeks after first BPD.

‡ In comparison to fetuses with average BPDs those with larger BPDs are 1 week younger while those with smaller BPDs are 1 week older.

§ Gestation disc calculator is first rotated to show the date in relation to the 50th percentile fetal age accepted temporarily. If this fetal age is qualified by a plus or minus sign, the disc is rotated an average of 2 days to the left or right, respectively. The calculator will then show the date on which fetal age is approximately 30–33 weeks. (Sabbagha RE, Hughey M, Depp R: Obstet Gynecol 51:383, 1978)

with large BPDs (seen either as a normal biologic variation or secondary to maternal diabetes mellitus) and small BPDs (seen either as a normal biologic variation or secondary to growth retardation) are excluded. Knowing all the factual data pertaining to a given pregnancy, the obstetrician is in the best position to determine if a given fetus with a BPD of 8.4 cm is likely to be of average cephalic size (ie, fetal age is 31–35 weeks), or large (ie, fetal age is 29–31 weeks), or small (ie, fetal age is 35–37 weeks).

Sonographers should not assign fetuses a highly specific gestational age (such as 33.4 or 32.7 weeks) in relation to a third trimester BPD (3, 10), because such reporting conveys to the obstetrician an impression of marked accuracy and places him in a position of false security. Similarly, a single BPD of 8.9 cm or 9.0 cm does

FIG. 8-8. In the construction of the GASA chart (Table 8-3) showing the correlation between fetal BPDs and fetal age, the duration of pregnancy was ascertained from the first day of the last menstrual period as follows: 1) pregnancies that fell at the end of a whole week were assigned the exact fetal age corresponding to that week, for example, 20 weeks; 2) pregnancies that fell 1–3 days beyond a completed week were labeled with a plus sign, for example, 20+ weeks; and 3) pregnancies that fell 1–3 days short of a completed week were labeled with a minus sign, for example, 20− weeks.

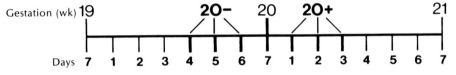

TABLE 8-5. RANGE OF GESTATIONAL AGE IN FETUSES WITH AVERAGE OR CLOSE TO AVERAGE CEPHALIC SIZE IN RELATION TO SINGLE BPDs OBTAINED AFTER 26 WEEKS' GESTATION

BPD	Range in gestational age (weeks)*
6.7	25—27
6.8	26—28
6.9	26—28
7.0	26—29
7.1	26—29
7.2	26—29
7.3	27—30
7.4	27—30
7.5	28—31
7.6	28—31
7.7	28—31
7.8	28—31
7.9	29—32
8.0	29—33
8.1	29—33
8.2	30—34
8.3	30—34
8.4	31—35
8.5	31—35
8.6	31—35
8.7	31—35
8.8	31—36
8.9	32—36
9.0	33—37
9.1	33—37
9.2	35—38
9.3	35—38
9.4	35—39
9.5	35—39

* Only applicable to approximately 2/3 of normal pregnancies. (Modified from Sabbagha RE, Barton FB, Barton BA: Am J Obstet Gynecol 126:479, 1976)

not indicate attainment of fetal maturity in all pregnancies and should not be reported as such.

SERIAL BPDS

The best intervals for serial BPD measurements are the following: 1) 20–24 weeks; 2) 30–33 weeks; and 3) 35–38 weeks. The first two readings are used to assign fetuses a GASA and a specific BPD percentile growth rank. The third BPD is used to evaluate growth attained in relation to each fetus's growth potential (see Ch. 10). In this way the risk for IUGR can be defined and the pregnancy managed appropriately.

The accuracy of fetal age prediction by a GASA is enhanced from ±11 days to approxi-

mately ±1–3 days (2 SD). However, many gravidas assume a GASA means that spontaneous labor will occur within ±1–3 days of the sonar EDD. Obviously, this is not true, and delivery takes place within ±2 weeks in about 84% of normal gravidas (26), with established dates (incidence of prematurity is 10% and of postmaturity is 6%).

Finally, interpretation of all BPD data and assessment of fetal age and growth should be shared by the pregnant woman's obstetrician, because of his familiarity with all the data pertaining to that pregnancy.

REFERENCES

1. BEAZLEY JM, UNDERHILL RA: Fallacy of the fundal height. Br Med J 4:404, 1970

2. BENSON RC, BERENDES H, WEISS W: Fetal compromise during elective Cesarean section. Am J Obstet Gynecol 105:579, 1969

3. BROWN RE: Ultrasonography: Basic Principles and Clinical Applications, p. 116. St. Louis, Warren H. Green, 1975

4. CAMPBELL S: The prediction of fetal maturity by ultrasonic measurement of the biparietal diameter. J Obstet Gynaecol Br Commonw 76:603, 1969

5. CAMPBELL S: The assessment of fetal development by diagnostic ultrasound. Clin Perinatol 1:2, 507, 1974

6. COWCHOCK FS: Use of alph-fetoprotein in prenatal diagnosis. Clin Obstet Gynecol 19:871, 1976

7. CRUZ AC, BUHI WC, SPELLACY WN: Comparison of the fetogram and L/S ratio for fetal maturity. Obstet Gynecol 45:147, 1975

8. DEWHURST CJ, BEAZLEY JM, CAMPBELL S: Assessment of the fetal maturity and dysmaturity. Am J Obstet Gynecol 113:147, 1972

9. GRUENWALD P: Infants of low birth weight among 5,000 deliveries. Pediatrics 34:157, 1964

10. HOBBINS JC, WINSBERG F: Ultrasonography in Obstetrics and Gynecology. Baltimore, Williams & Wilkins, 1977

11. HUGHEY M, SABBAGHA RE: Cephalometry by realtime imaging: a critical evaluation. Am J Obstet Gynecol 131:825, 1978

12. MERKATZ I, SOLOMON S: The fetoplacental unit. Clin Obstet Gynecol 13:665, 1970

13. PITKIN RM: Fetal maturity: nonlipid amniotic fluid assessment. In Spellacy WN (ed): Management of the High-Risk Pregnancy. Baltimore, University Park Press, 1976

14. QUEENAN JT: Amniotic fluid analysis. Clin Obstet Gynecol 14:505, 1971

15. SABBAGHA RE: Ultrasound in managing the high-risk pregnancy. In Spellacy WN (ed): Management of the High-Risk Pregnancy. Baltimore, University Park Press, 1976

16. SABBAGHA RE: Intrauterine growth retardation: antenatal diagnosis by ultrasound. Obstet Gynecol 52:252, 1978

17. SABBAGHA RE, BARTON BA, BARTON FB, KINGAS E, ORGILL J, TURNER JH: Sonar biparietal diameter. II. Predictive of three fetal growth patterns leading to a closer assessment of gestational age and neonatal weight. Am J Obstet Gynecol 126:485, 1976

18. SABBAGHA RE, BARTON FB, BARTON BA: Sonar biparietal diameter. I. Analysis of percentile growth differences in two normal populations using same methodology. Am J Obstet Gynecol 126:479, 1976

19. SABBAGHA RE, HUGHEY M: Standardization of sonar cephalometry and gestational age. Obstet Gynecol 52:402, 1978

20. SABBAGHA RE, HUGHEY M, DEPP R: Growth adjusted sonographic age (GASA): a simplified method. Obstet Gynecol 51:383, 1978

21. SABBAGHA RE, TURNER JH, CHEZ RA: Sonar BPD growth standards in the rhesus monkey. Am J Obstet Gynecol 121:371, 1975

22. SABBAGHA RE, TURNER JH, ROCKETTE H, MAZER J, ORGILL J: Sonar BPD and fetal age: definition of the relationship. Obstet Gynecol 43:7, 1974

23. SPELLACY WN: Monitoring of high-risk pregnancies with human placental lactogen. In Spellacy WN (ed): Management of the High-Risk Pregnancy. Baltimore, University Park Press, 1976

24. TULCHINSKY D: The value of estrogens in the high-risk pregnancy. In Spellacy WN (ed): Management of the High-Risk Pregnancy. Baltimore, University Park Press, 1976

25. VARMA TR: Prediction of delivery date by ultrasound cephalometry. Br J Obstet Gynaecol 80:316, 1973

26. YERUSHALMY J: Relation of birth weight, gestational age, and the rate of intrauterine growth to perinatal mortality. Clin Obstet Gynecol 13:107, 1970

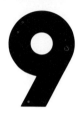

9

Assessment of fetal weight

RALPH K. TAMURA, RUDY E. SABBAGHA

Perinatal morbidity and mortality can be related to both fetal age and fetal weight. For example, Yerushalmy (56) reported an eightfold increase in the perinatal mortality of small-for-gestational-age (SGA) neonates as compared with normally grown fetuses, Figure 9–1. Usher and McLean (52) found a tenfold increase in perinatal mortality in infants whose birth weight fell below 2 SD of the mean for gestational age. As to perinatal morbidity Gruenwald (19), Naeye and Kelly (33), Scott and Usher (47), Neligan et al (34), and Fitzhardinge and Steven (13) have described the nature of both immediate and long-term physical and neurologic sequelae of the SGA or intrauterine growth-retarded (IUGR) infant.

Similarly, there are data that clearly show an increase in perinatal morbidity and mortality of the large-for-gestational-age (LGA) neonate. Chase (10) has shown that, when birth weight is 5001 g, perinatal mortality is increased approximately three times over that of infants weighing 4501 to 5000 g. Gellis and Hsia (16) and Freeman (14) have reported an increase in morbidity of LGA infants born to mothers with diabetes mellitus. Further, long-term neurologic disability in LGA infants is not uncommon (46). In one report Nelson et al (35) have also shown an increase in maternal morbidity in association with macrosomia.

It is generally accepted that a simple, accurate, and universally applicable method of assessing in utero fetal weight leads to an improved prospective management of high-risk pregnancies and a possible reduction in perinatal morbidity and mortality. To achieve this end, many workers have attempted birth weight predictions by both clinical and laboratory means. In one of the largest clinical series using examinations of the maternal abdomen Loeffler (29) found that approximately 80% of birth weight estimates were within ±454 g of the infant's actual birth weight, Table 9–1. Other workers (1, 23, 28, 36, 37, 39) have published similar results. Thus the clinical ability to determine fetal weight in utero entails a significant margin of error (4, 31).

Clearly, another, more precise method for fetal weight and growth assessment is needed. The simplicity, noninvasiveness, safety, and accuracy of diagnostic ultrasound make it, at present, the best available tool for obtaining certain fetal dimensions that correlate with fetal weight and growth—the subject of this chapter.

ULTRASONIC CEPHALOMETRY AS A TOOL FOR FETAL WEIGHT ESTIMATION

CEPHALOMETRY

Ultrasonic measurement of the fetal biparietal diameter (BPD) was first reported by Donald and Brown (12). Subsequently, a number of studies relating sonar cephalometry to birth weight (Table 9–2) showed that, for a specific BPD measurement, fetal weight can vary from a

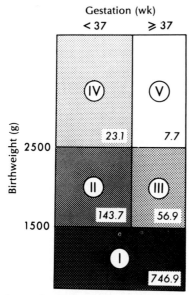

FIG. 9-1. Perinatal mortality/1000 live births for each of five fetal categories, grouped in accordance with birth weight and gestational age. (Yerushalmy J: Clin Obstet Gynecol 13:107, 1970)

discrepancy regarding the length of the BPD that corresponds to the attainment of this minimal fetal weight—the range extending from 8.7 to 9.4 cm (40), Table 9–2. Since the explanations for this observed variance in BPDs are now clear (Ch. 7) investigators are accepting the larger length of 9.4 cm.

SERIAL CEPHALOMETRY VERSUS FETAL WEIGHT

Sabbagha et al (42, 43) have shown that by employing serial cephalometry it is possible to place fetuses in large, average, or small cephalic categories (Ch. 10). A general relationship between BPD percentile rank and birth weight is apparent (Fig. 10–2). For example, 91% of fetuses with BPDs ≥ 75th percentile weigh more than 3000 g. By comparison, only 37% of fetuses with BPDs < 25th percentile weigh more than 3000 g; that is, the majority are small. Although in an individual pregnancy it is not possible to predict birth weight precisely on the basis of BPD rank, it is helpful to know antenatally each fetus's growth bracket and the weight probabilities expected for each BPD growth category (41).

CEPHALOMETRY IN CONJUNCTION WITH MEASUREMENTS OF OTHER FETAL PARAMETERS

The inadequacy of BPD measurements alone for exact fetal weight predictions prompted studies combining BPD with other fetal dimensions, Table 9–3. Thompson and Makowski (51), using A-mode scan for BPD measurements and

low of ± 638 g to a high of ± 980 g in 95% of the populations studied (40). In short, the BPD should not be used to predict exact fetal weight, because such predictions are as inaccurate as estimates made from clinical or radiologic examinations. A general assessment of fetal weight and growth can still, however, be made in relation to single or serial BPD values (3, 6, 45, 54).

SINGLE BPD VERSUS FETAL WEIGHT

Of significance is the observation that a specific BPD value can be used to indicate attainment of a minimal fetal weight of 2500 g with an accuracy of 97% to 100%. Unfortunately there is a

TABLE 9-1. BIRTH WEIGHT ESTIMATIONS ASSESSED BY EVALUATION OF UTERINE FUNDAL GROWTH, MATERNAL ABDOMINAL EXAMINATION, OR RADIOLOGIC METHOD

Author	Reference	No pts	Date	Mode of evaluations	Error margin of estimates
Poulos & Langstadt	(39)	45	1953	Uterine volume	± 250 g in 68%
Johnson & Tosach	(23)	200	1954	Fundal height	± 454 g in 80%
Loeffler	(29)	585	1967	Abdominal exam	± 454 g in 79.9%
Lind	(28)		1970	Clinical exam at 3300 g	± 454 g in 70%
Ong & Sen	(37)	506	1972	Clinical exam	± 454 g in 82.5%
Beazley & Kurjak	(1)		1973	Abdominal exam	± 500 g in 75%
Ogita et al	(36)	54	1977	Radiologic technique	Fetal weight of 2500 g attained with correlation coefficient of 0.86–0.91

TABLE 9-2. CORRELATION OF CEPHALOMETRIC VALUES (BPD) AND BIRTH WEIGHT

Author(s)	Reference	Date	Mode of Evaluation	Absolute mean error‡ (g) or 95% weight margin(±)*	BPD† and attainment of weight of 2500 g (% of cases)
Willocks et al	(55)	1964	A-scan	±900	9.0 (97.6)
Thompson et al	(50)	1965	A-scan	±960	9.0 (97)
Hellmann et al	(20)	1967	B-scan	392‡	
Kohorn	(25)	1967	A-scan	±980	8.5 (96)
Brown	(2)	1971	A-scan	±638	
Ianniruberto & Gibbons	(22)	1971	B-scan	368‡	8.7 (100)
Lee et al	(27)	1971	B-scan		8.7 (100)
Cohen	(11)	1972	B–A scan		8.7 (97)
Sabbagha & Turner	(44)	1972	B-scan	404‡	9.4 (97.5)
Stocker et al	(48)	1974	B real time	±652	
Campbell	(5)	1974	B–A scan	±840	

* Normal distribution being assumed.
† In all cases BPD ≥ the figure given.
‡ Absolute mean error.

TABLE 9-3. CORRELATION OF FETAL TRUNK DIMENSIONS AND BIRTH WEIGHT

Author	Reference	Date	No pts	Mode of evaluation	Error margin of estimates
Thompson et al	(50)	1965	50	A-scan for BPD, B-scan for cross-section of fetal thorax	±660 g (2 SD)
Garrett & Robinson	(15)	1971	11	A-scan for cross-sectional area of head and thorax	None given
Thompson & Makowski	(51)	1971	1079	BPD, chest A-P diameter	±580 g (2 SD)
Campbell	(4)	1974	82	B-scan for abdominal circumference*	±560 g (2 SD)
Campbell & Wilkin	(8)	1975	140	B-scan, abdominal circumference*	±160 g in 95% if predicted wt 1 kg ±290 g in 95% if predicted wt 2 kg ±450 g in 95% if predicted wt 3 kg ±590 g in 95% if predicted wt 4 kg
Higginbottom et al	(21)	1975	50	B-scan, abdominal circumference*	±145 g (2 SD)
Kurjak & Breyer	(26)	1976	830	B-scan, abdominal circumference*	±250 g (2 SD)
Lunt & Chard	(30)	1976	68	B-scan, STAM index†‡	±430 g (2 SD)
Morrison & McLennan	(32)	1976	20	A-scan, BPD, fetal volume*	±214 g (2 SD)
Picker & Saunders	(38)	1976	50	BPD, body height, thigh diameter & limb length§	±400 g (2 SD)
Campogrande et al	(9)	1977	50	A–B scan, BPD, abdominal circumference*	±200 g in 46%, ±300 g in 56% ±400 g in 82%
Gohari et al	(17)	1977	96	Total intrauterine volume	None given
Warsof et al	(53)	1977	32	Gray-scale, BPD, abdominal circumference & TIUV	±636 g (2 SD) in 3000-g infant
Kearney et al	(24)	1978	58	Abdominal circumference¶	±15% of total fetal weight in 82% of patients

* Scans obtained within 48 hours of delivery.
† STAM: Skull Thoracic Area Multiple.
‡ Scans obtained within 7 days of delivery.
§ Scans obtained 24 hours prior to delivery.
¶ Scans obtained within 2 to 5 days of delivery.

B-mode scan for cross-sectional views of the fetal thorax, estimated birth weight within ±660 g (2 SD). A possible reason for their margin of error may be the lack of a specific plane of the fetal thorax that can be consistently identified ultrasonically.

Lunt and Chard (30) measured the cross-sectional area of the fetal skull at the level of the BPD and the cross-sectional area of the fetal thorax at the level of the heart where there seemed to be maximal movement of one of the valves (probably either mitral or tricuspid). Their most significant parameter for birth weight prediction was the skull thoracic area multiple or STAM index. The range of error in 95% of the population was ±430g (2 SD). Campogrande et al (9) measured fetal BPD, transverse thoracic diameter, abdominal circumference (A-C) and abdominal area in 50 women at term 48 hours prior to delivery. With multiple regression analysis the error in prediction was ±400 g in 82% of the population. Warsof et al (53) obtained BPD, A-C, and total intrauterine volume (TIUV) data on 85 pregnancies; subsequently they used the BPD and A-C to estimate fetal weight by computer analysis in 32 patients prospectively and reported an error of ±636 g (2 SD) for fetuses with an average weight of 3000 g, Table 9–3. Interestingly in this study the A-C was shown to be superior to TIUV as an estimator of fetal weight.

In comparison to cephalometry alone the data derived by combining BPD with other fetal trunk measurements appear to be more accurate for prediction of fetal weight. However, this accuracy is still not superior to that of the A-C alone.

FETAL TRUNK DIMENSIONS FOR FETAL WEIGHT ESTIMATIONS

Campbell and Wilkin (8) obtained fetal abdominal measurements at the level of the umbilical vein. The latter was used as an ultrasonic marker (Fig. 9–2) because it could be readily localized by sonar. As a result, the reproducibility of fetal A-C measurements was improved. In addition the A-C is more likely to reflect the small size of the fetal liver known to occur in association with IUGR and to indicate the extent of accumulation of subcutaneous tissue overlying the abdominal area—also known to be diminished in association with IUGR.

In analyzing their results these authors found that when a second-degree polynomial regression formula was fitted to the data, the confidence limits for birth weight predictions de-

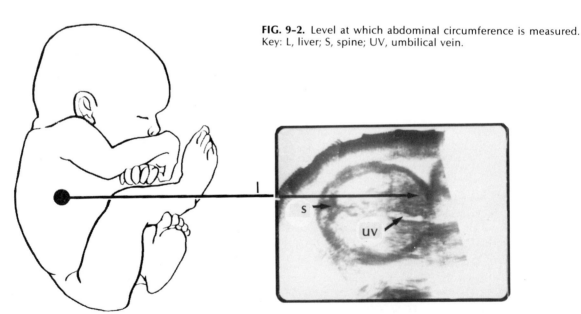

FIG. 9–2. Level at which abdominal circumference is measured. Key: L, liver; S, spine; UV, umbilical vein.

pended on the absolute size of the measurement, Table 9–3. At a predicted weight of 1 kg, 95% of birth weights fell within ± 160 g of the estimated value, while at 2, 3, and 4 kg, the corresponding values were ± 290 g, ± 450 g, and ± 590 g respectively. When this method was extrapolated to infants below the 5th percentile for weight between the 32nd and 38th weeks of gestation, the maximum yield in detecting the SGA fetus was achieved at 32 weeks. The successful diagnosis of babies born below the 5th percentile fell with increasing fetal maturity to 63% at 38 weeks. The false-positive diagnosis rate remained constant between 32–38 weeks at just over 1%.

Since IUGR may often begin after 32 weeks' gestation (19), fetuses who manifest growth retardation in the third trimester of pregnancy may be overlooked because the maximal detection period is at 32 weeks. Furthermore, even if fetal weight is predicted to fall within 1000 to 2000 g by their method, differentiation between a normal premature fetus (appropriate-for-gestational-age) and an SGA fetus is not possible unless gestational age is defined.

Other reports (21, 26) have claimed better fetal weight predictions from A-C measurements at the liver area as described by Campbell. These improvements are interesting to note but difficult to explain.

OTHER ULTRASONIC METHODS FOR FETAL WEIGHT AND GROWTH ASSESSMENT

HEAD TO ABDOMEN CIRCUMFERENCE RATIOS

Campbell (4) first reported the value of head-to-abdomen circumference ratios for the assessment of fetal growth and nutrition. In normal pregnancies, during and prior to the second trimester, this ratio was noted to be greater than 1. However, by 36 to 37 weeks' gestation, owing presumably to the accumulation of subcutaneous fat and soft tissue around the fetal abdomen, the abdominal circumference first equaled then surpassed the head circumference. In most cases

TABLE 9-4. MEAN HEAD-ABDOMEN (H-A) CIRCUMFERENCE RATIO VERSUS GESTATIONAL AGE (GA)

GA (weeks)	Mean H–A ratio	+2 SD
28	1.13	1.21
32	1.075	1.17
34	1.04	1.13
36	1.02	1.12
38	0.99	1.06
40	0.97	1.05

of asymmetric IUGR, however, the head-to-abdomen circumference ratio remained > 1.0. In a later study Campbell and Thoms (7) determined the mean head-to-abdomen circumference ratio and its 95% confidence limits in 568 normal pregnancies, Table 9–4. With these data, IUGR was predicted in 71% of fetuses, and all those detected were asymmetrically undergrown.

TOTAL INTRAUTERINE VOLUME (TIUV)

Gohari et al (17) proposed sonar measurement of TIUV for predicting fetal weight and IUGR (Ch. 2). This is an indirect method of estimating fetal weight because the fetus is not examined. Nonetheless, these authors correctly diagnosed SGA fetuses in 75% of patients, with a 15% false-positive rate. Later, Warsof et al (53) showed that determination of fetal weight by BPD and A-C was not improved by using TIUV determinations.

ASSESSMENT OF INDIVIDUAL FETAL GROWTH POTENTIAL

From the previous discussion it is apparent that, although fetal A-C is the best predictor of fetal weight, the biologic correlation is still less than ideal. For example, if fetal weight is estimated to be 3000 g (by an A-C value obtained at 38 weeks' gestation), the neonate may still be undergrown, and its birth weight could be as low as 2550 g (range in birth weight error in relation to A-C is +450 g). Further, the A-C value alone is meaningless unless gestational age is well defined by C-R-L (Ch. 6) or serial BPD (GASA) measurements of the fetus (Ch. 8).

We believe that A-C and TIUV determinations should not be used as estimators of mean birth weight, because the margin of error is wide; rather these measurements should be used during the third trimester of pregnancy, as additional parameters to assess the dynamics of growth in relation to each fetus's potential established by serial cephalometry and to delineate the population of fetuses at high risk for symmetric or asymmetric IUGR in relation to BPD size. Such fetuses should then be carefully monitored by bioelectric and biochemical means to determine the optimal time and mode of delivery of the affected fetus. Specifically fetuses at high risk for IUGR are identified by the following steps:

1. serial BPDs
2. A-C measurements at 34–36 weeks' gestation
3. TIUV determinations in fetuses likely to be undergrown by steps 1 and 2.

These three steps will be discussed further.

SERIAL BPDS

In a series of 463 high-risk pregnancies Sabbagha (41) defined the risk for IUGR by serial BPD measurements in four populations (Ch. 10):

1. In fetuses with BPDs consistently ≥ 75th percentile the risk for asymmetric IUGR is 3.5% (symmetric IUGR is virtually nonexistent in this group).
2. In fetuses with BPDs falling between the 25th–75th percentiles the risk for asymmetric IUGR is 10% (again symmetric IUGR is virtually nonexistent in this group).
3. In fetuses with BPDs <25th percentile the risk for symmetric or near symmetric IUGR is approximately 50%.
4. In fetuses who drop their BPD from an upper to a lower percentile rank the risk for IUGR (asymmetric or symmetric) is 20%.

Although the risk for IUGR is defined in all these groups, a method is still needed to help separate the normal from the affected fetus in an attempt to reduce the number of pregnancies that would require additional monitoring by bioelectric and biochemical means (Ch. 10 and 11).

A-C AND TIUV

Sonar measurement of A-C (see Addendum) between 34–36 weeks is useful in further separating the normal fetus from the one at high risk for IUGR. For example, a fetus with a BPD > 75th percentile, at 37 weeks' gestation but with an A-C value falling at the 10th percentile is at a much greater risk for asymmetric IUGR than another fetus in whom both BPD and A-C values are > 75th percentiles (exact risk still under study). When the A-C falls below the 25th percentile, TIUV may be used to further confirm IUGR.

We (49) have derived, prospectively, the A-C percentile measurements (percentiles 2.5–97.5) from the 18th to the 41st week of pregnancy, Table 9–5. Thus, by relating the three BPD growth patterns of fetuses (ie, large, average, or small) to a specific A-C percentile rank, nine fetal growth combinations are possible, Figure 9–3. Preliminary data indicate the following:

1. LGA fetuses are likely to fall in growth patterns 1 and 4.
2. Asymmetric IUGR fetuses are likely to fall in growth patterns 3 and 6; TIUV determinations (CH. 12) in these two growth patterns may lend further credence to the diagnosis.
3. Symmetrically undergrown fetuses are likely to fall in growth pattern 9. Again, if TIUV (Ch. 12) is low, the diagnosis is more likely to be accurate.
4. AGA fetuses are likely to fall in growth patterns 2, 5, 7, and 8.

SUMMARY

In summary the authors believe that estimates of mean fetal weight by A-C values should not be reported. Instead, a population of fetuses at high risk for IUGR or macrosomia may be identified as follows:

1. Gestational age should be assigned by C-R-L (Ch. 6) or GASA (Ch. 8).
2. If only C-R-L is used, a BPD should be obtained at 30–33 weeks' gestation to define the cephalic growth pattern of the fetus.
3. Sonar measurement of BPD and A-C should be obtained at 34–36 weeks' gestation to re-

TABLE 9-5. FETAL ABDOMINAL CIRCUMFERENCE MEASUREMENTS (CM)*

Weeks of gestation	PERCENTILE								
	2.5	5	10	25	50	75	80	95	97.5
18	9.8	10.3	10.9	11.9	13.1	14.2	14.5	15.9	16.4
19	11.1	11.6	12.3	13.3	14.4	15.6	15.9	17.2	17.8
20	12.1	12.6	13.3	14.3	15.4	16.6	16.9	18.2	18.8
21	13.7	14.2	14.8	15.9	17.0	18.1	18.4	19.8	20.3
22	14.7	15.2	15.8	16.9	18.0	19.1	19.4	20.8	21.3
23	16.0	16.5	17.1	18.2	19.3	20.4	20.7	22.1	22.6
24	17.2	17.7	18.3	19.4	20.5	21.6	21.9	23.3	23.8
25	18.0	18.5	19.1	20.2	21.3	22.4	22.7	24.1	24.6
26	18.8	19.3	19.9	21.0	22.1	23.2	23.5	24.9	25.4
27	20.4	20.9	21.5	22.6	23.7	24.8	25.1	26.5	27.0
28	22.0	22.5	23.1	24.2	25.3	26.4	26.7	28.1	28.6
29	23.6	24.1	24.7	25.8	26.9	28.0	28.3	29.7	30.2
30	24.1	24.6	25.2	26.3	27.4	28.5	28.8	30.2	30.7
31	24.7	25.2	25.8	26.9	28.0	29.1	29.4	30.8	31.3
32	25.4	25.9	26.5	27.6	28.7	29.8	30.1	31.5	32.0
33	25.7	26.2	26.8	27.9	29.0	30.1	30.4	31.8	32.3
34	26.8	27.3	27.9	29.0	30.1	31.2	31.5	32.9	33.4
35	28.9	29.4	30.0	31.1	32.2	33.3	33.6	35.0	35.5
36	30.0	30.5	31.1	32.2	33.3	34.4	34.7	36.1	36.6
37	31.1	31.6	32.2	33.3	34.4	35.5	35.8	37.2	37.7
38	32.4	32.9	33.5	34.6	35.7	36.8	37.1	38.5	39.0
39	32.6	33.1	33.7	34.8	35.9	37.0	37.3	38.7	39.2
40	32.8	33.3	33.9	35.0	36.1	37.2	37.5	38.9	39.4
41	33.8	34.3	34.9	36.0	37.1	38.2	38.5	39.9	40.4

* Circumference measurements are obtained from the outer aspect of the fetal abdomen at the area of the liver, which shows the ductus venosus. (Tamura RK, Sabbagha RE: Obstet Gynecol [in press])

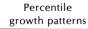

Percentile growth patterns

FIG. 9-3. Nine fetal growth patterns noted by using both biparietal diameter (BPD) and abdominal circumference (A-C) percentiles (P).

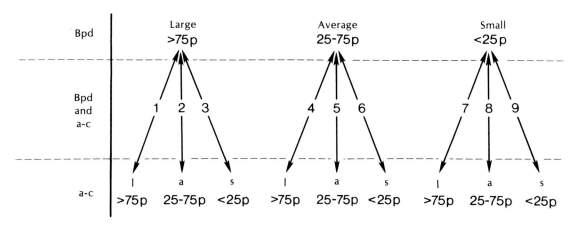

late actual growth to expected growth and to delineate fetuses at increased risk for IUGR or macrosomia, Figure 9–3.

4. TIUV determinations in fetuses at increased risk for IUGR (growth patterns 3, 6, 9, Fig. 9–3)

Once the obstetrician identifies a small population of fetuses at increased risk for asymmetric or symmetric IUGR, additional testing by bioelectric and biochemical methods becomes mandatory (Ch. 10 and 11). Such monitoring is cost effective because of the small number of fetuses involved (41). By managing high-risk pregnancies in this way, the optimal time for delivery of the affected fetus may be determined, and it is hoped that perinatal morbidity and mortality can be reduced.

ADDENDUM

The abdominal circumference (AC) is measured by using a digitizer (Fig. 9–4). The outer margin of the circumference is outlined by a colored felt-tip pen and the starting point is marked. The reading head of the digitizer (Fig. 9–4) is then used to measure the abdominal perimeter. Subsequently the actual distance of the 1-cm marker dots on the photograph are measured by the digitizer. Usually the distance between 5 or 10 markers is recorded; this measurement is used to delineate the extent to which the photograph is reduced.

The A-C measurement recorded by the digitizer is inversely proportional to the reduction in the size of the photograph. For example, if the A-C (recorded by the digitizer) measures 11 cm and the distance between the 10 markers is 0.3 cm (recorded by the digitizer), the actual A-C is $11 \times 1/0.3 = 36.6$ cm.

By using this methodology, the error in the A-C measurement is <2%.

REFERENCES

1. BEAZLEY JM, KURJAK A: Nursing Times, June 14, 1973, p 23
2. BROWN RE: Ultrasound fetal cephalometry. Proceedings of the First World Congress on Ultrasonic Diagnostics in Medicine, Vienna, 1969. Ultrasound Med Biol 3:193, 1971

FIG. 9-4. Shown below is a Model 237 Graphics Calculator. It functions as a digitizer and free-standing electronic planimeter with scale and multiplier. Each Graphics Calculator is available with magnifying or pointer-type cursor. Other types are also available.

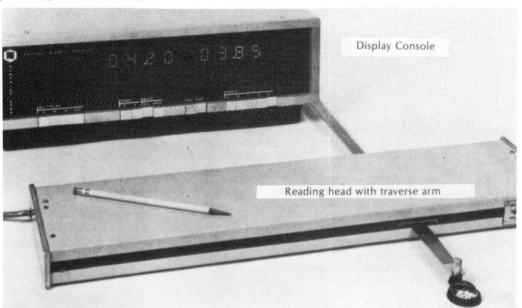

3. CAMPBELL S: An improved method of foetal cephalometry by ultrasound. Br J Obstet Gynaecol 75:518, 1968

4. CAMPBELL S: The assessment of fetal development by diagnostic ultrasound. Clin Perinatol 1:504, 1974

5. CAMPBELL S: The assessment of fetal development by diagnostic ultrasound. Clin Obstet Gynecol 1:41, 1974

6. CAMPBELL S, DEWHURST CJ: Diagnosis of the small-for-dates foetus by serial ultrasonic cephalometry. Lancet 2:1002, 1971

7. CAMPBELL S, THOMS A: Ultrasound measurement of the fetal head to abdomen circumference ratio in the assessment of growth retardation. Br J Obstet Gynaecol 84:165, 1977

8. CAMPBELL S, WILKIN D: Ultrasonic measurement of fetal abdominal circumference in estimation of fetal weight. Br J Obstet Gynaecol 82:689, 1975

9. CAMPOGRANDE M, TODROS, BRIZZOLARA M: Prediction of birth weight by ultrasound measurements of the fetus. Br J Obstet Gynaecol 84:175, 1977

10. CHASE HC: Perinatal mortality overview and current trends. Clin Perinatol 1:3, 1974

11. COHEN WN: The prenatal determination of fetal maturity by B-scan ultrasound—Comparison with a radiologic method. Radiology 103:171, 1972

12. DONALD I, BROWN TG: Demonstration of tissue interfaces within the body by ultrasonic echo-sounding. Br J Radiol 34:539, 1961

13. FITZHARDINGE PM, STEVEN EM: The small-for-dates infant. II. Neurological and intellectual sequelae. Pediatrics 50:50, 1972

14. FREEMAN RK: Obstetric management of the diabetic patient. Contrib Gynec Obstet 1:58, 1973

15. BARRETT WJ, ROBINSON DE: Assessment of fetal size and growth rate by ultrasonic echoscopy. Obstet Gynecol 38:525, 1971

16. GELLIS SS, HSIA DY: The infant of the diabetic mother. J Dis Child 97:1, 1959

17. GOHARI P, BERKOWITZ RL, HOBBINS JC: Prediction of intrauterine growth retardation by determination of total intrauterine volume. Am J Obstet Gynecol 127:255, 1977

18. GRUENWALD P: Chronic fetal distress and placental insufficiency. Biol Neonate 5:215, 1963

19. GRUENWALD P: Infants of low birth weight among 5,000 deliveries. Pediatrics 34:157, 1964

20. HELLMANN LM, KOBAYASHI M, FILLISTI L et al: Sources of error in sonographic fetal mensuration and estimation of growth. Am J Obstet Gynecol 99:662, 1967

21. HIGGINBOTTOM J, SLATER J, PORTER G, WHITFIELD CR: Estimation of fetal weight from ultrasonic measurement of trunk circumference. Br J Obstet Gynaecol 82:698, 1975

22. IANNIRUBERTO A, GIBBONS JM: Predicting fetal weight by ultrasonic B-scan cephalometry. An improved technique with disappointing results. Obstet Gynecol 37:684, 1971

23. JOHNSON RW, TOSACH CE: Estimation of fetal weight using longitudinal mensuration. Am J Obstet Gynecol 68:891, 1954

24. KEARNEY K, VIGNERSON N, FRISCHMAN P, JOHNSON JWC: Fetal weight estimation by ultrasonic measurement of abdominal circumference. Obstet Gynecol 51:156, 1978

25. KOHORN ES: An evaluation of ultrasonic fetal cephalometry. Am J Obstet Gynecol 97:553, 1967

26. KURJAK A, BREYER B: Estimation of fetal weight by ultrasonic abdominometry. Am J Obstet Gynecol 125:962, 1976

27. LEE BO, MAJOR FJ, WEINGOLD AB: Ultrasonic determination of fetal maturity at repeat cesarean section. Obstet Gynecol 38:294, 1971

28. LIND T: Estimation of fetal growth and development. Br J Hosp Med 3:501, 1970

29. LOEFFLER FE: Clinical weight prediction. Br J Obstet Gynaecol 74:675, 1967

30. LUNT RM, CHARD T: A new method for estimation of fetal weight in late pregnancy by ultrasonic scanning. Br J Obstet Gynaecol 83:1, 1976

31. MACLAURIN J: Methods of monitoring the fetus in pregnancy and labour. In Beard RW (ed): Proceedings of the Second Study of the Royal College of Obstetricians and Gynaecologists. Edinburgh, E. S. Livingstone, 1971, p 92

32. MORRISON J, MCLENNAN MJ: The theory, feasibility and accuracy of an ultrasonic method of estimating fetal weight. Br J Obstet Gynaecol 83:833, 1976

33. NAEYE RL, KELLY JA: Judgment of fetal age. III. The pathologist's evaluation. Pediatr Clin North Am 13:835, 1966

34. NELIGAN GS, ROBSON E, WATSON J: Hypoglycemia in the newborn: a sequelae of intrauterine malnutrition. Lancet 1:1282, 1963

35. NELSON JH, ROVNRE IW, BARTER RH: The large baby. South Med J 51:23, 1958

36. OGITA S, KAMEI T, SUGAWA T: Estimation of fetal weight by fetography. Am J Obstet Gynecol 127:37, 1977

37. ONG HC, SEN DK: Clinical estimation of fetal weight. Am J Obstet Gynecol 112:877, 1972

38. PICKER RH, SAUNDERS DM: A simple geometric method for determining fetal weight in utero with the compound gray scale ultrasonic scan. Am J Obstet Gynecol 124:493, 1976

39. POULOS PP, LANGSTADT JP: The volume of the uterus during labor and its correlation with birth. I. A method for the prediction of birth weight. Am J Obstet Gynecol 65:233, 1953

40. SABBAGHA RE: Biparietal diameter: an appraisal. Clin Obstet Gynecol 20:297, 1977

41. SABBAGHA RE: Intrauterine growth retardation: ante-

natal diagnosis by ultrasound. Obstet Gynecol 52:252, 1978

42. SABBAGHA RE, BARTON BA, BARTON FB, KINGAS E, ORGILL J, TURNER HJ: Sonar Biparietal diameter. II. Predictive of three fetal growth patterns leading to a closer assessment of gestational age and neonatal weight. Am J Obstet Gynecol 126:485, 1976

43. SABBAGHA RE, HUGHEY M, DEPP R: The assignment of growth adjusted sonographic age (GASA): a simplified method. Obstet Gynecol 51:383, 1978

44. SABBAGHA RE, TURNER HJ: Methodology of B-scan sonar cephalometry with electronic calipers and correlation with fetal birth weight. Obstet Gynecol 40:74, 1972

45. SABBAGHA RE, TURNER HJ, ROCKETTE H, MAZER J, ORGILL J: Sonar BPD and fetal age. Definition of the relationship. Obstet Gynecol 43:7, 1974

46. SACK RA: The large infant: a study of maternal, obstetric and newborn characteristics, including a long term pediatric followup. Am J Obstet Gynecol 104:195, 1969

47. SCOTT KE, USHER R: Fetal malnutrition: its incidence, causes and effects. Am J Obstet Gynecol 94:951, 1966

48. STOCKER J, MAWAD R, DELEON A, DESJARDINS P: Ultrasonic cephalometry—Its use in estimating fetal weight. Obstet Gynecol 45:275, 1974

49. TAMURA RK, SABBAGHA RE: Percentile ranks of sonar fetal abdominal circumference measurements (work in progress)

50. THOMPSON HE, HOLMES JH, GOTTESFELD KR, TAYLOR ES: Fetal development as determined by ultrasonic pulse echo techniques. Am J Obstet Gynecol 92:44, 1965

51. THOMPSON HE, MAKOWSKI EL: Estimation of birth weight and gestational age. Obstet Gynecol 37:44, 1971

52. USHER R, MCLEAN F: Normal fetal growth and the significance of fetal growth retardation. In Davis JA, Dobbing J (eds): Scientific Foundations of Paediatrics. London, Heinemann, 1974, p 69

53. WARSOF S, GOHARI P, BERKOWITZ RL, HOBBINS JC: The estimation of fetal weight by computer-assisted analysis. Am J Obstet Gynecol 128:881, 1977

54. WILLOCKS J, DONALD I, CAMPBELL S, DUNSMORE IR: Intrauterine growth assessed by ultrasonic foetal cephalometry. Br J Obstet Gynaecol 74:639, 1967

55. WILLOCKS J, DONALD I, DUGGAN TL et al: Fetal cephalometry by ultrasound. Br J Obstet Gynaecol 71:11, 1964

56. YERUSHALMY J: Relation of birth weight, gestational age and rate of intrauterine growth to perinatal mortality. Clin Obstet Gynecol 13:107, 1970

10

Intrauterine growth retardation

RUDY E. SABBAGHA

Antenatal diagnosis of intrauterine growth retardation (IUGR) by clinical means is possible in approximately one-third of such pregnancies (19). The reasons for this low yield are related to inaccurate assessment of gestational age and fetal weight by parameters such as menstrual dates and height of the uterine fundus (4, 5, 8, 12, 13).

In this chapter the rationale for serial ultrasonic study is presented, and the sequence of events leading to antenatal recognition of the population of fetuses at high risk for both symmetric and asymmetric IUGR is outlined. Then, the management of these fetuses is discussed and emphasis is placed on use of multiple diagnostic modalities for determining the affected fetus (6) and the optimal time for delivery, prior to the onset of severe asphyxia or intrauterine fetal death (IUFD) (19).

CONVENTIONAL DEFINITION OF INTRAUTERINE GROWTH RETARDATION (IUGR)

The diagnosis of IUGR is generally made at birth by pediatricians who relate the infant's weight to its gestational age (3). The length of pregnancy at birth is estimated retrospectively by analysis of one or more parameters, including menstrual dates, sonar fetal crown–rump length

(CRL) (Ch. 6), biparietal diameter (BPD) measurements (Ch. 7), and a pediatric examination (9, 22). Each of these parameters has its own biologic and measurement errors (Ch. 6, 7 and 8). As a result, on certain occasions, dating of pregnancies is difficult and inaccurate. Nonetheless, infants are classified as IUGR when birth weight falls at or below the 10th percentile for a given gestational age. Additionally, the diagnosis of IUGR is made if tissue wasting or fetal malnutrition (FM) is evident on physical examination of the neonate. A malnourished fetus is one whose birth weight may be above the 10th percentile for its age, and yet it clearly shows evidence of loss of subcutaneous tissue and a decrease in the muscle mass over its extremities. By either of these definitions IUGR can occur not only at term but also in preterm and post-term pregnancies.

OTHER DEFINITIONS OF IUGR

As we continue to learn about the entity of growth retardation it becomes apparent that the conventional definition of IUGR is simplistic and other diagnostic indices should be considered, namely: 1) length of the fetal body (2); 2) evaluation of the chronicity of the disorder and the pathophysiology of organ growth at the cellular level (24); 3) a comparison between actual

103

weight attained at birth versus weight expected at birth (11, 21); 4) a comparison between actual cephalic size attained at birth and cephalic growth potential (16); and 5) differentiation between symmetric and varying degrees of asymmetric IUGR (15). These parameters will be discussed separately.

LENGTH OF FETAL BODY

Although there are some controversies about the accuracy of body length measurements in neonates, it is generally agreed that reduction in both body length and birth weight is a manifestation of a moderately severe form of IUGR (2).

CHRONICITY OF IUGR

A number of factors may adversely influence fetal growth:

> Genetic
> Chromosomal aberrations
> Antigenic relationships
> Chronic fetal infections
> Maternal ingestion of cytotoxic agents
> Maternal smoking
> Maternal diseases
> (cardiovascular, metabolic)
> Poor maternal nutrition
> High altitude
> Multiple pregnancy
> Irradiation

If these factors operate from early pregnancy, organ growth is retarded secondary to a decrease in both cell number and cell size (24, 25). Winick (24) has shown that organ growth takes place first by cell hyperplasia or cell division. This is followed by cell hypertrophy or increase in cell size. Finally, hyperplasia ceases and growth continues by cellular hypertrophy alone.

Because hyperplasia normally ceases at some time during fetal life, the early onset of growth retardation is likely to affect cell division adversely and lead to an irreversible diminution in organ size and possibly function (24). By contrast, delayed onset of growth retardation (after organ cell number is completed) is known to decrease only cell size—an insult that is reversible (25). Thus, chronic IUGR results in a pathophysiologic environment, altering the nature of organ growth at the cellular level and possibly producing long-term central nervous system (CNS) deficits (10).

ACTUAL VERSUS POTENTIAL BIRTH WEIGHT

Turner (21) has shown that, whereas the majority of infants with congenital rubella are clearly growth retarded in comparison to their unaffected siblings, less than half of these neonates are considered undergrown in relation to the whole population. Thus, it can be assumed that birth weight in the unaffected siblings represents the normal growth potential unattainable by those who contracted the viral infection in utero. On the basis of these findings it may be helpful for physicians to estimate the potential birth weight of a given fetus in relation to that of its siblings.

ACTUAL VERSUS POTENTIAL BPD GROWTH

Evaluation of serial cephalic ultrasonic measurements in the rhesus monkey (17) and in the human fetus (16) has shown that, as early as 20 weeks' gestation, the biparietal diameter (BPD) (in at least 90% of the population studied) falls into one of three growth divisions, namely: 1) large, with BPDs $\geq$75th percentile; 2) average, with BPDs ranging between the 25th to the 75th percentiles; and 3) small, with BPDs $\leq$25th percentile, Figure 10–1. This means that BPD growth normally remains within one of three defined growth brackets, Figure 10–1.

In the antenatal assessment of a given fetus, if the BPD growth bracket is known, for instance by 30 weeks' gestation, growth potential can be defined for the remainder of pregnancy. In this way BPD growth attained can be compared to that expected, rather than to a mean value derived from a heterogeneous population of fetuses (16).

For example, a single BPD value of 9.0 cm is considered normal if the length of pregnancy is 36 weeks because it represents the 50th growth percentile, Table 10–1. In addition, the risk for IUGR in such a fetus is only 10% (15), Figure 10–2. If, however, the growth potential of the same fetus (defined by early cephalic readings) indicates that the BPD measurement at 36 weeks' gestation should be 9.4 cm rather than 9.0 cm (ie, at the 80th percentile rather than at the 50th percentile), the risk for IUGR is now doubled to 20%, Figure 10–3.

This concept of comparing actual to potential cephalic growth (by using serial cephalometry) is similar to that proposed by Turner (21), who compared the birth weight of infants affected by congenital rubella to the birth weight attained by their normal siblings (discussed previously). However, the assessment of fetal status by means of defining the cephalic growth potential is more useful because it represents an antenatal prospective method of fetal evaluation that may

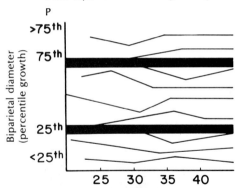

FIG. 10-1. Growth of the biparietal diameter (BPD) between 20-40 weeks' gestation falls in one of three growth patterns: 1) BPDs ≥ 75th percentile; 2) BPDs ranging between the 25th-75th percentiles; and 3) BPDs ≤ 25th percentile.

TABLE 10-1. BPD PERCENTILE RANGES AND MEASUREMENTS FOR BOTH BLACK AND WHITE FETUSES

Fetal age (wk)	BPD percentile values from 16–40 weeks							
	BPD percentiles							
	5	10	25	50	75	80	95	N
16	3.1	3.2	3.4	3.7	4.0	4.1	4.5	12
17	3.4	3.5	3.7	4.0	4.3	4.4	4.7	15
18	3.7	3.8	4.0	4.3	4.5	4.6	4.9	22
19	3.9	4.2	4.3	4.5	4.8	4.9	5.1	33
20	4.2	4.5	4.6	4.7	5.0	5.1	5.3	39
21	4.5	4.8	4.9	5.0	5.3	5.4	5.5	40
22	4.9	5.0	5.2	5.3	5.6	5.7	5.8	48
23	5.2	5.3	5.5	5.6	5.9	6.0	6.2	57
24	5.5	5.6	5.8	5.9	6.2	6.3	6.6	50
25	5.8	5.9	6.0	6.2	6.5	6.6	7.0	47
26	6.1	6.2	6.3	6.6	6.8	6.9	7.3	43
27	6.4	6.5	6.7	6.9	7.1	7.2	7.6	51
28	6.6	6.7	7.0	7.2	7.4	7.5	7.9	51
29	6.8	6.9	7.3	7.5	7.8	7.9	8.3	53
30	7.1	7.2	7.6	7.8	8.0	8.2	8.6	50
31	7.3	7.4	7.8	8.0	8.2	8.4	8.8	48
32	7.5	7.6	8.0	8.3	8.4	8.6	9.0	47
33	7.7	7.8	8.3	8.5	8.6	8.8	9.1	50
34	7.9	8.0	8.5	8.7	8.9	9.1	9.3	50
35	8.2	8.3	8.7	8.8	9.1	9.3	9.6	49
36	8.3	8.5	8.9	9.0	9.3	9.4	9.7	48
37	8.4	8.8	9.0	9.2	9.4	9.5	9.8	43
38	8.5	8.9	9.1	9.3	9.5	9.6	9.9	42
39	8.7	9.0	9.2	9.4	9.6	9.7	10.0	29
40	8.9	9.3	9.4	9.5	9.7	9.8	10.1	15

(Sabbagha RE, Barton BA, Barton FB et al: Am J Obstet Gynecol 126:485, 1976)

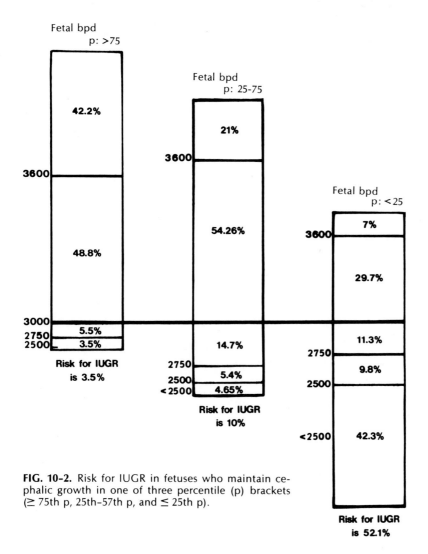

FIG. 10-2. Risk for IUGR in fetuses who maintain cephalic growth in one of three percentile (p) brackets (≥ 75th p, 25th–57th p, and ≤ 25th p).

FIG. 10-3. The risk for IUGR in fetuses who show a drop in the biparietal diameter from an upper to a lower percentile rank is 20%. (Sabbagha RE: Obstet Gynecol [in press])

Fetal biparietal diameter growth patterns

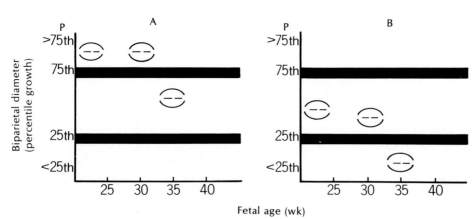

influence not only the management but also the outcome of pregnancy.

SYMMETRIC VERSUS ASYMMETRIC GROWTH RETARDATION

It is well established in the literature that IUGR in neonates can be classified into two groups. In the first group there is symmetric reduction in cephalic size and body weight to or below the 10th percentile; in this type of growth retardation the adverse influence on growth is prolonged, resulting in reduction of both cell number and cell size of all organs—an abnormality that may lead to CNS deficits (10, 24).

In the second group there is asymmetric IUGR, whereby cephalic size is relatively spared in comparison to body weight. However, the extent to which head size is affected has not received the attention it deserves and will be clarified. In asymmetric IUGR, whereas birth weight is reduced to the 10th percentile, cephalic size may vary between the 95th and the 15th percentiles, depending on the severity of IUGR.

Thus, asymmetric IUGR fetuses with BPDs falling close to the 10th percentile should be compared to symmetrically undergrown fetuses, because in both groups the "insult" is prolonged and long-term CNS deficits are more likely to occur. By contrast, asymmetric IUGR infants in whom BPD remains at the 50th or 90th percentiles are not subjected to prolonged growth retardation, and cell size rather than cell number is diminished—an abnormality that is more readily remediable by institution of proper nutrition postnatally (24).

The distinction between symmetric and various degrees of asymmetric growth retardation is possible only when serial BPD measurements are performed. First, fetuses are assigned a gestational age (by CRL or GASA or both). Second, they are placed in a BPD growth bracket by 31–33 weeks' gestation (Ch. 7 and 9). Finally, a third sonar examination is used to clarify the dynamics of growth. As an illustration, consider two IUGR fetuses, A and B. Let us assume that, in both fetuses, birth weight is 2400 g at 40 weeks' gestation and BPD obtained 10 days prior to delivery fell at the 20th percentile rank. The physician who is equipped with knowledge

of these two parameters can only make a diagnosis of asymmetric IUGR in both fetuses.

If, however, the results of serial BPD measurements are available, an appreciation of the dynamics of growth becomes possible and the degree of asymmetric IUGR in each fetus can then be defined. For example, if the BPD growth pattern in fetus A had continually fallen to the 20th percentile level, IUGR is considered to be chronic. By contrast, if the BPD growth in fetus B had fallen from the 70th to the 20th percentile in the last few weeks of pregnancy, the "insult" is considered to be of recent onset, and cell size rather than cell number is reduced. As a result the likelihood of fetus B developing long-term CNS complications is minimal, unless the perinatal period is associated with severe asphyxia.

DIAGNOSIS OF IUGR

A number of studies have appeared in the literature regarding the usefulness of serial cephalometry in the antenatal diagnosis of IUGR (1, 8, 14, 23). In these studies the investigators report varying degrees of success in the antenatal diagnosis of IUGR and different rates of false-positive and false-negative results, Table 10–2. The reasons for the discrepancy in these results may be related to the following (15): 1) nonuniformity in the method of obtaining sonar BPDs; 2) insufficient BPD data acquired prior to 26 weeks' gestation (during the interval that best correlates with fetal age); 3) evaluation of biweekly BPD growth increments in relation to a mean value derived from a heterogeneous population of fetuses rather than to the growth potential of each fetus; and 4) similarity in the mean BPD growth rate between IUGR and small but normal fetuses. Because of these discrepancies it appears that in a given pregnancy cephalometry should not be used to diagnose IUGR definitively; rather, it should be employed to identify fetuses at high risk for IUGR—with the understanding that a certain proportion of such fetuses may be normal. The final distinction between normal and affected fetuses is best arrived at by use of multiple diagnostic modalities, including the following:

TABLE 10-2. DIAGNOSIS OF INTRAUTERINE GROWTH RETARDATION (IUGR) BY SERIAL CEPHALOMETRY—FIVE STUDIES

	No of IUGR infants*	Correct IUGR Diagnosis by BPD	Percent false positive	Percent false negative
Dewhurst et al (8)	146	71%	28%	17%
Whetham et al (23)	23	70%	—	30%
Queenan et al (14)	16	50%	50%	9%
Arias (1)	12	43%	57%	—
Crane et al (7)	9	100%	36%	—

BPD, Biparietal diameter.
* Below the 10th percentile of birthweight (Sabbagha RE: Obstet Gynecol, 52:252, 1978)

1) measurement of fetal abdominal circumference and total intrauterine volume; 2) bioelectric methods of assessing fetal well-being—nonstress tests and oxytocin challenge tests (OCT) (6)—and biochemical tests reflecting fetoplacental or placental function, namely, maternal levels of estriol (20) and human placental lactogen (HPL) (18), respectively.

SERIAL CEPHALOMETRY VERSUS RISK FOR IUGR

The author used serial cephalometry to evaluate a large series of high-risk pregnancies with the intent of defining the risk for IUGR in fetuses with different BPD growth patterns (15). In this study, gestational age was defined by the method of GASA, Chapter 8, and birth weight analyzed in relation to two fetal BPD parameters. In one, cephalic size fell consistently in one of three growth BPD percentile brackets—large, average, or small. In the other, BPDs dropped from an upper to a lower percentile rank. The incidence of IUGR in fetuses with BPDs falling chronically below the 25th percentile as well as in those with BPDs dropping to lower percentile ranks is 50% and 20%, respectively (15), Figures 10–2 and 10–3. In these fetuses IUGR is either symmetric or close to being symmetric because the reduction in cephalic size is either at or close to the 10th percentile for age. In both groups, fetuses at high risk for IUGR are readily identified by serial cephalometry, and because their number is small (approximately 20% of a high-risk population), it is cost-effective for the physician to employ additional bioelectric and bio-chemical methods to determine the affected fetus and the most appropriate time for delivery.

By contrast, the incidence of IUGR in fetuses with BPDs falling either consistently above the 75th percentile or between the 25th and 75th percentiles is 3.5% and 10%, respectively (15), Figure 10–2. These IUGR fetuses are asymmetrically undergrown because cephalic size is quite spared while birth weight is at or below the 10th percentile. Obviously, these fetuses cannot be detected by serial cephalometry. Further, because of the very large number of normal fetuses with similar BPD growth patterns, it is neither feasible nor cost-effective for physicians to employ a battery of antenatal tests for detection of the affected fetus.

HOW TO IDENTIFY ASYMMETRIC IUGR FETUSES

Since, as previously mentioned in Chapter 8, a third ultrasound examination is recommended near term to compare BPD growth attained versus BPD growth expected, the author suggests that the third ultrasound examination include measurements such as circumference of fetal abdomen at the liver area. This additional ultrasonic fetal dimension is useful for estimating fetal weight and distinguishing normal from asymmetrically undergrown fetuses, Chapter 9.

ANTENATAL MANAGEMENT OF IUGR

As already shown, the physician who knows how to use diagnostic ultrasound antenatally can define a population of fetuses at high risk for

TABLE 10-3. OXYTOCIN CHALLENGE TEST IN IUGR

	OCT positive No. (%)	OCT not positive No. (%)
Perinatal Mortality	5/27 (18)	*1/67 (1) p 0.05
Low Apgar	8/24 (33)	14/68 (20) NS
Fetal distress	6/8 (75)	14/58 (24) p 0.01
Abnormal E_3	21/24 (87.5)	40/63 (63) p 0.01

*Corrected (Cetrulo C, Freeman R: Clin Obstet Gynecol 20:4, 979, 1977)

symmetric or asymmetric IUGR. Once this is accomplished, it becomes feasible, cost-effective, and mandatory to monitor all this high-risk group by bioelectric and biophysical means to detect the affected fetus and determine the most appropriate time for delivery, prior to the onset of severe asphyxia or intrauterine fetal death.

Cetrulo and Freeman (6) studied a large group of fetuses at risk for IUGR and compared the results of bioelectric and biochemical tests, Table 10-3. They outlined a schema suggesting intervention if both OCT and estriol levels are abnormal regardless of pulmonary maturity (see Ch. 11).

Most obstetricians agree with this mode of management. However, the question of when to deliver an IUGR fetus who has attained pulmonary maturity but in whom OCT and serial estriol levels are normal has not been scientifically answered yet. Some physicians feel that, under these circumstances, delivery should be effected by 37–38 weeks' gestation in the hope of preventing long-term CNS deficits (19). Others are not yet convinced of the benefits of such early delivery (6), and only further research can help solve this dilemma.

REFERENCES

1. ARIAS F: The diagnosis and management of intrauterine growth retardation. Obstet Gynecol 49:293, 1977

2. BARD H: Intrauterine growth retardation. Clin Obstet Gynecol 13:3, 511, 1970

3. BATTAGLIA FC, LUBCHENCO LO: A practical classification of newborn infants by weight and gestational age. J Pediatr 71:159, 1967

4. BEAZLEY JM, UNDERHILL RA: Fallacy of the fundal height. Br Med J 4:404, 1970

5. CAMPBELL S: The assessment of fetal development by diagnostic ultrasound. Clin Perinatol 1:507, 1974

6. CETRULO C, FREEMAN R: Bioelectric evaluation in intrauterine growth retardation. Clin Obstet Gynecol 20:4, 979, 1977

7. CRANE JP, KOPTA MM, WELT SI, SAUVAGE JP: Abnormal fetal growth patterns: ultrasonic diagnosis and management. Obstet Gynecol 50:205, 1977

8. DEWHURST CJ, BEAZLEY JM, CAMPBELL S: Assessment of fetal maturity and dysmaturity. Am J Obstet Gynecol 113:141, 1972

9. FINNSTROM O: Studies on maturity in newborn infants. II. External characteristics. Acta Paediat Scand 61:24, 1972

10. FITZHARDINGE PM, STEVEN EM: The small-for-date infant. II. Neurological and intellectual sequelae. Pediatrics 50:50, 1972

11. JONES MD, BATTAGLIA FC: Intrauterine growth retardation. Am J Obstet Gynecol 127:540, 1977

12. LIND T: The estimation of fetal growth and development. Br J Hosp Med 3:501, 1970

13. ONG HC, SEN DK: Clinical estimation of fetal weight. Am J Obstet Gynecol 112:877, 1972

14. QUEENAN JT, KUBARYCH SF, COOK LN, ANDERSON GD, GRIFFIN LP: Diagnostic ultrasound for detection of intrauterine growth retardation. Am J Obstet Gynecol 124:865, 1976

15. SABBAGHA RE: Intrauterine growth retardation: antenatal diagnosis by ultrasound. Obstet Gynecol 52:252, 1978

16. SABBAGHA RE, BARTON BA, BARTON FB, KINGAS E, ORGILL J, TURNER JH: Sonar biparietal diameter. II. Predictive of three fetal growth patterns leading to a closer assessment of gestational age and neonatal weight. Am J Obstet Gynecol 126:485, 1976

17. SABBAGHA RE, TURNER JH, CHEZ RA: Sonar biparietal diameter growth standards in the rhesus monkey. Am J Obstet Gynecol 121:371, 1975

18. SPELLACY WN: Monitoring of high-risk pregnancies with human placental lactogen. In Spellacy WN (ed): Management of the High-Risk Pregnancy. Baltimore, University Park Press, 1976

19. TEJANI N, MANN LI, WEISS RR: Antenatal diagnosis and management of the small-for-gestational-age fetus. Obstet Gynecol 47:31, 1976

20. TULCHINSKY D: The value of estrogens in the high-risk pregnancy. In Spellacy WN (ed): Management of the High-Risk Pregnancy. Baltimore, University Park Press, 1976

21. TURNER G: Recognition of intrauterine growth retardation by considering comparative birth weights.
Lancet 2:1123, 1971

22. USHER R, MCCLEAN F, SCOTT KE: Judgment of fetal
age. II. Clinical significance of gestational age and an
objective method for its assessment. Pediatr Clin
North Am 13:835, 1966

23. WHETHAM JCG, MUGGAH H, DAVIDSON S: Assessment
of intrauterine growth retardation by diagnostic ultrasound. Am J Obstet Gynecol 125:577, 1976

24. WINICK M: Fetal malnutrition. Clin Obstet Gynecol
13:3, 527, 1970

25. WINICK M, BRASEL JA, VELASCO EG: Effects of prenatal nutrition upon pregnancy risk. Clin Obstet Gynecol 16:1, 185, 1973

11

Dynamics of fetal growth

RICHARD DEPP

Appropriate action in the management of a high-risk pregnancy (Figure 11–1) requires proper interpretation not only of maternal and fetal risk factors but also of gestational age. Consideration of gestational age assumes secondary importance in only a few instances when there is severe maternal or fetal deterioration. In most cases, however, the length of pregnancy and, indirectly, organ maturity, are the major considerations. Certainly, Yerushalmy has demonstrated that both gestational age and birth weight correlate with perinatal mortality (32). In common high-risk situations such as maternal diabetes, preeclampsia, intrauterine growth retardation, premature labor, or premature rupture of membranes, management decisions may hinge on a gestational age assignment where a difference of 1 to 2 weeks may be crucial.

Only recently has the clinician begun to question the validity of previous clinical practices. Goldenberg and Nelson have indicated that 15% of all cases of respiratory distress syndrome (RDS) are the result of unwarranted physician intervention, largely a function of imprecise establishment of gestational age (11); many are the result of elective inductions or repeat cesarean section (C/S). Farrell and Wood estimate that 12,000 babies die yearly from RDS (7). Thus the possibility of eliminating 1800 (15% of 12,000) RDS deaths per year and reducing the morbidity inevitably associated with prematurity makes antenatal testing a cost-effective consideration.

At the other extreme many pregnancies are incorrectly assumed to be prolonged and are labeled "postdate" or "prolonged" because of inaccurate menstrual dates (4). Thus definition of gestational age with certainty enables the physician to limit management efforts to a smaller number of truly prolonged pregnancies and distinguish between benign prolonged pregnancy (greater than 42 weeks) and true postmaturity (growth retardation in a prolonged pregnancy). Incorrect assignment of gestational age greater than 42 weeks leads not only to unnecessary patient anxiety but also to unwarranted costs attributed to antenatal fetal heart rate (FHR) testing, estriol determinations, prolonged inductions, and cesarean sections for failure to progress.

Hertz et al have recently completed a critical evaluation of traditional tools to establish gestational age that include onset of fetal movement (FM), first detection of audible FHR and last menstrual period (LMP). They found that, to be only 90% sure (10% unsure) that a patient is ⪖38 weeks, a reliable LMP must have been 42 weeks prior to birth, first fetal heart tones heard for 21 weeks, and FM felt for 25 weeks. Further, if the LMP were unreliable, it must be at least 45 weeks prior to birth (14). Obviously, reliance solely on clinical data, particularly those gained after the fact, has inherent risks. Additional data concerning the limitation of the LMP are provided by Campbell, who noted that approximately 40% of patients have suspect dates (2).

111

Dewhurst and associates reported a 22% incidence (6). Sabbagha, in a prospective study, found that 28% of patients had uncertain dates; an additional 15% who reported the LMP with certainty were later determined to be in error by 3–4 weeks as evaluated by pediatric exam (28). It is thus clear that more precise patient data must be available if correct decisions are to be made.

The author does not propose that past practices be discarded in favor of biophysical and biochemical testing. In fact the reverse is true; the physician should approach each pregnancy as one with the potential to develop high-risk characteristics and gather gestational-age-related data (history, record of onset of FM, date heart tones first detected, method of detection) accurately in prospect rather than near term in retrospect when elicited dates are very suspect.

FETAL CEPHALOMETRY: AN OVERVIEW

Sonographic cephalometry, when properly applied, is useful in the prediction of gestational age (1, 3, 29–31). When additional information regarding functional pulmonary maturity is necessary, the determination of the lecithin-sphingomyelin (L/S) ratio of amniotic fluid is necessary.

Although ultrasound is useful in the prediction of gestational age, there are definite limitations in its use because the biologic variation in the biparietal diameter increases in range with gestation. As a result the predictive value of ultrasound in the third trimester is limited (Ch. 8). Unfortunately, awareness of this phenomenon is not widespread.

Table 11-1 summarizes pertinent literature that illustrates the predictive limitations of single ultrasound determinations, according to the trimester obtained, versus paired ultrasound determinations (GASA) obtained at 20–24 weeks and 30–33 weeks.

The significant increase in predictive accuracy provided by GASA offers an added dimension in obstetric care, namely, the ability to assess fetal head growth by percentiles for weeks' gestation (Ch. 8). In general, head growth maintains a predicted percentile pattern (rank) established by the second scan at 30–33 weeks. If, however, the intrauterine milieu is significantly altered by a condition such as preeclampsia, the associated decrease in uterine blood flow may modify fetal nutrition to such an extent that ce-

FIG. 11-1. Overall flow diagram of high-risk pregnancy evaluation and management. **Arrow** width reflects relative frequency of pathways: intervention for maternal indications; no evidence of maternal or fetal deterioration; intervention for fetal indication.

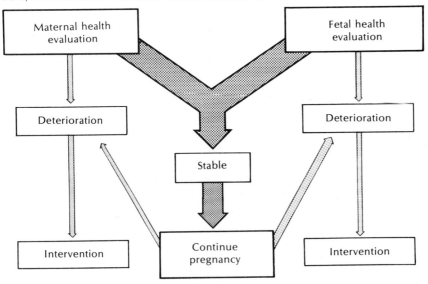

TABLE 11-1. PREDICTION OF GESTATIONAL AGE BY ULTRASONIC DETERMINATION OF CROWN-RUMP LENGTH AND BIPARIETAL DIAMETER

Author	Interval	Predictive range	Confidence limits
Campbell (1)	2nd trimester	±9 days	84%
Varma (31)	2nd trimester	±9 days	91%
Sabbagha et al (30)	20–26 weeks	±11 days	90%
	27–28 weeks	±14 days	90%
	≥ 29 weeks	±21 days	90%
Sabbagha et al (29)	GASA*	±1–3 days	95%
Robinson and Fleming (26)	Crown–rump		
	7–14 weeks	±1–4 days	95%

* Paired scans: First at 20–26 weeks; second at 30–33 weeks.

phalic growth may deviate below its predicted course in the latter part of the third trimester. In contrast, the fetus of the gestational diabetic may deviate above the predicted course, usually after 32 weeks' gestation, as a result of provision of excess nutrients.

CEPHALOMETRY: PATIENT APPLICATION

Unfortunately, present practice habits do not allow the physician to employ the GASA method. Instead, the first ultrasound determination may not be ordered until a high-risk situation is identified late in the third trimester. To use GASA to full advantage, ultrasound should be ordered routinely at 20–26 weeks in high-risk pregnancies, especially where there is increased risk of inaccurate menstrual data (Table 11–2); it will then be possible to obtain a growth-adjusted sonographic age. Patients scanned at 20–26 weeks may be divided into four groups (Table 11–3), depending on the correlation of sonographic and menstrual age and the presence of high-risk characteristics that imply increased risk of deviant fetal cephalic growth. In this way some patients will not require a second scan to determine GASA (Table 11–3—Group 1). Similarly pregnancies requiring both GASA and additional serial third-trimester scans (Table 11–3—Group 4) can be better evaluated. Such considerations are important to avoid overwhelming the sonography service with unnecessary scans while at the same time ensuring time for urgent scans (amniocentesis, placenta previa) and serial third-trimester scans.

The following is an analysis of the four groups of patients listed in Table 11–3:

Group 1: a group of patients, predominantly low risk (Table 11–2), who have increased likelihood of menstrual data inaccuracy (Table 11–2A) or are candidates for elective pregnancy termination (Table 11–2B). The single-scan gestational age (SSGA) at 20–26 weeks agrees (confirms ±8–11 days) with menstrual age (MA). The MA should be accepted; a second scan to establish GASA, or additional third-trimester scans, are not indicated unless the previously low-risk patient develops third-trimester complications known to be associated with reduced uteroplacental blood flow and abnormal fetal growth (Group 3 in this list), such as preeclampsia.

Group 2: a group like Group 1, but with menstrual-age-versus-SSGA discrepancy greater than 8–11 days (95% confidence limits of single scan at 20–26 weeks); a repeat scan should be performed at 30–33 weeks to define gestational

TABLE 11-2. INDICATIONS FOR ROUTINE EARLY CEPHALOMETRY*

A. Gestational age confirmation
  1. Irregular menses
  2. Recent discontinuation oral contraceptives
  3. Discrepancy between fundal height and LMP†
  4. Maternal age >35
  5. Obesity
B. Consideration of elective intervention
  1. Prior cesarean section
  2. Candidate for induction
C. GASA plus serial scan candidate
  1. High risk for uteroplacental insufficiency

* Indications for subsequent scan at 30–33 weeks plus additional biweekly scans are included in Table 11–3. All patients at risk for uteroplacental insufficiency (Table 11–4 B and 11–5) should have GASA plus serial scans.
† LMP = last menstrual period.

TABLE 11-3. CEPHALOMETRY FOLLOWUP SCHEME AFTER INITIAL SCAN AT 20-26 WEEKS

	MA SSGA discrepancy	High risk	GASA indicated	Serial scans‡
Group 1	<8–11 days	No	No	No
Group 2	>8–11 days	No	Yes	No
Group 3	<8–11 days	Yes*	Yes	No
Group 4	—	Yes†	Yes	Yes

* See Table 11–4a.

† See Table 11–5.

‡ Serial scans: biparietal diameter measurements after assignment of GASA at 30–33 weeks. Serial abdominal circumference determinations provide additional information.

MA = menstrual age.

SSGA = single-scan gestational age.

age precisely ±1–3 days; no serial scans are indicated after the establishment of GASA unless a high-risk complication develops.

Group 3: a group of patients, previously included in Group 1, who develop third-trimester high-risk characteristics (Table 11–4A) where gestational age is a critical factor in the clinical plan of management; the second scan at 30–33 weeks is indicated to define more precisely (±1–3 days) gestational age by GASA.

Group 4: a group in which gestational age is clinically significant but one in which the major concern is the risk of abnormal fetal growth (Table 11–5A). Establishment of GASA is essential; subsequent serial scans at 10- to 14-day intervals are then used to evaluate fetal cephalic growth.

Even by use of this scheme the indication for a scan at 20–26 weeks will not be apparent in many patients. For example, women who present with rupture of the membranes or premature labor at 27–34 weeks' gestation cannot have a GASA assignment. The limitations of ultrasound in the assessment of gestational age are most evident in this group because the predictive value of SSGA decreases with each week of gestation after 26 weeks. Nonetheless, ultrasound does provide useful information: a difference between menstrual age and SSGA by 3 or more weeks provides the most meaningful information. If SSGA is less than menstrual age by 3 or more weeks, the fetus is either more premature than suspected clinically or is growth retarded. Clinical information relative to accuracy of menstrual data, maternal weight gain, fundal height growth patterns, presence of factors known to be associated with uteroplacental insufficiency, and prior pregnancy outcome (prior premature labors) must be considered in

TABLE 11-4. LATE GESTATION INDICATIONS FOR THIRD-TRIMESTER SCANS*

A. Third-Trimester scan†
   1. Premature labor
   2. Premature rupture of membranes
   3. Hydramnios
B. Serial Third-trimester scans*
   1. Poor maternal weight gain
   2. Poor fundal height growth
   3. Oligohydramnios
   4. Preeclampsia
   5. Hypertension

* Pregnancy complications first noted in the third trimester

† Only a few patients will have an earlier scan at 20–26 weeks (Table 11–2). Most patients will not; GASA and serial percentile followup will not be possible. Serial scans are most helpful when both biparietal diameters and abdominal circumferences are performed.

TABLE 11-5. EARLY GESTATION INDICATIONS FOR MANDATORY GASA AND PROBABLE SERIAL THIRD-TRIMESTER SCANS*

A. At risk for altered fetal growth†
   1. Prior SGA neonate
   2. Diabetes
   3. Hypertension
   4. First-trimester bleeding
   5. First-trimester viral infection
   6. Drug addiction
   7. GI malabsorption
   8. Family history diabetes
   9. Family history of hypertension
B. Consideration of indicated induction
   1. Prior unexplained stillborn
   2. Rh isoimmune disease

* All are recognizable in early gestation when a prospective sonographic game plan is feasible.

† Preeclampsia is not included, since its prediction is not reliably possible prior to 26–28 weeks; the list is not intended to be all-inclusive.

balance with the predicted gestational age based on sonographic and clinical data.

On the other hand, if the SSGA is 3 or more weeks greater than menstrual age, the fetus may either be more mature or simply large for gestational age. The impact of differentiating these two possibilities is of great importance. For example, clinical fetal distress in a 28-week fetus requires more aggressive care than might be indicated in a 24-week fetus where the prospect of salvageability is small. Similarly, sonographic assignment of gestation as 39 weeks versus 36 weeks by menstrual data in a Class B diabetic with a prior cesarean delivery should arouse suspicion of an LGA fetus rather than an error in age assignment.

Even though establishment of precise gestational age is difficult in many instances, management decisions in preterm pregnancies must be made relative to intervention versus prolongation of pregnancy and use of corticosteroids to induce fetal surfactant activity if fetal lung maturity is unlikely. Unfortunately in most hospitals a significant number of patients have no indication for a scan at 20–26 weeks. Until routine sonography is accepted as a cost-effective and absolutely safe practice, patients will be scanned for the first time when a problem arises. It is then difficult for the clinician to define a rational basis for interpretation of sonographic and menstrual data, each with varying limitations; those clinicians unaccustomed to such a process are most likely to make serious judgment errors. To standardize the gestational age assignment process, the author has devised a scheme (Table 11–6) that considers the relative predictive ability of GASA versus a single-scan gestational age (SSGA). The scheme considers the impact of progressive loss of predictive ability of a single scan with increasing gestation beyond 26–28 weeks. Thus the sonographic determination of GASA or crown–rump length is highly predictive; SSGA determined at 20–26, 27–28, and 29–40 weeks have progressively larger confidence limits and must be interpreted with caution. Clinically, the scheme relies on use of the LMP (Boxes 6–10) as a reliable source of gestational age assignment when the sonographic age is within 7 days of the menstrual age. Similarly the menstrual age is considered when the discrepancy is only 8–14 days (Boxes 12, 17); menstrual age is used because it is a universal standard and the close correlation between sonographic and menstrual data suggests a pop-

TABLE 11-6. BASIS FOR CLINICAL ASSIGNMENT OF GESTATIONAL AGE WHEN THE LIMITATIONS OF CLINICAL AND SONOGRAPHIC DATA ARE CONSIDERED*

Sonographic age by scan at:	No/poor LMP	MA (±7)	MA (±8–11)	MA (±12–14)	MA (±15–21)
7–14 weeks	1) SSGA	6) MA	11) SSSA	16) SSGA	21) SSGA
20–26 weeks	2) SSGA	7) MA	12) Avg	17) Avg	22) SSGA
27–28 weeks	3) SSGA	8) MA	13) MA	18) Avg	23) Avg
29–40 weeks	4) Clinical and SSGA	9) MA	14) MA	19) MA	24) Avg
GASA	5) GASA	10) MA	15) GASA	20) GASA	25) GASA

CRL	Crown–rump length (2 SD = ± 1–4 days)
SSGA	Single–scan gestational age (BPD or CRL origin)
GASA	Growth-adjusted sonographic age (paired 20–24 weeks plus = 30–33 weeks)—2 SD = ± 1–3 days
MA	Menstrual age
MA (±7)	EDC by LMP agrees with EDC by scan ±7 days; menstrual dates probably highly reliable
MA (±8–11)	EDC by LMP agrees with EDC scan + 8–11 days
MA (±12–14)	EDC by LMP agrees with EDC by scan + 12–14 days
Clinical	Early assessment of uterine size plus onset of fetal movement (FM) plus fundal height
BPD probability	Gestational age is assigned for the fetus of average cephalic size. The probability of this occurrence should be stated (Ch. 8)
Average	MA plus SSGA divided by two

* BPD, Biparietal diameter—2 SD = ± 11 days (20-26 weeks), ± 14 days (27-28 weeks), and ± 21 days (29-40 weeks)

ulation of gravidas less prone to error in their menstrual dates. When a single scan is performed late in gestation (Box 24), the 6 weeks' confidence limits lead to a greater reliability on menstrual age. As a compromise an average of the two is reasonable.

In contrast, when GASA and LMP differ by 8–11 days (Box 15), GASA is more heavily weighted because of its ±1–3 days, 95% confidence limits. As the discrepancy increases (Boxes 20, 25) GASA assumes prime importance.

Finally, two points should be emphasized. First, advancement of menstrual gestational age with ultrasound should be done with caution, particularly in Boxes 22–24. Secondly, if a decision for intervention must be made where organ maturity is an issue, interpretation of L/S data is critical. Clinical and ultrasound data must be considered in all cases. Table 11–6 is nothing more than a device for standardization of data interpretation. It was designed for implementation by residents and private attending physicians in current prospective protocols.

SERIAL CEPHALOMETRY

Establishment of a prospective game plan to select the group of patients (Table 11–3) who will benefit from a single scan at 20–26 weeks has last-trimester dividends. It is possible both to define precisely gestational age (±1–3 days) and to project an individualized course of cephalic growth. Suboptimal deviations from the predicted growth curve imply increased risk. In contrast, serial third-trimester scans (Table 11–4B), without the benefit of growth-adjusted sonographic age (GASA) and percentiles, have a limited though definite value. Clinical observations such as poor maternal weight gain, poor fundal height growth in an otherwise normal pregnancy, or development of preeclampsia or other third-trimester conditions associated with uteroplacental insufficiency imply risk of intrauterine growth retardation (IUGR). Fetal growth should average at least 2mm/week up to week 34 and at least 1 mm/week thereafter over a 2 to 3 week interval even in the lowest percentile rank (29). Less or no growth over a 3-

week interval in the presence of fetal lung maturity is a reasonable indication for intervention, particularly if there have been three scans in that period to minimize measurement errors. A nonreactive NST and/or positive CST would provide confirmatory evidence and increase the urgency of delivery (see later discussion).

FETAL-PLACENTAL UNIT EVALUATION

The major problem in the management of third-trimester complications such as preeclampsia or premature rupture of the membranes is the determination of the optimal time of delivery. The decision involves the consideration of the relative benefits and cost of prolongation versus termination of pregnancy to fetus and mother (Fig. 11–1).

The contraction stress test (CST) (9, 10, 15, 24, 25) and nonstress test (NST) (8, 13, 15–17, 21, 27) are currently the most commonly used tools to evaluate fetal cardiovascular and placental function. Other tools to evaluate fetal placental unit integrity include serum or urinary estriols and human placental lactogen. In most instances the result of such testing is reassurance; the pregnancy from the fetal viewpoint may be allowed to continue. Occasionally, however, maternal risk, that is, sepsis or severe progressive preeclampsia, takes precedence, requiring intervention regardless of fetal status. With few exceptions data obtained from such procedures must be considered in balance with sonographic and fetal pulmonary surfactant assessment (L/S) before decisions regarding fetal care are finalized, because the management of high-risk pregnancies frequently involves a patient with unsure dates, potential uteroplacental insufficiency, and fetal growth retardation, as well as some jeopardy to maternal health. Essential hypertension or mitral stenosis are two examples.

Figure 11–2 summarizes the specifics of a scheme to evaluate fetal placental respiratory (NST–OCT) and nutritive (estriol) function. Use of this scheme allows prolongation of the majority of high-risk pregnancies to term. Prior practice, particularly in maternal diabetes, required uniform intervention at 36–37 weeks to

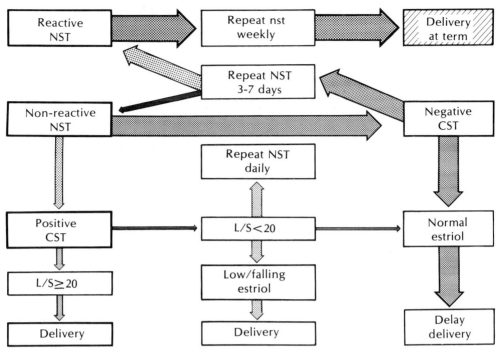

FIG. 11-2. Detection and management scheme for uteroplacental insufficiency. Arrow width reflects relative pathway frequencies. Nonstress Test (NST) is screening procedure for the contraction stress test (CST). A reactive NST is simply repeated weekly. A nonreactive NST requires final evaluation by the CST; most CSTs done after a nonreactive NST will be negative. Objective is delivery at term unless uteroplacental insufficiency is detected by NST/OCT testing. An L/S greater than 2, which predicts fetal pulmonary maturity, can be achieved in most instances.

maximize fetal survival; frequently the consequence was neonatal death from respiratory distress syndrome (RDS). Currently only 10%–15% of diabetics require delivery prior to term (nonreactive NST and/or positive CST), while the remainder derive the benefits of 3–4 additional weeks of intrauterine maturation prior to birth.

Although discussion of the specifics of antenatal fetal cardiovascular function is beyond the scope of this chapter, some discussion is indicated to place the various testing tools in proper clinical context for the reader whether obstetrician, radiologist, or technologist.

THE CONTRACTION STRESS TEST

The contraction stress test (CST), sometimes called the oxytocin challenge test (OCT) was introduced separately by Pose (1969) (24) and Kubli (1969) (15). Freeman subsequently popu-

larized the procedure in the United States (9). The induction of three uterine contractions over a period of 10 min provides a standard objective stress to the fetus at risk and is useful in separating the fetus with normal versus abnormal uteroplacental respiratory function. Uterine contractions reduce uterine and intervillous blood flow; the normal fetoplacental unit should tolerate this "stress," whereas a compromised unit cannot. Failure to tolerate the "stress" is reflected by the presence of repetitive uniform late decelerations related to fetal myocardial hypoxia—a positive CST. Until recently the CST (Fig. 11–3) was the most extensively used technique used antenatally to evaluate uteroplacental insufficiency.

Approximately 2%–10% of patients tested, (depending on the high-risk characteristics,) will have a positive test (abnormal). In contrast, a negative (reassuring) CST (Fig. 11–3) shows no uniform late decelerations in association with uterine contractions (a minimum frequency of

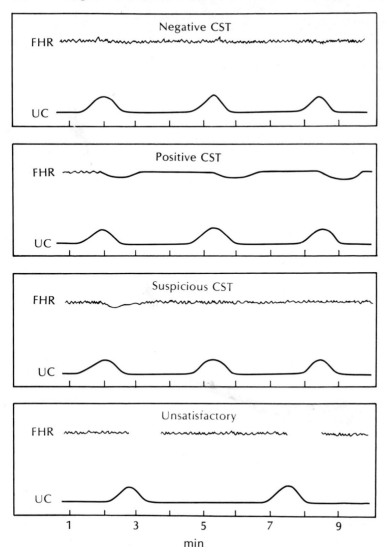

FIG. 11-3. Diagrammatic representation of possible Contraction Stress Test (CST) outcomes. Upper channel of each strip is fetal heart rate; lower channel reflects uterine contractions in a 10-min time interval.

three in 10 min and approximately 50–60 sec in duration). The CST is normal in 85%–95% of pregnancies tested. In some situations (5%–10%) the CST may be unsatisfactory (poor recording or less than three contractions over 10 min) or equivocal or suspicious (only occasional late decelerations).

Clinically, a negative CST is the most predictive of all results. While the incidence of false/positive results is high (30%–60%) false-negative results have been reported only sporadically. Parer and Afonso, for example, reported an incidence of 5/1000 false-negative results (22). In an extremely high-risk population Paul

and Miller (23) noted a 10/1000 incidence of false-negative results. It is thus obvious that these procedures have a large margin of safety, erring more in the direction of overdiagnosis of uteroplacental insufficiency.

THE NONSTRESS TEST

Despite its established effectiveness, the CST has definite limitations. The nonstress test developed by a number of investigators (8, 13, 16, 17, 21, 27) is, however, advantageous because: 1) it is less complex to perform; 2) it requires only

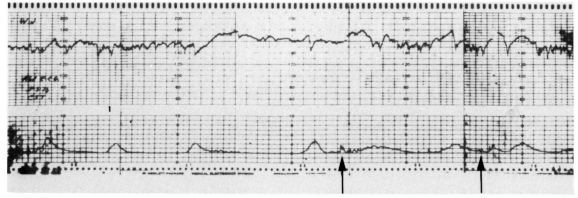

FIG. 11-4. Contraction stress test using abdominal ECG as source. Lower channel reflects uterine contractions of 40- to 60-sec duration. Small superimposed peaks represent fetal movement. Fetal heart rate (FHR) baseline (upper channel) is 145–150. Note accelerations of FHR in response to fetal movement **(arrows)** on lower channel. The estimated magnitude of accelerations is 25–30 bpm.

20–30 min versus 90–180 for CST; 3) no IV oxytocin is needed; and 4) no relative contraindications to its use exist.

A reactive (reassuring) interpretation (Fig. 11–4) depends on detection of at least two FHR accelerations, 15 bpm above baseline, in a 20-min test period (5); some authors insist on four or five accelerations (8). Other possible indicators of well-being proposed by the author include a FHR baseline below 150 bpm and long-term variability greater than 6 bpm. Evaluation of variability is, however, possible only in tracings of excellent quality (30%). It is not possible to evaluate short-term variability with external techniques.

A nonreactive NST is one in which the magnitude of acceleration above the FHR baseline is less than 15 bpm. Observance of diminished variability, even with use of ultrasound, is significant. Ultrasound introduces noise in the baseline; although ultrasound does average RR intervals, it does not artificially reduce baseline variability to such an extent as to be reflected by a flat baseline (absent variability). The presence of late deceleration in association with spontaneous contractions of any frequency is ominous.

The NST has been used as the primary tool for fetal assessment at Prentice Women's Hospital (Northwestern Perinatal Center) since July 1975 and by the author for 6 months prior to that time in parallel with CSTs (5). The ease of performing the procedure, its apparent reliability, and its low incidence of false-positive (normal outcome in presence of abnormal test) make it a very useful clinical tool.

In the past 3 years we have evaluated approximately 1800 high-risk patients. Although evaluation of data is not complete, only 2 unexplained deaths have occurred within a week of a reactive result; 2 additional deaths were observed, one in a hypertensive patient who presented with an abruption, the other in a severely toxic hyperthyroid patient within 24 hours after a very difficult amniocentesis. The time saved and the apparent reliability have encouraged our clinicians to use the CST as a final arbiter of a nonreactive NST, but not as the front-line screening procedure (Fig. 11–2). Indications for NST–OCT testing are included in Table 11–7. The most common indications are: "postdate"

TABLE 11-7. INDICATIONS FOR NST–OCT TESTING

1. Diabetes mellitus
2. Preeclampsia
3. Chronic hypertension
4. Intrauterine growth retardation
5. Postdatism versus postmaturity
6. Narcotic addiction
7. Sickle cell hemoglobinopathy
8. Chronic pulmonary disease
9. Heart disease
   a. Cyanotic
   b. Mitral stenosis (decreased cardiac output)
10. Rh isoimmune disease
11. Meconium-stained amniotic fluid
12. History of prior stillborn
13. History of prior SGA neonate

pregnancies and patients with suspected fetal growth retardation.

Martin and Schifrin have completed an analysis of patients managed in a manner identical to our proposed technique (20). In their series of 1169 cases (2422 NST tests), reactive patterns constituted approximately two-thirds of cases; only 2% of tests were unsatisfactory versus 5%–10% in many CST series. The incidence of stillbirth in the patients with a reactive NST was 4/1000; in contrast the stillborn mortality for the group who required a CST as a result of a nonreactive NST was 7/1000. The percentage of negative and positive CST results in the series of 851 nonreactive tests was 91 and 3 respectively. The authors concluded that a negative CST and reactive NST are equally predictive. It should also be obvious that the vast majority of tests are normal and thus reassure both patient and physician that the pregnancy may progress with minimal fetal risk.

CEPHALOMETRY AND NST–CST PROTOCOL

The place of ultrasound in the described scheme is not totally resolved. The author has worked in close collaboration with Rudy Sabbagha for the past 6 years in an attempt to link sonographic and fetal heart rate analysis in a meaningful manner. Total reliance on one to the exclusion of the other is not reasonable. Certainly, if one remembers that in those cases of IUGR where fetal jeopardy occurs late in pregnancy (approximately 35%), cephalic growth is compromised last (12). The observation that cephalic growth is deviating below the predicted course or is totally absent is disturbing no matter how negative the CST or reactive the NST. In contrast, observation that there is minimal or no growth over a 2-week period has not been a totally satisfactory indicator of increased risk in our hands. The possibility of overestimation of the BPD followed 2 weeks later by accurate or underestimation is a potential problem, especially in the hands of an inexperienced technician. For this reason we generally require three serial measurements over a 21-to-24-day period and in-

TABLE 11-8. SCHEME FOR USE OF SONOGRAPHIC AND AMNIOTIC FLUID L/S DATA IN THE PRESENCE OF A REACTIVE NST*

Reactive NST

BPD growth	L/S	Action
Good	—	NST, weekly
Poor	—	NST, weekly BPD and AC in 7–10 days
None	>2.0	Deliver soon
(21–24 days)	<2.0	NST in 5–7 days

* BPD = biparietal diameter.
AC = abdominal circumference.

TABLE 11-9. SCHEME FOR USE OF SONOGRAPHIC AND AMNIOTIC FLUID DATA IN THE PRESENCE OF A NONREACTIVE NST

Nonreactive NST

1. Negative contraction stress test (91%)			
BPD growth	L/S	Estriol	Action
Good	—	—	NST, weekly
Poor	—	Baseline	NST, weekly
None	<2.0	Daily	NST, weekly
None	>2.0	—	Deliver soon

2. Positive contraction stress test (3%)			
BPD growth	L/S	Estriol	Action
*	<2.0	Rising	NST, daily
*	<2.0	Falling	Deliver soon
*	>2.0	—	Deliver soon

* Positive CST interpretation takes precedence in decision; sonographic data, though useful, are not essential.

clude the abdominal circumference (Ch. 9) before considering intervention solely on the basis of sonographic data.

Tables 11–8 and 11–9 present our current protocol, which varies according to the presence of a reactive versus nonreactive NST. In general, serial BPDs are ordered at 2-week intervals. The detection of suboptimal or no growth in that interval is an indication for a repeat evaluation in 7–10 days. Growth over a 28-day period should be at least 5 mm at any percentile rank. Errors of that magnitude averaged over a 4-week period are unlikely; no growth would be difficult to explain on a random basis. Although the scheme reflects use of estriols, the final pathway of evaluating the fetal placental unit is virtually always determined by the NST–CST. Prolongation of pregnancy in the face of a nonreactive NST positive CST because of rising estriols is very rare.

CASE PRESENTATIONS

The previous discussion, though simplified, is abstract relative to actual application. The following are case studies that are useful in emphasizing techniques previously described. Cases are presented that use ultrasound as it is currently employed nationally rather than as proposed earlier. Additional information provided by our routine protocols emphasizes the benefits of GASA as well as serial scanning in the third trimester.

CASE 1

M.P. is an obese gravida 8 para 4 abortus 3 Class B diabetic with LMP 3/1/77 (EDC 12/6/77). Pertinent past history includes prior cesarean deliveries and prior newborn birth weights at term of 8 lb; 5 lb 6 oz; 10 lb; and 9 lb 13 oz. New problems encountered in this pregnancy include vaginal bleeding at 21 weeks' gestation and average early third-trimester pressure of 160/100 (thigh cuff). Since she is a Class B diabetic with hypertension and a prior cesarean, one would ordinarily plan delivery at 39 weeks' gestation; only the presence of uteroplacental insufficiency would dictate earlier intervention. In anticipation of delivery, an amniocentesis was attempted unsuccessfully by an experienced clinician on November 22 and 23. A BPD obtained on November 30 to document gestational age was 8.5 cm; this indicates either a 33-week fetus at the 50th percentile or, if dates are correct, a 39-week fetus at less than the fifth percentile. Over the ensuing 7 days, progressive decrease in insulin demands was noted by the en-

docrinologist, who was concerned that the change suggested decreasing insulin antagonism by a failing fetoplacental unit. Identified late gestation problems include 1) Class B diabetes; 2) hypertension; 3) questionable failing placental function as reflected by both suspect subnormal cephalic growth, as well as decreasing insulin demands; 4) inability to obtain amniotic fluid, suggesting oligohydramnios.

In reality, our protocol as advocated earlier was followed, providing more detailed information upon which to act. The case presented is, however, typical either of cases referred to Northwestern Perinatal Center or of histories obtained relative to infants of diabetic mothers transferred to our special care nursery with respiratory distress, hypoglycemia, hyperbilirubinemia, etc. Such cases cannot be justified if one properly employs serial cephalometry (GASA), NST–OCT testing, and amniotic fluid surfactant assessment.

More detailed data required by our perinatal team included 1) a history of irregular menses; 2) prospective recording of fetal movement onset on August 2 (22 weeks by LMP rather than the expected 17–19 weeks' gestation). A single scan performed on September 13 was 5.3 cm (22 weeks ±11 days), which was more consistent with her fetal movement history.

Table 11–10 summarizes the laboratory findings, which dramatically illustrate the value of GASA plus serial scans in a high-risk pregnancy. By luck alone, a single scan on November 30 was at the 50th percentile. However, the benefit of observing the dynamics of fetal growth in this individual fetus is obvious. The progressive fall in percentile rankings with gestation reflects a deficiency in the intrauterine milieu; it does not predict a small for dates newborn, only a small-for-self neonate whose

TABLE 11–10. CASE 1 SUMMARY. SINGLE-SCAN GESTATIONAL AGE (SSGA) (CASE M.P.)

	11/17	11/25	11/30	12/13	12/28	1/3
Fetal age (weeks)	37	38	39	41	43	44
BPD	8.3→	8.3→	8.5→	8.6→	8.8→	9.0→
GASA	31	32	33	35	37	38
Percentile	>75	50	50	<25	10	10–25
SSGA	32	32	33	34	35	36
NST–OCT	OK	OK	OK	OK	OK	OK
L/S	—	—	—	1.7→	2.4→	—

cephalic growth curve has failed to meet its potential.

Further, the growing discrepancy between fetal age in weeks by LMP (Row 1, Table 11–10) and fetal age predicted by a single scan (Row 5) underscores the limitations of single third-trimester scans in predicting gestational age. The transition of the L/S ratio from 1.7 to 2.4 at 36–37 weeks is common; errors in gestational age assignment in diabetics may be partially responsible for the proposed delay in lung maturation noted in infants of diabetics.

Delay of delivery until January 4 (38 weeks' gestation by GASA and 44 weeks' by LMP) was possible because of continued reassurance presented by reactive NST, negative OCT testing. We have not noted a correlation between falling insulin needs and evidence of placental insufficiency. The benefit in terms of reduction of neonatal morbidity that resulted from reassignment of EDC to early January rather than early December is evident.

CASE 2

J.L. is a 24-year-old gravida 2 para 1 with LMP 6/12/77 (EDC 3/19/78); she presented with premature rupture of membranes on January 22. Initial examination confirmed the presence of amniotic fluid in the vaginal vault; the cervix was 1 cm/50% effaced. A single scan done that day revealed: a BPD of 8.7 cm (34 weeks ±3 weeks) and an anterior left placenta with a pocket of fluid localized in the right lower quandrant. Analysis done on amniotic fluid revealed a strongly positive shake test and an L/S ratio of 2:1.

Plan of management included the following 1) observe for onset of amnionitis; 2) take cervical culture for group B streptococcus and N. gonococcus; 3) do not inhibit labor; 4) give no steroid to induce surfactant.

Spontaneous labor ensued 56 hours later; a viable 1800-g newborn, Apgar 7, 9, delivered vaginally. Nursery course was unremarkable.

This case illustrates a common problem, the management (Fig. 11–5) of premature labor and/or premature rupture of membranes in the presence of an apparent discrepancy between menstrual age (32 weeks) and single-scan gestational age (34 weeks). Assigned gestational age (Table 11–6, Box 19) was 32 weeks because of wide confidence limits of a single scan. If the assignment is correct, then the 8.7 reading indicates a BPD greater than the 80th percentile. Psychologically this is an important decision in that many clinicians opt to terminate all pregnancies complicated by premature rupture of membranes at 34 weeks; assignment of 32 weeks' gestation has the impact of arousing greater concern regarding lung maturity, which must be considered in balance with amnionitis and maternal sepsis.

Probable mature pulmonary function indicated by an L/S ratio of 2:1 occurs in 20% of our population at 28–34 weeks. The amniocentesis is justified because it determines the need for corticosteroid therapy to induce pulmonary surfactant (18, 19), and the need for inhibition of labor. Cortico steroid induction of surfactant activity is justified only when there is reasonable certainty of immaturity; the potential short- and long-term side effects of cortico steroids must be considered and explained to the patient in balance to possible benefit.

The 2-week discrepancy between LMP and BPD assignments is also common. In another case the L/S could easily be significantly less than 2. The correct clinical decision is derived from accumulation of factual data, taken in context with inherent limitations.

Ultimately, the crucial decisions depend on functional maturity more than on gestational age. For this reason the ultrasonographer should report the BPD value and the gestational age at the 50th percentile ±3 weeks. It is not reasonable for the sonographer, at this time in the evolution of the technique, to expect that all users will understand the problems of biologic variation in BPD at various times in gestation. It is the sonographer's responsibility to state the limits of his result. Otherwise, undue reliance may be placed on interpretation of sonographic data. Factors that may tip the decision in the direction of pregnancy intervention include patient noncompliance (uncooperative, unable to understand patient responsibilities), a 3-cm dilated cervix, and gestation of 37 or more weeks, when pulmonary maturity is highly likely.

CASE 3

G.R. is a 39-year-old gravida with LMP 1/21/77 (EDC 10/28/77). Pertinent history includes the following: 1) no contraceptive use since marriage 3 years earlier; 2) light spotting on 1/10/77 for 3 days; 3) menstrual periods every 26–34 days; 4) a husband who is executive vice president of local bank.

A single scan on 10/1/77 (36 weeks by LMP) was 9.5 cm (40 weeks at 50th percentile). The patient has been very anxious throughout pregnancy and has uterine contractions sporadically. After learning the scan results, she is insistent that her true EDC is 10/18/77 and is now sure that the bleeding on 1/10/77 was a "real" period. Physical examination revealed a 37-cm fundus, estimated fetal weight of 3500 g, and a long, closed cervix with a floating vertex. The knife is sharpened!

Assessment is that she is probably at 38 weeks' gestation (see Table 11–6, Box 24). The patient was reassured. The plan was to obtain an additional scan in 2 weeks (38 weeks by LMP; 42 weeks by first scan) and consider induction at that time. The BPD on 10/18/77 was 9.7 cm (good growth). The pelvic findings were unchanged.

At this point the clinician is faced with the following choices: 1) difficult induction and probable cesarean delivery; 2) NST–OCT protocol (Fig. 11–3) to distinguish: a) inaccurate date assignment, b) prolonged pregnancy, and 3) postmaturity (growth retardation in true postdate pregnancy).

This sequence of events is all too common. The principles outlined earlier eliminate

FIG. 11–5. Management scheme of premature rupture of membranes. Decisions are influenced by the following: results of gestational age determined according to relative predictive ability of ultrasound and historical data; presence of pulmonary maturity as indicated by the L/S ratio; and clinician's assessment of cost–benefit ratio of steroid administration to induce pulmonary maturity. Important variables in decision are the L/S ratio and gestational age. The scheme acknowledges equal clinical acceptance of option to administer steroids followed by 48- to 72-hour response time or option not to give steroids and wait until onset of spontaneous labor or until intervention is indicated.

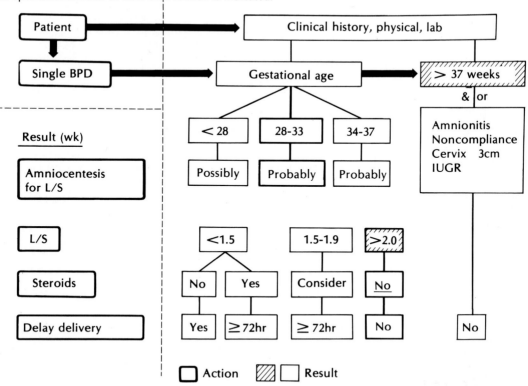

TABLE 11-11. CASE 3 SUMMARY; (SSGA) SINGLE-SCAN GESTATIONAL AGE; TEMPORARY ASSIGNMENT OF GESTATIONAL AGE UNTIL GASA ESTABLISHED AT 30-33 WEEKS*

Serial BPD (9 week interval): elderly primigravida

Date	7/1	9/3	9/17	10/1	10/18
MA	23	32	34	36	38
BPD	5.4→	8.0→	8.8→	9.5→	9.7→
SSGA	22	31	35	>40	>40
GASA	—	31	33	35	37
Percentile	—	50	80	>80	>95

* In this case the first two SSGA determination are identical to GASA (growth-adjusted age).

40%–60% of such cases, which are simply a function of inaccurate assignment of gestational age (5). Clinically, this is extremely important, for it eliminates a large percentage of NST–OCT testing in community hospitals where postdatism is the primary indication.

As indicated earlier, in reality, there were additional data (Table 11–11). A second-trimester scan was indicated (Table 11–2). Surprisingly the second scan on 9/3/77 was 8.0, which indicates high correlation between menstrual age, single-scan gestational age, and GASA (31, 32, and 31 weeks respectively). However, subsequent scans emphasize the problem of single third-trimester scans; the discrepancy between SSGA and MA grows from 1 to 3 weeks by the 37th menstrual week.

The additional information provided by GASA and subsequent serial sonography in the absence of clinical indication of growth retardation and maternal complications confirms the original EDC of 10/28/77, allays physician and patient anxiety, and delays the need for institution of the NST–OCT protocol until 42 weeks (11/10/77). The patient subsequently spontaneously delivered a 3975-g Apgar 8, 9 newborn on 11/2/77.

REFERENCES

1. CAMPBELL S: The prediction of fetal maturity by ultrasonic measurement of the biparietal diameter. Br J Obstet Gynaecol 76:603, 1969
2. CAMPBELL S: The assessment of fetal development by diagnostic ultrasound. Clin Perinatol 1:507, 1974
3. CAMPBELL S, NEWMAN GB: Growth of the fetal biparietal diameter during normal pregnancy. Br J Obstet Gynaecol 78:513, 1971
4. DEPP R: The puzzle of postmaturity. Contemp Obstet Gynecol 3:109–113, 1974
5. DEPP R: Unpublished data
6. DEWHURST CJ, BEAZLEY JJ, CAMPBELL S: Assessment of fetal maturity and dysmaturity. Am J Obstet Gynecol 106:676, 1970
7. FARRELL PM, WOOD RM: Epidemiology of hyaline membrane disease in the United States: analysis of national mortality statistics. Pediatrics 58:167, 1976
8. FLYNN AM, KELLY J: Evaluation of fetal well being by antepartum fetal heart monitoring. Br Med J 1:936, 1977
9. FREEMAN RK: The use of the oxytocin challenge test for antepartum clinical evaluation of uteroplacental respiratory function. Am J Obstet Gynecol 121: 481–489, 1975
10. FREEMAN RK, GOEBELSMAN U, NOCHIMSON D, CETRULO C: An evaluation of the significance of a positive oxytocin challenge test. Obstet Gynecol 47:8–13, 1976
11. GOLDENBERG RL, NELSON K: Iatrogenic respiratory distress syndrome. An analysis of obstetric events preceding delivery of infants who develop respiratory distress syndrome. Am J Obstet Gynecol 123:617, 1975
12. GRUENWALD P: Chronic fetal distress and placental insufficiency. Biol Neonate 5:215, 1963
13. HAMMACHER K: The clinical significance of cardiotocography. In Huntingford PS, Huter EA, Saling E (eds): Perinatal Medicine. New York, Academic Press, 1969
14. HERTZ RH, SOKOL RJ, KNOKE JD et al: Clinical estimation of gestational age: rules for avoiding preterm delivery. Am J Obstet Gynecol 131:395–402, 1978
15. KUBLI FW, KAESER O, HINSELMAN M: Diagnostic management of chronic placental insufficiency. In Pecile A, Finzi C (eds): The Foetal-Placental Unit. Amsterdam, Exerpta Medical Foundation, 1969
16. KUBLI F, RUTTGERS H: Semiquantitative evaluation of antepartum fetal heart rate. Int J Gynaecol Obstet 10:180, 1972
17. LEE CY, DILORETTO PC, LOGRAND B: Fetal activity acceleration determination for the evaluation of fetal reserve. Obstet Gynecol 48:19, 1976
18. LIGGINS GC: Prenatal glucocorticoid treatment: prevention of respiratory distress syndrome. In Lung Maturation and the Prevention of Hyaline Membrane Disease. Report of the Seventieth Ross Conference on Pediatric Research, Columbus, 1976
19. LIGGINS GC, HOWIE RN: A controlled trial of antepartum glucocorticord treatment for prevention of respiratory distress syndrome on premature infants. Pediatrics 50:515, 1972
20. MARTIN CB JR, SCHIFRIN BS: Prenatal fetal monitor-

ing. In Aladjem S, Brown AK (eds): Perinatal Intensive Care. St. Louis, CV Mosby, 1977

21. NOCHIMSON DJ, TURBEVILLE JS, TERRY JE et al: The non-stress test. Obstet Gynecol 51:419, 1978

22. PARER JT, AFONSO JF: Validity of the weekly interval between oxytocin challenge tests. Am J Obstet Gynecol 127:204, 1977

23. PAUL RH, MILLER FC: Antepartum fetal heart rate monitoring. Clin Obstet Gynecol 21:375, 1978

24. POSE SV, CASTILLO JB, MORA-ROJAS EO, SOTO-YANCES A, CALDEYRO-BARCIA R: In Perinatal Factors Effecting Human Development. Test of fetal tolerance to induced uterine contractions with a diagnosis of chronic distress. Washington DC, Pan-American Health Organization, 1969, pp 96–103

25. RAY M, FREEMAN RK, PINE S, HESSELGESSER R: Clinical experience with the oxytocin challenge test. Am J Obstet Gynecol 114:1–9, 1972

26. ROBINSON HP, FLEMMING JEE: A critical evaluation of sonar "crown-rump length" measurements. Br J Obstet Gynaecol 82:702, 1975

27. ROCHARD F, SCHIFRIN BS, GOUPIL F et al: Nonstressed fetal heart rate monitoring in the antepartum period. Am J Obstet Gynecol 126:699, 1976

28. SABBAGHA RE: Ultrasound in managing the high-risk pregnancy. In Spellacy WN (ed): Management of the High Risk Pregnancy. Baltimore, University Park Press, 1976

29. SABBAGHA RE, BARTON BA, BARTON FB et al: Sonar biparietal diameter. II. Predictive of three fetal growth patterns leading to a closer assessment of gestational age and neonatal weight. Am J Obstet Gynecol 51:383, 1978

30. SABBAGHA RE, TURNER HS, ROCKETTE H et al: Sonar BPD and fetal age-determination of the relationship. Obstet Gynecol 43:7, 1974

31. VARMA JR: Prediction of delivery date by ultrasound cephalometry. Br J Obstet Gynaecol 80:316, 1973

32. YERUSHALMY J: Relation of birth weight, gestational age, and the rate of intrauterine growth to perinatal mortality. Clin Obstet Gynecol 13:107, 1970

Management decisions in obstetrics

JOHN C. HOBBINS

Obstetric ultrasonography has exploded in the past 5 years, and not only has the quality of ultrasound imagery improved appreciably, but also companies are now producing low-cost portable real-time units that have utility in doctors' offices and hospital delivery suites. Since sales of these machines are increasing exponentially, more and more physicians are being exposed to ultrasound, and the potential for its use is limited only by one's experience.

This chapter will deal with ultrasound used adjunctively in critical and often emergent obstetric situations. It is hoped that it will provide readers with information that will aid in making some "11th hour" decisions on the delivery floor.

FETAL LIE

There are many occasions, for example, in the obese patient, where the classic Leopolds' abdominal maneuvers fail to diagnose fetal presentation. In some cases even a pelvic examination does not reveal which fetal pole is in the pelvis. In these cases a quick scan with any ultrasound unit will provide the physician with exact knowledge of fetal presentation (Fig. 12–1). For example, in a transverse lie, one can tell whether the back is up or down, and with a quick scan of the lower uterus it is possible to diagnose the often responsible placenta previa. Since cesarean section is the method of delivery for a viable fetus in a transverse lie, information about the exact position of the placenta is extremely useful to the physician about to enter the uterus through the lower uterine segment. In fact, to eliminate surprises, we often scan any intrapartum patient just prior to cesarean section.

PREMATURE RUPTURE OF MEMBRANES (PROM)

Today there is a trend toward conservative management of premature rupture of membranes (1) in patients who are at less than 33 weeks' gestation. For example, after documentation by speculum examination that the patient has ruptured membranes, she is put to bed and delivered only if labor or infection ensues. In these cases it has been emphatically stated by some that the patient should have one "baseline" pelvic examination to determine the following: 1) what the fetal presentation is, 2) whether prolapse of the cord has occurred, 3) whether cervical dilatation is a "starting point." One can argue, however,

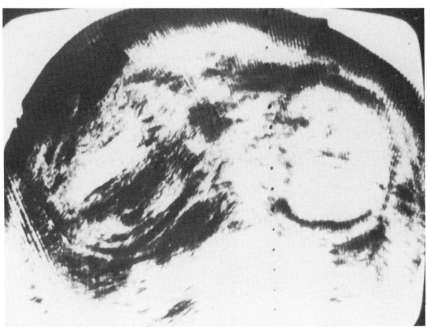

FIG. 12-1. Transverse scan of fetus in transverse lie.

that this examination is not only unnecessary but dangerous, because of the infectious potential of a digital examination. The incidence of prolapsed cord in PROM is no greater in these cases than the overall incidence of this condition, and if it does occur, it will be noted by external monitoring of fetal heart rate. If the patient is not in labor, and the cervix does not appear dilated on speculum examination, then it is unlikely the cervix will change before the patient is in labor. With an ultrasound unit convenient to the delivery floor, not only can fetal presentation be confirmed but also a careful BPD will help to confirm the patient's dates, since management of this condition depends on gestational age. If a transverse lie is noted with ultrasound, then it would be injudicious to allow the patient to labor once contractions commence.

BREECH PRESENTATIONS

EXTERNAL VERSION

Breech presentation occurs in about 4% of term pregnancies. Because breech deliveries are associated with higher morbidity and mortality, physicians are using cesarean section liberally. Some physicians (7) are, however, trying to avoid cesarean section in these patients by attempting to convert these breeches to vertices by external version in the mid and late third trimester. Using this technique, one author reports a reduction of breech presentations in labor to 1% (7).

Real-time ultrasound is extremely useful during the version because the exact fetal position can be ascertained throughout the procedure. Moreover, valuable ultrasonic information prior to the procedure may help the obstetrician to determine possible risks to the fetus. For example, if an anterior placenta is noted, then the version is performed with great gentleness (some will not even attempt it). Furthermore, if the umbilical cord is located in the nuchal area, the procedure is performed with caution and abandoned at the slightest sign of fetal heart rate deceleration. If the umbilical cord is entangled during the manipulation, fetal bradycardia will occur, which can be seen on real time. By knowing the long axis of the fetus and the position of the spine, the physician can best decide in which direction to move the fetus.

THE PREMATURE BREECH

There is now a trend to refer laboring patients with premature babies to institutions with fully staffed and equipped newborn special care units. Because of suggestions in the literature of higher morbidity in premature breeches delivered vaginally (8, 10), it is now the policy at many of these referral institutions to deliver all premature breeches by cesarean section.

Occasionally the intrapartum patient referred to the level-three hospital arrives with undocumented dates, and, unfortunately, decisions concerning the use of tocolytic agents and/or route of delivery depend heavily on the age of the fetus. The best way to confirm the patient's dates is by an ultrasound examination. We have found portable real-time scanners to be invaluable in this situation because the patient need not be moved from the delivery area. The accuracy of BPDs performed with a real-time scanner is acceptable when compared with measurements with contact equipment (2). It must be remembered, however, that the accuracy of prediction of gestational age by BPD with any technique diminishes as pregnancy progresses. Certainly, if the BPD is within 2 weeks of the patient's dates before the 34th week of gestation, the dates are probably correct. If there is a larger discrepancy, the dates may be assigned in accordance with Table 11–6. At present, at Yale–New Haven High-Risk Service, we are performing cesarean section on all patients with breech presentations who are in labor between 27 and 35 weeks.

TERM BREECH

If there is a place for vaginal delivery in a patient with a breech presentation, it is in the term breech. Circumstances must, however, be ideal, and it is the task of the responsible physician to weigh all the variables carefully before deciding on the route of delivery. First, fetal weight must be estimated, along with the size of the aftercoming head. There are many ultrasonic formulas for estimation of the fetal weight, but it is not sufficient to invoke a one-variable formula, since fetuses have a rather complex shape. In some techniques, however, measurement of so many dimensions are included, making the method impractical. We have found a computerized formula (11) based on head size (BPD) and body size (abdominal circumference at the level of umbilical vein) to be useful in patients with term breeches. It is accurate to within 100 g/kg (1 SD). It must be remembered, however, that in a 4000-g fetus, a two-standard deviation splay would be equivalent to ±800 g.

Since most of the morbidity in breeches is associated with trauma to the aftercoming head, an estimation of head size is essential. At Yale, if the BPD is more than 9.6 cm, we deliver all patients by cesarean section, no matter how capacious the maternal pelvis. If the BPD is of moderate size (less than 9.6), then the capacity of the pelvis is quantitated by x-ray pelvimetry, and if any of the measurements are not adequate, cesarean section is performed. In breech presentations the BPD reported should represent the outer aspects of the fetal head (Ch. 7).

Occasionally, an extended head is noted on x-ray pelvimetry. This alone is an indication for cesarean section, since transection of the spinal cord can result from vaginal delivery when the fetal head is extended. Unlike the flexed fetus in a vertex presentation, the fetal head will often be at about 90° angle with the body in a breech (military position). Abnormal extension occurs when the head-to-body angle is more than 90°. With ultrasound this angle can be determined by scanning across the body until most of the abdominal aorta can be seen in one sagittal plane (Figs. 12–2A and B). This plane represents the long axis of the fetal body. The head is then scanned at varying angles to the long axis of the body until the head appears as an elongated ellipse (Fig. 12–3). This represents the long axis of the fetal head. The angle between these two axes is the angle of inclination of the head. The maneuver is possible only when the back is on the side. If an extended head is suspected by this ultrasound maneuver, then it can be confirmed with x-ray. With or without the x-ray these patients should be sectioned because of the possibility of neurologic damage.

TWINS

It is not unusual for twins to be missed on ultrasound examination in the second trimester if

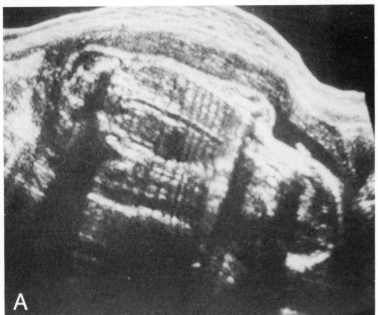

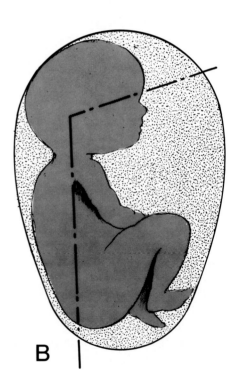

FIG. 12-2. A. Representative scan of long axis of fetus—notice fetal aorta. **B.** Schematic of transducer position in determining angle of inclination of head—dotted line refers to scan through fetal body at level of aorta.

FIG. 12-3. A. Representative scan of long axis of fetal head. **B.** Schematic of transducer position in determining angle of inclination of head—dotted line refers to long axis of fetal head.

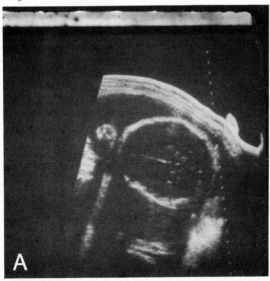

the diagnosis is not suspected and the patient is referred for another reason such as dating or placental position. This should not, however, happen if a systematic scanning technique is employed. It is particularly important to detect twins early so that the pregnancy can be accurately dated and baseline information obtained for subsequent ultrasonic monitoring of growth and development.

Since this chapter deals with the value of ultrasound in making last-minute assessments, let us discuss the all too frequent case of undiagnosed twins at term. Clinically, the uterus appears large for dates. With ultrasound it is relatively easy to piece heads and bodies together to determine fetal presentation. The most common combinations encountered (in order of frequency) are vertex–vertex; vertex–breech; breech–vertex; breech–breech. When a breech–vertex presentation is noted, one should always keep in mind the remote possibility of locking of twins. If the first twin is a breech, then all previously stated criteria for singleton breeches apply. The BPDs of twins are no different than those of singletons of the same gestational age until the 28th week of gestation, after which twin BPDs tend to be somewhat smaller (6). The discrepancies become clinically meaningful after about 32 weeks.

Because marked discrepancies in size can occur between twins, it is very useful to attempt to estimate fetal size by measurements of BPD, head circumference, and abdominal circumference (Fig. 12–4). When monozygotic twins share the same blood supply, the plethoric recipient and the scrawny growth-retarded donor are both at grave risk of intrauterine demise. When these ultrasonic measurements indicate a marked discrepancy in fetal mass, the twins should be delivered as soon as there is a reasonable chance of extrauterine survival.

In the twin delivery there are distinct advantages to having a portable real-time machine in the delivery room. For instance, the position of twins can change so that prelabor evaluations of twin position may be misleading, especially after the birth of Twin *A*. One is never sure which fetal pole (or other presenting part) will enter the pelvis first after the delivery of the first twin. If possible, one would prefer to avoid an internal podalic version. If the fetus is in a vertex oblique presentation, the head can be gently guided into the pelvis once the physician is aware of the exact position of the head. If the second twin presents as an oblique breech, then the same external manipulation can be accomplished with the help of ultrasound.

Real-time ultrasound is of greatest benefit when the second twin remains in a transverse lie with the back facing up. It is possible to direct the operator's hand with real-time through intact membranes to both feet of the fetus. Internal podalic version can then be accomplished expeditiously after artificial rupture of membranes.

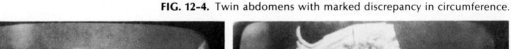

FIG. 12-4. Twin abdomens with marked discrepancy in circumference.

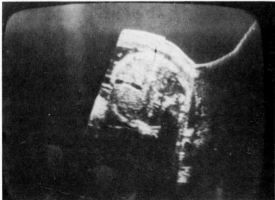
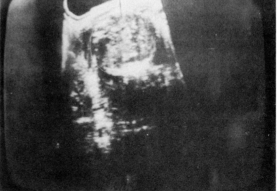

This technique has been so useful that a real-time machine is brought into our delivery room in all twin deliveries.

INTRAUTERINE FETAL DEMISE (IUFD)

About 1% of all pregnancies result in intrauterine fetal death. This condition not only is emotionally devastating to the patient but also represents a significant physical threat to her if the pregnancy is not terminated within a month of the fetal demise. Today it is possible to effect delivery with prostaglandin E_2 suppositories as soon as the condition is appreciated. For these reasons, it is preferable to make the diagnosis as early as possible. Today, with compact doppler devices, one should hear the fetal heart by the 12th week of gestation. Failure to hear a fetal heart does not preclude a viable pregnancy but strongly suggests fetal death. The diagnosis is easily confirmed by noting an absence of fetal heart motion with real time. There will also be no fetal limb motion. Other signs of fetal death often quoted in the literature are the finding of gas in the abdomen (Robert's sign), overlapping skull bones (Spaulding's sign), a skull halo, and a distorted fetal configuration. These findings can be demonstrated with x-ray or ultrasound. Their presence is, however, academic, since all are late sequelae of IUFD, and fetal death can be diagnosed with real time as soon as the heart stops beating.

A note of caution should be injected here. Occasionally, one can identify low-level artifactual echoes in the area of the heart. Since the physician is often eagerly hoping to see fetal heart motion, he should not be misled into diagnosing fetal life by wishful thinking.

AMNIOCENTESIS

Amniotic fluid is a rich source of fetal information, and there are many occasions, some emergent, where management of the patient is based on this information. For example, if a laboring patient is febrile on admission, amnionitis should always be considered as a possible source, even in the absence of rupture of membranes. Once other sources of infection have been excluded, an amniocentesis can often be accomplished with the aid of ultrasound and the fluid examined for the presence of bacteria. A positive tap is always associated with amnionitis, but the absence of bacteria does not always preclude the patient's developing the condition.

Amniotic fluid plays an important role in other clinical situations. It is very useful to know the status of the fetal lungs by lecithin-sphingomyelin (L/S) ratio, shake test, or any other index of pulmonic maturity in a high-risk patient whose condition is worsening. In an unregistered patient whose history is compatible with postterm pregnancy, the best indicator of postmaturity syndrome is meconium-stained amniotic fluid. This fluid must, however, be safely obtained, and since amniotic fluid volume normally decreases in late gestation, the procedure is potentially dangerous. With ultrasound, however, it is possible to identify a pocket of fluid away from vital fetal parts even in the presence of oligohydramnios.

It is preferable to avoid the placenta, and in 50% of cases where the placenta is anteriorly implanted, one can find a placenta-free window through which to insert a needle. If placental penetration is unavoidable because of the location of amniotic fluid pockets, then an area is selected away from the ultrasonically demonstrated umbilical cord insertion.

Available pockets of amniotic fluid depend on the position of the fetus. In most cases the fetus at term is on its side. There is very little fluid in the area of the fetal back, but there is almost always fluid in the area of the arms and legs (Fig. 12–5). Even in the presence of ruptured membranes, one can often find a small pocket of fluid beneath the fetal chin or lateral to a thigh. The umbilical cord must, however, be assiduously avoided. Little fluid accumulates in the often-used nuchal area. Here, if the cord is around the neck, it can be penetrated more easily than when it is floating freely in the amniotic cavity. For these reasons the nuchal tap is hazardous. The suprapubic approach is very useful if the head is not deep in the maternal pelvis and the bladder is empty. The head must be elevated with one hand while the needle is inserted with the other. We have often used a vacutainer in these cases to

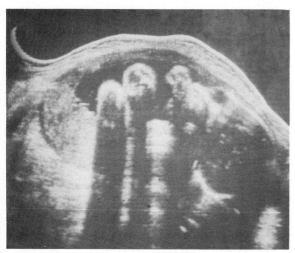

FIG. 12-5. Scans through fetal limbs—normal amount of amniotic fluid.

diminish the need for syringe manipulation, which requires another hand.

If bloody fluid is encountered, it is almost always maternal blood that enters the cavity from the penetrated intervillous space. This blood clots rapidly on the fetal surface, and with a little patience, clear fluid can be obtained once syringes are changed and more fluid aspirated. If the amniotic fluid in the uterine cavity does not clear rapidly, then the fetal heart should be monitored and a sample of fluid analyzed for the presence of fetal cells. Although fetal exsaguination has been reported (9), this is an unlikely complication if the amniocentesis is performed carefully and if fetal heart rate monitoring is done after a traumatic tap.

With experience one can carefully weigh the risk of the procedure against the benefits obtained from an amniocentesis, especially in the patient on the delivery floor. Armed with ultrasonically derived information, the physician can best decide when *not* to tap.

EVALUATION OF POSSIBLE INTRAUTERINE GROWTH RETARDATION (IUGR) IN THE PREVIOUSLY UNSTUDIED PATIENT

Since a growth-retarded fetus is at greater risk of intrapartum asphyxia, stillbirth, and neonatal problems, it is extremely important to identify these fetuses before labor (5). In many cases the fetus should be delivered rather than be subjected to further time in an alien intrauterine environment. In the third trimester the BPD alone is of little help as a single examination to diagnose IUGR, simply because a smaller than expected BPD could indicate erroneous dates, and an appropriate for dates BPD could mislead the physician into excluding the diagnosis of IUGR in a growth-retarded fetus with head-to-body disproportion (a phenomenon inappropriately labeled "brain sparing"). Since in most cases of IUGR, oligohydramnios is the rule and since by definition the body mass of a growth-retarded fetus is diminished, measurements of total intrauterine volume (TIUV) reflect these changes. The TIUV is calculated by measuring ultrasonically the longest diameter between the fundus and a point at the level of the internal cervical os (length), the greatest distance between side walls (width), and the largest dimension between anterior and posterior uterine walls (thickness). The TIUV is calculated from a formula appropriate for an ellipse (L × W × Th × 0.5233). A nomogram has been constructed from data in normal pregnancies (3). Thus far, in patients where the TIUV has been within one standard deviation of the mean for gestation as indicated by simultaneous BPD, there has been no evidence of IUGR at birth (Fig. 12-6). Conversely, it is rare for an infant not to have IUGR when the TIUV has been more than two standard deviations below the mean for gestation indicated by simultaneous BPD. This screening test has been very accurate in including or excluding the diagnosis. More information about the cause and severity of IUGR can, however, be ascertained from measurement of head circumference, abdominal circumference, serial BPDs, and ultrasonic evaluation of fetal organs and spine.

DETERMINATION OF FETAL MATURITY THROUGH ULTRASONIC GRADING OF PLACENTAL MORPHOLOGY

On occasion a pregnant woman may be admitted to the delivery floor in early labor but with-

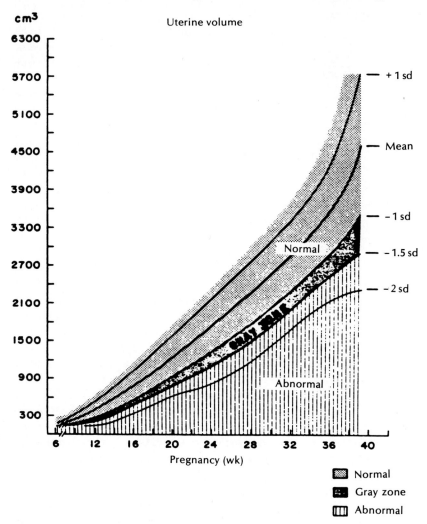

cm³

Uterine volume

FIG. 12-6. Total intrauterine volume. (Gohari P, Berkowitz RL, Hobbins JC: Am J Obstet Gynecol 127:250, 1977)

out reliable historic information regarding gestational age. If the L/S ratio indicates that the fetal pulmonary system is not mature the physician should attempt to inhibit labor with tocolytic agents. However, in a pregnancy associated with oligohydramnios or a large anterior placenta, withdrawal of amniotic fluid for determination of L/S ratio may be impossible. Under these circumstances knowledge of fetal pulmonary status may be indirectly derived from the placenta.

Based on ultrasonically derived information, a classification of placental maturity has been designed (4). Placental grading (grade 0 through grade III) is based on morphologic changes in the region of the chorionic plate, the basal plate, and the intervening placental substance. These criteria are summarized in Table 12–1 and are schematically represented in Fig. 12–7.

In correlating placental grading with demonstration of fetal pulmonic status by L/S ratio obtained at the time of the scan, it has been noted thus far that in all cases where grade III placentas were noted, the L/S ratios were indicative of fetal pulmonic maturity (greater than 2) and the infants did not develop RDS. This cor-

TABLE 12-1. SUMMARY OF PLACENTAL GRADING

	Grade O	Grade I	Grade II	Grade III
Chorionic plate	Straight and well-defined	Subtle undulations	Indentations extending into but not to the basal layer	Indentations communicating with the basal layer
Placental substance	Homogeneous	Few scattered echogenic areas	Linear echogenic densities (comma-like densities)	Circular densities with echo-spared areas in center; large irregular densities which cast acoustic shadowing
Basal layer	No densities	No densities	Linear arrangement of small echogenic areas (basal stippling)	Large and somewhat confluent basal echogenic areas; can create acoustic shadows

(Grannum PAT, Berkowitz RL, Hobbins JC: Am J Obstet Gynecol 133(8):915, 1979)

FIG. 12-7. Ultrasonic classification of placental maturity, grade 0 through grade III. (Grannum PAT, Berkowitz RL, Hobbins JC: Am J Obstet Gynecol 133[8]:915, 1979)

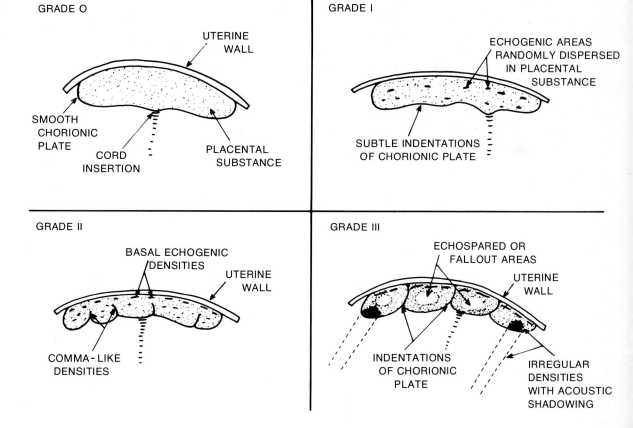

relation was noted to occur as early as 33 weeks in pregnancies complicated by fetal growth retardation and/or hypertension. Although grade II placentas were often associated with L/S ratios of greater than 2, the association was by no means invariable.

If further studies continue to demonstrate a consistent correlation between the finding of a grade III placenta and the absence of RDS, then in those cases where the patient's dates are unknown and delivery is desired, it may be possible to circumvent the need for an invasive procedure if a grade III placenta is noted during ultrasound examination.

CONCLUSION

It is feasible that soon in most obstetric services an ultrasound machine will be available for 24-hour use. It is imperative that physicians be properly trained in ultrasound so that these machines will be used responsibly. Five-day ultrasound courses do not provide sufficient experience. Some residency programs are now incorporating "on-the-job" training courses, so that within a few years physicians will be comfortable in ordering and sometimes performing and interpreting scans. The scans will provide the physicians with the information needed to help them with the obstetric dilemmas discussed in this chapter, and the uses for this modality will then be limited only by one's imagination.

REFERENCES

1. BERKOWITZ RL: Premature rupture of membranes: a review and treatment plan. Contemp Ob/Gyn 10:35, 1977

2. COOPERBERG PL, CHOW T, KITE V, AUSTIN S: Biparietal diameter: a comparison of real-time and conventional B scan techniques. J Clin Ultrasound 4:421, 1976

3. GOHARI P, BERKOWITZ RL, HOBBINS JC: Prediction of intrauterine growth retardation by determination of total intrauterine volume. Am J Obstet Gynecol 127:250, 1977

4. GRANNUM PAT, BERKOWITZ RL, HOBBIN JC: The ultrasonic changes in the maturing placenta and their relation to fetal pulmonic maturity. Am J Obstet Gynecol 133(8): 915, 1979

5. HOBBINS JC, WINSBERG F: Ultrasound in Obstetrics and Gynecology. Baltimore, Williams & Wilkins, 1977

6. LEVENO KJ, SANTOS-RAMOS R, WHALLEY PJ, DUENHOELTER JH: Sonar cephalometry in twins: a comparison with singleton fetuses and an evaluation of twin discordancy. SGI Abstract 153, presented at Society for Gynecologic Investigation, Atlanta, March, 1978

7. RANNEY B: The gentle art of external cephalic version. Am J Obstet Gynecol 116:239, 1973

8. ROVINSKY JJ, MILLER JA, KAPLAN S: Management of breech presentation at term. Am J Obstet Gynecol 115:497, 1973

9. RYAN ET, FACO G, IVY R: Fetal bleeding as a major hazard of amniocentesis. Obstet Gynecol 40:702, 1972

10. THOMPSON JF: Perinatal mortality in breech presentation. Obstet Gynecol 15:415, 1960

11. WARSOF SL, GOHARI P, BERKOWITZ RL, HOBBINS JC: Estimation of fetal weight by computer-assisted analysis of fetal dimensions. Am J Obstet Gynecol 128:881, 1977

13

A comparison of antenatal tests

Y. B. GORDON, J. G. GRUDZINSKAS

The basic aim of modern perinatal medicine is the prevention of mortality and morbidity. Antenatal care is geared to achieving this aim by the identification of patients at risk and the institution of the appropriate diagnostic and therapeutic measures. During the past two decades there has been an explosion in the use of biochemical (22, 30) and ultrasonic (5) methods for monitoring fetal well-being. The aim of the present review is to compare biochemical tests with ultrasonic measurements of the conceptus and placenta with a view to highlighting the advantages and limitations of the two methods. This review is divided into four sections: methodology, the diagnosis of pregnancy, the detection of congenital abnormalities, and fetal risk in late pregnancy.

METHODOLOGY

The measurement of biologic parameters by biochemical, electronic, or biophysical means has an inherent methodologic source of error. If the variation in the method is added to the biologic variation, the range of "normal" becomes wide; thus in all but the most gross abnormalities, there is likely to be overlap between normal and abnormal. The potential sources of error have been well described for biochemical tests of fetal well-being (9, 22), and it is incumbent on the investigator to reduce the imprecision to a minimum.

The biochemical tests of fetal well-being currently performed on maternal blood involve the measurement of protein and steroid molecules produced by the fetus and placenta. The selection of a marker of fetoplacental function is determined by the available laboratory expertise and facilities and the type of molecule, its range in normal pregnancy, its physiologic variations, and the ease of access to the compartment in which it is present. Since the development of specific steroid assays the measurement of maternal plasma levels of estrogens is likely to supersede the traditional determination of 24-hour urinary estrogen levels (13, 30). In addition fetoplacental protein molecules in the maternal circulation are commonly used as an index of fetal well-being (Fig. 13–1). The technique of measurement of these molecules is primarily radioimmunoassay (RIA). The technique involves no risk to the patient, and the major advantages are the following: 1) High sensitivity can be achieved because full advantage is taken of the avidity of the antibody. 2) The specificity of RIA is due to the close "fit" essential for the antigen–antibody interactions; thus an assay for the β-subunit of chorionic gonadotrophins (hCG) permits a clear distinction from pituitary gonadotrophins, though luteinizing hormone is chemically similar (45); likewise it is possible to

Placental proteins

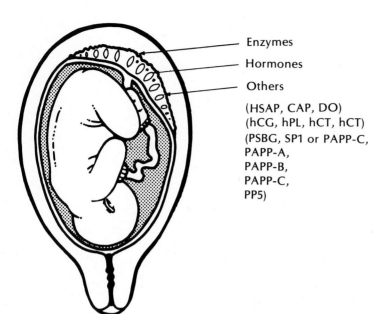

Enzymes

Hormones

Others

(HSAP, CAP, DO)
(hCG, hPL, hCT, hCT)
(PSBG, SP1 or PAPP-C,
PAPP-A,
PAPP-B,
PAPP-C,
PP5)

FIG. 13-1. Proteins produced by the human placenta: heat-stable alkaline phosphatase (HSAP); cystine amino peptidase (CAP); diamine oxidase (DO); human chorionic gonadotrophin (hCG); human placental lactogen (hPL); human chorionic thyrotrophin (hCT); pregnancy-specific β_1 glycoprotein (PSβG, SP$_1$); pregnancy-associated plasma proteins A, B, and C (PAPP-A, PAPP-B, PAPP-C); placental protein 5 (PP5).

distinguish between estradiol (E_2) and estriol (E_3) when specific antisera are used. 3) RIA can be automated; this permits a sample throughput of 20,000 tests/technician/annum at low unit cost. The major disadvantages of RIA are first, the interassay variation, which may exceed 15% and thus make interpretation of results difficult (7, 22). The second and more important disadvantage of RIA is the dissociation between biologic and immunologic activity, because the antigenic sites on a protein are often unrelated to that portion of the molecule responsible for its biologic potency (22). The molecule may be partly degraded (16), or bound to a protein (4), or it may circulate in a precursor form and retain its antigenicity (41). The other difficulty in the interpretation of circulating levels of pregnancy-"specific" molecules is that their biologic activity is unknown (9).

Biochemical tests of fetal well-being performed on amniotic fluid can be divided into a number of groups. These include the following measurements: of specific enzymes in cultured cells in the diagnosis of metabolic disorders (14), of α-fetoprotein (AFP) by RIA for neural tube defects (3, 24), of bilirubin in Rhesus isoimmunisation (35), and of amniotic phospholipids in the assessment of fetal lung maturation (19). The major problem associated with the use of amniotic fluid is that amniocentesis is an invasive procedure and there is a risk of abortion, premature labour, fetomaternal transfusion, and injury to the fetus (21, 37), and mother. In addition, enzyme and chromosomal analyses are expensive, time consuming, and occasionally unreliable, and the vast majority of fetal abnormalities are not detected, because they occur in women with a clinical history that does not indicate the need for amniocentesis.

The major advantages of ultrasonography are as follows: 1) It is noninvasive, and there is no evidence at present that intracellular function is altered after multiple exposures to ultrasound at diagnostic power levels during pregnancy (43); 2) Recent technical advances such as the scan converter have permitted better definition of fetal structures (5); 3) With the advent of real-time scanning, a dynamic assessment of fetal function can now be made (Ch. 18, 28). The major disadvantages are that the equipment is expensive and the technique is time consuming, particularly when used to assess fetal breathing.

THE DIAGNOSIS OF PREGNANCY

Since the development of specific radioimmunoassays for the β-subunit of hCG (45), pregnancy can be diagnosed within 12 days of conception (Fig. 13–2). Radioreceptor assays are more sensitive but less specific because there is cross-reaction with luteinizing hormone (31). There are several major potential uses of these systems. The first is to quantitate the incidence of unrecognized abortions and thus define the role of abortion as a filter mechanism for fetal abnormalities. Second, termination of pregnancy by menstrual regulation can now be selectively performed within days of the first missed menstrual period; thus unnecessary interference is avoided in up to 30% of subjects with prolonged menstrual cycles who have not conceived (15). The measurement of circulating levels of pregnancy-specific β_1-glycoprotein

(SP$_1$, PSβG, or PAPP-C) is a recent addition to the biochemical armamentarium in early pregnancy (25, 26) (Fig. 13–3), and, though SP$_1$ is detectable later than hCG, its measurement is valuable in subjects who have received gonadotrophins during the luteal phase of the conceptual cycle.

A variety of biochemical parameters have been used in the assessment of patients with a threatened abortion. These include maternal plasma levels of hCG, AFP, and human placental lactogen (hPL) (18, 38). Although depressed hPL levels provide the most accurate biochemical prediction of inevitable abortion (38), the high incidence of false-positive and false-negative results indicates that ultrasonographic evaluation of the conceptus is the method of choice.

The gestation sac can be reliably visualized by use of ultrasound from 3 weeks after conception

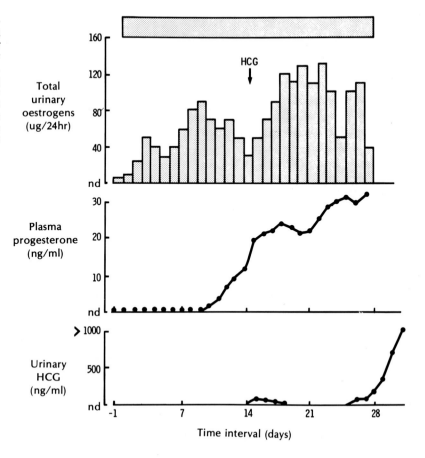

FIG. 13–2. Diagnosis of pregnancy in patient with anorexia nervosa using a specific RIA for hCG. Ovulation was induced by use of LH/FSH-RH and hCG. Conception occurred, resulting in delivery at 40 weeks' gestation. Immunoreactive hCG was detected transiently in the urine after the initial injection; it subsequently reappeared on the 11th day after ovulation.

and the increase in size of the embryo monitored throughout the first trimester by measurement of the crown–rump length (40). The technique is useful in determining the gestational age, fetal life, and multiple pregnancy, as well as abnormalities of early pregnancy such as anembryonic and ectopic gestation.

THE DETECTION OF CONGENITAL ABNORMALITIES

Perinatal mortality has been declining progressively during the past two decades, and congenital abnormalities of the fetus now account for an increasing proportion of perinatal deaths (8). Congenital abnormalities are the major cause of severe mental retardation (27), a condition that represents a massive financial and sociologic burden, both for the family unit and the state.

At present it is technically possible to diagnose chromosomal and biochemical abnormalities of the fetus by means of specific assay systems using amniotic fluid. However, because amniocentesis is an invasive procedure that is potentially hazardous (21, 37) and time consuming, universal screening is limited to ultrasonic assessment of the fetus or to biochemical tests performed on maternal blood. The ultrasonic diagnosis of congenital abnormalities is described in Chapter 19.

Central nervous system abnormalities are the commonest cause of perinatal mortality associated with fetal malformations in Britain (8). With the advent of specific RIA for AFP it is now possible to screen all pregnant subjects for an open neural tube defect of the fetus, anencephaly, or spina bifida by use of a maternal blood sample (11, 15, 34, 39). In the presence of an open neural tube defect, large quantities of AFP and other larger proteins escape into the amniotic fluid from the fetal circulation via capillaries exposed on the surface of the defect (4, 24) (Fig. 13–4). A similar mechanism exists in exomphalos, where the vessels surrounding the bowel are exposed (10). The amniotic fluid AFP is then transferred in excessive concentrations into the maternal circulation.

FIG. 13-3. Plasma concentrations of SP$_1$ in nine subjects after conception.

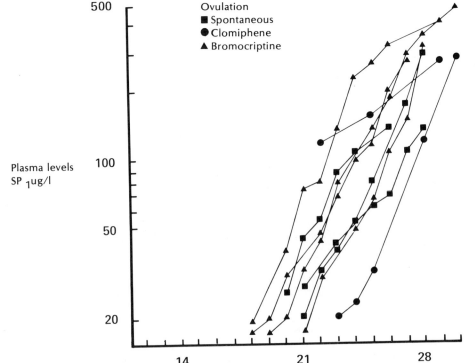

The optimal time to perform a maternal plasma AFP estimation is between the 16th and 20th weeks of pregnancy (Fig. 13–5). At this time the false-negative rate (ie, normal AFP levels in the presence of a neural tube defect) is lowest at about 10% (34, 39), and termination of pregnancy is still feasible. However, elevated maternal plasma AFP levels also occur in a variety of other conditions, including 2% of normal pregnant subjects (34), 50% of multiple pregnancies (11), threatened and missed abortion (11), and abnormalities of the fetal gastrointestinal tract (10), kidney (29), and skin (47). All these conditions constitute false-positive results (ie, raised AFP levels in the absence of a neural tube defect), and the diagnosis must be proved either by the measurement of AFP in amniotic fluid obtained after amniocentesis or by use of Gray-scale ultrasound to outline the fetal head, spinal column, and abdomen. The noninvasive nature of ultrasonography and the potential to diagnose exomphalos make this procedure the method of choice, but false-negative results may occur (Ch. 19). If Gray-scale ultrasound facilities are not available, an amniocentesis must be performed and the amniotic fluid AFP level measured, after the gestational age has been confirmed and multiple pregnancy and intrauterine death excluded by use of conventional ultrasonic techniques. The incidence of open neural tube defect in Britain is around 4/1000 births, and 20/1000 normal pregnant subjects have consistently elevated AFP levels (34), so that 1–6 patients undergoing amniocentesis could be expected to have a neural tube defect (21).

In our recent survey of 102 amniocenteses performed on the basis of elevated maternal serum AFP levels, there were 16 neural tube defects and two cases with exomphalos, one of whom had multiple abnormalities, and the second was surgically correctable (21). However, three spontaneous abortions of unaffected fetuses followed the amniocenteses, some of which were performed without ultrasonic direction. Placental puncture occurred in two of the three subjects who aborted. Since efficient ultrasonic examination is essential to exclude other causes of raised maternal AFP levels, the availability of an experienced ultrasound unit must be re- garded as a sine qua non of any program for the detection of congenital abnormalities of the fetus in which amniocentesis is performed. It is unlikely, however, that ultrasonic diagnosis of neural tube defects will replace maternal plasma AFP screening because visualization of the fetal spine is time consuming and expensive, whereas AFP estimations are inexpensive, and a single laboratory can test up to 50,000 samples per year.

FETAL RISK IN LATE PREGNANCY

Although perinatal mortality has now fallen below 20/1000 in Britain, this is substantially above the theoretic minimum, and for every child who dies there will be others who are severely and permanently damaged. Antenatal care is geared to the prevention of morbidity and mortality by identifying patients at risk and instituting diagnostic and therapeutic measures. The cornerstone of antenatal care remains the clinical examination, but with the advent of biochemical and biophysical methods for monitoring fetal well-being (5, 22), the precision of antenatal diagnosis has been considerably improved. The two main questions that these ancillary diagnostic aids must answer are, first, whether it is possible to detect high-risk patients and second, when delivery should be undertaken in the high-risk group. The identification of high-risk subjects involves the detection of subclinical obstetric disease by the use of routine screening programmes and also the confirmation of a clinical suspicion of fetal risk. Once the high-risk group has been identified, continuing surveillance of the fetus is essential because the timing of delivery is critical to ensure that the risks of prematurity do not outweigh the risk of intrauterine asphyxia and malnutrition.

The cornerstone of biochemical tests of fetal well-being was the elucidation of the pathways of estrogen synthesis and metabolism (12). Specific radioimmunoassays now allow the specific measurement of circulating estrogens in maternal plasma, but the controversy about urinary versus blood estrogen determination continues, and the question of the appropriate blood estrogen to be measured remains unresolved (44).

Dynamic tests of fetoplacental function such as the dehydroepiandrosterone sulfate loading test require further evaluation (32). Knowledge of estrogen metabolism, the development of inexpensive assays, and the attractive concept of measuring fetoplacental rather than placental function have resulted in widespread use of estrogen assays. Their use has, however, not yet been justified by prospective studies.

THE PREDICTION OF FETAL RISK

There is still widespread scepticism about the real value of biochemical tests in screening for the detection of high-risk pregnancies. Published studies are unhelpful, presenting a retrospective assessment in which high-risk groups are compared with a test rather than the test with the entire obstetric population (9). Rarely, if at all, is the test described in the context in which it is presented to the clinician, namely, as one of a number of potential risk parameters in an individual patient in whom the risk cannot be determined until the child is delivered. Even more rarely is the biochemical test directly compared with other clinical or biophysical parameters of fetal risk. For example, is the observation of low serum hPL or estrogens more or less ominous than the observation that the mother has low weight or hypertension or that the fetus has poor growth on ultrasonic examination?

To study the value of one biochemical parameter, maternal plasma hPL levels, we have recently completed a prospective survey of the entire obstetric population who delivered at St. Bartholomew's Hospital during 1976 (23). The analysis was confined to 1029 singleton deliveries after the 28th week of gestation. The population was divided into two groups: the high fetal risk group consisted of 104 (10.1%) babies with a birthweight below the 5th centile for gestation, or a perinatal death, or a major congenital abnormality, or an Apgar score of 3 or less at 1 min; the remaining 925 (89.9%) subjects served as controls. The relative fetal risk for each parameter was computed by use of the ratio of true-positive results as a fraction of all the positive results to false-negative results as a fraction of all the negative results (Table 13–1). The analysis

showed that high hPL values were associated with a low relative risk factor (0.2), whereas consistently depressed values were associated with increased risk (2.9). In comparative terms the observation of low hPL indicated a higher risk than any other parameter with the exception of a severely elevated diastolic blood pressure (> 110 mm Hg) and fetal distress in labor. Absolute maternal weight measurement at 32 weeks was a useful indicator of high fetal risk, whereas weight gain in the second half of pregnancy was of minimal diagnostic value. In this study the ultrasonic assessment of the fetal biparietal diameter was performed only between 18 and 22 weeks' gestation and was not useful in predicting fetal risk; however, the biparietal measurement was crucial in the assessment of the gestational age in 20% of subjects with uncertain dates. The major advantage of hPL, like AFP, is that the test can be performed inexpensively on all pregnant subjects, and though some subjects with depressed levels delivered normal babies, it is a valuable addition to the antenatal diagnosis of fetal risk.

Pregnancy-specific β_1 glycoprotein (SP$_1$, PSβG) is a placental "specific" protein synthesized by the syncytiotrophoblast throughout pregnancy (20, 25). It has been evaluated in the prediction of intrauterine growth retardation of the fetus, and up to 70% of subjects show depressed levels (Fig. 13–6) (20, 42). It will be of interest to compare the clinical use of SP$_1$ with that of hPL because the two molecules differ in

---

FIG. 13-4. Levels of AFP and FgE after chromatography of amniotic fluid from a normal pregnancy and pregnancies associated with open spina bifida and anencephaly on a 2.5- × 100-cm Agarose (Biogel A 1.5m) column. The void volume and the expected elution patterns of fibrinogen, AFP, and FgE standards are indicated by arrows. In the presence of a neural tube defect, intact fibrinogen escapes into the amniotic fluid via exposed capillaries on the surface of the defect, whereas in normal pregnancy only smaller sized degradation fragments are present.

FIG. 13-5. Median and 95th centile of maternal plasma AFP throughout normal pregnancy (**solid lines**). Single or serial levels of maternal AFP are shown for patients with a fetus having either anencephalus (•) or open spina bifida (o). Serial levels in individual cases are joined by interrupted lines.

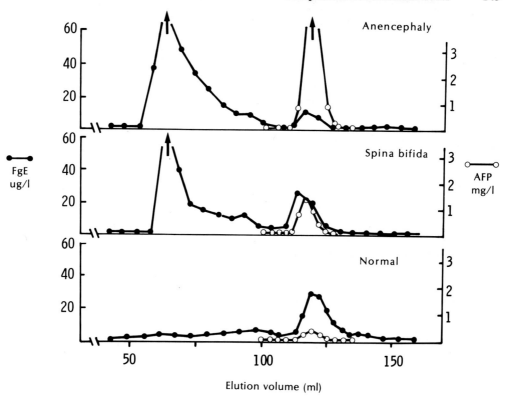

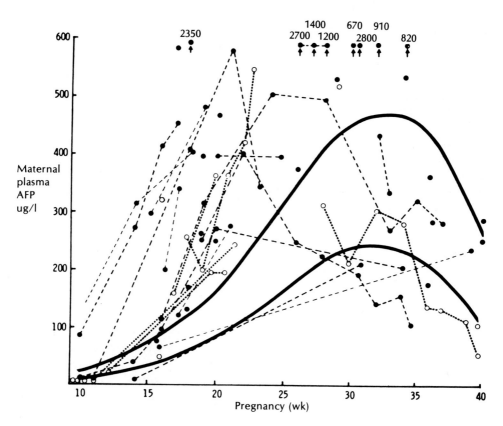

TABLE 13-1. THE RELATIVE RISK AS AN INDEX OF FETAL WELL-BEING

Parameter studied	Relative risk
hPL levels after 30 weeks >90th centile	0.2*
Mild essential hypertension (diastolic blood pressure 90–110 mm Hg)	0.5
Average weekly weight gain (20–40 weeks) >90th centile	0.5
Maternal weight at 32 weeks >90th centile	0.6
Nonsmokers	0.6†
Threatened abortion	0.6
Average weekly weight gain (20–40 weeks) <10th centile	0.7
Previous perinatal death (multiparous subjects)	0.7
Maternal age <20 years	1.0
Mild preeclampsia (diastolic blood pressure 90–110 mm Hg, no albuminuria)	1.0
Biparietal diameter (weeks 18–22)	1.1
Non-Caucasian ethnic origin	1.3
Elevated maternal AFP levels (weeks 16–20)	1.3
Antepartum hemorrhage	1.3
Maternal cardiac, renal, gastrointestinal diseases	1.3
Meconium-stained amniotic fluid in labor	1.7
Maternal weight at 32 weeks <10th centile	1.8*
Smoking >15 per day at booking	2.0†
Maternal age >34 years	2.4†
hPL levels after 30 weeks <10th centile	2.9‡
Fetal heart abnormality (in 1st stage of labor)	3.2‡
Severe preeclampsia and essential hypertension	8.6‡

Chi-squared test: significant at 5% level*, 1% level†, 0.1% level‡.

size and half-life, and the circulating levels of SP_1 are 50-fold greater than hPL in the third trimester.

Comparative studies (6, 46) evaluating serial ultrasonic cephalometry and urinary estrogen estimations in the assessment of "at risk" pregnancies showed that serial ultrasonography was superior to estrogen assays in the detection of growth retardation of the fetus and the prediction of perinatal asphyxia. At present, however, there are no prospective studies comparing the use of ultrasonic parameters with biochemical parameters in the prediction of fetal risk in an obstetric population. In our prospective survey midtrimester biparietal diameter measurements were less reliable than third-trimester hPL values on fetal risk prediction; however, it will be of interest to see whether ultrasonic measurement of fetal head and abdominal circumferences and fetal breathing patterns will increase the rate of prediction of the high-risk group (23).

THE TIMING OF DELIVERY

The timing of delivery in high-risk pregnancies is one of the most difficult problems in antenatal care. With the advent of amniotic fluid phospholipid determinations it is now possible to predict the likelihood of development of the respiratory distress syndrome after delivery, and this represents a major advance in antenatal diagnosis (19). A fall in circulating levels of hPL of SP_1 cannot be used as an aid, because the levels fall only after actual or incipient fetal demise. The clinical usefulness of these two tests ends after the diagnosis of fetal risk has been made. For many years falling estriol levels have been used as a parameter of incipient fetal demise (1). However, the measurement of a true fall is very difficult, particularly when urinary estriol levels are measured, because the day-to-day variation is 30% in normal subjects and a drop from 15 mg to 10 mg/24 hours may merely reflect problems of urine collection and assay variation. The variation in plasma estrogen values, measured by radioimmunoassay, is lower than that found in the urine (1, 30), but the assays showing lowest day-to-day variation are hPL and SP_1 (36). It should therefore be possible to detect falling estriol levels with greater accuracy by use of plasma assays. However, in a randomized study of high-risk pregnancies, plasma estriol levels were found to be of limited

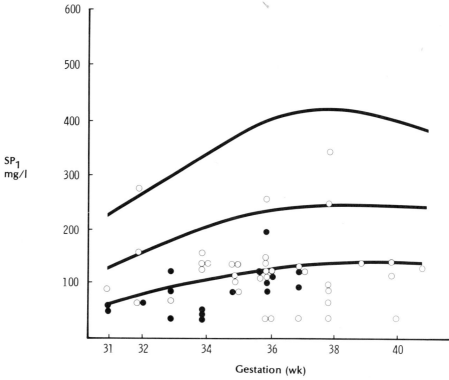

FIG. 13-6. Median, 10th, and 90th centiles of maternal plasma SP_1 (PSβG) after the 30th week of normal pregnancy **(solid lines).** The SP_1 concentrations are shown for pregnancies with (•) and without (o) maternal hypertension in which there was IUGR of the fetus.

value in the timing of delivery and a significant number of false-positive results occurred in the control group (13).

Measurement of fetal growth by ultrasound does not provide the answer about when delivery should be undertaken. A reduction in the rate of growth of the biparietal diameter of the fetal skull or abdominal or head circumferences merely highlights the group at risk. With the introduction of real-time ultrasound it is now possible to monitor fetal breathing patterns (2). It is likely that this technique will be a valuable adjunct to the management of high-risk pregnancies, because an alteration in fetal breathing has been shown to be an accurate predictor of incipient fetal death in lambs. At present, however, the most widely used parameter is antenatal cardiotography with or without the aid of an oxytocin challenge test (17, 33).

The two major criteria of any test of fetal well-being are accuracy of prediction and ease and safety of performance. Ultrasonography has the advantages of safety and ease of performance; however, apart from the determination of fetal life and the measurement of the biparietal diameter, the quantitation of other vital parameters may be time consuming. With the exception of hCG determinations in early pregnancy, the most accurate biochemical parameters are those performed on the amniotic fluid. This compartment is in closest proximity to the fetus, but amniocentesis is an invasive and potentially hazardous procedure. When the investigation moves from the amniotic fluid into the maternal compartment, tests of fetal well-being compromise the accuracy of their predictive value because of maternal metabolism of the circulating molecules. But tests on maternal blood form the basis for safe, inexpensive screening procedures. There can be little doubt that the quality and precision of antenatal care has been substantially improved as a result of the introduction of biochemical and biophysical techniques for the assessment of fetal well-being.

REFERENCES

1. BEISCHER NA, BROWN JB: Current status of estrogen assays in obstetrics and gynaecology. Obstet Gynaecol Rev 27:303, 1972

2. BODDY K: Fetal circulation and breathing movements. In Beard RW, Nathanielsz PW (eds): Fetal Physiology and Medicine. Philadelphia, Saunders, 1976, p 302

3. BROCK DJH, SUTCLIFFE RG: Alphafetoprotein in the antenatal diagnosis of anencephaly and spina bifida. Lancet 2:197, 1972

4. BURKE CW: Accurate measurement of steroid-protein binding by steady state gel filtration. Biochim Biophys Acta 176:403, 1969

5. CAMPBELL S: Fetal growth. In Beard RW, Nathanielsz PW (eds): Fetal Physiology and Medicine. London, Saunders, 1976, p 271

6. CAMPBELL S, KURJAK A: Comparison between urinary estrogen assay and serial ultrasonic cephalometry in the assessment of fetal growth retardation. Br Med J 4:336, 1972

7. CHALLAND GS, CHARD T: Quality control in a radioimmunoassay: observations on the operation of a semi-automated assay for human placental lactogen. Clin Chim Acta 46:133, 1973

8. CHAMBERLAIN R: Illness of the baby. In British Births, 1970, Vol 1. London, William Heinemann, 1975, p 118

9. CHARD T: Normality and abnormality. In Klopper A (ed): Plasma Hormone Assays in Evaluation of Fetal Wellbeing. Edinburgh, Churchill Livingstone, 1976, p 1

10. CLARKE PC, GORDON YB, KITAU MJ, MCNEAL AD, CHARD T: Alphafetoprotein levels in pregnancies complicated by gastro-intestinal abnormalities of the fetus. Br J Obstet Gynaecol 84:285, 1977

11. CLARKE PC, GORDON YB, LETCHWORTH AT, KITAU MJ, CHARD T: A pilot study of screening for neural tube defects by maternal blood alphafetoprotein determination in a complete population. Br J Obstet Gynaecol 84:568, 1977

12. DICZFALUSY E: Steroid metabolism in the fetoplacental unit. In Pecile A, Finzi C (eds): The Fetoplacental Unit. Amsterdam, Excerpta Medica Foundation, 1969, p 65

13. DUENHOELTER JH, WHALLEY PJ, MACDONALD PC: Analysis of the utility of plasma immunoreactive estrogen measurements in determining the delivery time of gravidas with a fetus considered to be at high risk. Am J Obstet Gynecol 125:889, 1976

14. EMERY AEH: Biochemical tests for enzymes in amniotic fluid cell cultures. In Emery AEH (ed): Antenatal Diagnosis of Genetic Disease. Edinburgh, Churchill Livingstone, 1973, p 1

15. Family Planning Digest 2, No. 4, Publ No. (HSM) 73–1600, 1973, p 13. Department of Health, Education and Welfare, Rockville, MD. 20852

16. FORSLING ML, BOYD NRH, CHARD T: The dissociation of the immunological and biological activity of oxytocin: in vivo studies. In Kirkham KE, Hunter WM (eds): Radioimmunoassay Methods. Edinburgh, Churchill Livingstone, 1971, p 549

17. FREEMAN RK: The use of the oxytocin challenge test for antepartum clinical evaluation of uteroplacental respiratory function. Am J Obstet Gynecol 121:481, 1975

18. GAROFF L, SEPPALA M: Prediction of fetal outcome in threatened abortion by maternal serum placental lactogen and alphafetoprotein. Am J Obstet Gynecol 121:257, 1975

19. GLUCK L, KULOVICH MV: Lecithin/sphingomyelin ratios in amniotic fluid in normal and abnormal pregnancy. Am J Obstet Gynecol 115:539, 1973

20. GORDON YB, GRUDZINSKAS JG, JEFFREY D, LETCHWORTH AT, CHARD T: Concentrations of pregnancy specific β_1 glycoprotein in maternal blood in normal pregnancy and in intrauterine growth retardation. Lancet 4:331, 1977

21. GORDON YB, GRUDZINSKAS JG, KITAU MJ, USHERWOOD M MCD, LETCHWORTH AT, CHARD T: Fetal wastage as a result of an alpha-fetoprotein screening programme. Lancet 1(8066):677, 1978

22. GORDON YB, LANDON J: Applications of radioimmunoassay in perinatal medicine. In Scarpelli EM, Cosini EV (eds): Reviews in Perinatal Medicine. New York, Raven Press, 1978, p 173

23. GORDON YB, LEWIS JD, PENDLEBURY DJ et al: Is the measurement of placental function and maternal weight worthwhile? Lancet 1(8072):1001, 1978

24. GORDON YB, RATKY SM, LEIGHTON PC, KITAU MJ, CHARD T: Amniotic fluid levels of fibrin(ogen) degradation fragment E and alphafetoprotein in normal pregnancy and fetal neural tube defects. Br J Obstet Gynaecol 83:77, 1976

25. GRUDZINSKAS JG, GORDON YB, JEFFREY D, CHARD T: Specific and sensitive determination of pregnancy specific β_1 glycoprotein by radioimmunoassay. Lancet 1:333, 1977

26. GRUDZINSKAS JG, LENTON EA, GORDON YB, KELSO IM, JEFFREY D, SOBOWALE O, CHARD T: Circulating levels of pregnancy specific β_1 glycoprotein in early pregnancy. Br J Obstet Gynaecol 84:740, 1977

27. HAGBERG B: Pre-, Peri-, and postnatal prevention of major neuropediatric handicaps. Neuropediatrics 6:331, 1975

28. HULL MGR: The clinical applications of plasma estrogen assays in human late pregnancy. Bibliog Reprod 26:1, 1975

29. KJESSLER B, SHERMAN M, JOHANSSON SGO, GUSTAVSIN K, HULTQVIST G: Alphafetoprotein in antenatal diagnosis of congenital nephrosis. Lancet 1:432, 1975

30. KLOPPER A: Criteria for the selection of steroid assays in the assessment of fetoplacental function. In Klopper A (ed): Plasma Hormone Assays in Fetal Wellbeing. London, Churchill Livingstone, 1976, p 20

31. LANDESMAN R, SAXENA BB: Results of the first 1000 radioreceptorassays for the determination of human chorionic gonadotrophin: a new rapid, reliable and sensitive pregnancy test. Fertil Steril 27:357, 1976

32. LAURITZEN G, STRECKER J, LEHMANN WD: Dynamic tests of placental function: some findings on the conversion of DHAS to estrogens. In Klopper A (ed): Plasma Hormone Assays in Evaluation of Fetal Wellbeing. London, Churchill Livingstone, 1976, p 113

33. LEE CY, DI LORETO PC, LEGRAND B: Fetal activity acceleration determination for the evaluation of fetal reserve. Obstet Gynecol 48:19, 1976

34. LEIGHTON PC, GORDON YB, KITAU MJ, LEEK AE, CHARD T: Levels of alphafetoprotein in maternal blood as a screening test for fetal neural tube defect. Lancet 2:1012, 1975

35. LILEY A: Liquor amnii analysis in management of pregnancy complicated by Rhesus sensitization. Am J Obstet Gynecol 82:1359, 1961

36. MASSON GM, KLOPPER AI, WILSON GR: Plasma estrogens and pregnancy associated plasma proteins. Obstet Gynecol 50:435, 1977

37. MILUNSKY A: Risk of amniocentesis for prenatal diagnosis. N Engl J Med 293:932, 1975

38. NIVEN PAR, LANDON J, CHARD T: Placental lactogen levels as a guide to outcome of threatened abortion. Br Med J 3:799, 1972

39. Report of UK Collaborative Study on Alpha-fetoprotein in relation to neural tube defects. Lancet 1:1323, 1977

40. ROBINSON JP: Sonar measurements of fetal crown-rump lengths as a means of assessing maturity in the first trimester of pregnancy. Br Med J 4:28, 1973

41. STARR IJ, RUBENSTEIN AH: Insulin, proinsulin and C peptide. In Jaffe BM, Behrman HR (eds): Methods of Hormone Radioimmunoassay. New York, Academic Press, 1974, p 239

42. TATRA G, PLACHETA P, BREITENECKER G: Pregnancy specific β_1 glycoprotein (SP$_1$): clinical aspects. Wien Klin Wochenschv 87:279, 1975

43. TAYLOR KJW: Current status of toxicity investigation. J Clin Ultrasound 2:149, 1974

44. TULCHINSKY D: The value of estrogen assays in obstetric disease. In Klopper A (ed): Plasma Hormone Assays in Evaluation of Fetal Wellbeing. London, Churchill Livingstone, 1976, p 72

45. VAITUKAITIS J, BRAUNSTEIN GD, ROSS GT: A radioimmunoassay which specifically measures human chorionic gonadotrophin in the presence of human luteinizing hormone. Am J Obstet Gynecol 113:751, 1972

46. VARMA YR: Prediction of delivery date by ultrasound cephalometry. Br J Obstet Gynaecol 80:316, 1973

47. YACOUB T, CAMPBELL CA, GORDON YB, MANNUCCI N: Maternal serum and amniotic fluid levels of alpha-fetoprotein in epidermolysis bullosa dystrophica 1978, (in preparation)

14

Abnormal pregnancy

ALAN V. CADKIN, RUDY E. SABBAGHA

The gravida who presents with a poor obstetric history, vaginal bleeding, and low abdominal cramping is at high risk of carrying an abnormal pregnancy. With this background, a number of diagnostic possibilities should be considered, Figure 14–1. Although the history, pelvic examination, and laboratory tests may often be useful in excluding some of these possibilities, in many patients, the exact disorder remains obscure. The use of diagnostic ultrasound will, however, lead to a correct diagnosis in the majority. For example, a single ultrasound examination can demonstrate the following: 1) fetal life, 2) placental size and characteristics, and 3) location of the pregnancy, ie, intrauterine or ectopic.

In the evaluation of abnormal pregnancy the sonographer should obtain a good clinical history because this will help in making a definitive diagnosis. Questions should pertain to menstrual dates, results of Doppler examination, and pregnancy test if done. In addition a history of uterine anomalies, infertility, previous abortions, and major medical diseases should be elicited—all of which may predispose to fetal wastage.

This chapter deals with the ultrasonic characteristics of threatened abortions, blighted ova, missed abortions, and hydatidiform moles.

THREATENED ABORTION

In the first trimester of pregnancy a history of vaginal bleeding suggests threatened abortion.

In the ultrasonic examination of such a patient the sonographer should evaluate:

1. Gestational sac: location, appearance, and size in relation to uterus (19).
2. Fetus: presence of fetal echoes, crown–rump length (CRL) (22), and detection of fetal life by real-time or time–motion (T–M) mode (17) imaging, or both. If a live intrauterine pregnancy is demonstrated, the prognosis is favorable, for more than 80% will progress normally (6, 14, 24).
3. Placenta: location, size, and appearance.

A number of abnormalities may be detected by ultrasound in threatened abortion; some of these are characteristic and lead to a definitive diagnosis from the initial ultrasound examination, while others may require later confirmation.

ULTRASONIC FINDINGS PATHOGNOMONIC OF ABNORMAL PREGNANCY

Certain sonographic findings are virtually pathognomonic of an abnormal pregnancy at the initial ultrasound examination.

BLIGHTED OVUM

The diagnosis of blighted ovum is made by demonstrating an intrauterine gestational sac

149

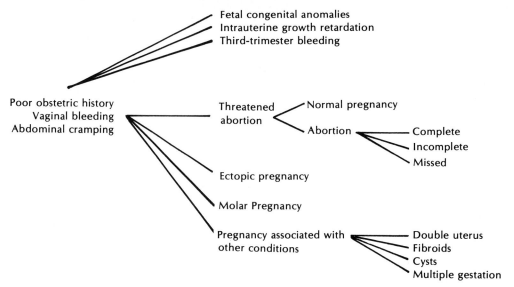

FIG. 14-1. Diagnostic possibilities in high-risk pregnancies (Cadkin AV, Sabbagha RE: COG 20 [2]:266, 1977)

small or appropriate for dates without fetal echoes (20) (anembryonic pregnancy), Figure 14–2. The wall of the gestational sac may appear to be thin, broken, fragmented, or acoustically invisible (Fig. 14–3) because of poor development, degeneration, or necrosis. Note that in many gravidas with a blighted ovum the pregnancy test (urine HCG) remains positive up to the second trimester. Additionally, if by visual inspection of the echogram the gestational sac is 5–7 weeks in size, an interval during which fetal echoes are not normally present, the scan should be repeated in 1–2 weeks before a diagnosis of blighted ovum is made.

FETAL DEATH

The diagnosis of fetal death is made by demonstrating a fetus commensurate with at least a 7 weeks' gestation (mean CRL = 10 mm) without evidence of motion or cardiac activity on real-time imaging or T–M mode (20), or both. Using T–M mode, Robinson demonstrated fetal life with 100% accuracy in patients after 7 weeks of amenorrhea (17). Nonetheless, we feel that inability to trace cardiac motion on T–M mode early in pregnancy necessitates another ultrasound examination at least 1 week later for confirmation of fetal death.

Clinically, in fetal death, spontaneous abortion (incomplete or complete) or missed abortion will follow. Ultrasound can play an important role in the diagnosis and proper management of these patients.

MISSED ABORTION

The sonographic findings in missed abortion vary with the duration of pregnancy and with the time that has elapsed since fetal death, Figure 14–4. The uterus is usually small for dates. There may be degeneration and necrosis of the gestational sac, placenta, or fetus, alone or in combination, and decrease or absence of amniotic fluid, Figure 14–5. If the fetus is acoustically invisible, blighted ovum may be diagnosed. If a fetus is not seen and there is a decrease or absence of amniotic fluid, the ultrasonic picture may be indistinguishable from molar pregnancy, especially if there is hydropic degeneration of the placenta, Figure 14–6.

INCOMPLETE ABORTION

The diagnosis can be established by demonstrating retained products of conception in utero (18).

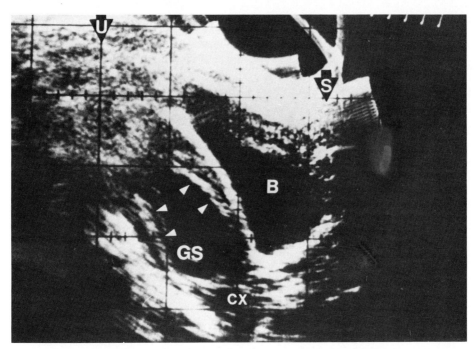

FIG.14-2. U, umbilicus; S, symphysis pubis; Cx, cervix; B, bladder. Blighted ovum in a patient with 14 weeks of amenorrhea, recent onset of bleeding, and a uterus small for dates. Longitudinal midline scan shows a large, empty gestational sac (GS) with a well defined wall **(arrowheads)** occupying the entire uterine cavity. The uterus is about 8–10 weeks' size. Thorough scanning of the sac failed to demonstrate fetal echoes. (Cadkin AV, Motew M: Clinical Atlas of Gray-Scale Ultrasonography in Obstetrics & Gynecology. Springfield IL, CC Thomas, 1979)

FIG. 14-3. UF = uterine fundus; B, bladder. Blighted ovum in a patient with 19 weeks of amenorrhea and a uterus slightly enlarged by pelvic examination. There were no bleeding and no fetal heart tones. Longitudinal scan of the uterus shows a collection of amniotic fluid (A) in the lower portion of the uterus. No fetal structures are seen. (Cadkin AV, Motew M; Clinical Atlas of Gray-Scale Ultrasonography in Obstetrics & Gynecology. Springfield, IL, CC Thomas, 1979)

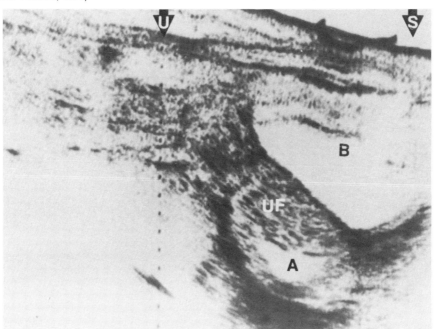

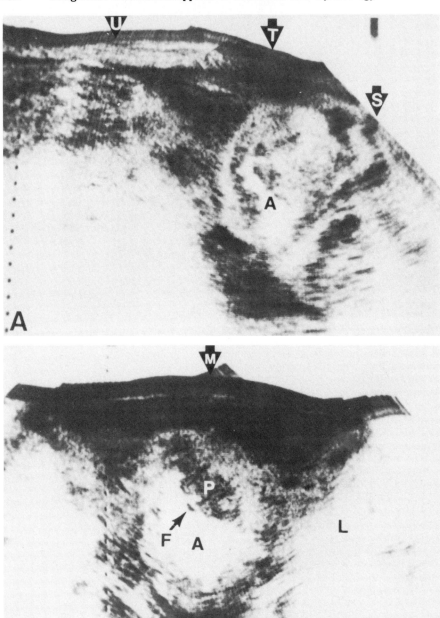

FIG. 14-4. U, umbilicus, S, symphysis pubis; M, midline; T, point at which transverse scan is obtained; L, left. Missed abortion in a patient with amenorrhea of 12 weeks' duration, vaginal spotting, and a positive pregnancy test. **A.** Longitudinal scan at M shows an enlarged uterus containing some amniotic fluid. There is an irregular collection of strong echoes along the anterior aspect of the uterus that represents a poorly defined placenta. **B.** Transverse scan at T shows a large amniotic cavity (A) and a shaggy looking placenta (P) along the antero-left lateral uterine wall. There is an 8-mm strong linear echo that represents a nonviable fetus. A normal fetus should have a CRL of at least 50 mm at this stage of pregnancy. (Cadkin AV, Motew M: Clinical Atlas of Gray-Scale Ultrasonography in Obstetrics & Gynecology. Springfield IL, CC Thomas, 1979)

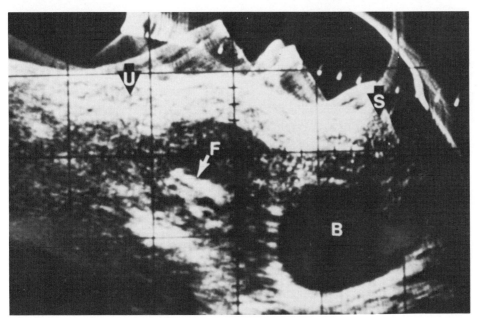

FIG. 14–5. T–M, time–motion study for recording fetal heart motion. Missed abortion in a patient with amenorrhea of 18 weeks' duration and no uterine growth in 4 weeks. Pregnancy test was negative. Longitudinal scan shows a small uterus for dates. Strong fetal echoes (F) are seen. There is marked decrease in the amount of amniotic fluid, and placental echoes cannot be identified. No heart sounds were heard by doppler, and T–M mode study was negative. Pathologic examination showed a markedly necrotic fetus and placenta. (Cadkin AV, Motew M: Clinical Atlas of Gray-Scale Ultrasonography in Obstetrics & Gynecology. Springfield IL, CC Thomas, 1979)

FIG. 14-6. UF, uterine fundus; UCG, urinary chorionic gonadotropin. Missed abortion in a patient with amenorrhea of 15 weeks' duration and a poor obstetric history (four previous abortions). Uterus is normal for dates and UCG is positive. Longitudinal scan at midline shows uterine size corresponding to dates but filled with diffuse echoes. The posterior uterine wall (PW) is clearly defined. Scans at low sensitivity show disappearance of the intrauterine echoes and a strong posterior uterine wall echo. There is no evidence of amniotic fluid or fetal echoes. *The scan findings are indistinguishable from those of molar pregnancy.* Pathologic examination showed hydropic degeneration of the placenta with a microscopic fetus. (Cadkin AV, Motew M: Clinical Atlas of Gray-Scale Ultrasonography in Obstetrics & Gynecology. Springfield IL, CC Thomas, 1979)

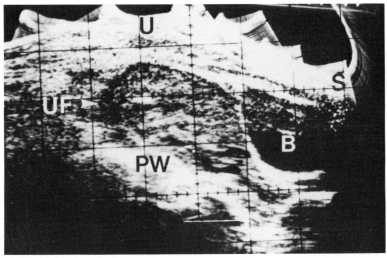

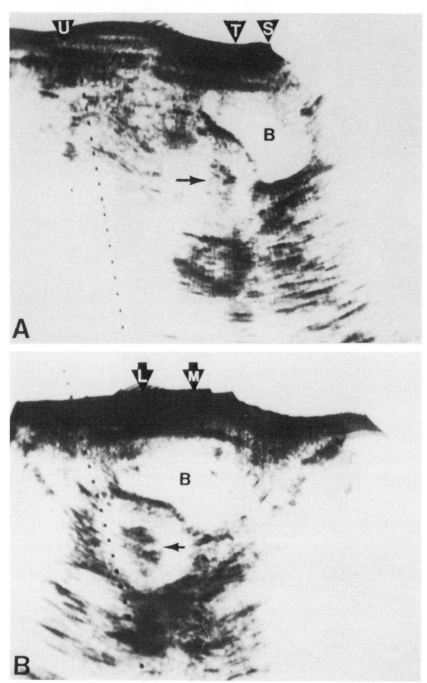

FIG. 14-7. L, midline; T, point at which transverse scan is obtained. Missed abortion in a patient with amenorrhea of 12 weeks' duration and recent onset of vaginal bleeding. **A.** Longitudinal scan at L. **B.** Transverse scan at T shows a 7 weeks' size uterus containing a central clump of strong echoes **(arrow).** The ultrasonic findings are compatible with a missed abortion but similar to the findings seen with chorio-carcinoma (see Fig. 14-14). Pathologic examination showed decidua and immature chorionic villi with degenerative necrosis. (Cadkin AV, Motew M: Clinical Atlas of Gray-Scale Ultrasonography in Obstetrics & Gynecology. Springfield IL, CC Thomas, 1979)

COMPLETE ABORTION

The diagnosis can be confirmed by demonstrating an empty uterus, which may have a thin, central, linear echo.

ENLARGED UTERUS WITH CENTRAL CLUMP OF ECHOES

This pattern is nonspecific and requires clinical correlation for accurate diagnosis, Figure 14–7. In pregnant patients the sonographic differential diagnosis includes the following: residuum of blighted ovum, missed abortion, choriocarcinoma, and rarely, molar pregnancy.

ULTRASONIC FINDINGS SUGGESTIVE OF ABNORMAL PREGNANCY

Some ultrasonic findings are suggestive of abnormal pregnancy but require follow-up examination at least 1 week later to establish the diagnosis. If the pregnancy is abnormal, a follow-up ultrasound examination will show lack of sufficient growth or actual decrease in volume of the gestational sac. It may also show absence of fetal echoes or fetal life (10, 20). Ultrasonic findings suggestive of abnormal pregnancy include the following:

1. Gestational sac that is small for dates (10, 20). Note, if by visual inspection of echogram the gestational sac size is equivalent to 5–7 weeks and shows no fetal echoes, a follow-up examination will differentiate an abnormal pregnancy from a normal but incorrectly dated one, Figure 14–8.

2. Small ratio of sac volume to fetal CRL with a viable fetus (20). This occurs in only 5% of normal pregnancies.

3. Low implantation of the gestational sac. Although most of these patients progress normally, the incidence of abortion (5, 6, 10) and placenta previa may be increased, Figure 14–3 (13).

FIG. 14–8. Blighted ovum in a patient with amenorrhea of 10 weeks' duration and vaginal bleeding of 2 days' duration. Longitudinal scan through the largest portion of the gestational sac shows what appears to be a normal 6-week gestational sac **(arrow)** in the center of the uterus. Gestational sac volume measured 1.3 cc and fetal echoes were not seen. Repeat scans 4 weeks later showed no evidence of growth of the sac, and fetal echoes were not present. (Cadkin AV, Motew M: Clinical Atlas of Gray-Scale Ultrasonography in Obstetrics & Gynecology. Springfield IL, CC Thomas, 1979)

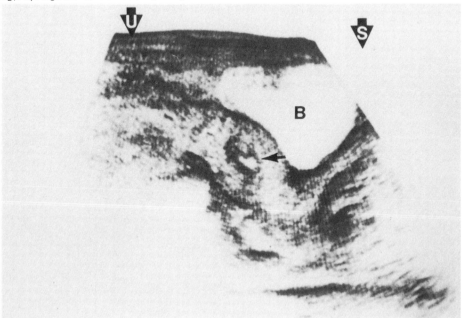

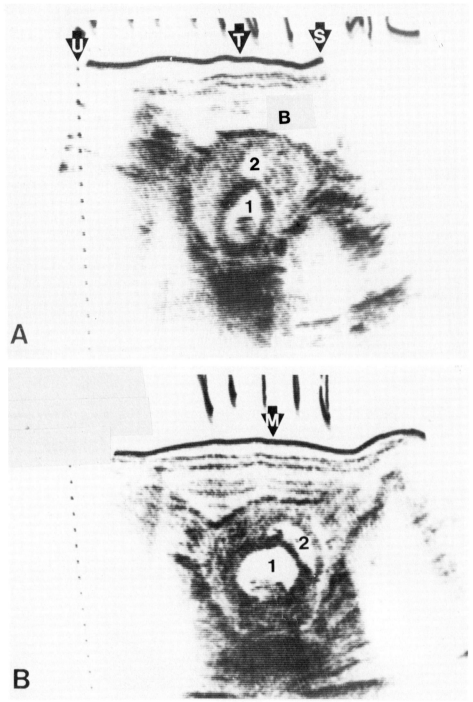

FIG. 14-9. T, point at which transverse scan is obtained. **A.** Longitudinal midline scan shows two gestational sacs. Sac one is well defined and shows a fetal echo with a crown–rump length of 1.8 cm corresponding to 8+ weeks' gestation. Sac two shows a poorly defined wall and is small. **B.** Transverse scan at T confirms the findings seen in A. There is a normal 8 weeks' gestation in the posterior aspect of the uterus (1). The second gestational sac (2) appears small and the fetus is smaller. Time–motion study of fetus one showed normal cardiac activity, while fetus two was dead. Follow-up examination at 14 weeks showed a single gestation with complete disappearance of the second sac and fetus. A singleton pregnancy was delivered at 38 weeks' gestation. (Courtesy of Carlos Reynes, M.D., Loyola Hospital, Maywood, IL)

4. Double or multiple gestational sacs (10, 16, 21). Each sac must be evaluated separately, Figure 14–9. Reexamination may be needed to determine if one or more of the sacs disappear or fail to grow or if multiple gestation persists.

5. A fragmented or incomplete sac. If this is the only abnormal finding, it is of little diagnostic value. Interference with sound propagation by intervening bone or bowel or improper scanning techniques may make a gestational sac appear incomplete or broken when, in fact, it is intact. The shape of the gestational sac is of little importance in diagnosis, since deformity or flattening is frequently due to an overdistended bladder or normal variation.

HYDATIDIFORM MOLE

Hydatidiform mole (molar pregnancy) is usually a benign lesion of the developing placenta in which the terminal aspects of the chorionic villi are converted into transparent cysts (hydropic villi) of varying size. A molar pregnancy may on occasion (incidence 16% [2] become locally invasive and is referred to as chorioadenoma destruens. Rarely (incidence 2.5% [2] molar tissue is transformed into frankly malignant choriocarcinoma. Choriocarcinoma may develop not only in abnormal pregnancies (threatened abortion, ectopic pregnancy, hydatidiform mole) but also in apparently normal gravidas.

Vassilakos (25) described two categories of molar pregnancy: partial and complete. His description of the pathology in this disease entity is helpful in understanding the sonographic appearance of hydatidiform mole.

PARTIAL MOLES

Partial moles constitute 75% of molar pregnancies. They are characterized by the presence of small hydropic villi (0.5 mm–5 mm), particularly prior to 10–12 weeks' gestation. This anatomic finding is the reason behind our inability, on certain occasions, to diagnose hydatidiform mole definitively early in the first trimester. In partial moles fetal tissue is always present (usually a stunted embryo is noted but on occa-

sion a live fetus is found) but shows cytogenic abnormalities—specifically chromosomal aberrations such as trisomies and tetraploidy are noted. Partial moles rarely progress to invasive trophoblastic disease.

COMPLETE MOLES

By contrast, complete moles constitute only 25% of molar pregnancies and are characterized by having *large* hydatid villi, with a characteristic 46XX chromosome configuration, no fetal tissue, and a 2.5% chance of transformation into choriocarcinoma.

SYMPTOMS AND SIGNS OF MOLAR PREGNANCY

In general, physicians consider the diagnosis of molar pregnancy when fundal height in a gravida is larger than expected by menstrual dates and if one or more of the following manifestations are noted: 1) vaginal bleeding; 2) hyperemesis; 3) pregnancy-induced hypertension associated with proteinuria and edema; 4) presence of pelvic mass or masses in association with pregnancy, usually attributed to theca-lutein cysts; 5) symptomatology consistent with hyperthyroidism, attributed to very high levels of HCG (12); and 6) pulmonary symptoms related to trophoblastic embolization.

DIAGNOSIS OF MOLAR PREGNANCY

It is imperative that the diagnosis of molar pregnancy be made as soon as possible and therapy instituted for morbidity and prognosis appear to be time related. In the majority of gravidas chorionic gonadotropin (HCG titer) is elevated over normal pregnancy values, and fetal heart tones are absent.

At present, ultrasound is the method of choice for making the diagnosis of hydatidiform mole. It is preferred over both amniography and arteriography because it is highly accurate and noninvasive. Because the majority of hydatidiform moles are partial moles, hydatid villi are small (0.5 mm–5 mm) by 8–10 weeks' gestation, as discussed elsewhere. Thus, the echo pattern produced by molar changes early in pregnancy are nonspecific, and a repeat examination in 2–3 weeks will often be necessary to clinch the diagnosis.

In the remaining discussion we focus on the ultrasonic characteristics of hydatidiform mole and the differential diagnosis that should be considered.

CLASSIC ECHOGRAM PATTERN

Many hydatidiform moles exhibit what may be described as a classic echogram pattern, in which the uterus is diffusely filled with echoes of moderate strength (snowstorm appearance). These echoes disappear at low sensitivity settings (8, 15). The posterior uterine wall remains, however, clearly visible at low gain because of the sonolucent nature of the fluid-filled vesicles. When the vesicles are small (0.5 mm–5 mm) the ultrasonic appearance may be similar to that of a normal placenta, but careful analysis of high-quality scans usually reveals the vesicular pattern, Figure 14–10. When the vesicles are large, the uterus shows multiple small cystic spaces separated by strong echoes from interfaces between adjacent vesicles. In a patient known to be pregnant, the diagnosis is usually straightforward; however, missed abortion and, rarely, choriocarcinoma may produce a similar ultrasonic picture.

Occasionally, a myoma with degeneration, a teratoma, a granulosa cell tumor, or a fibroma of the ovary may produce molar-like echoes. The use of a high-frequency transducer (5 MHz) may help differentiate solid masses from molar tissue. In the presence of a solid mass there may be attenuation of the high-frequency ultrasonic beam with loss of visualization of the posterior aspect of the mass. By contrast, the posterior wall of the uterus in molar pregnancy is clearly visible. Further, in the case of ovarian tumors the adnexal origin of these masses is readily appreciated once the uterine outline is evident on the sonogram.

ATYPICAL ECHOGRAM PATTERN

This pattern results from the presence of bleeding within the mole. The blood clots are frequently seen as echo-free spaces within or about the periphery of the mole (4). If the clots are large and central, they may simulate an amniotic cavity, Figure 14–11. When this happens, the possibility of a missed abortion with molar degeneration of the placenta must be considered. In either case, however, the treatment is evacuation of uterine contents.

FETUS IN CONJUNCTION WITH MOLAR PREGNANCY

The visualization of a fetus by ultrasound does not rule out coexisting trophoblastic disease (1, 3). Although the diagnosis of hydatidiform mole with coexisting fetus is rare (less than 2% of moles), the diagnosis can be suggested when characteristic ultrasonic findings are present, Figures 14–12 and 14–13. The diagnosis can be made by sonography at a time when the fetus is not yet visible on plain film of the abdomen. In addition fetal age and viability can be established by ultrasound; this knowledge will assist the physician in choosing the most appropriate therapeutic approach. Suction curettage is the preferred modality of treatment if the fetus is under 12 weeks' gestation. In the presence of a second trimester fetus the abnormal pregnancy is terminated by means of pitocin stimulation, amnioinfusion of prostaglandin F_2 alpha, vaginal prostaglandin E_2 suppositories (23), hysterotomy, or hysterectomy, depending on the clinical exigencies.

A LARGE PLACENTAL MASS

A large placental mass, if seen in the first trimester, should not be readily accepted as evidence of trophoblastic disease, because it may be secondary to multiple pregnancy. The recent advent of real-time imaging has proved to be useful in the quick and accurate diagnosis of twin gestation.

THECA LUTEIN CYSTS

These cysts may be seen in as many as 40% of molar pregnancies (7) and must be carefully searched for when this diagnosis is considered. They are usually large, multilocular, and frequently bilateral (Figs. 14–10, 14–12) but may

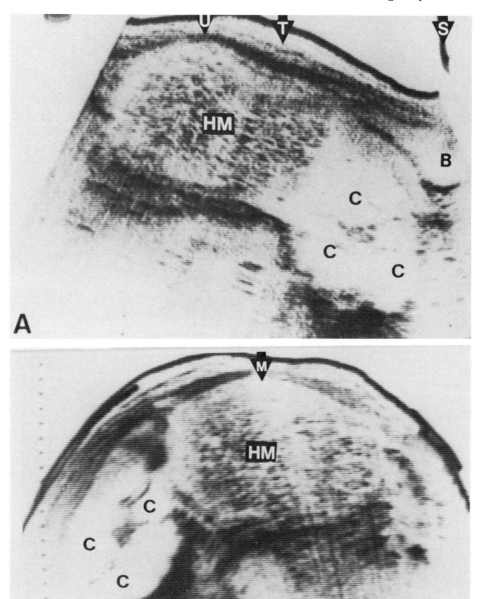

FIG. 14–10. T, point at which transverse scan is obtained. Hydatidiform mole with theca-lutein cysts in a gravida, at 20 weeks' gestation, presenting with nausea and vomiting. **A.** Longitudinal midline scan shows a complex multilocular cyst (C) in the cul-de-sac displacing the lower aspect of the uterus to the left side. The upper portion of the uterus is filled with echoes consistent with a hydatidiform mole (HM). **B.** Transverse scan at T shows the echo pattern of hydatidiform mole and the cystic structure (C) (theca-lutein cysts) on the right side. (Courtesy of Carlos Reynes, M.D., Loyola Hospital, Maywood, Illinois)

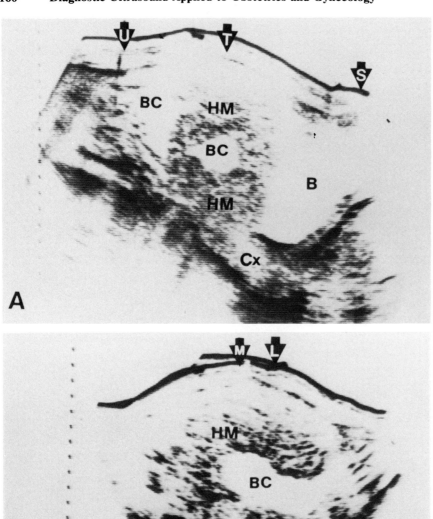

FIG. 14–11. T, point at which transverse scan is obtained. Hydatidiform mole with blood clots in a gravida at 17 weeks' gestation. **A.** Longitudinal midline shows a uterus compatible with dates containing a complex mass consisting of cystic (BC) and solid (HM) areas. **B.** Transverse scan at T through the uterus shows the molar tissue (HM) with a large central echo-free space due to blood clots (BC). At surgery, there was a hydatidiform mole containing large blood clots. (Courtesy of Tom Grant, D.O., Chicago Osteopathic Hospital, Chicago, Illinois)

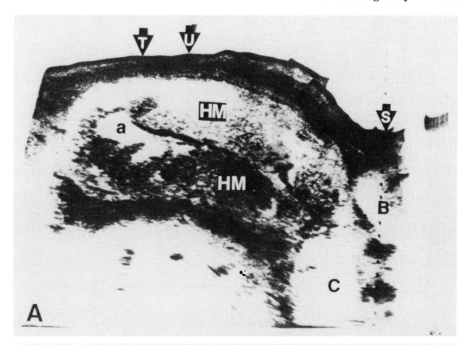

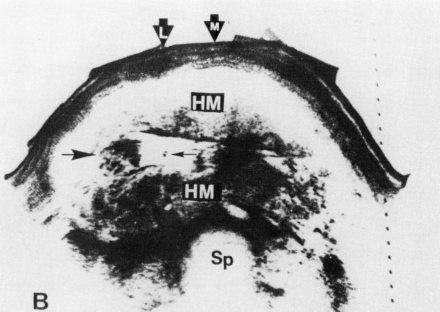

FIG. 14-12. U, umbilicus; T–M, time–motion study; Sp, maternal spine; T, point at which transverse scan is obtained. Hydatidiform mole with coexisting missed abortion in a gravida at 15 weeks' gestation. Clinically, uterus is large for dates and no fetal heart sounds are heard by doppler. **A.** Longitudinal midline scan shows a uterus markedly enlarged for dates containing placental or molar-type echoes (HM) and a small amount of amniotic fluid (a). There is a large cyst (C) in the cul-de-sac. **B.** Transverse scan at T shows the molar tissue (HM) covering the entire inner surface of the uterus. There is a central amniotic space with definite cord echo **(small arrow)** and fetal echoes **(large arrow).** The T–M exam of the fetus showed no cardiac activity. The ultrasonic diagnosis was a hydatidiform mole with coexisting missed abortion, and this was confirmed at surgery.

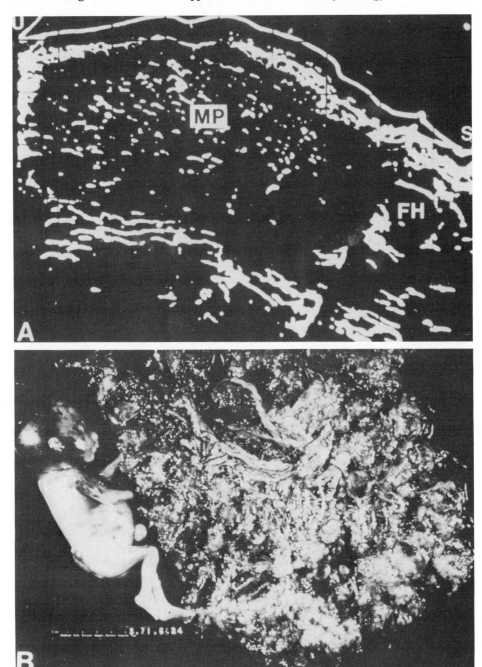

FIG. 14–13. Hydatidiform mole with coexistent fetus. **A.** Longitudinal scan shows a molar pregnancy (MP) in conjunction with a 15- to 16-week fetal head (FH). This scan was done by use of bistable technique. **B.** Mole and fetus at hysterotomy (Sabbagha RE: In Spellacy WN (ed): *Management of the High-Risk Pregnancy.* Baltimore, University Park Press, 1976)

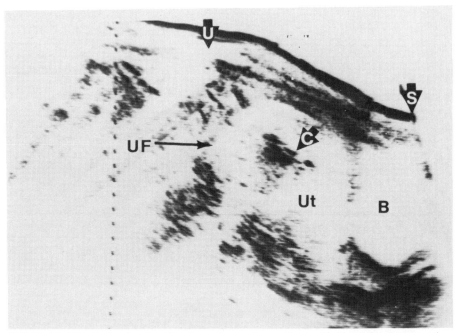

FIG. 14-14. UF, uterine fundus. Choriocarcinoma in a patient with 12 weeks of amenorrhea who presented with vaginal bleeding and a markedly elevated HCG titer. Longitudinal scan of the uterus at low sensitivity shows an enlarged uterus (Ut) with a relatively echo-free thick uterine wall. There is a central collection of strong echoes (C) that were proved to be a choriocarcinoma on pathologic examination.

occasionally present as a simple cyst. After evacuation of a molar pregnancy, these cysts should regress in size and can be followed by ultrasound. The development or increase in size of these cysts may be evidence for the presence of an invasive mole or choriocarcinoma. We are aware of two tragic cases of hydatidiform mole associated with large bilateral theca-lutein cysts in which unnecessary oophorectomy was performed prior to ultrasonic evaluation of the uterine contents. Both gravidas were subsequently shown to have molar pregnancies.

SONOGRAPHIC FINDINGS IN CHORIOCARCINOMA

There are no characteristic ultrasonic findings in choriocarcinoma. The sonographic picture may be indistinguishable from molar pregnancy (7). When the tumor presents as a somewhat raised nodular tumor involving the uterine wall, there may be localized unorganized echoes in the uterus, Figure 14–14. At times, the sonographic picture is identical to a missed abortion, adenomyosis, or endometrial carcinoma.

REFERENCES

1. BARONE CM: Ultrasonic diagnosis of hydatidiform mole with a coexistent fetus. Radiology 124:798, 1977

2. BREWER JI, TOROK EE, WEBSTER AI, DOLKART RE: Hydatidiform mole: a follow-up regimen for identification of invasive mole and choriocarcinoma and for selection of patients for treatment. Am J Obstet Gynecol 101:557, 1968

3. CUNNINGHAM ME, WALLS WJ, BURKE MF: Gray-scale ultrasonography in the diagnosis of hydatidiform mole with a coexistent fetus. Br J Obstet Gynaecol 84:73, 1977

4. DEWBURY KC, POLL V: An unusual ultrasound appearance of a hydatidiform mole. Br J Radiol 50:443, 1977

5. DONALD I, MORLEY P, BARNETT E: The diagnosis of blighted ovum by sonar. Br J Obstet Gynaecol 79:304, 1972

6. DUFF GB: Prognosis in threatened abortion: a comparison between predictions made by sonar, urinary

hormone assays and clinical judgment. Br J Obstet Gynaecol 82:858, 1975

7. FLEISCHER AC, JAMES AE, KRAUSE DA, MILLIS JB: Sonographic patterns in trophoblastic diseases. Radiology 126:215, 1978

8. GOTTESFELD KR, TAYLOR SE, THOMPSON HE, HOLMES JH: Diagnosis of hydatidiform mole by ultrasound. Obstet Gynecol 30:163, 1967

9. GRAHAM MF: First trimester abdominal pregnancy. J Clin Ultrasound 5:321, 1977

10. HELLMAN LM, KOBAYASHI M, CROMB E: Ultrasonic diagnosis of embryonic malformation. Am J Obstet Gynecol 115:615, 1973

11. HELLMAN LM, KOBAYASHI M, FILLISTI L, LAVENHAR M: Growth and development of the human fetus prior to the twentieth week of gestation. Am J Obstet Gynecol 103:789, 1969

12. HIGGINS HP, HERSHMAN JM, KENIMER JG, PATILLO RA, BAILEY TA, WALFISH P: The thyrotoxicosis of hydatidiform moles. Ann Intern Med 83:307, 1975

13. HORGER EO, KREUTNER KA, UNDERWOOD PB: Ultrasonic diagnosis of low implantation preceding placenta previa. Am J Obstet Gynecol 120:1119, 1974

14. JOUPPILA P, PIIROINEN O: Ultrasonic diagnosis of fetal life in early pregnancy. Obstet Gynecol 46:616, 1975

15. LEOPOLD GR: Diagnostic ultrasound in the detection of molar pregnancy. Radiology 98:171, 1971

16. LEVI S, Ultrasonic assessment of the high rate of

human multiple pregnancy in the first trimester. J Clin Ultrasound 4:3, 1976

17. ROBINSON HP: Detection of fetal heart movement in the first trimester of pregnancy using pulsed ultrasound. Br Med J 4:466, 1972

18. ROBINSON HP: Sonar in the management of abortion. Br J Obstet Gynaecol 79:90, 1972

19. ROBINSON HP: "Gestation sac" volumes as determined by sonar in the first trimester of pregnancy. Br J Obstet Gynaecol 82:100, 1975

20. ROBINSON HP: The diagnosis of early pregnancy failure by sonar. Br J Obstet Gynaecol 82:849, 1975

21. ROBINSON HP, CAINES JS: Sonar evidence of early pregnancy failure in patients with twin conceptions. Br J Obstet Gynaecol 84:22, 1977

22. ROBINSON HP, FLEMING JEE: A critical evaluation of sonar "crown-rump length" measurements. Br J Obstet Gynaecol 82:702, 1975

23. SOUTHERN EM, GUTKNECHT GD: Management of intrauterine fetal demise and missed abortion using prostaglandin E_2 vaginal suppositories. Obstet Gynecol 47:602, 1975

24. VARMA TR: The value of ultrasonic B-scanning in diagnosis when bleeding is present in early pregnancy. Am J Obstet Gynecol 114:607, 1972

25. VASSILAKOS P, RIOTTON G, KAJII T: Hydatidiform mole: two entities a morphologic and cytogenetic study with some clinical considerations. Am J Obstet Gynecol 127:167, 1977

15

Ultrasound and amniocentesis

SHERMAN ELIAS, JOE LEIGH SIMPSON

Second-trimester amniocentesis for the prenatal diagnosis of genetic disorders is a relatively safe and reliable procedure that has become an integral part of modern obstetrics. Although ultrasonography is usually considered standard practice (2), its efficacy and safety preceding amniocentesis remain unproved. In this chapter we review the indications for genetic amniocentesis, describe the technique and risks of amniocentesis, and evaluate the potential benefits and risks of ultrasonography used in conjunction with amniocentesis. Ultrasonography for prenatal diagnosis of fetal abnormalities is reviewed elsewhere in this volume (Ch. 19).

GENETIC INDICATIONS FOR SECOND-TRIMESTER AMNIOCENTESIS

A proper genetic evaluation should be a routine part of obstetric practice. Ideally, couples should have the opportunity to discuss their risks of having a child with a congenital anomaly either before pregnancy or before the end of the first trimester. Some genetic counseling problems are sufficiently complex to warrant consultation with a fully trained geneticist; however, many common problems may be handled by well-informed obstetricians.

The following prerequisites for genetic counseling have been enunciated by Milunsky (39):

1. An accurate diagnosis must first be established.

2. The mode of inheritance of the disorder must be known. Knowledge of the recurrence risk is vital.

3. An insight into the variations of the disease in life is important (for example heterogeneity, infantile and juvenile forms of the disease etc.), together with knowledge of the prognosis, the quality of life anticipated and the therapy available.

4. Methods to determine the carrier state, where possible, must be known by the counselor, who should then be able to arrange such testing for other family members.

5. A knowledge of methods and risks of therapeutic abortion and an insight into contraceptive methods as well as the problems of adoption and artificial insemination should all be available.

6. Experience and sensitivity in counseling would be desirable (recognition of parental anxieties, use of simple terms, need for repetition and an ability to communicate with people).

In evaluating the risks of various disorders, the physician should recall that congenital anomalies may result from 1) changes in chromosome number or structure, 2) changes at a single genetic locus (Mendelian disorders), 3) cumulative effects of genes at several loci (polygenic or multifactorial inheritance), or 4) environmental (teratogenic) factors.

CHROMOSOMAL ABNORMALITIES

The incidence of a chromosomal abnormality is about 1:200 newborn infants (28). Situations known to be associated with an increased likelihood of having offspring with a chromosomal abnormality include 1) advanced maternal age; 2) a parent with a balanced translocation, inversion, or other chromosomal abnormality; and 3) a previous child with a chromosomal abnormality, particularly autosomal trisomy.

ADVANCED MATERNAL AGE

The most common indication for genetic amniocentesis is advanced maternal age. Autosomal trisomies and X-chromosomal polysomies (eg, 47, XXY and 47, XXX) are usually associated with an increased mean maternal age (11, 23, 53). For example, if a mother is 35–39 years of age, the risk of her offspring having Down's syndrome is about 1:300 (9). Between ages 40 and 44 years the risk is about 1:100, and after age 44 the risk is about 1:50. Women aged 35 years and older comprise only 13.5% of the pregnant population, yet produce 50% of infants with Down's syndrome (46). Moreover, between ages 35 and 39 years the likelihood that a chromosomal abnormality of any type will occur is 1:70; between ages 40 and 45 the risk is about 1:62 (35). However, some of the latter risks are the result of sex chromosome polysomies (e.g., 47, XXX), which may or may not be associated with severe phenotypic abnormalities. Because of these increased risks, women aged 35 and older should be counseled regarding amniocentesis for prenatal diagnosis.

PARENT WITH A TRANSLOCATION OR OTHER CHROMOSOMAL ABNORMALITY

Any parent may unwittingly be a carrier (heterozygote) for a balanced translocation. From 2% to 3% of individuals with Down's syndrome have a translocation, usually between chromosomes 14 and 21. Translocations associated with Down's syndrome also occur between chromosomes 13 and 21, 15 and 21, 21 and 21, 21 and 22, and occasionally between 21 and a nonacrocentric chromosome. About 25% of these translocations are inherited, the remainder occurring de novo (i.e., not detected in either parent) (58). The likelihood that future progeny of parents who have had a child with a de novo translocation will similarly be affected is probably no higher than for the general population. In about 25% of individuals who have Down's syndrome as the result of a translocation, one parent is a balanced translocation carrier. If so, the empiric recurrence risk depends on the type of translocation and on the sex of the parent carrying it (58). If the mother carries a D/G translocation (usually 14/21), the risk is about 10% (38). If the father carries the same translocation, the risk is only 2%–3% (38). These empiric figures are less than the theoretic risk (33%), possibly because of selection against chromosomally abnormal gametes or embryos. Although less than theoretically expected, these risks are sufficiently high to justify antenatal diagnosis. A different situation exists if a parent has a 21/21 translocation. Pregnancies lead either to nonviable monosomic zygotes or to zygotes with Down's syndrome; thus, all living offspring of a parent with a 21/21 translocation will be chromosomally abnormal.

Amniocentesis for prenatal diagnosis may also be considered for other parental chromosomal abnormalities. Individuals with a chromosomal inversion (a chromosome aberration in which a segment of a chromosome is reversed end to end) may also produce unbalanced gametes that result in chromosomally abnormal offspring. Other examples might include a father with a known 47, XYY chromosomal complement, a parent with chromosomal mosaicism, or families that apparently show a predisposition toward aneuploidy. Counseling in such situations is usually complex and should best be offered by experienced geneticists.

PREVIOUS CHILD WITH A CHROMOSOMAL ABNORMALITY

Following the birth of one child with autosomal trisomy or sex chromosome trisomy, the likelihood that subsequent offspring will have a chromosomal abnormality is increased, irrespective of the parental ages or their chromosomal complements. The likelihood of liveborn Down's syndrome (47, XX, +21 or 47, XY, +21) recurring in subsequent progeny is perhaps 1% assuming both parents have normal chromosomal complements (38). Indeed, pooled data (20) indicate that 1.2% (24 of 1970) of pregnancies monitored because a previous child was trisomic (47, XX, +21 or 47, XY, +21) showed aneuploidy. The etiology of recurrent trisomy (aneuploidy) is unknown.

MENDELIAN DISORDERS

Mendelian disorders result from mutations at a single genetic locus. The locus may be on an autosome or on a sex chromosome, and it may be dominant or recessive. An autosomal dominant trait can be recognized by its ability to be transmitted from generation to generation. If a person has a completely penetrant autosomal dominant trait and his (her) mate lacks the trait, the likelihood of passing the trait to any given child is 50%. In autosomal recessive inheritance two phenotypically normal parents are heterozygous for the same recessive allele; the likelihood that their offspring will be affected is 25%. This type of inheritance is usually recognized by presence of multiple affected sibs of both sexes, without other affected relatives.

If a gene is recessive and located on the X chromosome, the trait controlled by that gene is expressed by all males (46, XY) carrying the allele. Affected males are termed hemizygous. Females will usually be affected only if homozygous. Usually, therefore, X-linked recessive disorders occur only in males; thus, the trait appears to be transmitted through phenotypically normal yet actually heterozygous females. In practice, distinguishing an X-linked recessive gene from a sex-linked dominant gene is sometimes difficult, though several approaches are theoretically possible. Male-to-male transmission would, for example, exclude X-linked recessive inheritance.

Most inborn errors of metabolism are autosomal recessive, but a few X-linked recessive and autosomal dominant enzyme abnormalities have been identified. Inborn errors include metabolic disorders of amino acids, carbohydrates, lipids, mucopolysaccharides, and porphyrins. Although individually rare, inherited metabolic disorders occur with an estimated frequency of

1%. Among the 1200 or more Mendelian disorders, only 60–80 enzymatic deficiencies can be diagnosed in utero. The prenatal diagnosis of a metabolic disorder usually requires assay of amniotic fluid cultures for a specific enzyme activity or metabolic product. The success of these assays rests on the premise that the cultured cells accurately reflect the fetal status with respect to the presence or absence of the metabolic disorder in question. In addition, sex determination may be useful in X-linked recessive disorders, and linkage analysis may occasionally be diagnostically helpful.

POLYGENIC (MULTIFACTORIAL) INHERITANCE

Some disorders result from the cumulative effects of several genes (polygenic) or from interactions between genes and environment (multifactorial). After the birth of one child with a disorder believed inherited in polygenic or multifactorial fashion, the likelihood of recurrence is usually 2%–5%. Because the recurrence risk is relatively low, most individuals with these disorders have no affected relatives. Examples of disorders inherited in polygenic or multifactorial fashion include cleft palate, certain cardiac defects, pyloric stenosis, talipes equinovarus, and the neural tube defects (anencephaly myelomeningocele, and spina bifida).

Any couple delivered of a child with a neural tube defect should be offered antenatal detection in future pregnancies. If one parent has spina bifida, the pregnancy should likewise be monitored. There is no unanimity about whether spina bifida occulta in a parent or first-degree relative is an indication for amniocentesis. Assay for amniotic fluid alpha-feto protein for the prenatal diagnosis of meningomyelocele is 90% reliable; 10% of affected fetuses have lesions covered with skin and thus are not amenable to diagnosis by this approach (40). Amniotic fluid alpha-feto protein is essentially 100% reliable for the antenatal diagnosis of anencephaly. False-positive values occur, though the most experienced laboratories report the phenomenon rarely (0.1%–0.2%). Some false-positive values are associated with fetal demise, twins, or anomalies; however, often no explanation is available.

Ultrasonographic surveillance of the fetal head and vertebral column can also be used for diagnosis of neural tube defects (Ch. 19).

ENVIRONMENTAL (TERATOGENIC) FACTORS

Unfortunately, the antenatal diagnosis of either acquired congenital infections or other teratogenic effects is rarely feasible. At present amniocentesis is not helpful diagnostically for women exposed during early pregnancy to rubella, cytomegalovirus, or toxoplasmosis. Likewise, analyzing amniotic fluid is of no value in determining whether a fetus has been damaged by X-irradiation or maternal drug ingestion. However, other diagnostic procedures, for example, fetoscopy, may prove useful in detecting structural abnormalities in the fetus.

TECHNIQUE OF AMNIOCENTESIS

Transabdominal amniocentesis for prenatal diagnosis is best performed between 15 and 16 weeks after the last menstrual period. At this time a sufficient volume of amniotic fluid volume is present (approximately 180 ml) and an adequate sample (20–30 ml) can safely be aspirated. Before the 12th week of pregnancy the uterus has not extended beyond the pelvic brim, and transabdominal amniocentesis is difficult. Transvaginal amniocentesis during the late first trimester is possible but not recommended (17), because it is associated with a relatively high risk of abortion and infection. Amniocentesis should be performed sufficiently early so that pregnancy interruption for abnormal results remains an option for the parent.

Amniocentesis may be performed in any outpatient facility. The arguments for and against routine ultrasonography are discussed later. If ultrasonography is to precede amniocentesis, the bladder should be emptied immediately before the procedure. Fetal life should be documented before and after amniocentesis, either by Doppler ultrasound or direct visualization of fetal activity or heart movements by real-time ultrasonography.

Strict aseptic conditions being used, the lower abdomen is cleansed with povidone–iodine solution and 70% isopropyl alcohol and draped with a sterile fenestrated towel. A 1% lidocaine hydrochloride solution is infiltrated into the insertion site. A 20- or 22-gauge 3½-in. spinal needle with stylet is then directed transabdominally into the amniotic cavity. After the stylet is removed, a 5-ml syringe is attached to the trocar, and several milliliters of amniotic fluid are aspirated. This initial sample is theoretically most likely to contain maternal cells derived from the abdominal wall or the myometrium; therefore, this sample is often not analyzed. This fluid may, however, be used to differentiate amniotic fluid from inadvertently obtained maternal urine (discussed later). After approximately 30 ml of amniotic fluid has been aspirated into sterile, disposable plastic syringes, the needle is withdrawn. Amniotic fluid is either transferred into sterile, disposable plastic screw-capped tubes or kept in the syringes, which are tightly capped. The specimens are properly labeled and then transported to the appropriate laboratory. The patient may resume her normal activities and is instructed to report any complications immediately (discussed later, "Risks of Amniocentesis").

Urine and amniotic fluid are often indistinguishable in appearance, and analysis of cells derived from the former could obviously lead to erroneous interpretations of fetal status. Inadvertent aspiration of maternal urine is a particular risk if a suprapubic site is chosen. If the origin of aspirated fluid is in doubt, tests should be performed to determine its origin. Pirani et al (47) recommend use of Labstix reagent strips (Ames) to differentiate amniotic fluid from urine. This test depends on the presence of albumin and glucose in amniotic fluid and their absence in urine. This test is, however, unreliable if the pregnancy is complicated by diabetes mellitus, renal disease, or possibly polyhydramnios. Guibaud et al (22) advocate analyzing fluid for urea and potassium, both present in much higher levels in urine than in amniotic fluid. Urea and potassium levels indeed differentiate amniotic fluid from urine, but in most institutions these tests cannot be performed quickly. Elias et al (16) found that the crystalline arborization pattern characteristic of amniotic fluid

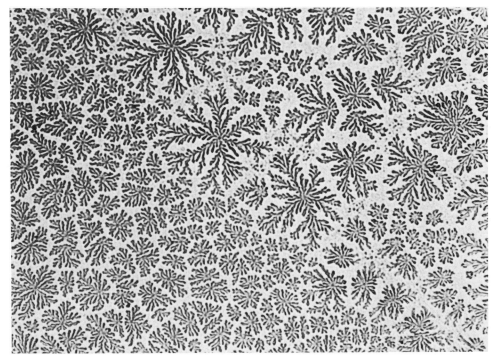

FIG. 15-1. Characteristic crystalline arborization pattern of amniotic fluid when fluid is allowed to dry on an acid-cleaned slide and examined under low-power X100 magnification.

(Fig. 15-1) is observed if the fluid is allowed to dry on an acid-cleaned slide and examined under low power (× 100) magnification. This test differentiates amniotic fluid from urine with a high degree of accuracy.

RISKS OF AMNIOCENTESIS

Amniocentesis carries both maternal and fetal risks. Potential maternal risks include hemorrhage secondary to puncture of uterine or other intraabdominal vessels, puncture or laceration of a viscus, infection, and Rh immunization. Whether routine ultrasonography reduces the incidence of Rh immunization is considered in greater detail later. Occasionally women complain of lower abdominal pressure or soreness following amniocentesis, but these complaints usually abate within 24 hours without treatment.

Potential fetal risks include bleeding, injuries directly caused by the needle (see section entitled "Fetal Puncture"), injuries indirectly caused by withdrawal of amniotic fluid, and death. In a prospective study coordinated by the National Institute of Child Health and Human Development (NICHHD) (44) and comprising 1040 subjects and 992 controls, the incidence of immediate complication (e.g., leakage of amniotic fluid, bleeding, abortion) was about 2%, a figure slightly higher than in the control sample. However, only a few of the immediate complications were serious; 3.5% of pregnant women who underwent amniocentesis experienced fetal loss subsequent to the procedure, whereas an almost identical percentage (3.2%) of pregnant controls experienced fetal loss. In conclusion, amniocentesis probably carries some risk of fetal complications, but this risk can be estimated at 0.5% or less.

POTENTIAL BENEFITS OF ULTRASONOGRAPHY IN GENETIC AMNIOCENTESIS

Whether ultrasonography should be employed routinely as an adjunct to amniocentesis is controversial. Two major questions must be considered: 1) Does routine ultrasonography increase the safety and accuracy of amniocentesis? 2) What are the known and potential dangers of ultrasound exposure during early pregnancy?

MODES OF ULTRASOUND

Various modes of ultrasound are currently employed. These include 1) Doppler ultrasound, 2) A-mode, 3) B-mode, 4) gray-scale, 5) real-time, and 6) M-mode. If more than one mode is used, considerable diagnostic information can be obtained.

Two major forms of ultrasound are routinely employed in obstetrics: a continuous beam of low intensity in which echoes returning from moving structures are altered in frequency (so-called Doppler techniques) and short repetitive ultrasonic pulses of microsecond duration in which the transducer is used for both transmitting and receiving (so-called pulse-echo techniques). The former is most commonly used in monitoring the fetal heart rate, whereas the latter is used for diagnostic examinations. Whether the Doppler regimen or the pulse-echo regimen is employed is of particular relevance in evaluating studies that explore the safety of ultrasound exposure. Doppler instruments transmit continuous ultrasound and monitor simultaneously with separate crystals. By contrast, in the pulsed-echo regimen the target is isonated by short pulses of microsecond duration, the transducer listening for the returning echos 99.9% of the time. Thus, Doppler regimens deliver a much higher dosage of isonation energy to target structures than pulsed-echo ultrasound does.

DETECTION OF MULTIPLE GESTATION

Although multiple gestation may be suspected if uterine size is larger than expected on the basis of the last menstrual period, the diagnosis may be missed, especially in an obese woman. By the early second trimester multiple gestation is readily detectable by ultrasonography.

Amniocentesis of each amniotic sac would be necessary to determine the chromosomal complement of each fetus. If twins are detected, separate sacs may be distinguished by injecting a dye (e.g., indigo carmine) following aspiration of first fluid sample. Following ambulation, a second amniocentesis is performed in the ultrasonographically determined location of the other fetus. Aspiration of colorless fluid indicates that the second sac was entered, whereas aspiration of fluid colored with dye indicates that the original sac was reentered. Occasionally twins share a common sac, in which case separate chromosomal analysis of each fetus is not possible. Multiple needle insertions undoubtedly carry a higher risk than a single amniocentesis attempt; however, no risk figures are available. Finally, the parents and physician may be faced with the dilemma of having one normal fetus and one abnormal fetus.

CONFIRMATION OF GESTATIONAL AGE

The date of the last normal menstrual period may be uncertain, or a discrepancy between uterine size and dates may exist. Ultrasonographic determination of the biparietal diameter of the fetal skull correlates well with gestational age, especially during the second trimester (Ch. 8). Thus, ultrasonography may be correlated with the clinical examination to determine the optimal time for amniocentesis.

PLACENTAL LOCALIZATION TO DECREASE "BLOODY TAPS"

Placental location can be accurately and quickly determined by use of ultrasonography. In one series 46.8% of placentas were implanted in the posterior portion of the uterus, whereas 51.4% were implanted in the anterior portion (55); 30%–50% of placentas occupied a large portion of the intrauterine surface. In 43.3% of patients a portion of the placenta was seen in the lower uterine area; however, this low placental position in the second trimester apparently does not carry the same prognosis as at term because the large majority of these patients neither require intervention for bleeding nor develop placenta previa at term (Ch. 16).

Routine ultrasonographic placental localization preceding amniocentesis should theoretically reduce the incidence of bloody taps, decrease the likelihood of Rh immunization in women at risk, and minimize the risk of placental injury and possibly abortion (19, 24, 41). Some investigators have, however, been unable to confirm the benefits of routine placental localization (30).

Miskin et al (42) studied 73 women undergoing genetic amniocentesis between 16 and 18 weeks of pregnancy. The first 32 patients underwent amniocentesis without ultrasonography; 7 taps were bloody (22%). The next 41 patients underwent amniocentesis preceded by ultrasonographic placental localization using a B-mode scanner; only 1 tap was bloody ("minor blood staining"). These investigators concluded that ultrasonographic placental localization reduced the incidence of bloody taps tenfold. However, the reduction in the number of bloody taps in the second group could have resulted from increasing experience gained by the obstetrician, rather than from introduction of ultrasonography.

Harrison et al (24) studied 133 amniocenteses performed during the second trimester. A group of 44 amniocenteses not using ultrasonography were compared to 89 subsequently performed over the next 2 years. The first group was performed for midtrimester abortion, whereas the second was performed for genetic reasons and used B-mode ultrasonography. The frequency of grossly bloody taps was 11% (5:44 patients) without ultrasonography and only 4% (3:89 patients) with ultrasonography. The shortcomings of this study include the following: 1) the control group (without ultrasonography) was ascertained over a different time period than the experimental group (with ultrasonography), 2) the procedures were performed at different hospitals with different techniques, and 3) the indications for amniocentesis were different in the two groups studied.

Finally, in a retrospective study of second-trimester amniocenteses for prenatal diagnosis, Kerenyi and Walker (31) reported that 14.4% (123:856 cases) of all amniotic fluid samples were contaminated with blood, both grossly and microscopically. The frequency of blood-contaminated fluid was 11.6% (21 of 181 cases) if ultrasonography was employed, compared to 23.6% (43 of 182 cases) if ultrasonography was not used. The best results (2.0% grossly bloody

taps) were obtained if the procedure was performed by an operator not only experienced in performing second-trimester amniocentesis but also knowledgeable in ultrasonography. Unfortunately, the control and amniocentesis groups were dissimilar. Most amniocentesis procedures performed without ultrasonography were prior to 1974, whereas those with ultrasonography were after 1974. The authors also describe differences in techniques between the various operators. For example, the "inexperienced" operators frequently did not clear the needle of the initial several milliliters of amniotic fluid, whereas experienced operators routinely cleared the needle. This initial sample not infrequently contains blood from either the abdominal wall or myometrium. Such differences in techniques were not taken into consideration in the evaluation of a "bloody tap." In addition, there was no mention of other attempts to standardize techniques, such as using the same size needles.

In contrast to the studies just cited a reduction in bloody taps by using ultrasonography could not be demonstrated in other reports. Gerbie and Shkolnik (19) reported a 6% incidence of grossly bloody amniotic fluid in tests performed before the routine use of ultrasonography, compared to 10% after introduction of ultrasonography. Nevertheless, these investigators recommend routine ultrasonography because "in theory, avoiding the placenta should decrease placental trauma, with an attendant decrease in the number of bloody taps." They describe several instances in which ultrasonography was felt to be helpful by revealing a "window" through which the needle was inserted and clear fluid obtained. Such areas would presumably not be chosen unless ultrasonography were used.

In a retrospective study of 242 patients undergoing second-trimester amniocentesis for prenatal diagnosis, Young et al (59) were unable to demonstrate a significant reduction in bloody taps by use of ultrasonography. The incidences were 13.8% and 16.0%, with and without ultrasonography respectively. Moreover, most amniocenteses preceded by ultrasonography (70 of 87) were performed at a university medical center by two obstetricians, whereas those without ultrasonography (139 of 156) were performed by "miscellaneous operators" outside the medical center. In addition, if ultrasonography was used, the obstetrician received a Polaroid photograph of the scan along with an interpretative report. The amniocentesis procedure itself was, however, performed at an unspecified later time rather than immediately following ultrasonography. It is therefore difficult to compare this study with other series in which ultrasonographic studies were performed immediately prior to amniocentesis.

Karp et al (30) compared 32 patients undergoing genetic amniocentesis with prior B-mode ultrasonographic placental localization to 50 patients who had no prior ultrasonography. Patients were not randomly assigned to groups using and not using ultrasonography, because of "ethical considerations." Patients who were selected for ultrasonographic studies included 1) those with fetuses at risk for neural tube defects (so chosen because anencephaly may be diagnosed by ultrasonography), 2) Rh-negative women with Rh-positive husbands, 3) individuals in whom the diagnosis of twins might itself constitute a reason for abortion, and 4) any other woman who requested that ultrasonography be used. All amniocenteses were performed by either an obstetrician/geneticist or three resident trainees; however, the number of procedures actually performed in each group by the more experienced senior investigator was not reported. The authors concluded that ultrasonographic placental localization neither significantly reduced incidence of bloody taps (21.9% with and 14% without ultrasonography) nor affected the erythrocyte count in the amniotic fluid sample. In addition, ultrasonography did not significantly reduce the incidence of multiple puncture attempts. Because long-range hazards of in utero exposure to ultrasound cannot be excluded, Karp et al (30) recommend that ultrasonography should be used selectively rather than as a routine procedure.

PLACENTAL LOCALIZATION TO PREVENT RH IMMUNIZATION

Whether ultrasonographic localization of the placenta decreases the likelihood of fetomaternal transfusion, which presumably would increase the risk of Rh immunization in unsensi-

tized women with Rh-positive fetuses, is also controversial (24). Fetomaternal transfusion by disruption of the fetoplacental circulation may have an immunizing effect; however, the magnitude of this risk has not been determined. One must also consider such factors as ABO compatibility, the number of needle insertions, the placental location, and the amount of fetal blood transfused into the maternal circulation. Nonetheless, many investigators have clearly documented Rh sensitization following third-trimester, and occasionally following second-trimester, amniocentesis (34, 45, 49, 61). Henry et al (26) recommended administration of Rh-immune globin in cases of potential Rh-incompatability; however, both short and long term fetal consequences of administering this drug during the second trimester have yet to be established.

In a series of 28 patients between 22 and 24 weeks of pregnancy, Curtis et al (13) showed a significant fetomaternal transfusion in 50% of women in whom an amniocentesis was performed through an anterior placenta (B-mode ultrasound).

Harrison et al (24) obtained maternal venous samples before and 5 minutes after amniocentesis to detect fetal cells by using the Betke–Kleihaur test. A fetomaternal transfusion of 2 ml or greater, defined by at least 35 fetal red cells counted in 2 min under low-power microscopy, was considered "significant" in the postamniocentesis specimen. If ultrasonography did not precede amniocentesis, 4 of 44 cases (9%) showed significant fetomaternal transfusion, whereas if ultrasound preceded amniocentesis, only 4 of 87 (4.5%) had a significant transfusion. Thus, ultrasonographic placental localization prior to amniocentesis appeared to reduce the incidence of fetomaternal transfusions.

DETERMINATION OF FETAL POSITION

Fetal puncture is a recognized hazard of third-trimester amniocentesis (3, 10, 12, 15). The NICHD (44) prospective midtrimester amniocentesis study showed no significant risk of fetal injury that could be attributed to needle puncture, but isolated reports of serious injuries following amniocentesis have included gangrene of the arm (33), ileocutaneous fistula (50), temporary neurologic damage (29), and umbilical cord puncture (60). Karp and Hayden (29) and Broome et al (7) believe that the risk of puncture is 1%–4%, though usually fetal puncture produces only a small punctate lesion or linear scars. We suspect that the fetus is often inadvertently touched by the needle tip and probably moves away in most cases; however, if the fetus is entrapped between the needle and the uterine wall, a potentially serious puncture could occur. Whether delineation of the fetal position immediately prior to amniocentesis reduces the risk of needle puncture has not yet been determined.

Some investigators advocate use of an ultrasonic aspiration-biopsy transducer during the actual amniocentesis procedure (21). Such transducers lie on the maternal abdomen and have a central lumen through which a needle can be passed. An A-mode display can be obtained in which an echo representing the needle tip can be produced, enabling the depth of the needle tip to be monitored throughout the procedure. Use of such an instrument might theoretically reduce the hazard of needle puncture, but no data concerning its efficacy are available.

FETAL ANOMALIES

A number of fetal abnormalities may be ultrasonographically detected during the second trimester (eg, anencephaly, hydrocephalus, meningomyelocele, and omphalocele). As newer high-resolution techniques are employed, the accuracy for the prenatal detection of anomalies will undoubtedly increase (Ch. 19).

UTERINE AND ADNEXAL ABNORMALITIES

Some women undergoing genetic amniocentesis may also have uterine or adnexal abnormalities detectable by ultrasonography. Uterine leiomyomata are especially common and of importance because the uterus appears larger than expected by dates. Such confusion might result in premature and, hence, inevitably unsuccessful attempts at amniocentesis. In addition, the amniotic cavity may be distorted by submucous leiomyomata. Another infrequently encountered abnormality is a bicornuate uterus. How-

ever, amniocentesis is rarely a problem because the nonpregnant horn is usually only minimally enlarged. Finally, if an adnexal tumor is discovered, careful evaluation is mandatory.

POTENTIAL RISKS OF ULTRASONOGRAPHY

In using ultrasonography either before amniocentesis or during the actual procedure there are the following major concerns: 1) Will ultrasound exposure interfere with amniotic fluid cell growth? 2) Is ultrasound exposure teratogenic?

FAILURE OF AMNIOTIC FLUID CULTURES

In 1973 Robinson et al (52) reported growth failure in 39 of 65 (60%) amniotic fluid cultures obtained from women who underwent ultrasonography prior to amniocentesis, compared to only 13 of 106 (12%) cases not preceded by ultrasonography. Despite this fivefold difference in the number of culture failures, these investigators stated at that time that ". . . the number of uncontrollable factors make the significance of these observations in relation to ultrasound being the cause of the difference somewhat dubious." Indeed, the same group later failed to observe continuation of the phenomenon (51). Other studies have been unable to demonstrate adverse effects on the success rate of amniotic fluid cell cultures as a result of ultrasound exposure (43, 59). By contrast, Young et al (59) indicated that cultures initiated from grossly bloody amniotic fluid samples have a significantly higher rate of failure, though in our laboratory we do not have this impression. If ultrasonography decreases so-called bloody taps, preliminary ultrasonography would secondarily diminish the likelihood of culture failure.

TERATOGENIC EFFECTS

X-irradiation and possibly other forms of energy may be hazardous to the developing embryo. It is reasonable, therefore, to question the safety of sonar, a physical and mechanical form of energy. Donald (14) identifies three potential mechanisms of damage by ultrasound: 1) heating, 2) cavitation, and 3) unequal spatial target response to radiation pressure, resulting in shearing stresses and "streaming" phenomena in particle-containing fluids. Determination of the "margin of safety" between the effective dose of ultrasound required to obtain sufficient diagnostic information and the dosage of deleterious effects is necessary. In evaluating the numerous studies that have dealt with the possible adverse biological effects of ultrasound, it is useful to recall the following six basic principles of teratology (56):

1. Susceptibility to teratogenesis depends on the genotype of the conceptus and the manner in which this interacts with adverse environmental factors.

2. Susceptibility to teratogenesis varies with developmental stage at the time of exposure to an adverse influence.

3. Teratogenic agents act in specific ways (mechanisms) on developing cells and tissues to initiate sequences of abnormal develmental events (pathogenesis).

4. The access of adverse influences to developing tissues depends on the nature of the influence (agent).

5. The four manifestations of deviant development are death, malformation, growth retardation, and functional deficit.

6. Manifestations of deviant development increase in frequency and degree as dosage increases, from the no effect to the totally lethal level.

EXPERIMENTAL STUDIES OF ULTRASOUND EXPOSURE

Many experimental systems have been used to evaluate the effects of ultrasound exposure. Macintosch and Davey (37) reported that Doppler ultrasound emitted from commercially available fetal pulse detectors significantly increased the number of chromosome aberrations in exposed human blood cultures, compared to unexposed control cultures. These aberrations consisted of chromatid breaks, achromatic lesions or gaps, chromosome (isochromatid) gaps, and chromosomes fragments. In addition, two dicentric chromosomes and one ring chromosome were detected in two of the treated cul-

tures. However, many other investigators failed to confirm the Macintosch–Davey findings (1, 5, 6, 8, 27).

Kunze-Mühl (32) showed that, when x-ray-damaged cells from human venous blood were exposed to an ultrasound fetal heart detector, the number of chromosomal aberrations was significantly lower than that of controls. However, ultrasound exposure with the same instrument performed before x-ray treatment increased chromosome damage, compared with controls. On the basis of these experiments, Kunze-Mühl recommended that radiographic studies be performed prior to ultrasonographic investigations, if both diagnostic procedures are to be undertaken. Vicissitudes of cell selection and uncertainty concerning cell losses in vitro may or may not invalidate this conclusion.

Other investigations have yielded conflicting results. For example, Galperin-Lemaitre and Kirsch-Volders (18) reported that doses of ultrasound exposure commonly used in obstetrics (i.e., 20 mW/cm^2, 1 MHz) had no effect on mammalian deoxyribonucleic acid (DNA) as determined by fragmentation of purified DNA examined by electronmicroscopy. By contrast, Prasad et al (48) found that HeLa cells exposed to 4 mW/cm^2, 1 MHz ultrasound intensity showed up to 14% less DNA synthesis, determined by ^{3}H-thymidine-methyl incorporation.

Considerable experimental data are also available on the threshold intensities of ultrasound exposure necessary to produce structural or functional alterations in tissues. Among these changes are mitochondrial swelling, disruption of cristae, change in transport capacity across membranes, lyosomal changes, centrilobular liver necrosis, and hemorrhagic spinal cord and brain injuries (see review by Taylor and Dyson [54]). Of particular interest are studies by Lyon and Simpson (36). Mice exposed to either continuous-wave or pulsed ultrasound were compared to mice exposed to 100 rad x-rays and to controls. For up to 8 weeks after treatment there was no evidence of decreases in testicular weight or sperm counts, sterility in males, increases in dominant lethal mutations, or translocations or chromosome fragments in spermatocytes. There was, however, a significant increase in sterile matings among females treated either with 30-sec pulsed ultrasound 1 to several days prior to mating or with continuous-wave ultrasound on the day of mating. These doses were, however, near the maximum that could be administered without sterilizing the animals. By contrast, overt genetic damage was observed in the x-ray-treated animals. Lyon and Simpson (36) concluded that the use of ultrasound in antenatal diagnosis was unlikely to be a genetic hazard to either mother or fetus. These findings were consistent with those of an earlier study by Woodward et al (57), who similarly failed to demonstrate any difference in the incidence of abnormalities in offspring of pregnant mice exposed to pulsed ultrasound intensities well above that commonly used in clinical practice (490 Wcm^2).

CLINICAL STUDIES

To date, no clinical studies have shown teratogenic effects as a result of diagnostic ultrasound. In one retrospective series of 720 obstetric patients undergoing ultrasonic Doppler inspection of the fetus at varying times during pregnancy, Bernstine (4) reported no adverse effects on fetal survival. The incidence of prematurity or congenital anomalies was also not significantly different than expected on the basis of United States Navy statistics over the same period of time. However, the study group and the control group were not necessarily comparable, because such important variables as maternal age, race, socioeconomic status, and previous obstetric history were not considered.

In a collaborative study of 3297 pregnancies from three different centers, Hellman et al (25) attempted to assess the effect of ultrasound on the fetus; 1114 or the 3297 patients considered to have "completely normal pregnancies" at the time of initial examination were selected for analysis. Except for abortions, which amounted to 10.1% of cases examined before 20 weeks' gestation, the frequency of fetal abnormalities in all 3297 cases was 3.7%, compared to 2.7% fetal abnormalities in the "normal group." If ultrasound were teratogenic, exposure prior to 10 weeks' gestation would be expected to show the highest frequency of anomalies. In fact, the lowest frequency of fetal abnormalities (2 of 145 or 1.4%) occurred in the group first exposed to ultrasound before 10 weeks' gestation. Interpre-

tation of these data is difficult, however, because 1) there were no true controls, i.e., cases not exposed to ultrasound, and 2) the group studied was selected by excluding all pregnancies thought to be abnormal (66%).

Donald (14) attempted to determine possible hearing defects as a result of in utero exposure to diagnostic ultrasound. Of 160,000 births in Glasgow between 1966 and 1974, 216 children with hearing defects were ascertained through a registry. Of these 216 children, 7 were offspring of women who had had ultrasonographic examinations during pregnancy. Donald (14) found multiple reasons other than ultrasound for all except one child's deafness. Among the obvious methodologic shortcomings in this study are the following: 1) lack of controls, 2) failure to obtain audiometric tests to determine the type of deafness in the affected children, 3) failure to exclude heritable deafness, 4) failure to confirm normal audiograms in those considered unaffected, and 5) biases of ascertainment made inevitable by including only those deaf children listed in the registry.

CONCLUSIONS

Objective considerations of possible benefits and risks of ultrasonography prior to second-trimester amniocentesis do not permit definitive conclusions at this time. The consensus among geneticists and obstetricians is that routine ultrasonography should logically be useful in confirming fetal age, detecting twin gestations, and avoiding the placenta. No well-designed study has, however, verified that these possible benefits are in fact realized. Similarly, the consensus is that ultrasound is relatively safe, but detailed long-term evaluations of fetuses exposed in utero have not been performed. Moreover, pulsed ultrasound in quantities used diagnostically indeed has effects on DNA, and without question nonpulsed ultrasound can be deleterious. Nonpulsed ultrasound apparently does not cause chromosomal breakage, but breakage is a relatively insensitive indicator of genetic damage.

Having concluded that neither the efficacy nor the safety of ultrasound is proved, some investigators believe that ultrasonography should not be employed routinely before amniocentesis. Although cognizant of such reasoning, we prefer a less nihilistic approach. If confusions concerning gestational age or uterine size exist, the possible benefits accrued by ultrasound surely seem to outweigh the possible risks. No firm conclusions concerning usefulness of ultrasonographic placental localization in avoiding the placenta are possible; however, until more definitive data verify the deleterious effects of nonpulsed ultrasound, we shall continue to use ultrasonography routinely in hopes of minimizing placenta puncture. If ultrasound should prove harmful, the benefits/risks ratio may be altered so that ultrasonography for placental localization is not warranted routinely. On the basis of available data, however, we conclude that routine ultrasonography prior to amniocentesis is justified.

REFERENCES

1. ABDULLA U, CAMPBELL S, DEWHURST CJ, TALBERT D, LUCAS M, MALLARHEY M: Effect of diagnostic ultrasound on maternal and fetal chromosomes. Lancet 2:829, 1971

2. Antenatal diagnosis of genetic disorders. American College of Obstetricians and Gynecologists Technical Bulletin No. 39, 1976

3. BERNER HW, SEILER EP, BARLOW J: Fetal cardiac tamponade, a complication of amniocentesis. Obstet Gynecol 40:599, 1972

4. BERNSTINE RL: Safety studies with ultrasonic Doppler technique. A clinical follow-up of patients and tissue culture study. Obstet Gynecol 34:707, 1969

5. BOBROW M, BLACKWELL N, UNRAU AN, BLEANEY E: Absence of any observed effect of ultrasonic irradiation on human chromosomes. Br J Obstet Gynaecol 78:730, 1971

6. BOYD E, ABDULLA U, DONALD I, FLEMING JEE, HALL AJ, FERGUSON-SMITH MA: Chromosome breakage and ultrasound. Br Med J 2:501, 1971

7. BROOME DL, WILSON MG, WEISS B, KELLOGG B: Needle puncture of fetus: a complication of second trimester amniocentesis. Am J Obstet Gynecol 126:247, 1976

8. COAKLEY WT, HUGHES DE, SLADE JS, LAURENCE KM: Chromosome aberrations after exposure to ultrasound. Br Med J 1:109, 1971

9. COLLMAN RD, STOLLER A: A survey of mongoloid births in Victoria, Australia, 1942–1957. Am J Public Health 52:813, 1962

10. COOK LN, SHOTT RJ, ANDREWS BF: Fetal complications of diagnostic amniocentesis: a review and report of a case with pneumothorax. Pediatrics 53:421, 1974

11. COURT BROWN WM, LAW P, SMITH PG: Sex chromosome aneuploidy and parental age. Ann Hum Genet 33:1, 1969

12. CROSS HE, MAUMENEE AE: Ocular trauma during amniocentesis. N Engl J Med 287:993, 1972

13. CURTIS JD, COHEN WN, RICHERSON HB, WHITE CA: The importance of placental localization preceding amniocentesis. Obstet Gynecol 40:194, 1971

14. DONALD I: The biological effects of ultrasound. In Donald I, Levi S (eds): Present and Future of Diagnosis Ultrasound. New York, John Wiley & Sons, 1975

15. EGLEY CC: Laceration of fetal spleen during amniocentesis. Am J Obstet Gynecol 116:582, 1973

16. ELIAS S, MARTIN AO, PATEL VA, GERBIE AB, SIMPSON JL: Analysis for amniotic fluid crystallization in second-trimester amniocentesis. Am J Obstet Gynecol 133:401, 1979

17. FUCHS F: Amniocentesis and abortion: methods and risks. Birth Defects: Original Article Series 7:18, 1971

18. GALPERIN-LEMAITRE H, KIRSCH-VOLDERS M: Ultrasound and mammalian DNA. Lancet 2:662, 1975

19. GERBIE AB, SHKOLNIK AA: Ultrasound prior to amniocentesis for genetic counseling. Obstet Gynecol 46:716, 1975

20. GOLBUS MC: Prenatal diagnosis of genetic defects. Where it is and where it is going. Birth Defects, 432:330, 1978

21. GOLDBERT BB: Amniocentesis with ultrasonic guidance. In Sanders RC, James AE (eds): Ultrasonography in Obstetrics and Gynecology. New York, Appleton-Century-Crofts, 1977

22. GUIBAUD S, BONNET M, DURY A: Amniotic fluid or urine? Lancet 1:746, 1976

23. HAMERTON JL: Human Cytogenetics, Vol I. New York, Academic Press, 1971

24. HARRISON R, CAMPBELL S, CRAFT I: Risks of fetomaternal hemorrhage resulting from amniocentesis with and without ultrasound placental localization. Obstet Gynecol 46:389, 1975

25. HELLMAN LM, DUFFUS GM, DONALD I, SUNDEN B: Safety of diagnostic ultrasound in obstetrics. Lancet 1:1133, 1970

26. HENRY G, WEXLER P, ROBINSON A: Rh-immune globin after amniocentesis for genetic diagnosis. Obstet Gynecol 48:557, 1976

27. HILL CR, JOSHI GP, REVELL SH: A search for chromosome damage following exposure of Chinese hamster cells to high-intensity, pulsed ultrasound. Br J Radiol 45:333, 1972

28. HOOK EB, HAMERTON JL: The frequency of chromosome abnormalities in consecutive newborn stud-

ies—Differences between studies—Results by sex and by severity of phenotypic involvement. In Hook EB, Porter IH (eds): Population Cytogenetics. New York, Academic Press, 1977

29. KARP LE, HAYDEN PW: Fetal puncture during midtrimester amniocentesis. Obstet Gynecol 49:115, 1977

30. KARP LE, ROTHWELL R, CONRAD SH, HOEHN HW, HICKOCK DE: Ultrasonic placental localization and bloody taps in midtrimester amniocentesis for prenatal diagnosis. Obstet Gynecol 50(5):589, 1977

31. KERENYI TD, WALKER B: The preventability of "bloody taps" in second trimester amniocentesis by ultrasound scanning. Obstet Gynecol 50:61, 1977

32. KUNZE-MÜHL E: Chromosome damage in human lymphocytes after different combinations of x-ray and ultrasonic treatment. In Kazner E, de Vlieger M (eds): Proceedings of 2nd European Congress on Ultrasonics in Medicine. Int Congr Ser No. 363, New York, American Elsevier, 1975

33. LAMB MP: Gangrene of a fetal limb due to amniocentesis. Br J Obstet Gynaecol 82:829, 1975

34. LAWRENCE M: Diagnostic amniocentesis in early pregnancy. Br Med J 2:191, 1977

35. LUBS HA, RUDDLE FH: Chromosomal abnormalities in the human population: estimation of rates based on New Haven newborn study. Science 169:495, 1970

36. LYON MF, SIMPSON GM: An investigation into the possible genetic hazards of ultrasound. Br J Radiol 47:712, 1974

37. MACINTOSCH IJC, DAVEY DA: Chromosome aberrations induced by an ultrasound fetal pulse detector. Br Med J 4:92, 1970

38. MIKKELSEN M: Down's syndrome: current stage of cytogenetic research. Humangenetik 12:1, 1971

39. MILUNSKY A: The Prenatal Diagnosis of Hereditary Disorders. Springfield, IL, CC Thomas, 1973

40. MILUNSKY A, ALPERT E: Prenatal diagnosis of neural tube defects. I. Problems and pitfalls: analysis of 2495 cases using the alphafetoprotein assay. Obstet Gynecol 48:1, 1976

41. MISKIN M, DORAN TA, RUDD NL, BENZIE RJ, MALONE RM: Ultrasound in prenatal genetics. In Sanders RC, James AE (eds): Ultrasonography in Obstetrics and Gynecology. New York, Appleton-Century-Crofts, 1977

42. MISKIN M, DORAN TA, RUDD N, GARDNER HA, LIEDGREN S, BENZIE RJ: Use of ultrasound for placental localization in genetic amniocentesis. Obstet Gynecol 43:872, 1974

43. NELSON LH, GOODMAN HO, BROWN SH: Ultrasonography preceding diagnostic amniocentesis and its effect on amniotic fluid cell growth. Obstet Gynecol 50:65, 1977

44. NICHD National Registry for Amniocentesis Study Group: Midtrimester amniocentesis for prenatal diagnosis. Safety and accuracy. JAMA 236:1471, 1976

45. PEDDLE LJ: Increase of antibody titer following amniocentesis. Am J Obstet Gynecol 100:567, 1968

46. PENROSE LS, SMITH GF: Down's Anomaly. London, J and A Churchill, 1966

47. PIRANI BBI, DORAN TA, BENZIE RJ: Amniotic fluid or maternal urine? Lancet 1:303, 1967

48. PRASAD N, PRASAD R, BUSHONG SC, NORTH LB, RHEA E: Ultrasound and mammalian D.N.A. Lancet 1:1181, 1976

49. QUEENAN JT, ADAMS DW: Amniocentesis: a possible immunizing hazard. Obstet Gynecol 24:530, 1964

50. RECKWOOD AM: A case of ileal atresia and ileocutaneous fistula caused by amniocentesis. J Pediatr 91:312, 1977

51. ROBINSON A: Intrauterine diagnosis and ultrasound. Lancet 2:1504, 1973

52. ROBINSON A, BOWES W, DROEGENMUELLER W, PUCK M, GOODMAN S, SHIKES R, GREENSHUR A: Intrauterine diagnosis: potential complications. Am J Obstet Gynecol 116:937, 1973

53. SIMPSON JL, MORILLO-CUCCI G, HORWORTH M, STEIFEL FH, FELDMAN F, GERMAN J: Abnormalities of human sex chromosomes. VI. Monozygotic twins with the complement 48,XXY. Hum Genet 21:301, 1974

54. TAYLOR KJW, DYSON M: Experimental inosation of animal tissues and fetuses. In Sanders RC, James AE (eds): Ultrasonography in Obstetrics and Gynecology. New York, Appleton-Century-Crofts, 1977

55. WEXLER P, GOTTESFELD KR: Second trimester placenta previa: an apparently normal placentation. Obstet Gynecol 50:706, 1977

56. WILSON JG: Environment and Birth Defects. New York, Academic Press, 1974

57. WOODWARD B, POND JB, WARWICK R: How safe is diagnostic ultrasound? Br J Radiol 43:719, 1970

58. WRIGHT SW, DAY RW, MULLER H, WEINHOUSE R: Frequency of trisomy and translocation in Down's syndrome. J Pediatr 70:420, 1967

59. YOUNG PE, MATSON MR, JONES OW: Amniocentesis for prenatal diagnosis. Review of problems and outcomes in a large series. Am J Obstet Gynecol 125:495, 1976

60. YOUNG PE, MATSON MR, JONES OW: Fetal exsanguination and other vascular injuries from midtrimester genetic amniocentesis. Am J Obstet Gynecol 129:21, 1977

61. ZIPURSKY A, POLLOCK J, CHOWN B, ISRAELS LG: Transplacental fetal hemorrhage after placental injury during delivery or amniocentesis. Lancet 2:493, 1963

16

The Placenta

DANIEL I. EDELSTONE

Ultrasound has been used for the past decade to localize the placenta during pregnancy (10, 13, 17, 23, 24). Accurate localization of the placenta is important in the management of patients with third-trimester vaginal bleeding. Placental localization has also proved useful when performed prior to diagnostic amniocentesis (4, 15, 18).

Ultrasound placentography involves the use of high-frequency sound waves to define the size, shape, and location of the placenta within the uterus (10). This is in contrast to other techniques of placental localization such as soft-tissue placentography, arteriography, and isotope placentography, all of which require ionizing radiation (34). Ultrasound is the ideal method of placental localization because it is accurate, is safe for mother and fetus, involves no maternal discomfort, and is effective at any point in gestation. In addition, because of the safety of ultrasound, evaluation of the placenta can be repeated many times during pregnancy. This has recently enabled investigators to study the structure and function of the placenta during normal and abnormal pregnancies (6, 9, 14, 19, 42).

In this chapter primary attention is given to the use of ultrasound for placental localization, including a brief comparison between sonographic and radiographic methods for placental localization. In addition this chapter describes the application of ultrasound in evaluating growth, development, and function of the placenta throughout normal and abnormal pregnancies.

PLACENTAL LOCALIZATION

METHODS OF PLACENTAL LOCALIZATION

SOFT-TISSUE PLACENTOGRAPHY

Of all the techniques for placental localization, soft-tissue placentography (plain film radiography) is by far the easiest to perform. Nevertheless, the information obtained is frequently unsatisfactory (2). In this method the uterine outline appears as a soft tissue shadow around the fetus, and the placenta is visualized as a crescentic shadow between fetus and uterus. The radiodensity of the placenta is slightly higher than amniotic fluid; this may be related to calcium deposits scattered within the placenta (34).

Using soft-tissue placentography, the radiologist frequently encounters confusing placenta-like shadows in pregnancies under 32 weeks in duration or in pregnancies complicated by hydramnios (in which amniotic fluid volume is relatively large compared to fetal volume). Furthermore, an abnormal fetal lie (transverse or oblique) can present similar diagnostic difficulties (2, 34). Yet it is in all these clinical conditions that placenta previa is more common and accurate localization of the placenta is essential.

ARTERIOGRAPHY

Although arteriography can accurately define the limits of the placenta, it remains technically complex and potentially dangerous for the mother (39). The radiologist injects a water-soluble contrast material into a maternal femoral artery by means of a catheter whose tip is placed 3 cm above the aortic bifurcation. A single lateral or oblique roentgenogram taken 2 sec after the injection demonstrates the placental sinusoids as ill-defined collections of contrast material within the uterus.

ISOTOPE PLACENTOGRAPHY

Isotope placentography requires the intravenous injection of a radioisotope that will remain in the maternal circulation for a reasonable length of time. The radiologist uses a scintillation counter to detect increased radioactivity over the highly vascular placental site (1, 12, 26, 34). Radiation exposure is minor when compared with either soft-tissue placentography or arteriography (12, 34). Unlike soft-tissue placentography, however, an abnormal fetal presentation or the presence of hydramnios does not influence the accuracy of placental localization.

ULTRASOUND PLACENTOGRAPHY

The reliability and accuracy of ultrasound for placental localization compare favorably with those of arteriography and isotope placentography (1, 12, 24, 26, 39). However, the advantages of ultrasound are the following: 1) mother and fetus are not exposed to ionizing radiation (34), 2) placental localization can be performed at any time after the ninth week of pregnancy (14, 28), 3) the entire placenta is visualized, and 4) the limits of the lower uterine segment and the site of the internal cervical os are defined (13, 24, 26, 34). The relationship between the lower placental margin and the cervix is of utmost importance in the accurate diagnosis of placenta previa.

TECHNIQUES OF ULTRASOUND PLACENTOGRAPHY

The sonographer has available three techniques for placentography: 1) B-scan sonography, 2) gray-scale sonography, and 3) real-time imaging. Conventional B-scan sonography uses a threshold detection mechanism by which strong echoes appear on the oscilloscope screen while weak echoes (those below threshold) do not. Images produced are therefore only black and white without intervening shades of gray. The major disadvantage of this method is that it fails to show the internal fine structure of the placenta (13). Gray-scale ultrasound adds a scan converter to the sonographic system, making possible the simultaneous display of both strong and weak echoes. This results in an image with various shades of gray, which differs dramatically from the all-black-and-white image obtained with conventional B-scanning (27, 28). The third ultrasound technique, real-time imaging, uses an array of transducers to emit high-frequency sound waves in rapid overlapping sequence; real-time imaging provides, therefore, a constantly updated gray-scale display and is particularly suited for evaluating structures in motion. The resolving power of real-time imaging is not, however, nearly as good as that of static gray scale ultrasound.

CHARACTERISTICS OF NORMAL PLACENTAL ECHOES

Regardless of the technique used, ultrasound identification of the placenta depends on the presence of two characteristic images, the fetal chorionic plate and multiple internal placental echoes (24, 28). In a typical sonogram (longitudinal plane) (Fig. 16–1), the placenta appears as a semilunar area composed of multiple echoes bordered on the maternal side by the uterine wall and on the fetal side by a generally continuous line representing the fetal chorionic plate. The chorionic plate is demonstrated best when it is not in contact with the fetus and when there is amniotic fluid adjacent to it. The multiple internal echoes (placental speckles) probably represent pools of blood within cotyledons. The extent to which a placenta speckles depends on the location of the placenta as well as the sensitivity (gain) setting of the instrument. In general, a placenta on the posterior uterine wall displays fewer internal echoes than one on the anterior uterine wall, because the ultrasound beam is attenuated in traversing an overlying fetus (Fig.

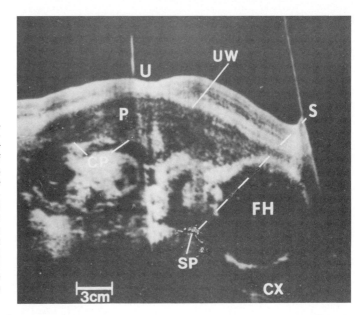

FIG. 16-1. Anteriorly implanted placenta, 36 weeks. The fetal head (FH) closely applied to the anterior uterine wall (UW) near the symphysis eliminates the possibility of anterior placenta previa. All ultrasonograms are longitudinal scans in approximately the midline sagittal plane; all figures are gray-scale sonograms except Figures 16–5 and 16–8, which are B-mode scans. The 3-cm scale applies to each scan. Abbreviations: AF, amniotic fluid; B, bladder; CP, chorionic plate; CX, cervix; FH, fetal head; FT, fetal trunk; P, placenta; S, symphysis; SP, sacral promontory; U, umbilicus; UW, uterine wall. The dashed line divides the uterus into upper and lower segments.

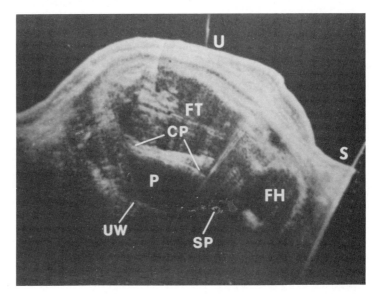

FIG. 16-2. Posteriorly implanted placenta, 36 weeks. There are fewer internal placental echoes than with an anterior placenta (compare to Fig. 16-1). The fetal head (FH) closely applied to the sacral promontory (SP) excludes the possibility of posterior placenta previa.

16-2). Increases in sensitivity typically increase internal placental speckling, whereas decreases in sensitivity decrease them, a characteristic that is extremely important in accurately identifying the placental site.

INDICATIONS FOR PLACENTAL LOCALIZATION

ANTEPARTUM HEMORRHAGE

Placenta Previa. Gray-scale ultrasound is clearly the technique of choice for the evaluation of placenta previa since it provides better resolution than either B-scan or real-time imaging (27, 28). Real-time imaging can, however, be used as a screening technique to exclude those placentas situated entirely in the upper uterine segment.

Sonography can correctly diagnose placenta previa more than 95% of the time (24, 28). The false-negative rate is usually less than 5%, which surpasses the false-negative rates for isotope placentography (5%–13%) and for soft-tissue placentography (7%–25%) (12, 24, 34). The lower uterine segment and internal cervical os (Fig. 16–1) must be identified if placental previa

181

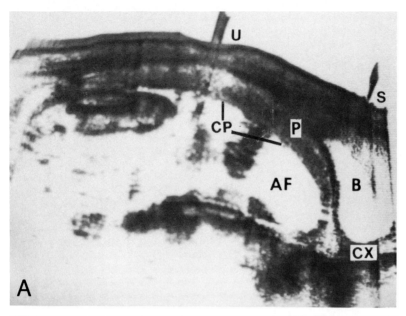

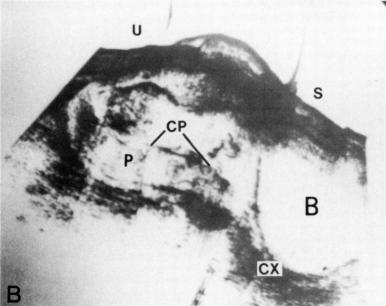

FIG. 16–3. A. Anterior partial placenta previa, 34 weeks (transverse fetal lie). Placental tissue displaces fetus and amniotic fluid from bladder and anterior surface of lower uterine segment. The cervix is partially occluded by placental tissue. **B.** Posterior partial placenta previa, 30 weeks. Placental tissue partially obstructs the cervical os. **(Continued)**

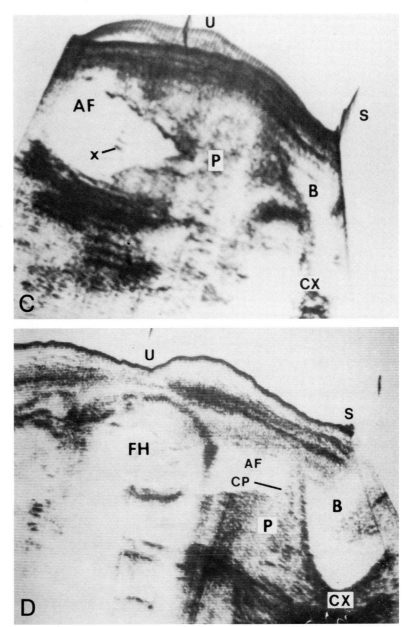

FIG. 16–3. (*Continued*) C. Complete placenta previa, 34 weeks. **D.** Complete placenta previa, 38 weeks; in these latter two sonograms placenta fills the entire lower uterine segment and obstructs the cervix (CX). B, bladder, x, umbilical cord.

is to be accurately diagnosed. A partially distended bladder helps delineate these structures. The lower uterine segment is defined arbitrarily as that area below a line that joins the symphysis pubis and the sacral promontory, that is, the inlet of the true pelvis (13, 23, 34, 35). This is an approximation, since during the third trimester the lower uterine segment lengthens from 1.0 cm to as much as 10 cm at term (32). The cervix appears rectangular prior to term and contains a few echoes within its outline. When the cervix begins to efface near term, it is no longer identifiable and its approximate position is then defined as the area of junction between the vaginal canal and the uterus.

Anatomic and ultrasound diagnoses of placenta previa depend on identifying placental tissue covering some (partial placenta previa, Figs. 16–3A, B; see [13] for additional sonograms) or all of the internal cervical os (complete placenta previa, Figs. 16–3C, D). A placenta that lies within the lower uterine segment but only approaches the cervix without covering it is defined as a low-lying placenta (Figs. 16–4A, B).

An anterior placenta previa (Fig. 16–3A) displaces the fetus and amniotic fluid away from the anterior surface of the lower uterine segment, cervix, and bladder. In the normal patient in the third trimester, the presenting part of the fetus descends into the pelvis to fill the anteroposterior diameter of the pelvic inlet. When the fetal presenting part is applied closely to the anterior uterine wall or to the distended maternal bladder, the possibility of anterior placenta previa is effectively eliminated (Fig. 16–1).

A posterior placenta previa (Fig. 16–3B) displaces the fetal presenting part away from the maternal sacral promontory. Therefore, demonstration of the fetal presenting part applied in close proximity to the maternal sacral promontory excludes posterior placenta previa (Fig. 16–2). Nevertheless, the accurate diagnosis of posterior placenta previa may be difficult early in the third trimester. In this instance the fetal presenting part may not be large enough to fill the entire anteroposterior diameter of the pelvic inlet, and thus a space is left between maternal sacral promontory and fetus. Either amniotic fluid or placenta may occupy this space. Increasing the sensitivity (gain) setting of the ultrasound instrument increases placental speckling when placenta is present. When amniotic fluid is present, however, there is no change in the echo pattern (Figs. 16–4A, B).

A placenta that is located posteriorly in the uterus is likely to extend to the lower uterine segment if the distance between the posterior fetal parietal bone and the adjacent sacral margin exceeds 15 mm (23) (Figs. 16–4A, B). In some cases, however, a low-lying posterior placenta cannot easily be distinguished from a partial posterior placenta previa. In these cases the sonographer reports the uncertainty of the diagnosis to the clinician, who will then manage the patient in accordance with established obstetric principles. In spite of these difficulties, the diagnosis of posterior placenta previa is accurately made in the vast majority of cases.

How Early Can Diagnosis of Placenta Previa Be Made? Evaluation of the placenta with ultrasound during the second trimester has shown that the placenta is a large organ whose implantation site can cover more than one-half of the intrauterine surface. Prior to 30 weeks' gestation, sonar examination of the placenta often demonstrates a low-lying placenta, and yet later reexamination (particularly late in the third trimester) often shows a normal implantation site (22). King has termed this phenomenon "placental migration," but this probably does not represent true movement of the placenta. This positional change probably reflects a more rapid growth of the uterus than of the placenta during the third trimester (22, 29). The lower uterine segment undergoes tremendous development during the last half of pregnancy. The length of the lower uterine segment increases from approximately 0.5 cm at 20 weeks to as much as 8–10 cm at term (32). During the third trimester, rapid development of the uterus (in particular the lower uterine segment) increases the distance between the inferior placental margin and the cervix. As a result many low-lying placentas are converted to normal implantations by term. Additionally, Buttery and Davis (8), using time-lapse echography, have recently offered convincing data to explain the reason for the sonar visualization of the placenta in the lower uterine area, at least in some women, during the

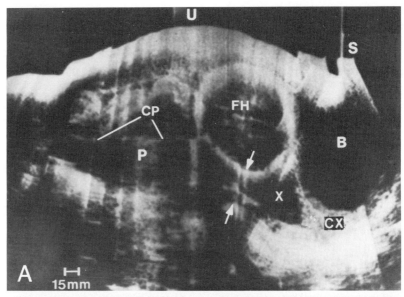

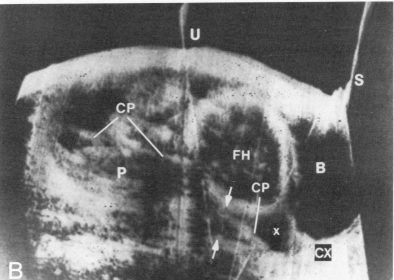

FIG. 16-4. A. Posterior low-lying placenta, 36 weeks—low sensitivity (gain). **B.** Posterior low-lying placenta, 36 weeks—high sensitivity (gain). A lower uterine segment (low-lying) placenta is documented since the placental edge extends below the sacral promontory and produces a separation **(arrows)** of greater than 15 mm between fetal head and maternal sacrum. Placenta previa does not, however, exist, because the increase in sensitivity (gain) does not result in an increase in multiple internal placental echoes near the cervix (X).

second trimester. In essence they have shown that Braxton–Hicks contractions occur periodically and displace the placenta toward the cervical area (Fig. 16–5); these physiologic contractions often produce a thickening along the posterior uterine wall simulating a myoma, Figure 16–5. Finally, excessive distention of the bladder has also been shown to displace the lower part of the placenta toward the cervix, leading to a false diagnosis of placenta previa. When the diagnosis of low-lying placenta is made in the second trimester or early in the third trimester, reexamination closer to term is essential (22, 29).

Since placental position in relation to the cervix appears to change dynamically during the last half of pregnancy, the question that arises is: how early in pregnancy can placenta previa be diagnosed definitively? To answer this question, Meyenburg (31) studied the placental site of 52 pregnant women serially beginning prior to the 20th week. One-half of these patients had placentas that were normally implanted. The other half had low-lying placentas diagnosed prior to the 20th week of gestation. Thirteen of these patients had experienced some second-trimester bleeding. Nevertheless, almost all of these 52 patients had placentas that were implanted nor-

mally by term, including 11 of the 13 patients who had been bleeding. In the remaining 2 patients, placental positions did not change by the third trimester and partial placental previas were confirmed at term. Wexler and Gottesfeld (41) have recently confirmed these observations in a larger series of patients.

In conclusion placenta previa should not be diagnosed definitively during the second trimester. The presence of placenta in the lower uterine segment during the second trimester should be reported as such, and a repeat examination should be requested at approximately 32–34 weeks' gestation.

Placental Abruption. In a patient with third-trimester vaginal bleeding the diagnosis of placental abruption may be supported by excluding the presence of placenta previa by ultrasound. Occasionally the sonographer identifies a retroplacental blood clot as a clear space between the basal plate and the uterine wall (Fig. 16–6). Tenderness over the area of the blood clot supports the diagnosis. In some patients, rupture of a marginal sinus has been diagnosed with ultrasound by observing a separation of the placental margin from the uterine wall (37).

ABNORMAL FETAL LIE

In the absence of vaginal bleeding in the third trimester, the presence of a transverse or an oblique fetal lie indicates the need for placental localization. A relatively large proportion of such pregnancies have some degree of placenta previa. Ultrasound placentography therefore aids in the clinical management of these patients as they approach term, particularly if antepartum hemorrhage develops.

AMNIOCENTESIS

Prenatal Genetic Diagnosis. Obstetricians perform amniocentesis for prenatal diagnosis of genetic disorders during the second trimester, a time when the normal placenta covers approximately one-half to two-thirds of the internal uterine surface (Fig. 16–7). At this point in gestation, ultrasound placentography should precede amniocentesis to reduce the incidence

FIG. 16–5. Longitudinal scan at 16 weeks' gestation, obtained during a Braxton–Hicks contraction. Note Placenta (P) extending to lower uterine area. Arrow is pointing at myoma-like mass that actually represents a thickened posterior uterine wall secondary to the contraction.

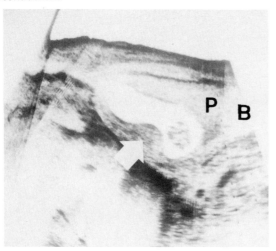

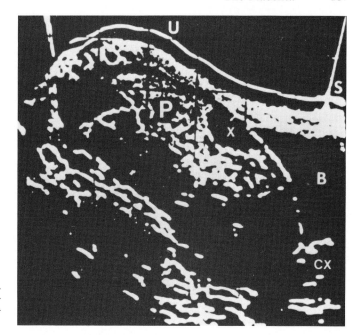

FIG. 16-6. Placental abruption, 27 weeks. The clear space (X) represents a retroplacental blood clot between the placental basal plate and the uterine wall.

FIG. 16-7. Normal growth and development of the placenta. **A.** Upper left, 10 weeks. Placenta has a uniform granular appearance. **B.** Upper right, 18 weeks. The normal placenta covers approximately two-thirds of the internal uterine surface. **C.** Lower left, 24 weeks. Placenta has a honeycombed appearance. Note the choriodecidual sinus (CDS) between uterine wall and placenta. **D.** Lower right, 32 weeks. Placenta has a reticular texture. Note the echo-free avillous spaces (AVS) within the placenta.

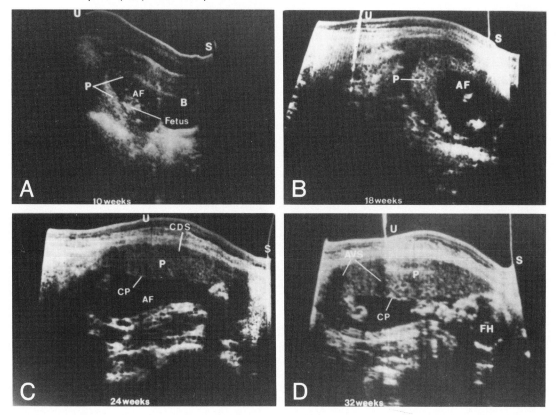

of bloody taps (18, 21, 38). Without prior localization, blood contaminates approximately 5%–10% of amniotic fluid samples obtained transabdominally (4, 18). The presence of maternal or fetal red blood cells in amniotic fluid can invalidate α-fetoprotein determinations or prevent fetal cell growth in tissue culture (11), which would necessitate a second amniocentesis.

The role of the sonographer is to define a pocket of amniotic fluid for aspiration in relationship to maternal surface landmarks such as the symphysis pubis or umbilicus. It is essential that the patient's bladder be empty at the time of ultrasound examination to ensure a good correlation between the fluid site identified and the eventual needle placement during amniocentesis. Additionally sonar examination of pregnancy before amniocentesis is mandatory to 1) confirm pregnancy length (optimal time for amniocentesis is 16 weeks' gestation), 2) exclude presence of twins, and 3) evaluate the normalcy of pregnancy (see Ch. 15). Amniocentesis via an ultrasound transducer equipped with an aspirating needle has been described (40). To date, no studies have shown that its use decreases the incidence of bloody taps when compared to amniocentesis performed by the method just described.

Amniocentesis in High-Risk Pregnancies. Obstetricians have used the analysis of bilirubin in amniotic fluid to improve fetal outcome in pregnancies complicated by rhesus sensitization. In these pregnancies it is essential to avoid penetrating the placenta because placental injury during amniocentesis may aggravate rhesus sensitization (18). In addition the presence of highly pigmented serum from an affected fetus can complicate interpretation of amniotic fluid results. Similarly, contamination of amniotic fluid with maternal serum or with serum from an unaffected fetus can alter bilirubin concentration (30).

Evaluation of the lecithin-sphingomyelin ratio in amniotic fluid as an index of fetal pulmonary maturity is reliable only when uncontaminated fluid is analyzed. With placental puncture, maternal or fetal red blood cells or serum can combine with the amniotic fluid to alter the assay of surfactant (7). If blood or serum enters the amniotic cavity, 2 weeks may be required for its complete removal.

PLACENTAL STRUCTURE AND FUNCTION

NORMAL PLACENTAL GROWTH AND DEVELOPMENT

Using gray-scale ultrasound, several investigators have defined the sonographic appearance of the normal placenta throughout pregnancy (9, 14, 28, 42). After 10 weeks of amenorrhea placental tissue has a uniform granular appearance (Fig. 16-7A). By 18–22 weeks the fetal membranes can be identified separating placental tissue from the surrounding echo-free amniotic fluid. Placental volume increases in relation to total intrauterine volume (19). The placenta takes on a honeycomb appearance and becomes less granular in texture (Fig. 16–7B). By 20–24 weeks it is also possible to identify echo-free choriodecidual sinuses between placenta and uterine wall (Fig. 16–7C).

At 28–30 weeks of gestation echo-free spaces within placental tissue (Fig. 16–7D) can be identified by gray-scale ultrasound. Histologic examination shows that these spaces are virtually free of villi and that their sizes range from 0.5 to 3.0 cm in diameter. These avillous spaces enlarge as pregnancy continues toward term.

During the last 6 weeks of pregnancy the texture of the placenta becomes more reticular and less honeycombed, corresponding to the increase in fibrous septae that separate placental lobules. Near term, ultrasound occasionally demonstrates echo-free spaces between the fetal membranes and the placenta; these spaces represent chorionic cysts.

Morphometric studies of the normal placenta throughout pregnancy have shown the thickness of the placenta to increase continually from the 16th week until the 36th week and then to decrease slightly until term (20). The average thickness of the placenta *in situ* in normal term pregnancies is approximately 3.6–3.8 cm. Placental volume calculated by ultrasound increases from approximately 60 ml at 10 weeks' gestation to 1000 ml by term. The doubling time for placental volume is much more rapid in the first 20 weeks than in the last 20 weeks of gestation. The volume of the placenta calculated by ultrasound averages approximately 35% more than placental volume measured postpartum. Blood lost from both the intervillous space and the umbilical cord at the time of delivery accounts for the differences measured between the two volumetric methods (19).

Ultrasound has also been used to evaluate how placental volume changes during labor (6). Uterine contractions increase the length, thickness, area, and therefore volume of the placenta.

ABNORMAL PLACENTAL GROWTH AND DEVELOPMENT

In some pregnancies avillous spaces and chorionic cysts, which generally do not appear until the last eight weeks of normal pregnancy, are seen earlier than one would expect (9, 14, 42) (Fig. 16–8). These pregnancies have resulted in infants that are small for gestational age at delivery. Premature appearance of avillous spaces may represent a need for greater placental blood

flow in situations in which the fetus is in jeopardy. This is related to the presumed role of the avillous space, which is to increase the amount of blood flowing through the intervillous space to keep pace with the rapid growth of the fetus (14). Since the appearance of the normal placenta changes in a consistent manner, abnormal maturation can aid in determining whether a fetus is small or large for gestational age, particularly in instances in which length of gestation is not known accurately.

SPECIFIC PLACENTAL ABNORMALITIES EVALUATED WITH ULTRASOUND

Rhesus Sensitization and Diabetes Mellitus. The placenta is a dynamic organ whose size changes in response to fetal needs (35). In pregnancies complicated by rhesus sensitization or diabetes mellitus, the thickness, length, and volume of the placenta increases (20). These increases in placental size may relate to fetal anemia in erythroblastosis and to a rapidly growing fetus in diabetes mellitus. Nevertheless, placentas that are large for gestational age have been observed ultrasonically by the 20th week of

FIG. 16–8. Chorionic cyst (CC), 28 weeks. Pregnancies associated with the early appearance of these cysts have resulted in infants that are small for gestational age.

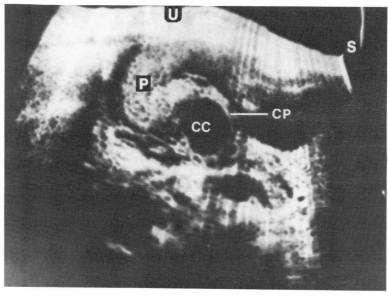

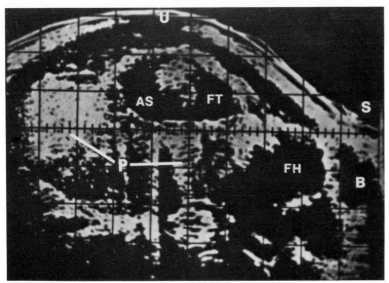

FIG. 16-9. Hydrops fetalis, 28 weeks. Greatly enlarged posterofundal placenta with the characteristic increase in internal placental echoes. Note the ascites (AS) in fetal trunk (FT).

rhesus-incompatible pregnancies, at a time when the degree of sensitization is not maximal. It is therefore possible that unidentified immunologic or endocrinologic factors are responsible for the observed increases in placental size. The edema and increased vascularity of placentas associated with fetal hydrops produce a characteristic ultrasound image (16, 20) (Fig. 16–9). Placental thickness of 5 cm or more is cause for concern in the patient with rhesus sensitization, and hydrops fetalis has often been associated with placentas thicker than 6 cm (16). A rapid increase in the thickness of the placenta in a rhesus-sensitized pregnancy generally indicates a poor prognosis for the fetus.

Molar Pregnancy. Ultrasound plays an important role in diagnosis and follow-up evaluation of molar pregnancies (3, 25, 36). This topic is discussed in detail in Chapter 14 of this book.

Other Placental Abnormalities. Ultrasound has been used to diagnose placenta membranacea antepartum (43), to evaluate retained products of conception in patients with postpartum bleeding (33), and to evaluate the patient with an intraabdominal pregnancy in whom the placenta has been left after delivery of the fetus (5).

CONCLUSIONS

Ultrasound visualization of the placenta is now an established diagnostic procedure in obstetrics. Its use defines the size, shape, and location of the placenta within the uterus and enables the clinician to make appropriate management decisions in patients with pregnancy-related complications. Furthermore, ultrasound has provided us with a better understanding of the normal growth and development of the placenta. By understanding normal structure and function, we are better able to evaluate and possibly (at some future date) treat those pregnancies associated with abnormal placentas.

REFERENCES

1. AIERS M, EVERED DC, SMITH AH: Placental localization by the use of ^{132}I-Human serum albumen and by ultrasonic scanning—A comparative study. J Obstet Gynaecol Br Commonw 76:220, 1969

2. BADRIA L, YOUNG GB: Correlation of ultrasonic and soft tissue x-ray placentography in 300 cases. J Clin Ultrasound 4:403, 1976

3. BALLAS S, PEYSER MR, TOAFF R: Diagnosis of hydatidiform mole with and without coexistent fetus by nonstored image echography. Obstet Gynecol 50:182, 1977

4. BARTSCH FK, LUNDBERG J, WAHLSTRÖM J: The technique, results and risks of amniocentesis for genetic reasons. J Obstet Gynaecol Br Commonw 81:991, 1974

5. BECKER DI, WICKSMAN RS: Retained abdominal placenta followed by angiography and ultrasound. Radiology 119:207, 1976

6. BLEKER OP, KLOOSTERMAN GJ, MIERAS DJ, OOSTING J, SALLE HJA: Intervillous space during uterine contractions in human subjects: an ultrasonic study. Am J Obstet Gynecol 123:697, 1975

7. BUHL WC, SPELLACY WN: Effects of blood or meconium on the determination of the amniotic fluid lecithin/sphingomyelin ratio. Am J Obstet Gynecol 121:321, 1975

8. BUTTERY B, DAVISON G: The dynamic uterus revealed by time-lapse echography. J Clin Ultrasound 6:19, 1978

9. CHEF R, CHEF-GLOTZ J: Étude morphologique par la méthode ultrasonoscopique du placenta in utero. Résultats préliminaries. J Gynecol Obstet Biol Reprod [Suppl] 15 (2):308, 1972

10. DONALD I, ABDULLA U: Placentography by sonar. J Obstet Gynaecol Br Commonw 75:993, 1968

11. DORAN TA, RUDD NL, GARDNER HA, LOWDEN JA, BENZIE RJ, LIEDGREN SI: The antenatal diagnosis of genetic disease. Am J Obstet Gynecol 118:314, 1974

12. DUNSTER GD, RHYS DAVIES E, ROSS FGM, JOHN AH: Placental localization: a comparison of isotopic and ultrasonic placentography. Br J Radiol 49:940, 1976

13. EDELSTONE DI: Placental localization by ultrasound. Clin Obstet Gynecol 20:285, 1977

14. FISHER CC, GARRETT W, KOSSOFF G: Placental aging monitored by gray scale echography. Am J Obstet Gynecol 124:483, 1976

15. GERBIE AB, SHKOLNIK AA: Ultrasound prior to amniocentesis for genetic counseling. Obstet Gynecol 46:716, 1975

16. GHORASHI B, GOTTESFELD KR: Recognition of the hydropic fetus by gray scale ultrasound. J Clin Ultrasound 4:193, 1976

17. GOTTESFELD KR, THOMPSON HE, HOLMES JH, TAYLOR ES: Ultrasonic placentography—a new method for placental localization. Am J Obstet Gynecol 96:538, 1966

18. HARRISON R, CAMPBELL S, CRAFT I: Risks of fetomaternal hemorrhage resulting from amniocentesis with and without ultrasound placental localization. Obstet Gynecol 46:389, 1975

19. HELLMAN LM, KOBAYASHI M, TOLLES WE, CROMB E: Ultrasonic studies on the volumetric growth of the human placenta. Am J Obstet Gynecol 108:740, 1970

20. HOLLÄNDER HJ, MAST H: Intrauterine dickenmessungen der plazenta mittels ultraschalls bei normalen schwangerschaften und bei Rh-inkompatibilität. Geburtshilfe Frauenheilkd 28:662, 1968

21. KERENYI TD, WALKER B: The preventability of "bloody taps" in second trimester amniocentesis by ultrasound scanning. Obstet Gynecol 50:61, 1977

22. KING DL: Placental migration demonstrated by ultrasonography. Radiology 109:167, 1973

23. KING DL: Placental ultrasonography. J Clin Ultrasound 1:21, 1973

24. KOBAYASHI M, HELLMAN LM, FILLISTI L: Placental localization by ultrasound. Am J Obstet Gynecol 106:279, 1970

25. KOBAYASHI M: Use of diagnostic ultrasound in trophoblastic neoplasms and ovarian tumors. Cancer 38:441, 1976

26. KOHORN EI, SECKER WALKER RH, MORRISON J, CAMPBELL S: Placental localization. Am J Obstet Gynecol 103:868, 1969

27. KOSSOFF G, GARRETT WJ: Ultrasonic film echoscopy for placental localization. Aust NZ J Obstet Gynaecol 12:117, 1972

28. KOSSOFF G, GARRETT WJ, RADOVANOVICH G: Gray scale echography in obstetrics and gynaecology. Australas Radiol 18:63, 1974

29. KURJAK A, BARSIC B: Changes of placental site diagnosed by repeated ultrasonic examination. Acta Obstet Gynecol Scand 56:161, 1977

30. LILEY AW: Errors in the assessment of hemolytic disease from amniotic fluid. Am J Obstet Gynecol 86:485, 1963

31. MEYENBURG M: Gibt es veränderungen des plazentasitzes im bereich kaudaler uterusabschnitte während der schwangerschaft? Geburtshilfe Frauenheilkd 36:715, 1976

32. MORRISON J: The development of the lower uterine segment. Aust NZ J Obstet Gynaecol 12:182, 1972

33. ROBINSON HP: Sonar in the puerperium, a means of diagnosing retained products of conception. Scott Med J 17:364, 1972

34. RUSSELL JGB: Radiology in Obstetrics and Antepartum Paediatrics. London, Butterworth, 1973

35. SABBAGHA RE: Ultrasound in managing the high-risk pregnancy. In Spellacy WN (cd): Management of the High-Risk Pregnancy. Baltimore, University Park Press, 1976

36. SAUVAGE JP, CRANE JP, KOPTA MM: Difficulties in the ultrasonic diagnosis of hydatidiform mole. Obstet Gynecol 44:546, 1974

37. SCHLENSKER KH: Zur diagnostik der vorzeitigen lösung der normalen sitzenden plazenta mit dem ultraschall-schnittbildverfahren. Geburtshilfe Frauenheilkd 32:773, 1972

38. SCHWARZ RH, MENNUTI MT: Antenatal diagnosis of genetic disorders. American College of Obstetricians and Gynecologists Technical Bulletin #39, May, 1976

39. SUTTON D: Arterial placentography and placental previa. Br J Radiol 39:47, 1966

40. WEINER S: An ultrasound aspiration transducer for diagnostic amniocenteses. Obstet Gynecol 47:113, 1976

41. WEXLER P, GOTTESFELD R: Second trimester placenta previa. An apparently normal placentation. Obstet Gynecol 50:706, 1977

42. WINSBERG F: Echographic changes with placental ageing. J Clin Ultrasound 1:52, 1973

43. WLADIMIROFF JW, WALLENBURG HCS, PUTTEN P, DROGENDIJK AC: Ultrasonic diagnosis of placenta membranacea. Arch Gynaekol 221:167, 1976

17

Intrauterine transfusions in the rh-negative patient

MARTIN N. MOTEW, ALLAN G. CHARLES

The management of fetuses affected by Rh disease has improved following: 1) introduction of amniocentesis, 2) development of reliable methodology for analysis of amniotic fluid components, and 3) use of sonography to evaluate fetal status and to enhance the procedures of amniocentesis and intrauterine transfusion.

In the management of gravidas at risk for Rh sensitization certain basic evaluations should be made. First, an antibody screen and titer to determine the presence and level of antibodies in the maternal serum should be obtained. In the presence of a high titer, amniocentesis should be performed and the fluid analyzed spectrophotometrically for bilirubin content—the result of excessive breakdown of fetal erythrocytes (1).

Yellow bile pigment in amniotic fluid causes a deviation from the normal spectrophotometric fluid curve at 450 mu. The extent of this deviation depends on the optical density of the yellow pigment—and is expressed at ΔOD 450 mμ. The greater the ΔOD at 450 mμ the more severe the red cell hemolysis and Rh disease.

In Rh-sensitized gravidas early ultrasonic examinations should be performed to define gestational age which is mandatory for the interpretation of the level of bilirubin in amniotic fluid and in turn the severity of Rh disease (Chs. 6 and 8). Specifically, a fetal CRL should be obtained before 14 weeks' gestation and fetal growth subsequently assessed as outlined in Chapters 9 and 10. Amniocentesis should be performed only under sonographic visualization, because a transplacental puncture may result in a fetomaternal bleed, increasing the degree of sensitization and worsening the disease (Chs. 15, 16).

The time of the first amniocentesis is based on maternal antibody titer and obstetric history (2).

MATERNAL ANTIBODY TITER

As soon as the critical maternal antibody titer is found (provided the patient is not at term and the cervix is not ripe enough to induce labor), amniocentesis should be performed. In our laboratory a titer of 1–16 or greater is significant. The physician should realize that what constitutes a significant antibody level is not uniform in all laboratories.

OBSTETRIC HISTORY

The relationship between past obstetric history and amniocentesis is as follows:

1. If the previous infant was mildly affected at term, the first amniocentesis can be performed at 28–30 weeks' gestation.

2. If the previous infant was severely affected, amniocentesis should be performed at about 26 weeks' gestation.

3. If the previous pregnancy resulted in fetal loss (due to hydrops fetalis), the first amniocentesis should be performed 8–10 weeks prior to the gestational age at which the previous fetal demise occurred.

Amniocentesis should be repeated in 1–3 weeks, depending on the severity of the disease. Once a pattern of the rate of change of ΔOD 450 is established, the frequency of performing amniocentesis may be altered. For example, if the rate of fall is 0.01 unit/week, amniotic fluid analysis may be performed at intervals of 2 weeks.

Before every amniocentesis the fetus should be examined by ultrasound for detection of changes known to occur with erythroblastosis

(4–7). These are as follows: 1) increase in amniotic fluid (polyhydramnios); 2) placental hypertrophy, Figure 17–1; 3) scalp edema, Figure 17–2; 4) fetal ascites (3, 4) or enlargement of fetal liver or spleen, Figure 17–3.

INTRAUTERINE TRANSFUSION (IUT)

The indication for an intrauterine fetal transfusion is a leveling or rise in the ΔOD at 450 mμ over three successive weekly analyses.

In the third trimester of pregnancy, the choice between intrauterine transfusion and immediate delivery is based on a number of factors: 1) the degree of fetal maturity (as determined by sonar fetal CRL measurements or serial BPDs—GASA), amniotic fluid values of the lecithin/sphingomyelin ratio, and creatinine; 2) professional skills of the neonatoligist and capabilities of the intensive care nursery; and 3) experience of the obstetric team performing IUTs.

Successful insertion of a needle into the fetal

FIG. 17–1. Fetal death—erythroblastosis. Clincial history: patient with known erythroblastosis with normal ultrasound examination 72 hours prior to this study. The patient had an intrauterine fetal transfusion, and no fetal heart tones were heard the past 24 hours. Twenty-eight weeks' gestation. Longitudinal scan shows a fetus in breech presentation. The placenta (P) is anterior. Notice the strong echoes in the fetal abdomen (FA), which are probably secondary to the transfusion (FH, fetal head).

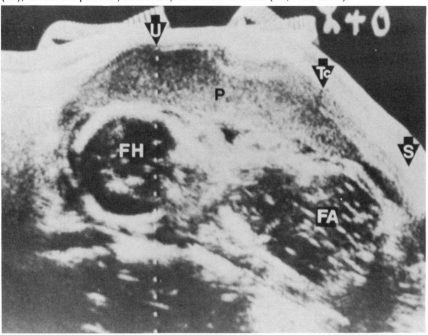

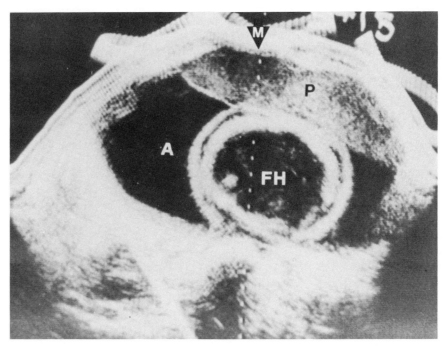

FIG. 17–2. Transverse scan shows marked edema surrounding the fetal head (FH). (A, amniotic fluid; P, anterior placenta). Comment: When there is severe scalp edema (more than 5 mm), this always indicates fetal death or severe erythroblastosis with impending fetal demise.

FIG. 17–3. Erythroblastosis fetalis—fetal ascites. Clinical history: Rh sensitization at 27 weeks' gestation. A coronal section of the fetal head (FH) and fetal abdomen with ascites (As). Note the echo-free ascitic fluid (As) between the fetal liver and anterior abdominal wall of the fetus. The posterior placenta (P) with its ground glass appearance is well seen. There is slight hydramnios (A). Comment: Fetal ascites signal a severely affected fetus, and the prognosis for survival is poor, even with IUT.

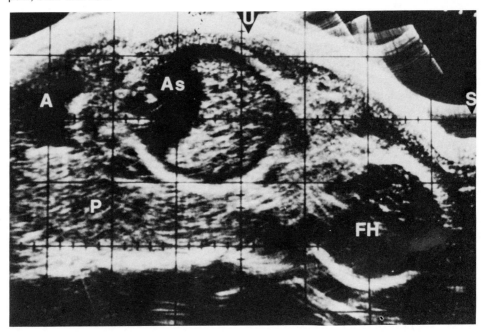

abdomen for an IUT necessitates fluoroscopic visualization of the fetus; such exposure to x-ray may be responsible for an increase in the incidence of leukemia observed in these children (9, 10). In an attempt to lower the relatively high radiation exposure to the fetus during IUT (8), real-time imaging has been incorporated into the procedure. By using the real-time scanner the fluoroscopic part of the transfusion procedure is eliminated, reducing the radiation exposure to both mother and fetus. It is hoped that further development of the technique may lead to the total elimination of x-ray from the procedure of IUT.

METHODOLOGY FOR IUT

Amniocentesis is performed in the morning and an aqueous solution of radiopaque dye is injected. Conray 400* is used by these authors in amounts of 10—40 ml, depending on the gestational age of the fetus. Since this is an iodine preparation, a careful history to rule out possible sensitization to iodine should be obtained. Four to five hours later, the patient is sedated with Demerol† (50–75 mg), Vesprin‡ (20 mg) and atropine (4 mg). Sedation is particularly important because it results in a decrease of fetal movement. As a result the IUT is more likely to be successful. The patient is then transported to the x-ray department and allowed to rest for 1 hour. Ten lead markers are placed on the abdomen (Fig. 17–4) over the uterus. The markers help to localize the fetal bowel pattern if fluoroscopy has to be used. A flat film of the abdomen is then taken to determine if dye is present in the fetal intestinal tract—an indication of whether fetal swallowing has occurred. Severely affected hydropic infants are unable to swallow the dye and are not candidates for an IUT.

Real-time scanning of the maternal abdomen is then performed to show fetal position, lie, and organs (bladder, stomach, and liver).

The physician using the real-time transducer selects the site for insertion of the transfusion needle and points the pathway of the needle

* Methylglucamine iothalamate, Mallinckrod.
† Meperidine, Breon.
‡ Triflupromazine, Squibb.

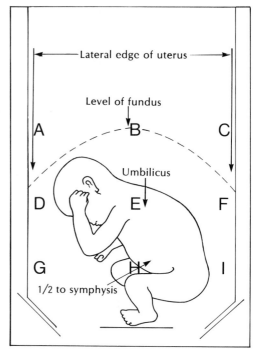

FIG. 17–4. Illustration of the placement of the lead markers to localize on x-ray fetal bowel patterns. The first line of markers, (A, B, and C) is placed at the level of the top of the uterine fundus. The second line of markers is placed at the level of the maternal umbilicus (D, E, F). The third line of markers is placed one-half way between the umbilicus and pubic symphysis. The lateral markers, A, D, G and C, D, I, are placed at the lateral edge of the uterus. Comment: The use of x-ray localization of fetal bowel by lead marker placement is now supplanted by real-time scanning in many cases.

(noting both the depth and angle of penetration into the fetal abdomen). The exact site of the desired puncture into the maternal abdomen is then marked. After sterile prepping and draping of the patient, local anesthesia is injected into the maternal abdomen over the marked area. The skin is incised and a 17-gauge Touhy needle is inserted through the maternal abdomen and uterine wall along the pathway previously outlined. The tip of the needle is visualized on the real-time screen by placing the transducer out of the sterile field on the side of the maternal abdomen parallel to the needle pathway (Fig. 17–5). Occasionally the needle is jiggled and its position confirmed by real-time imaging. The needle is then slowly advanced until it is abutting the fetal abdominal wall. With the fetal bladder as a landmark, the needle is inserted into the fetal

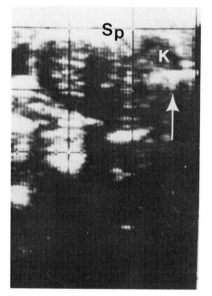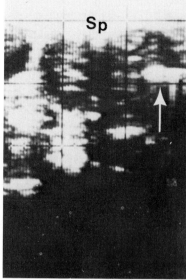

FIG. 17-5. Needle tip in intrauterine transfusion. Real-time examination at 29 weeks' gestation shows two scans of a cross-section of the fetal abdomen with the fetal spine (Sp) anterior against the maternal abdominal wall. The needle was inserted by use of real-time monitoring, and the needle tip **(arrow)** can be seen just below the fetal kidney (K) during intraperitoneal injection of blood.

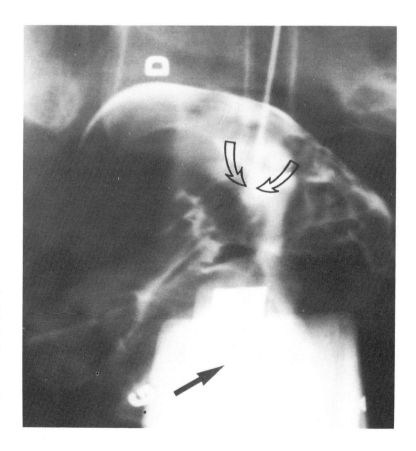

FIG. 17-6. Photograph of an x-ray film showing a 28-week-size fetus during an IUT with radiopaque dye in the fetal abdomen surrounding fetal bowel. The typical flow pattern ensures placement of the needle within the peritoneal cavity **(arrows).** The **black arrow** depicts the position of the real-time transducer at the side of the maternal abdomen with the transducer head parallel to the needle.

peritoneal cavity at a point superior and lateral to the bladder, which avoids both bladder and umbilical cord insertion. The fetal chest, liver, and back are identified with the real-time scanner before fetal puncture. The Touhy needle is then advanced through the abdominal wall and its intraabdominal position is confirmed by 1) aspiration of ascitic fluid and 2) observation of "waves of echoes" caused by injection of saline. If steps 1 and 2 fail, radioopaque dye may be injected and viewed fluoroscopically, Figure 17–6. The intraperitoneal position of the needle having been confirmed, Figure 17–5, transfusion with the appropriate packed red blood cells is performed. During transfusion the fetal abdomen is sonographically noted to distend. The fetal heart rate can be monitored with the real-time machine before, during, and after the transfusion.

Real-time imaging has dramatically improved the technique of intrauterine transfusion. To date, we have performed 14 IUTs (on 10 different patients) by using real-time imaging. In several cases no x-ray was used at all. In one case the fetal back was against the maternal abdomen, and we were unable to perform the transfusion; however, 24 hours later a successful transfusion was performed on that patient.

The overall fetal mortality rate in more than 200 cases of IUTs performed by these authors is more than 50% (excluding grossly hydropic infants). Approximately 30% of all fetuses, including a few with hydrops fetalis, survive. Fortunately Rho-Gam* prophylaxis has reduced

* Ortho Pharmaceutical Corporation

the incidence of Rh sensitization. Thus, at present only a few referral centers are capable of offering the highly specialized type of treatment necessary for the severely affected fetuses. In these centers the prospect for refining IUTs by real-time imaging is favorable.

REFERENCES

1. BEVIS DCA: Composition of liquor amnii in haemolytic disease of the newborn. Lancet 2:443, 1950
2. CHARLES AG: Management of the Rh-negative gravida. In Wynn RM (ed): Obstetrics and Gynecology Annual. New York, Appleton-Century-Crofts, 1976, p 167
3. COOPERBERG PL, CARPENTER CW: Ultrasound as an aid in intrauterine transfusions. Am J Obstet Gynecol 128:239, 1977
4. GHORASHI B, GOTTSEFELD KR: Recognition of the hydropic fetus by gray scale ultrasound. J Clin Ultrasound 4:193, 1976
5. HAMILTON EG: IUT safeguard or peril? Obstet Gynecol 50:255, 1977
6. HOBBINS JC, DAVIS CD, WEBSTER J: A new technique utilizing ultrasound to aid in intrauterine transfusion. J Clin Ultrasound 4:135, 1976
7. JONES M: Ultrasonic B-scanning in rhesus incompatibility. J Clin Ultrasound 2:185, 1974
8. PLATT L, MANNING FA, LEMAY M: Real-time B-scan directed amniocentesis. Am J Obstet Gynecol 130:700, 1978
9. STEWART A, KNEALE GW: Radiation dose effects in relation to obstetric x-rays and childhood cancers. Lancet 1:1185, 1970
10. TURNER HH, PETRICCIANI J: Intrauterine and/or exchange transfusion with the development of leukemia. Soc Gynecol Invest (presentation), 1976

18

Fetal breathing

HAROLD E. FOX

"The infant comes by his 'mind' in the same way that he comes by his body, that is, through the process of development. This growth process (the terms 'growth' and 'development' are virtually interchangeable) is in every phase, a process of morphogenesis. It creates new forms and configurations in the molecules of living tissues, in the anatomy of the constituent organs, and in the reactions of the total organism. It configures the basic patterns of behavior which are mediated by the nervous system" (28).

The application of linear-array ultrasound transducers to provide a constantly updated B-scan gray-scale display of moving images of fetal structures is a significant advance in diagnostic ultrasound (20). Ultrasound techniques allow visualization of fetal activity as early as 6 weeks' gestational age. Later in gestation, precise definition of fetal activities is possible. As the embryo, and subsequently the fetus, develops, differentiation of the activities such as body and limb movement becomes apparent. The study of the development of specific fetal movements may lead to an enhanced understanding of the functional development of the fetal central nervous system.

The research presented has been supported in part by The National Foundation March of Dimes Clinical Research Grant 6–42, and the DHEW, PHS, Bureau of Community Health Services, Maternal and Child Health Services Research Grant MC-R-350375-03-0.

The study of specific fetal movements such as fetal breathing activity has led to a basic understanding of the physiology of their control. Since breathing movements are under neural control, an understanding of the natural history of development of these movements and of their physiology may provide insight into functional development of the fetal midbrain and higher central nervous system (19). This chapter presents a basic overview of the physiology involved in fetal breathing movement control, the various ultrasound techniques used to record the movements, and data on our current understanding of fetal breathing movement development in the human fetus.

BASIC PHYSIOLOGY

A series of experiments carried out in 1969 at the Nuffield Institute for Medical Research confirmed an impression that had waxed and waned in popularity over the previous century that the normal fetus made breathing-like movements in utero (14). The observations that fetal breathing movements did occur in normal gestation were simultaneously made by a second group in Paris (42). The distinct periodic nature of the occurrence of these breathing movements in the fetal lamb suggested an association with fetal activity state. Simultaneous recording of the electrocorticogram of the fetus in chronic preparations demonstrated that the fetal breathing movements occurred only during periods of low-voltage fast electrocortical activity. This type of electrocortical activity can be seen in either an

199

awake, alert activity state or a state of sleep often termed "rapid eye movement" or "paradoxical sleep." To differentiate the point, eye movement recordings were done in the chronic fetal lamb preparations. These experiments demonstrated an increased incidence of eye movements during periods of rapid, irregular fetal movements and low-voltage fast electrocortical activity. Observations of exteriorized fetal lamb activity in a saline bath preparation confirmed the impression that rapid, irregular fetal breathing movements occurred during periods of rapid eye movement sleep (15). Further substantiating the relationship to fetal neural respiratory center control, observations by Bahoric and Chernick have indicated the association of phrenic nerve activity and diaphragmatic muscle activity with fetal breathing-like movements (2). Subsequently, fetal breathing movements were recorded in other species. Esophageal pressure recordings of intrathoracic pressure in fetal rabbits (24) and tracheal pressure recordings in fetal rhesus monkeys (39) have indicated the occurrence of rapid irregular breathing movements.

Animal models have provided information regarding the control of fetal breathing activity. Various species demonstrate breathing activity from 40%–60% of the time (15, 39). A diurnal variation in the occurrence of fetal breathing has been reported in the fetal lamb (13). The association of fetal breathing movements and rapid eye movement sleeplike states has been confirmed in the rhesus monkey preparation (39).

Hypercapnia has been shown to increase the frequency of occurrence of fetal breathing movements (8). On the other hand, hypoxia has been seen to decrease the occurrence of rapid fetal breathing movements (15, 8, 40). Asphyxia has been associated with gaspinglike movements. Hypoglycemia in the fetal lamb has been demonstrated to decrease the incidence of fetal breathing movements. In rhesus monkeys, however, no correlation between fetal and maternal plasma glucose levels and the amount of fetal breathing movements has been demonstrated (38).

Clinical interest in fetal breathing movements involves the predictive significance for defining fetal hypoxia, hypercapnia, or asphyxia. Dr. John Patrick and his colleagues have reported

on continuous observations in 16 fetal lambs many days prior to their death in utero from hypoxia, asphyxia, infection, or other causes (43). They report a consistent, prolonged period of apnea followed by continuous abnormal breathing in 6 fetal lambs and by gasping or brief episodes of abnormal breathing in the other 10. This report documents the complexity of fetal breathing patterns that may precede fetal death. Early human studies indicated that hypoxia was associated with the cessation of fetal breathing movements (6). Such a simple association of apnea or gasping with fetal hypoxia or asphyxia is not suggested by these animal studies. In the animal model, continuous fetal breathing, apnea, and gasping or apnea interrupted by brief episodes of breathing movements and gasping may be seen prior to fetal death. These observations being kept in mind, it may be expected that a complex array of breathing patterns will be observed in the human fetus associated with fetal hypoxia or asphyxia.

ULTRASOUND TECHNIQUES AND FETAL BREATHING

A useful technique for recording fetal breathing movements must be one that is easily applied, reliable, and safe. It must provide valid information that can be quantitated. It should be comfortable for the patient and inexpensive. Various ultrasound techniques have been applied to the study of human fetal breathing movements. These techniques include pulsed A-scan, real-time B-scan by linear transducer array or by mechanical sector scanner, and phased array transducer systems. Continuous-wave Doppler ultrasound systems have also been used. Under specified circumstances, all these techniques may provide valid information for interpretation of fetal breathing activities. The transmission of fetal breathing movements to the maternal abdominal wall has also been used as a technique to record fetal breathing activity (10, 45).

Each of these techniques has certain restrictions and benefits. Recording fetal breathing movements by transmission to the surface of the maternal abdominal wall is very dependent on fetal position. The amplitude of breathing movements transmitted to the abdominal wall is affected by maternal movements and fetal movements, and much fetal breathing activity may go unrecorded.

The first ultrasound technique to be applied to the problem of recording fetal breathing movements was pulsed A-scan with a one-dimensional display. Boddy and Robinson demonstrated fetal breathing in human subjects and validated the one-dimensional display technique in a fetal lamb preparation by simultaneously recording tracheal pressure changes (11). The A-scan technique has been applied extensively by many researchers in Europe for the study of fetal breathing movements. There are numerous limitations with this technique. Farman and his colleagues discussed several areas of concern regarding the application of this technique to the study of fetal breathing (17, 18). Artifactual movements of the ultrasound transducer on the abdominal wall or movements of the fetus and maternal abdominal contents may be confused with fetal breathing movements. Maintaining a consistent orientation to the fetal chest or abdominal wall proved to be a difficulty. Dr. Marsal has pointed out that the echo complex from a flattening concavity may be moving in the back portion and remains stationary at its leading edge, producing errors in recording. In this case, when a gating system is used to provide an indication of fetal chest wall movements, an erroneous recording of apnea may be generated. Flexibility in the adjustment of the equipment may allow for a failure to identify breathing movements from echos of small amplitude or may, in fact, allow for erroneous interpretation of artifactual movements as breathing (18).

In our experience A-scan recordings have proved to be difficult to quantitate. The precise definition of breathing patterns, apnea intervals, and the validity of prolonged recordings of fetal breathing activity are in question (20). An experienced operator using A-scan techniques can minimize the operating and interpretation errors only by eliminating substantial portions of the record, because of artifactual movements. Numerous attempts to improve the accuracy of A-

scan recording of fetal breathing movements have been made (35, 41). The performance of a static B-scan with directed application of the A-scan transducer oriented to the chest wall or abdominal wall has been helpful. The selection of one line of real-time two-dimensional B-scan display for interpretation as an A-scan has provided useful analogue records of fetal breathing activity by measuring chest wall movement (37).

The system we use to record fetal breathing activity is a linear array transducer real-time B-scan.* A videotape recording system adapted to the real-time scanner provides a continuous recording of the image of fetal activities. A longitudinal orientation to the fetus is maintained and both the fetal chest and abdomen visualized. Fetal breathing activity is recorded when paradoxical fetal chest wall and abdominal wall movements are seen. In order to process the videotaped fetal activities each videotape is viewed by an observer who controls a button system connected to the analogue input channels of a computer system (Interdata 7/32). As each button is pushed, an indication of the activity observed on the video screen is recorded on the magnetic tape system. Activities such as fetal breathing, gasping, general fetal movements, and hiccups, as well as transducer movement, are recorded. The information is blocked and transferred to a digital tape system for subsequent analysis. A second approach is computer interface, which has been designed in our laboratory to allow for the intake of static image from the ADR linear transducer array system (1). Real-time image acquisition is in progress and will allow for quantitative analysis of fetal movements.

Recently, continuous-wave Doppler systems have been applied to the problem of recording fetal breathing movements. With these systems, Doppler shift frequencies of ultrasonic echos returning from moving targets are used to generate audible signals that indicate the velocity of the movement. This technique is very useful for recording fetal heart movements. The first Doppler indication of breathing movements was described by Bishop in 1966 (3), though these were not then known to be associated with fetal

*ADR Model 2139, Tempe, Arizona or SKI Ekolife, Sunnyvale, California.

breathing movements. Boyce and his colleagues in 1976 (12) reported on these audible movements associated with fetal breathing activity. Simultaneous recording of tracheal pressures in the fetal lamb and Doppler indication of fetal breathing movements have been done. It is now felt that, though first thought to represent tracheal–bronchial fluid movements, the sounds generated indicate venous blood flow associated with altered intrathoracic pressures generated by the fetal breathing movements. It is felt that the target of the Doppler ultrasound system for recording human fetal breathing movements is the vena cava at the level of the diaphragm. Observations in human pregnancies suggest that good recordings of fetal breathing movements may be obtained by maintaining a consistent orientation of the Doppler transducer, despite movements of the fetus and mother. The consistent orientation may allow the production of an audible shift-peak frequency change associated with the breathing movements that can be relatively simply converted to signals that may be quantitatively analyzed. As with A-scan techniques the problem with the Doppler technique is continuous orientation to the target. It is quite possible that this technique will provide the most sensitive method of detecting very small changes in intrathoracic pressure.

A number of ultrasound techniques have been described that may provide an indication of fetal breathing movements. The simplest technique is the real-time ultrasound B-scan system, which allows a consistent orientation with the fetus to observe fetal chest and abdominal movements.

HUMAN FETAL BREATHING

A-SCAN OBSERVATIONS

The A-scan ultrasound technique for recording human fetal breathing movements has demonstrated that they occur about 70% of the time with a normal range of 50%–90% at rates between 30 and 70/min (6). With this technique most observations are performed after the 30th week of pregnancy. Diurnal variations have been observed, similar to those reported in animal models (9). An increase in fetal breathing

movements has been noted to occur after the intravenous administration of glucose (9).

Pharmacologic studies have shown a decrease in the occurrence of fetal breathing movements after maternal administration of sodium amytal and diazepam (5). At less than 30 weeks' gestation, the effect of diazepam seems to be prolonged.

Dr. Gennser has demonstrated that meperidine, in a dose of 1 mg/kgm given intramuscularly to the mother, causes a marked increase in the incidence of fetal apnea (27). Peak depression of fetal breathing occurs within 60 min after injection. It is tempting to assume that the meperidine had a direct effect on fetal breathing mediated via medullary control mechanisms. It is not possible, however, to infer this from measurements made in the human being. Boddy et al have shown that there is no effect on breathing movements in fetal lambs given large doses of meperidine (7). Transcutaneously measured maternal PO_2 falls after meperidine administration (32). This observation and the fact that fetal hypoxia significantly depresses fetal breathing movements (8) may explain the effect of meperidine seen in Dr. Gennser's study.

Valium (diazepam), administered in 5-mg intravenous or 10-mg intramuscular doses to patients not in labor, was shown to be followed by transient reduction in fetal breathing activity (5, 27). It has been shown that diazepam may cause hypoventilation in the newborn. The delayed effect on the respiratory movements of the fetus may be due to the main metabolite N-desmethyldiazepam, which has a more pronounced depressant effect on neonatal respirations than diazepam itself (33). As with meperidine it is not possible to dissociate the eventual direct effect on the fetus from the effects mediated by the metabolic and circulatory alterations in the mother.

Terbutaline, a beta stimulant used for control of premature labor, has been shown to increase the incidence of fetal breathing (27). It is possible that this increased fetal breathing activity is related to improved fetal–placental perfusion. The use of cortico steroids such as betamethasone to induce fetal pulmonary maturity has also been studied. Betamethasone treatment in 19 pregnant women reported by Gennser over a 3-day course in the last trimester did not change the pattern of fetal breathing. It has also shown that physical activity of the mother decreases the incidence of fetal breathing movements (27).

The study of the effect of Methyldopa on normal fetal breathing movements has produced an interesting observation. In a small number of patients Boddy has noted that patients requiring Methyldopa for control of hypertension and who also show a decrease in the occurrence of fetal breathing movements had a higher incidence of perinatal morbidity (5). It is unlikely, as mentioned by Boddy, that a central effect of Methyldopa on fetal central nervous system function accounts for this decrease in fetal breathing activity. It is more likely that the administration of Methyldopa decreases fetal breathing movements in a certain group of hypertensive patients because of the effect on fetal circulation and/or placental circulation.

According to the A-scan observations, prolonged apnea and apnea and gasping have been observed to precede fetal death on 12 occasions by 1976 (4). Boddy's data suggest that a mixed pattern of fetal breathing including irregular breathing movements and gasping activity has been seen in both normal and abnormal pregnancies and that this may be predictive of the fetus that later develops distress in labor (4, 6).

The observations that have been made by use of A-scan ultrasound techniques are valuable for our understanding of the occurrence of human fetal breathing movements. The technique is, however, difficult to apply, and obtaining optimal records for analysis frequently proves, therefore, frustrating.

REAL-TIME B-SCAN STUDIES

In 1975 the first application of real-time B-scan imaging to the study of fetal breathing began (26, 29). Independent studies by Fox and Patrick have indicated that fetal breathing movements after the 32nd week of pregnancy seem to occur approximately 31% of the time (20, 44). This is approximately half the incidence of fetal breathing movements recorded by use of A-scan techniques. With real-time B-scan imaging, gross body movements and other fetal activities can be separately interpreted (20, 29). Since this type of activity occupies 10%–30% of recording times, much of the discrepancy between real-time B-scan image interpretation and A-scan interpretation may be accounted for by this difference.

Carefully controlled observations of 45 obstetric patients with uncomplicated pregnancies has resulted in an increased understanding of the development of fetal breathing activity (23). In this group, patients underwent either morning or afternoon recording sessions, approximately 30 min in length. A linear-transducer array real-time B-scan system was used. All patients were placed in a semi-Fowler's position with no supine hypotension noted during the recording session. The transducer was oriented to show fetal chest and abdominal wall movements to allow for visual interpretation of fetal breathing activity. The results of the 142 examinations showed that there was no statistical difference between the results of the morning and the afternoon recording sessions. The results indicated that the longest apnea period recorded decreased with gestational age, with a rank-order correlation of −.21. There was no relationship between the longest apnea and serum glucose levels. A clear positive relationship is evident when one considers the proportion of time spent in breathing activity related to gestational age (Fig. 18–1). The rank-order correlation is 0.46.

The relationship of an oral glucose load to the occurrence of fetal breathing has also been studied (21, 31). At 36 weeks' gestation, 10 women were fasted from midnight to 9:00 a.m. A 75-g oral glucose load was given after fetal breathing had been recorded for a baseline period of one-half hour. Fig. 18–2 indicates the response and the percentage of time spent in fetal breathing activity following the oral glucose load in this fasted group. Five patients in a fasted control group given water rather than the glucola load showed no response (Fig. 18–3). Similar results were obtained in nonfasted patients administered the glucose load, though the baseline percentage of occurrence of fetal breathing was somewhat higher.

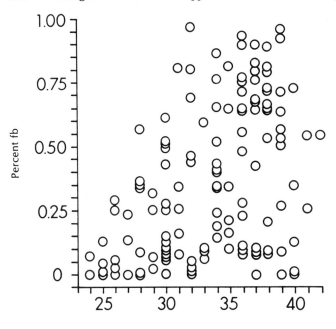

FIG. 18-1. Proportion of time spent in fetal breathing (fb) activity versus gestational age.

A diurnal variation in the occurrence of fetal breathing activity has been described (20, 30). At least one component of this activity seems to be related to the consumption of meals. The metabolic environment of the mother, which is related to glucose intake, may influence the observed incidence of fetal breathing movements in large population studies.

HIGH-RISK OBSTETRIC STUDIES

A-scan ultrasound techniques have noted that patterns of prolonged apnea or gasping and apnea precede fetal death. Of perhaps greater significance, the observation of normal fetal breathing movements with A-scan techniques is felt to be a reassuring sign in the presence of other indications of fetal distress (4, 5). The use of real-time B-scan imaging has shown long periods of apnea in gestations with normal perinatal outcome. The normal variation in the occurrence of fetal breathing, maternal exercise preceding fetal breathing movement recording, maternal smoking (34), and the general metabolic state of the mother all contribute to the occurrence of fetal breathing movements at any one time.

At our center, fetal breathing movements have been studied after a positive oxytocin challenge test (21). We have previously noted that the occurrence of accelerations with fetal movement seems to indicate relative fetal well-being, even in the presence of late decelerations with uterine contractions (25). We have noted that, in our series of 25 positive oxytocin challenge tests, accelerations were present in 14 and absent in 11. In the 11 cases where accelerations with fetal movement were absent, fetal movement was present in 3. In all 3 of these cases, increased perinatal morbidity of the newborn was noted. Gross measurements of fetal movements seem not, therefore, to be a good indicator of fetal well-being in patients showing signs of uteroplacental insufficiency. Observations of fetal breathing have been made in 12 patients following a positive oxytocin challenge test. In 5 of these patients, no accelerations with fetal movement were noted, and no fetal breathing was observed. In all 5, increased perinatal morbidity was noted. In patients with a positive oxytocin challenge test and accelerations with fetal movement (N = 7) 4 showed fetal breathing activity to be present and 3 showed an absence of fetal breathing movements. In those cases with

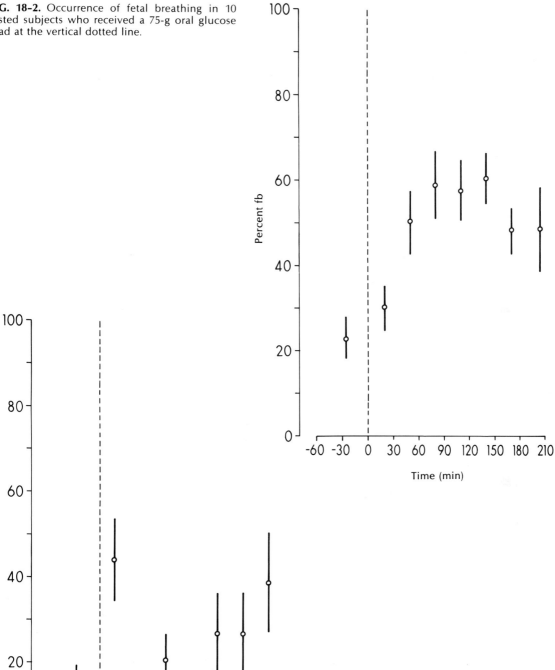

FIG. 18-2. Occurrence of fetal breathing in 10 fasted subjects who received a 75-g oral glucose load at the vertical dotted line.

FIG. 18-3. Occurrence of fetal breathing in 5 fasted subjects receiving a noncarbohydrate drink at the vertical dotted line (control).

fetal breathing movements present, no increased perinatal morbidity was noted.

The data from animal preparations examined prior to death indicate that various patterns of fetal breathing movements may be seen. Before fetal breathing observations can be applied to clinical use, detailed large-scale studies are necessary to document the significance of the presence of fetal breathing movements in high-risk obstetric situations.

NERVOUS SYSTEM MATURATION

Pharmacologic studies performed by Gennser, Boddy, and others have shown a relationship of medication use to the occurrence of fetal breathing movements. In many cases the etiology of the effect on fetal breathing movements is unclear. For example, the administration of meperidine to a gravid patient decreases the occurrence of fetal breathing movements, but this may be related to the hypoventilation that has been documented to occur in such circumstances with resultant fetal hypoxia. To define the relation of fetal breathing to central nervous system function, we have studied the effect of a social cocktail on the fetal breathing movements in 7 patients (22). One ounce of alcohol (80 proof vodka) was given in an 80-cc diet ginger ale carrier. But alcohol levels reached a concentration of approximately 10 mg%. Cessation of fetal breathing movements was noted in all cases. Fig. 18–4 is an example of fetal breathing movements in one patient, as they are affected by the consumption of alcohol. Dilts and others have studied the effects of alcohol on fetal blood gas status (16). There is no evidence to indicate any altered pH or PO_2 environment of the fetus at the levels of blood alcohol achieved in this study. No effect on fetal breathing was seen in the control group who received the nonalcoholic beverage. This evidence of direct central nervous system suppression by a small quantity of the ingested alcohol reflected in fetal breathing movement occurrence supports the concept that the study of fetal breathing activity may be an important index of fetal central nervous system development. Patterning of the occurrence of fetal breathing movements has been shown. Fig. 18–5 indicates the occurrence of fetal breathing activity during other movement-free periods of observation characteristic of various gestational ages. The precise definition of these developmental patterns may indicate functional central nervous system maturation.

SUMMARY

The application of ultrasound techniques to the study of fetal morphology and function is exciting. As a result an understanding of the dynamic processes of growth and development is now within the grasp of researchers of fetal physiology and behavioral maturation.

Animal studies have revealed the general physiology of control of fetal breathing movements. Using ultrasound techniques, studies are being accomplished in human gestation to increase our understanding of functional central nervous system maturation. Preliminary evidence from clinical studies indicates that the presence of normal fetal breathing movements may be a reassuring sign even in the presence of other indicators of fetal compromise.

Analysis of data on fetal breathing requires a careful consideration of the technique being used to record fetal breathing activities. With real-time B-scan ultrasound imaging, long periods of apnea have been noted in normal pregnancy. To allow clinical application of the observations of fetal breathing movements in high-risk obstetrics, detailed study of the patterns of the development of fetal breathing activity and an understanding of patterns of breathing in high-risk obstetric populations must be sought. Detailed studies of fetal breathing movement development promises to increase our understanding of developmental physiology and become a useful clinical tool in the evaluation of high-risk perinatal patients.

Acknowledgment: The collegial assistance of Edward Angel, Ph.D., David Pessel, Ph.D., and Ms. Margaret Steinbrecher is gratefully acknowledged. The research presented has been supported in part by The National Foundation March of Dimes Clinical Research Grant 6-42, and the DHEW, PHS, Bureau of Community

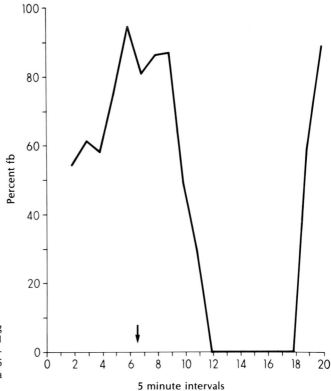

FIG. 18-4. Occurrence of fetal breathing movements in one patient who received 1 ounce of vodka (80 proof) in a noncarbohydrate-containing carrier at the **arrow.** In all 5 patients, fetal breathing activity ceased for a period of time.

FIG. 18-5. Character of the timing of the occurrence of fetal breathing movements in other fetal movement-free periods at various gestational ages.

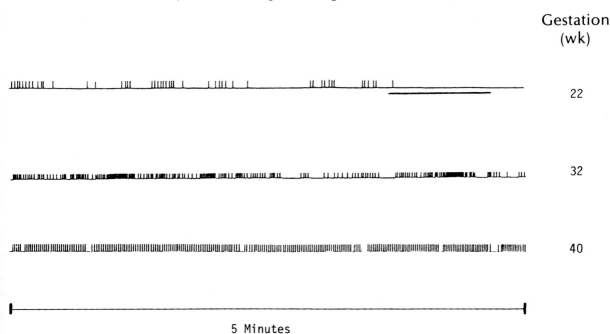

Health Services, Maternal and Child Health Services Research Grant MC-R-350375-03-0. The research was carried out at the University of Rochester Medical Center, Rochester, New York.

REFERENCES

1. ANGEL E, FOX HE, INGLIS J, LOGGHE S, PESSEL D, STEINBRECHER M: Computer analysis of fetal breathing movements recorded by real-time ultrasound imaging. Presented at American Institute of Ultrasound in Medicine 6th Annual Meeting, Dallas, 1977 (in press)

2. BAHORIC A, CHERNICK V: Electrical activity of phrenic nerve and diaphragm in utero. J Appl Physiol 39:513, 1975

3. BISHOP EH: Obstetric uses of the ultrasound motion sensor. Am J Obstet Gynecol 96:863, 1966

4. BODDY K: Fetal circulation and breathing movements. In Beard RW, Nathaniels PW (eds): Fetal Physiology in Medicine. Philadelphia, WB Saunders, 1976, p 302

5. BODDY K: The influence of maternal drug administration on human fetal breathing movements in utero. In Louis PJ (ed): Therapeutic Problems in Pregnancy. Baltimore, University Park Press, 1977, p 153

6. BODDY K, DAWES GS: Fetal breathing. Br Med Bull 31:3, 1975

7. BODDY K, DAWES GS, FISHER R, PINTER S, ROBINSON JS: The effects of pethidine on fetal breathing movements in sheep. Br J Pharmacol 57:311, 1976

8. BODDY K, DAWES GS, FISHER R, ROBINSON JS: Foetal respiratory movements, electrocortical and cardiovascular responses to hypoxaemia and hypercapnia in sheep. J Physiol (Lond) 243:599, 1974

9. BODDY K, DAWES GS, ROBINSON JS: Intrauterine fetal breathing movements. In Gluck L (ed): Modern Perinatal Medicine. Chicago, Yearbook, 1974

10. BODDY K, MANTELL CD: Observations of fetal breathing movements transmitted through maternal abdominal wall. Lancet 2:1219, 1972

11. BODDY K, ROBINSON JS: External method for detection of fetal breathing in utero. Lancet 2:1231, 1971

12. BOYCE ES, DAWES GS, GOUGH JD, POOR ER: Doppler ultrasound method for detecting human fetal breathing in utero. Br Med J 2:17, 1976

13. DAWES GS: Revolutions and cyclical rhythms in prenatal life: fetal respiratory movements rediscovered. Pediatrics 51:965, 1973

14. DAWES GS, FOX HE, LEDUC BM, LIGGINS GC, RICHARDS RT: Respiratory movements and paradoxical sleep in the foetal lamb. J Physiol (Lond) 210:47, 1970

15. DAWES GS, FOX HE, LEDUC BM, LIGGINS GC, RICHARDS RT: Respiratory movements and rapid eye movement sleep in the foetal lamb. J Physiol (Lond) 220:119, 1972

16. DILTS PV: Effect of ethanol on uterine and umbilical hemodynamics and oxygen transfer. Am J Obstet Gynecol 108:221, 1970

17. FARMAN DJ, THOMAS G: The use of ultrasound for monitoring fetal breathing movements. Biomed Eng 10:172, 1975

18. FARMAN DJ, THOMAS G, BLACKWELL RJ: Errors and artifacts encountered in the monitoring of fetal respiratory movements using ultrasound. Ultrasound Med Biol 2:1, 1975

19. FOX HE: Fetal breathing and ultrasound. Am J Dis Child 130: 127, 1976

20. FOX H, HOHLER C: Fetal evaluation by real-time imaging. In Sabbagha RE (ed): Clinical Obstetrics and Gynecology. Hagerstown, Harper & Row, 1977

21. FOX HE, HOHLER CW, JAEGER H, STEINBRECHER M, PECO N: A preliminary report of an alteration of human fetal breathing associated with the glucose tolerance test and oxytocin challenge test. In Gennser G, Marsal K, Wheeler T (eds): Proceedings of the Third Conference on Fetal Breathing. Malmo, 1976, p 56

22. FOX HE, INGLIS J, STEINBRECHER M: Maternal ethanol ingestion and the occurrence of human fetal breathing movements. Presented at the Society of Gynecologic Investigation Annual Meeting, Atlanta, March, 1978

23. FOX HE, INGLIS J, STEINBRECHER M: Fetal breathing movements in uncomplicated pregnancies. I. Relationship to gestational age and maternal blood glucose. Am J Obstet Gynecol (in press)

24. FOX HE, LEDUC BM: Unpublished observations

25. FOX HE, STEINBRECHER M, RIPTON B: Antepartum fetal heart rate and uterine activity study in high risk pregnancy. I. Accelerations and the OCT. Am J Obstet Gynecol 126:61, 1976

26. GENNSER G, MARSAL K: Real-time videotape demonstration. Fetal Breathing Conference, Oxford, 1975

27. GENNSER G, MARSAL K, LINDSTROM K: The influence of external factors on breathing movements in the human fetus. In Rooth G, Bratteby L (eds): Perinatal Medicine. Uppsala, Alqvist & Wiksell, 1976, p 18

28. GESELL A: The Embryology of Behavior. New York, Harper & Row, 1945, p vii

29. HOHLER CW, FOX HE: Real-time grey-scale B-scan ultrasound recording of human fetal breathing movements in utero. In White D, Barnes R (eds): Ultrasound in Medicine, Vol 2. New York, Plenum Press, 1976, p 203

30. HOHLER CW, FOX HE, INGLIS J, STEINBRECHER M: 24-hour continuous observation of the human fetal breathing using real-time B-scan. In White D, Brown

RE (eds): Ultrasound in Medicine, Vol 3a, Clinical Aspects. New York, Plenum Press, 1977, p 709

31. HOHLER CW, FOX HE, JAEGER H, INGLISH J, STEIN-BRECHER M: Real-time B-scan observations: effect of maternal glucose load on human fetal breathing. In White D, Brown RE (eds): Ultrasound in Medicine, Vol 3a, Clinical Aspects. New York, Plenum Press, 1977, p 721

32. HUCH A, HUCH R, LINDMART G, ROOTH G: Maternal hypoxemia after pethidine. Br J Obstet Gynaecol 81:608, 1974

33. LANGSLET A, UNDE PKM: Respiratory effects of diazepam medication in neonates. In Proceedings of the Fifth Nordic Congress of Perinatal Medicine, Gothenburg, 1975, p 8

34. MANNING FA, SEYERABEND C: Cigarette smoking and fetal breathing movements. Br J Obstet Gynaecol 3:262, 1976

35. MANTELL CD: Breathing movements in the human fetus. Am J Obstet Gynecol 125:73, 1976

36. MARSAL K, GENNSER G, HANSSON GA, LINDSTROM K, MAURITZSON L: New ultrasonic device for monitoring fetal breathing movements. Biomed Eng 11:47, 1976

37. MARSAL K, GENNSER G, LINDSTROM K: Real-time ultrasonography for quantified analysis of fetal breathing movements. Lancet 2:718, 1976

38. MARTIN CB, MURATA Y, IKENOUE T: Lack of effective hypo- and hyperglycemia on breathing movements in fetal rhesus monkeys. Gynecol Invest 6:68, 1975

39. MARTIN CB, MURATA Y, PETRIE RH, PARER JT: Respiratory movements in fetal rhesus monkeys. Am J Obstet Gynecol 119:939, 1974

40. MARTIN CB, MURATA Y, TSUYOMU I, ETTINGER BB: Effect of alterations of PO_2 and PCO_2 on fetal breathing movements in rhesus monkeys. Gynecol Invest 6:74, 1975

41. MEIRE HB, FISH P, WHEELER T: Ultrasound recording of fetal breathing. Br J Radiol 48:477, 1975

42. MERLET C, HOERTER J, DEVILLENEUVE C, TCHOBROUTSKY C: Mise en evidence de mouvements respiratoires chez le foetus d'agneau in utero au cours du dernier mois de la gestation. C R Acad Sci (Paris) 270:2042, 1970

43. PATRICK JE, DALTON KJ, DAWES GS: Breathing patterns before death in fetal lambs. Am J Obstet Gynecol 125:73, 1976

44. PATRICK J, FETHERSTON W, VICK H, BOEGELIN R: Human fetal breathing movements at 34–35 weeks gestation. Gynecol Invest 8:110, 1977

45. TIMOR-TRITSCH I, ZADOR I, HERTZ RH, ROSEN MG: Classification of human fetal movement. Am J Obstet Gynecol 126:70, 1976

19

Congenital Anomalies

RUDY E. SABBAGHA

Congenital anomalies, or birth defects, can be attributed to the following: 1) chromosomal aberrations (eg, Down's syndrome); 2) mendelian heritable disorders governed by mutations of recessive, dominant, or X-linked genes (eg, Tay–Sachs disease, a recessive disorder); 3) polygenic or multifactorial etiology (eg, anencephaly), and 4) environmental (teratogenic) causes (eg, cytomegalovirus; see Ch. 15).

Chromosomal aberrations are expressed in amniotic fluid cells exfoliated from the fetal surface; these cells may be obtained antenatally by amniocentesis. Likewise, more than 75 enzymatic or metabolic inherited disorders (27) are expressed in amniotic cells or fluid and may be detected during the second trimester of pregnancy.

A variety of congenital anomalies are diagnosed by ultrasound (13, 16). In addition ultrasound is becoming an essential tool both for localizing the best site for needle insertion in amniocentesis and for interpretation of elevated levels of α-fetoprotein (AFP) in maternal serum or amniotic fluid, Fig. 19–1. If truly elevated, AFP is predictive of a number of fetal abnormalities, as discussed elsewhere in this chapter.

Fetoscopy (1) can also be used to obtain fetal blood for the detection of some mendelian genetic diseases such as hemoglobinopathies (β-thalassemia, sickle-cell disease) and classic hemophilia (8, 12). Recently, ultrasonically guided fetoscopy has been successfully used, by 20 weeks' gestation, to obtain a fetal skin biopsy for ruling out autosomally inherited skin diseases such as ichthyosis congenita, a condition incompatible with life (10, 11).

Similarly, in the presence of a short-limb skeletal dysplasia the diagnosis may only be reached by ultrasound or fetoscopy or both (17, 22).

PREDICTORS OF HEREDITARY DISEASE AND CONGENITAL ANOMALIES

In early March 1979, the National Institute of Child Health and Development (NICHD) sponsored a consensus-development conference concerning predictors of congenital anomalies (27). These predictors encompassed amniocentesis, fetoscopy, AFP, and ultrasound. The safety, effectiveness, and proper use of these techniques or tests were discussed at length by health professionals, lawyers, ethicists, and consumer representatives. As a result the following guidelines were adopted for offering couples intrauterine evaluation, beginning with amniocentesis:

Maternal age equal to or greater than 35 years
Previous chromosomally abnormal child
History of three or more miscarriages

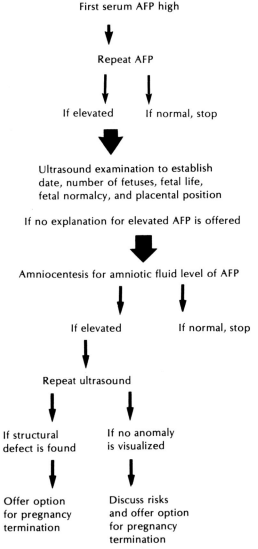

First serum AFP high

↓

Repeat AFP

↓   ↓

If elevated   If normal, stop

↓

Ultrasound examination to establish
date, number of fetuses, fetal life,
fetal normalcy, and placental position

If no explanation for elevated AFP is offered

↓

Amniocentesis for amniotic fluid level of AFP

↓   ↓

If elevated   If normal, stop

↓

Repeat ultrasound

↓   ↓

If structural   If no anomaly
defect is found   is visualized

↓   ↓

Offer option   Discuss risks
for pregnancy   and offer option
termination   for pregnancy
                     termination

FIG. 19–1. Schema for management of gravidas with elevated α-fetoprotein (AFP).

History of several miscarriages in a husband's previous wife

Chromosomal abnormality involving the pregnant woman, her family, or her spouse's family

Male relative of the gravida with Duchenne muscular dystrophy or severe hemophilia

Suspicion of the presence of a harmful gene on the X chromosome of the gravida

High risk for some hereditary error of metabolism detectable in utero

High risk for a neural tube defect

The participants emphasized that the physician's role was to inform the couple in question about the risks and benefits of intrauterine studies, whereas the final decision about implementation should be that of the gravida and her partner.

ROLE OF ULTRASOUND

While ultrasound occupies a central position in the diagnosis of fetal physical defects it is not yet widely used as a screening tool for the diagnosis of congenital anomalies in all gravidas. As a result the full potential of this modality for antenatal diagnosis of birth defects has not yet been achieved. The reasons for not using ultrasound routinely are related to the following:

Unknown long-term effects of sonic energy (see Ch. 3) and the consequent inability of many investigators to endorse the routine use of ultrasound, except in high-risk pregnancies

Cost:benefit ratio of the procedure; ie, the yield of congenital anomalies may be too small to justify the present cost of an ultrasound screening test

Lack of sufficiently trained personnel to conduct the examination and interpret the results (The use of ultrasound for the detection of congenital anomalies requires marked proficiency on the part of the sonographer and the availability of both static gray-scale and real-time equipment.)

Insufficient clinical research necessary for defining the sensitivity and specificity of ultrasound as a screening test

Interestingly, in Perth, Scotland, Millar has managed to carry out total antenatal population screening by sonar since 1974 (24). He finds that when ultrasound is used extensively in this manner it becomes economical and leads to the detection of almost all cases of anencephaly and serious spina bifida by 19 weeks' gestation, in time to offer the gravida the choice of terminating the pregnancy.

At present the indications for ultrasound examination of a gravida at high risk for harboring a fetus with a birth defect are:

Amniocentesis initiated in accordance with the NICHD guidelines, listed previously

Intrauterine orientation of the fetoscope, in conjunction with fetoscopy (22)

Elevated AFP values in serum or amniotic fluid

A uterine fundus that is large or small for dates

History of a heritable disorder which may be diagnosed by ultrasound

The last three indications and the birth defects which may be ultrasonically visualized are discussed further.

ELEVATED AFP

In amniotic fluid AFP is elevated in a number of conditions. These are:

Presence of a neural tube defect (NTD)

Pregnancy that is less mature or more advanced than estimated by menstrual dates. (Macri et al [21] reported elevated AFP in 156 gravidas, representing 4.3% of pregnancies screened for a NTD; of these women 41 [26.6%] were shown, using ultrasound, to have inaccurate menstrual dates and the AFP concentration fell to the normal range relative to the newly assigned sonar dates.)

Contamination of amniotic fluid by fetal blood

Fetal death

Multiple gestation

Rh disease

Fetal gastrointestinal anomalies

Fetal renal anomalies

Turner's syndrome and unbalanced D–G chromosomal translocation

False-positive elevations

In an individual gravida the interpretation of an abnormally elevated level of AFP rests on ultrasonic examination of the fetus to determine fetal life, fetal age, fetal number, and the presence or absence of a structural anomaly (Fig. 19–1). In some cases amniography may also be necessary to help interpret an abnormal AFP concentration because the presence of a NTD or a gastrointestinal anomaly such as duodenal atresia may remain questionable by ultrasound.

UTERINE FUNDUS AND DATES

Many gravidas are referred for ultrasound because the uterine fundus is either large or small for dates. Under these circumstances the physician may be clinically unable to distinguish the following entities: hydramnios, oligohydramnios, multiple gestation, inaccurate dates (Chs. 6 and 8), and pelvic mass associated with pregnancy (Ch. 20). By contrast, these entities are readily differentiated by ultrasound; as illustration, the first two conditions are discussed.

Hydramnios. This appears as a large cystic (fluid-filled) area (Fig. 19–2) surrounding the

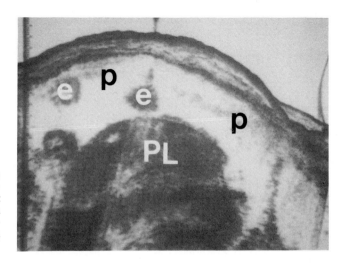

FIG. 19-2. Moderate polyhydramnios **(p)** seen in association with Rh disease. Note echo pattern of extremities **(e)** dispersed in amniotic fluid. Placenta **(PL)** is voluminous. (Sabbagha RE, Depp OR: Sonar: tool for detection of congenital anomalies. Clin Obstet Gynecol 20:279, 1977).

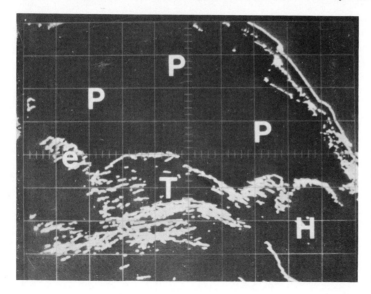

FIG. 19-3. Severe polyhydramnios (P) associated with absence of the characteristic echo pattern of the extremities in amniotic fluid. Note short extremity **(e).** The diagnosis of short-limb skeletal dysplasia (achondroplasia or decreased proliferation in the cartilage plate of tubular bone) was confirmed neonatally. Note fetal position along posterior uterine wall. **H,** Fetal head; **T,** fetal trunk. (Sabbagha RE, Depp OR: Sonar: tool for detection of congenital anomalies. Clin Obstet Gynecol 20:279, 1977).

fetus invariably located in close proximity to the posterior uterine wall, Figure 19–3. Additionally, in hydramnios fetal extremities are recognized as circular echo patterns (blotches) dispersed within the amniotic fluid, Figure 19–2; absence of these echoes (Fig. 19–3) is highly suggestive of short-limb skeletal dysplasias, discussed later in the chapter.

Although the diagnosis of hydramnios is usually evident on visual inspection of the echogram, it can be objectively confirmed by measurement of the total intrauterine volume (15) (TIUV; see Ch. 12). In hydramnios the TIUV is $\geq$ 2 SD (standard deviations) of the mean value, Table 19–1. Physicians quite readily refer women for ultrasound when the pregnancy is complicated by hydramnios. Because hydramnios is frequently associated with congenital anomalies (29, 32) sonographers have been able to see and diagnose a large number of birth defects antenatally (although some are more difficult to see than others). For example Horger and McCarter (18) discovered a fetus with a sacrococcygeal teratoma, Figure 19–4, and successfully delivered it by cesarean section; the pediatric surgeon was alerted prior to the delivery and was able to initiate definitive therapy without delay (13). Weiss et al (38) were able to diagnose conjoined twins in a gravida with hydramnios and elevated serum AFP, Figure 19–5.

Oligohydramnios. This is more difficult to appreciate echographically but fetal crowding is noted, Figure 19–6, and the TIUV is about 1.5–2 SD below the mean. Oligohydramnios is frequently associated with renal agenesis.

HERITABLE DISORDERS

CENTRAL NERVOUS SYSTEM

Anencephaly. The diagnosis is relatively easy to make sonographically even as early as 14–15

TABLE 19-1. RANGE OF TOTAL INTRAUTERINE VOLUME* (FROM MINUS −1.5 SD to +2 SD) IN RELATION TO GESTATIONAL AGE

Weeks' gestation	1.5 SD below mean	2 SD above mean
16	450	1800
18	600	2700
20	750	3300
22	900	3900
24	1100	4500
26	1250	5100
28	1500	5700
30	1750	6300
32	2000	6900
34	2350	7800
36		
	2550	9000
38	2850	10800
40	3000	12300

* Total intrauterine volume (TIUV) is derived by multiplication of sonar-derived uterine length × width × depth × 0.5233.

(Gohari P et al: Am J Obstet Gynecol 127:255, 1977)

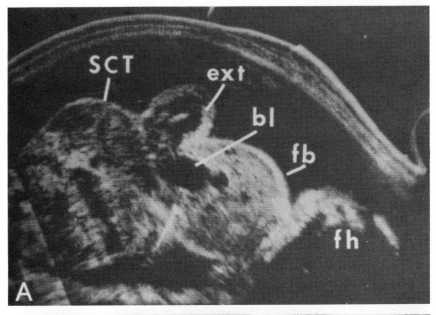

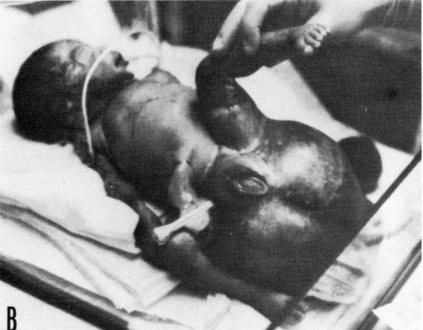

FIG. 19-4. A. Echogram of large sacrococcygeal teratoma **(SCT). Ext,** Extremity; **bl,** bladder; **fb,** fetal body; **fh,** fetal head. **B.** Neonate after birth. (Horger EO, McCarter LM: Am J Obstet Gynecol 134:228, 1979)

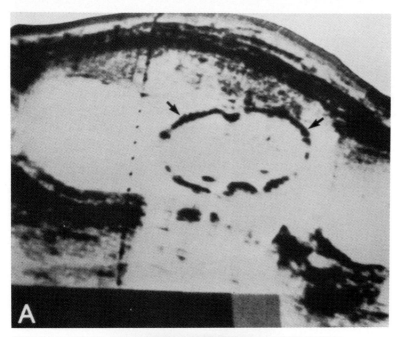

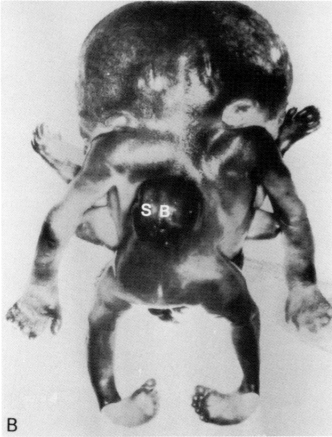

FIG. 19–5. A. Echogram showing fetal head **(arrows)** in a gravida with conjoined twins. **B.** Twins after birth. Note spina bifida **(SB).** (Weiss RR et al: Early prenatal diagnosis of unusual gestational abnormalities. E. Meadow, N.Y., Dept. OB/Gyn Nassau County Med. Ctr. Presented at ACOG, NY, 1979)

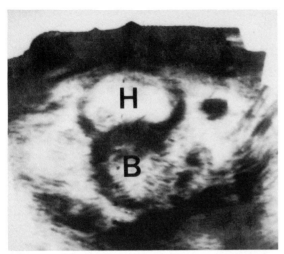

FIG. 19-6. Echogram of 19-week fetus showing severe oligohydramnios. No echo free area is seen around the fetal head **(H)** and body **(B)**. Fetal growth was retarded. The gravida elected to terminate the pregnancy and delivered a stillborn with multiple congenital anomalies, including congenital heart disease.

weeks' gestation. In this condition the fetal trunk is clearly visualized but only a portion of the head is seen, Figure 19–7. On occasion it may be necessary to perform a vaginal examination to make sure that the fetal head is not located deep in the pelvis.

Spina Bifida. This can be difficult to visualize by ultrasound, particularly if the defect is small and located in the lumbosacral area; however, most of these small lesions can be surgically corrected with minimal neurologic sequelae (3, 4, 5).

The spine should be examined in its entirety by ultrasound in both longitudinal and transverse planes; longitudinally the normal spine appears as a hollow tube, Figure 19–8, and in transverse planes the vertebral bodies are seen as circular structures, Figure 19–9.

In the presence of spina bifida an open U-shaped deformity is noted on transverse echograms. However, because the fetus may be either in the supine position or exhibiting excessive motion, evaluation of the vertebral column along multiple transverse planes may be difficult, frustrating, and time-consuming. Examination of the spine has been enhanced by real-time

imaging because the transducer is not attached to a scanning arm and can be angled to the appropriate plane reflecting echoes from the vertebral bodies. However, despite this advantage, on occasion spina bifida can only be diagnosed by gray-scale apparatus.

Meningocele, meningomyelocele, and encephalocele. These appear as cystic areas attached to the fetal head (25) or body and can be seen by real-time imaging to move concomitantly with the fetus.

The ultrasonic distinction between meningocele and meningomyelocele is difficult. Likewise, cranial meningocele and encephalocele cannot be differentiated with certainty. An occipitothoracic meningocele detected by ultrasound at 22 weeks' gestation is shown in Figure 19–10A. The pregnancy was terminated upon the request of the couple; the fetus is shown in Figure 19–10B.

Other fetal abnormalities such as marked edema of the fetal neck and hygroma colli (cystic lymphangioma of the neck) also appear as cystic areas adjacent to the spine and should be considered in the differential diagnosis of meningocele. Thus, if for any reason a NTD cannot be clearly visualized along the spine or if the fetus is in the supine position, amniography

FIG. 19-7. Anencephalus at 20 weeks' gestation. **a,** Anencephalus; **t,** boundaries of fetal trunk. (Sabbagha RE, Depp OR: Sonar: tool for the detection of congenital anomalies. Clin Obstet Gynecol 20:279, 1977).

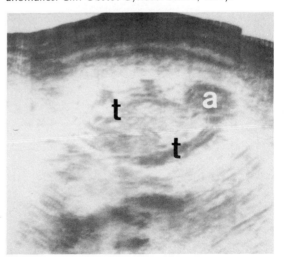

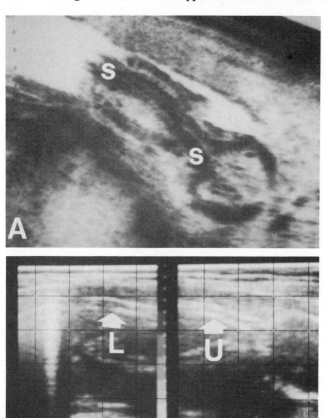

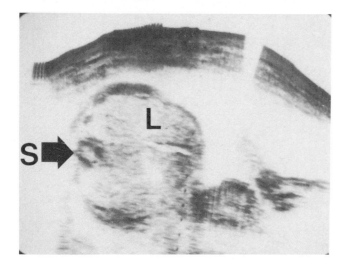

FIG. 19–8. Longitudinal echogram of fetal spine. **A.** By gray-scale apparatus. **B.** By real-time imaging. **S,** Spine; **L,** lower spine; **U,** upper spine.

FIG. 19–9. Cross section of the upper fetal abdomen showing the circular echo pattern of the vertebral body **(S→)** and liver **(L).**

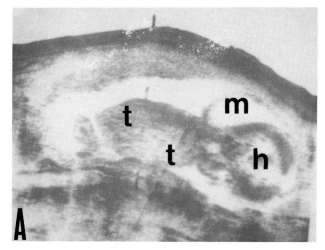

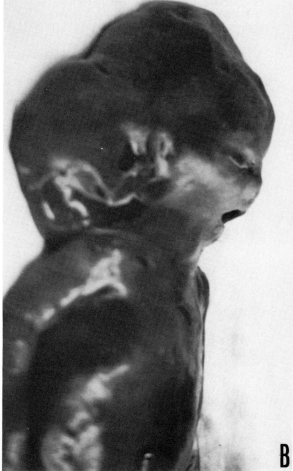

FIG. 19-10. **A.** Echogram of 22-week fetus with large occipitothoracic meningocele **(m). h,** Fetal head; **t,** fetal trunk. **B.** Actual appearance of meningocele. (Sabbagha RE, Depp OR, Grasse D, Kipper I: Am J Obstet Gynecol 131:113, 1978).

should be performed since it may lead to the correct diagnosis (23, 29, 34).

Hydrocephalus. This results from distention of the ventricular system of the brain secondary to obstruction in the flow of cerebrospinal fluid (CSF). In the newborn, the CSF is secreted into the lateral ventricles by the choroid plexus at the rate of approximately 650 ml/day (2); it then flows through the ventricles (lateral, third and fourth) to enter the subarachnoid space via the foramina of Luschka and Magendie.

The third and fourth ventricles are connected by the aqueduct of Sylvius. Aqueductal stenosis is the most common cause of hydrocephalus; however, the abnormality can result from a number of causes, listed in Table 19–2.

The ultrasound dimensions of the lateral ventricles in relation to each gestational week have not been firmly defined. Nonetheless, it is generally observed that the outer margins of the lateral ventricles normally extend only to 1/3 of the distance between the midline cerebral echo and the outline of the skull tables, Figure 19–11.

Campbell reports that the walls of the lateral ventricles recede, between 15 and 17 weeks' gestation, to the level just described (5). He correctly diagnosed hydrocephalus in four 17-week fetuses who failed to show a reduction in the size of the ventricles, even though the biparietal diameter (BPD) fell within the normal range for the duration of pregnancy. The author of this chapter has also noted temporary dilatation of the lateral ventricles in two large-for-gesta-

TABLE 19-2. CAUSES AND MECHANISMS OF HYDROCEPHALUS

Cause	Mechanism
Papilloma of choriod plexus	Overproduction of CSF
Fetal viral infection	Aqueductal stenosis
Autosomal recessive gene	Aqueductal stenosis (recurrence risk is 25% of offspring)
X-linked recessive gene	Aqueductal stenosis (recurrence risk is 50% of male offspring)
Aneurysum of vein of Galen	Pressure on ventricles Short and bowed
Dandy–Walker syndrome	Atresia, foramina of Luschka and Magendie
Arnold–Chiari syndrome	Obstruction to subarachnoid pathway (unknown etiology)
Infection (bacterial, toxoplasmal, viral)	Obliteration of subarachnoid space
Hurler's syndrome	Fibrous tissue proliferation in subarachnoid spaces
Achondroplasia	Small occipital skull and interference with flow of CSF in subarachnoid space
Vitamin A intoxication	Unknown

FIG. 19-11. Echogram demonstrating fetal head (35 weeks' gestation) and normal extension of the walls of the lateral ventricles **(arrows).**

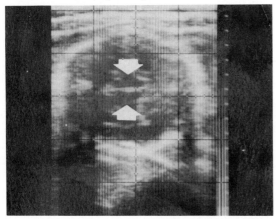

tional-age (LGA) fetuses in the interval of 31 to 35 weeks of pregnancy. Subsequently, ventricular size returned to normal, and neither infant had hydrocephalus.

Although, as described, the diagnosis of hydrocephalus can be made during the second trimester of pregnancy (4), it is more commonly

seen after the 30th week of gestation. Further, ventricular dilatation is rarely observed in its early stages. Rather, the full-blown picture of severe hydrocephalus is usually noted sonographically, Figure 19–12; ie, a distinct interface between the ventricular walls and the skull tables is not identifiable and the BPD is enlarged. When one considers the large amount of CSF formed each day it becomes apparent why, in the face of an obstruction, ventricular dilation occurs rapidly.

The diagnosis of advanced hydrocephalus should only be made if the following criteria are met:

1. BPD is very large in relation to gestational age.
2. The circumference of the fetal head markedly exceeds that of the abdomen.
3. The area of the fetal head is echo free.

The distinction between the different causes of hydrocephalus is not yet possible by ultrasound. However, there is preliminary evidence that a choroid plexus papilloma, which carries a more favorable prognosis than other forms of hydrocephalus, may have a characteristic ultrasound appearance. Similarly, the distinction between hydrocephalus and hydranencephaly (19) (congenital absence of the brain) or porencephaly (cavitation of the brain) may not always

FIG. 19-12. Advanced hydrocephalus. Note difference in size of head **(arrows)** and of fetal body **(B).** The ventricles extend to the skull tables (obvious posteriorly since reverberations are seen anteriorly).

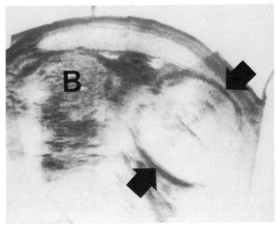

TABLE 19–3. CAUSES OF MICROCEPHALY

Heritable
Mendelian (recessive or x-linked genes)
Seckel's syndrome (recessive gene)
Chromosomal aberration (trisomies)
Maternal phenylketonuria
Other
Environmental
Intrauterine infection with TORCH*
Ionizing radiation

* TORCH = Toxoplasma, other (syphilis), rubella, cytomegalovirus, and herpes virus.

be feasible. It is theoretically possible that megalencephaly, an extremely rare disorder in which excessive brain growth results from proliferation of glial cells, would be distinguishable from hydrocephalus.

The mode and the most optimal time for delivery of the hydrocephalic fetus are difficult to ascertain. The reasons are related to two factors. First, the prognosis in a given fetus with hydrocephalus is difficult to estimate. Secondly, the correlation between degree of hydrocephalus and intellectual dysfunction is not uniform; up to 50% of children with a very thin cerebral mantle (<10 mm) can have normal intelligence. In general once pulmonary maturity is attained delivery by cesarean section should be considered because 1) the prognosis may be related to the duration of the disease process; and 2) surgical treatment (placement of a shunt between the cerebral ventricles and the right atrium or peritoneal cavity) is indicated in the majority of cases even if the cerebral mantle is <10 mm.

Microcephaly. A defect in the growth of the brain as a whole can result in microcephaly. The major specific causes of the abnormality are listed in Table 19–3. In microcephaly the occipitofrontal circumference of the head is reduced to 3 SD or more below the mean and the fetal BPD falls below the fifth percentile in relation to a specific gestational week. However, the ultrasonic differentiation between microcephaly and intrauterine growth retardation (IUGR) may be difficult because many of the factors predisposing to microcephaly also result in IUGR. In a particular gravida at high risk for microcephaly the finding of a normal BPD measurement virtually rules out the disorder.

GASTROINTESTINAL ANOMALIES

Omphalocele versus Gastroschisis. Abdominal wall defects are separated into two entities: omphalocele and gastroschisis (33). Omphalocele is more common than gastroschisis (1:5,000 versus 1:50,000); the abdominal defect is large, centrally located, and the herniated viscera are covered by a sac. The umbilical cord is inserted at the apex of the sac. In infants with omphalocele the birth weight distribution approaches normal; however, there is a high incidence of serious cardiac, gastrointestinal, and chromosomal abnormalities. Further, as many as 14% of infants with omphalocele exhibit organomegaly, macroglossia, and severe hypoglycemia, a conglomerate of findings known as Beckwith's syndrome.

In gastroschisis the abdominal defect is small (2–5 cm) and paraumbilical in location, and the herniated viscera are not covered by a sac; the defect is associated with a high incidence of prematurity, but congenital abnormalities are rarely observed.

Antenatal detection of omphalocele by ultrasound is possible because the defect is large and the viscera are located within a sac, Figure 19–13. Gastroschisis, however, may be missed sonographically because the defect is likely to be small.

In the presence of omphalocele delivery by cesarean section may be indicated, especially if fetal size is large, as in Beckwith's syndrome.

Fetal Ascites. Ordinarily the fetal bowel reflects a homogeneous echo pattern filling all of the abdominal cavity. In the presence of fetal ascites a fluid interface is readily apparent between the bowel and the abdominal wall, Figure 19–14.

The etiology of fetal ascites is protean. It can be attributed to immunologic hemolytic disease as well as to nonimmunologic factors (37). In the latter case the following causes are implicated: peritoneal inflammation (from bacterial or viral disease or toxoplasmosis), chorioangioma of the placenta, and severe cardiopulmonary malformations; on rare occasions, lymphatic obstruction can lead to chylous ascites.

Serial ultrasound measurements of the ab-

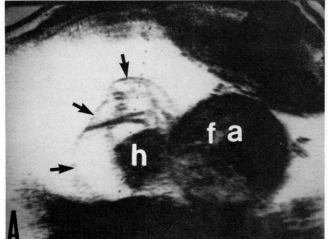

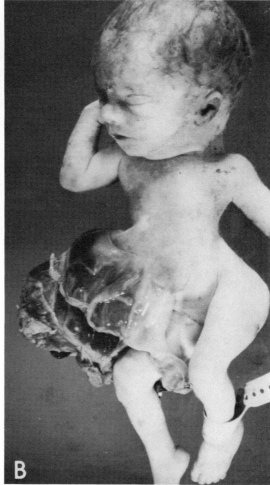

FIG. 19-13. A. Cross section of fetus with omphalocele. **Arrows** point to sac wall. **H,** herniated bowel; **fa,** fetal trunk. **B.** Neonate showing herniated gut (the sac is ruptured).

dominal circumference (Ch. 9) should be used to determine the severity of the condition. The disease is usually progressive and associated with multisystem anomalies. Interestingly, in one report (28) fetal ascites was ultrasonically seen to disappear gradually with advancing gestational age and subsequently a normal fetus was delivered.

Intestinal Anomalies. In intestinal obstruction secondary to duodenal atresia, the proximal aspect of the duodenum and the stomach are dilated and can be seen by ultrasound as two cystic areas ("double bubble" sign) adjacent to the liver (20), Figure 19–15.

In meconium ileus associated with cystic fibrosis and in obstruction of the lower intestinal tract, dilated loops of bowel can be ultrasonic-

ally visualized, Figure 19–16. However, in some normal LGA fetuses a similar dilatation of the bowel may be seen sonographically. Thus, in ruling out serious intestinal obstruction amniography should be used as an adjunct to ultrasound; the presence of contrast medium in the fetal gastrointestinal tract is evidence against intestinal obstruction.

ANOMALIES OF THE EXCRETORY SYSTEM

Renal Dysplasia. Approximately 50% of fetal abdominal masses can be attributed to a renal origin. Of these about half are related to renal dysplasia: multicystic kidneys (20%) and polycystic kidneys (5%). The other renal abnormalities include hydronephrosis, Wilms' tumor (5%), and other renal masses (14).

In multicystic kidney disease there is a lack of differentiation of both nephrotic and ductal elements and a replacement of collecting tubules by cystic dilatation, Figure 19–17. Additionally, because there is no urine production the fetal bladder is not visualized. The abnormality may be associated with chromosomal aberrations, imperforate anus, coarctation of the aorta, and Meckel's syndrome (encephalocele, eye abnormalities, cleft palate, polydactyly, and congenital heart disease).

In polycystic renal disease cortical and medullary differentiation is grossly preserved and the shape of the kidneys is recognized; although the collecting tubules are dilated to varying degrees, the cysts are usually smaller than those observed in multicystic renal dysplasia, and oligohydramnios is a characteristic feature. The disease is inherited as an autosomal recessive trait with a 25% recurrence risk. The neonate may exhibit abdominal enlargement, respiratory distress, congestive heart failure, and Potter's facies. The latter is characterized by low-set ears, hypertelorism, skin creases extending between the inner canthus of the eyes and the cheeks, a receded chin, and a wizened look.

Renal Agenesis. In renal agenesis both renal and bladder echoes are ultrasonically absent. However, because of oligohydramnios the renal area is often difficult to evaluate. Further, the bladder area should be examined over an inter-

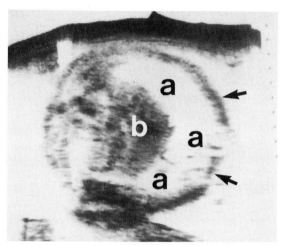

FIG. 19–14. Cross section of fetal abdomen showing ascites **(a). B,** Fetal bowel; **arrows** point to anterior abdominal wall.

FIG. 19–15. Cross section of upper fetal abdomen showing duodenal atresia. **1,** Dilated proximal part of stomach; **2,** dilated duodenum.

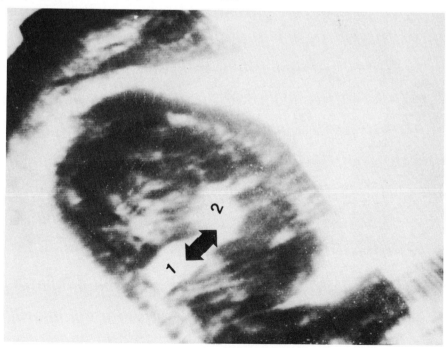

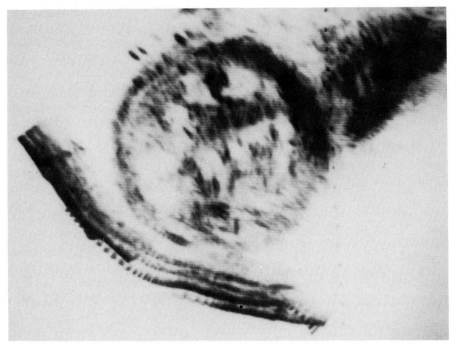

FIG. 19-16. Cross section of fetal abdomen showing dilated loops of bowel (see text).

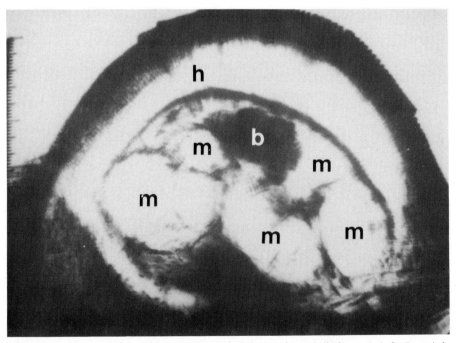

FIG. 19-17. Cross section of fetal abdomen showing multicystic kidneys **(m). b,** Bowel; **h,** hydramnios. From Sabbagha RE, Current concepts in obstetrics and gynecology (ed. Zuspar FP), Lea and Febiger, 1979.

TABLE 19–4. SOME CHARACTERISTICS OF FETAL SKELETAL DYSPLASIAS POTENTIALLY DIAGNOSABLE BY ULTRASOUND

Dysplasia	Limbs	Head and body
Achondrogenesis (AR)	Short	Increase in H:A ratio (one variety)
Achondroplasia (AD)	Short	Increase in BPD, AC, and H:A ratio
Campomelic (unknown mode of inheritance)	Short (most varieties)	Increase in BPD, AC, and H:A ratio (most varieties)
Chondroectodermal (AR) (Ellis–Van Creveld)	Short, with hexadactyly	Not characteristic
Diastrophic (AR)	Short, with contractures, "hitchhiker thumbs"	Not characteristic
Hypophosphatasia (AR)	Short, with fractures	Poorly visualized ribs and spine due to poor mineralization
Langer mesomelic (AR)	Short in middle segments	Micrognathia
Osteogenesis imperfecta (types I & IV) (AD)	Bowing	Not characteristic; occasional rib fractures
Osteogenesis imperfecta (types II & III) (AR)	Broad and angulated; short in type II	Thin cranium
Short rib–polydactyly (AR)	Short, with polydactyly	Narrow thorax
Spranger–Wiedemann (AD)	Proximal shortening	Barrel-shaped chest
Thanatophoric (unknown inheritance)		Increase in BPD, AC, and H:A ratio
Asphyxiating Thoracic (AR)	Variable shortening	Long, narrow chest

AC = abdominal circumference of fetus; AR = autosomal recessive; AD = autosomal dominant; BPD = biparietal diameter of fetus; H:A = ratio of circumference of fetal head and abdomen.
(Modified from Sillence DO et al: Pediatr Clin North Am 25:453, 1978).

val of a few hours before the diagnosis of anuria is made (3, 7). Neonates with this condition are stillborn or are delivered prematurely and die secondary to pulmonary hypoplasia and pneumothorax. Additionally, they exhibit Potter's facies, and frequently have other anomalies such as duodenal atresia and Meckel's diverticulum.

SKELETAL DYSPLASIAS

Fetal limbs are shortened in a variety of heritable disorders, Table 19–4. Sonographers are not infrequently called upon to examine the normalcy of fetal extremities in gravidas at high risk for skeletal dysplasia. As a result they have gained experience in detecting short-limb dysplasia and other related defects. Nonetheless these diagnoses remain difficult to make and may require repeated ultrasound examinations.

Mahoney and Hobbins (22) have recently defined the mean length of several limbs from autopsy data of premature neonates, Table 19–5. Using these data they were able to diagnose correctly, by both ultrasound and fetoscopy, a fetus with Ellis–van Creveld dysplasia in

which the length of the femur was reduced to 2.8 cm (normal 3.7 cm).

The fetal femur is usually the bone most accessible to ultrasound imaging, Figure 19–18. The fetal thigh is usually flexed, making an angle of 45°–90° with the lower part of the fetal body; thus, in outlining it the longitudinal axis of the fetus is first located and the real-time transducer is rotated until the femur is visualized, Figure 19–19.

In many forms of skeletal dysplasia the ratio of the circumference of the fetal head and abdomen (H:A ratio) is increased (Table 19–4); this finding may be useful in confirming the diag-

TABLE 19–5. POSTMORTEM MEASUREMENTS OF FETAL EXTREMITIES*

Extremity	Mean length (cm)	±2 SD (cm)
Femur	3.7	±0.2
Humerus	3.7	±0.3
Forearm	3.0	±0.5

* Measurements taken from 22 fetuses of gestational (menstrual) age of 16–20 weeks.
(Modified from Mahoney MJ, Hobbins JC: N Engl J Med 297:258, 1977)

nosis of short-limb defects even by 20 weeks' gestation because cephalic size may already be enlarged at midpregnancy (30). The normal variation in the H:A ratio is shown in Table 19–6.

Of interest is the progress made in the antenatal diagnosis of osteogenesis imperfecta (36, 39). Solomons and Gottesfeld (36) were able to identify fetal fractures ultrasonically by 19 weeks' gestation in 2 of 16 fetuses at risk for this disorder. In both cases, however, the diagnosis was made in conjunction with elevated levels of amniotic fluid pyrophosphate.

In a variety of multisystem congenital anomalies involving the skeleton the presence of short limbs can serve as a marker of the disease. For example, in Fanconi's anemia approximately 10% of infants have absent or hypoplastic radii. Similarly, in Robert's syndrome the anomalies include cleft palate, genital hypertrophy, tetraphocomelia, and nonfunctioning kidneys; the latter two can be diagnosed by ultrasound (16).

ANOMALIES OF INTEGUMENT

In pregnant women at high risk for giving birth to neonates with heritable skin disorders the combined use of ultrasound and fetoscopy has made it possible to obtain fetal skin biopsies by

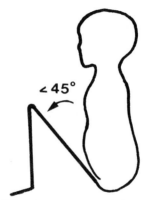

FIG. 19-19. To visualize the femur the ultrasound transducer should be rotated to an angle of 45°–90° from the longitudinal axis of the fetus.

midpregnancy (17). Using both diagnostic techniques concomitantly a number of investigators successfully diagnosed both the dominant and recessive forms of icthyosis congenita by 20 weeks' gestation (11). Newburger et al diagnosed chronic granulomatous disease in utero (26).

ULTRASOUND EXAMINATION AND REPORT

In looking for physical defects it is best to start the ultrasound examination by 16–18 weeks' gestation. A minimum time of 30 minutes should be allotted for the test.

In the search for some anomalies such as a small meningocele or spina bifida, a limb deformity, or renal agenesis the pregnant woman may have to be examined at weekly intervals before a report is issued. In some cases amniography should also be performed and the films evalu-

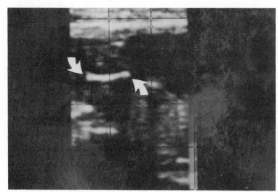

FIG. 19-18. Echogram of femus (arrows) at 16 weeks' gestation. The area of the knee joint is not visualized.

TABLE 19-6. HEAD: ABDOMEN (H:A) CIRCUMFERENCE RATIO VERSUS GESTATIONAL AGE

Gestational age (weeks)	H:A ratio	+2 SD
17–18	1.18	1.29
19–20	1.18	1.26
21–22	1.15	1.25
23–24	1.13	1.21
25–26	1.13	1.22

(Modified from Campbell S, and Thoms A: Br J Obstet Gynaecol 84:165, 1977)

TABLE 19-7. CONGENITAL ANOMALIES DETECTED BY ANTENATAL SONOGRAPHY

Neural tube defects	Anencephalus
	Spina bifida*
	Meningomyelocele
	Hydrocephalus
Cardiac defects	Bradycardia
Gastrointestinal defects	Omphalocele
	Gastroschisis
	Obstruction, upper bowel (duodenal atresia)
	Fetal Ascites
Renal defects	Multicystic kidneys
	Renal agenesis
	Bladder obstruction
Extremities	Short-limb dysplasia
Other	Conjoined twins
	Sacrococcygeal teratoma
	Hygroma
	Diaphragmatic hernia

* Small lesions in the lumbar area may not be visualized by Ultrasound.

ated in concert with the echograms before a final diagnosis is made.

At present, not all birth defects are detected by ultrasound. For example, the various forms of congenital heart disease cannot yet be discerned with any degree of certainty. Similarly, superficial skin lesions, craniofacial defects, and polydactyly are not visualized. When no anomaly is seen by ultrasound the report should indicate that the result is not all-inclusive; one way of phrasing the report is as follows: "None of the abnormalities which may be ultrasonically visualized are apparent at present." It may also be preferable to attach to the final report, a list of the congenital anomalies which may be detected echographically, Table 19–7.

REFERENCES

1. BENZIE PJ, DORAN TA: The "fetoscope"—A new clinical tool for prenatal genetic diagnosis. Am J Obstet Gynecol 121:460, 1975

2. BEHRMAN R: Textbook, Neonatal Perinatal Medicine. 2nd ed. St. Louis, Mosby, 1977

3. CAMPBELL S: The antenatal detection of fetal abnormality by ultrasonic diagnosis. Int Congress 310:240, 1973

4. CAMPBELL S: Early prenatal diagnosis of neural tube defects by ultrasound. Clin Obstet Gynecol 20:351, 1977

5. CAMPBELL S, PRYSE-DAVIES J, COLTART TM, SELLER MJ, SINGER JD: Ultrasound in the diagnosis of spina bifida. Lancet 1:1065, 1975

6. CAMPBELL S, THOMS A: Ultrasound measurement of the fetal head to abdomen circumference ratio in assessment of growth retardation. Br J Obstet Gynaecol 84:165, 1977

7. CAMPBELL S, WLADIMIROFF JW, DEWHURST CJ: The antenatal measurement of fetal urine production. Br J Obstet Gynaecol 80:680, 1973

8. CHANG H, HOBBINS JC, CIRIDALLI G et al: In utero diagnosis of hemoglobinopathies. N Engl J Med 290:1067, 1974

9. DUENHOELTER JH, SANTOS-RAMOS R, ROSENFELD ÇR, COLN CD: Prenatal diagnosis of gastrointestinal tract obstruction. Obstet Gynecol 47:618, 1976

10. ELIAS S, MAZUR M, SABBAGHA R, SIMPSON JC: The prenatal diagnosis of Ichthyosis congenita—submitted 1979

11. ESTERLY ND: The ichthysiform dermatoses. Pediatrics 42:900, 1968

12. FIRSHEIN SI, HOYER LW, LAZARCHICK J et al: Prenatal diagnosis of classic hemophilia. N Engl J Med 300:937, 1979

13. GARRETT WJ, KOSSOFF G: Selection of patients by ultrasonic echography for fetal and immediate neonatal surgery. Aust Paediatr J 12:313, 1976

14. GARRETT WJ, KOSSOFF G, OSBORN RA: The diagnosis of fetal hydronephrosis, megaureter, and urethral obstruction by ultrasonic echography. Br J Obstet Gynaecol 82:115, 1975

15. GOHARI P, BERKOWITZ RL, HOBBINS JC: Prediction of intrauterine growth retardation by determination of total intrauterine volume. Am J Obstet Gynecol 127:255, 1977

16. HOBBINS JC, GRANNUM PAT, BERKOWITZ RC, SILVERMAN R, MAHONEY MJ: Ultrasound in the diagnosis of congenital anomalies. Am J Obstet Gynecol 134:331, 1979

17. HOBBINS JC, MAHONEY MJ, GOLDSTEIN LA: New method of intrauterine evaluation by the combined use of fetoscopy and ultrasound. Am J Obstet Gynecol 118:1069, 1974

18. HORGER EO, MCCARTER LM: Prenatal diagnosis of sacrococcygeal teratoma. Am J Obstet Gynecol 134:228, 1979

19. LEE TG, WARREN BH: Antenatal diagnosis of hydranencephaly by ultrasound: correlation with ventriculography and computed tomography. J Clin Ultrasound 5:271, 1977

20. LOVEDAY BJ, BARR JA, AITKEN J: The ultrauterine demonstration of duodenal atresia by ultrasound. Br J Radiol 48:1031, 1975

21. MACRI JN, HADDOW JE, WEISS RR: Screening for neural tube defects in the United States. Am J Obstet Gynecol 133:119, 1979

22. MAHONEY MJ, HOBBINS JC: Prenatal diagnosis of

chondroectodermal dysplasia (Ellis-van Creveld Syndrome) using fetoscopy and ultrasound. N Engl J Med 297:258, 1977

23. MENNUTI MR, MORANZ JG, SCHWARZ RH, MELLMAN WJ: Amniography for the early detection of neural tube defects. Obstet Gynecol 49:25, 1977

24. MILLAR WG: Personal communication

25. MISKIN M, RUDD NL, DISCHE MR, BENZIE R, PIRANI BB: Prenatal ultrasonic diagnosis of occipital encephalocele. Am J Obstet Gynecol 130:585, 1978

26. NEWBURGER PE, COHEN JH, ROTHCHILD SB et al: Prenatal diagnosis of chronic granulomatous disease. N Engl J Med 300:178, 1979

27. NICHD Consensus Development Conference on Antenatal Diagnosis. Bethesda, Maryland. April, 1979

28. PLATT LD, COLLEA JV, JOSEPH DM: Transitory fetal ascites: an ultrasound diagnosis. Am J Obstet Gynecol 132:906, 1978

29. QUEENAN J, GODOW E: Amniography for detection of congenital anomalies. Obstet Gynecol 35:648, 1970

30. SABBAGHA RE, BARTON BA, BARTON FB, KINGAS E, ORGILL J, TURNER JH: Sonar biparietal diameter II. Predictive of three fetal growth patterns leading to a closer assessment of gestational age and neonatal weight. Am J Obstet Gynecol 126:485, 1976

31. SABBAGHA RE, DEPP R, GRASSE D, KIPPER I: Ultra-sound diagnosis of occipitothoracic meningocele at 22 weeks' gestation. Am J Obstet Gynecol 131:113, 1978

32. SANTOS-RAMOS R, DUENHOELTER JH: Diagnosis of congenital fetal abnormalities by sonography. Obstet Gynecol 45:279, 1975

33. SEASHORE JH: Congenital abdominal wall defects. Clin Perinatol 5:61, 1978

34. SHAFF MR, BLUMENTHAL B, COETZEE M: Meningoencephalocoele: pre-partum ultrasonic and fetoamniographic findings. Br J Radiol 50:754, 1977

35. SILLENCE DO, RIMOIN DL, LACHMAN R: Neonatal dwarfism. Pediatr Clin North Am 25:453, 1978

36. SOLOMONS CC, GOTTESFELD K: Prenatal biochemistry of osteogenesis imperfecta. In University of California at San Francisco National March of Dimes, Birth Defects Conference, 1978

37. TURSKI DH, SHAHIDI N, VISESKUL C, GILBERT E: Non-immunologic hydrops fetalis. Am J Obstet Gynecol 131:586, 1978

38. WEISS RR, CHATTERJEE S, VERMA U et al: Early prenatal diagnosis of unusual gestational abnormalities. Dept of Ob/Gyn Nassau County Med Ctr, E Meadow, NY. Presented at ACOG, NY, 1979

39. ZERVOUDAKIS IA, STRONGIN MJ, SCHROTENBOER KA, BEHAN M, KAZAM E, HAWKS GG: Diagnosis and management of fetal osteogenesis imperfecta congenita in labor. Am J Obstet Gynecol 131:116, 1978

20

Pelvic masses in pregnancy

ALEX A. BEZJIAN

Diagnostic sonography has become a very useful diagnostic tool in obstetrics and gynecology, for it is a noninvasive and harmless procedure both to the patient and the fetus. Its use in obstetrics and perinatology has been so well established (10–12) that the American College of Obstetricians and Gynecologists strongly recommended in a Newsletter statement on July 2, 1975, that every obstetric facility have a diagnostic ultrasound service available for its use (1).

The usefulness of ultrasonography in gynecology has, however, lagged behind obstetrics, since almost all persistent large pelvic masses are surgically removed and an additional diagnostic test with the additional cost and inconvenience to the patient is often felt unnecessary by the gynecologist. The situation is, however, different in cases of pelvic masses associated with pregnancy, for it is desirable to avoid surgery in pregnancy if the pelvic mass can definitely be shown to be benign and harmless.

Another factor contributing to the late development of gynecologic, as well as upper abdominal, ultrasonography has been technical. Whereas a pregnant uterus with a fetus surrounded by amniotic fluid has been ideal for sonographic scanning even with the old bistable imaging technics, the nonpregnant abdomen without such distinct interphases had not been so amenable to ultrasonography. With the introduction of gray-scale ultrasonography, how-

ever, interphases previously not seen can now be visualized in different shades of gray allowing much clearer differentiation between cystic, solid, mixed, and inflammatory masses (4).

More recently, real-time scanning has also been commonly used in obstetrics. Its use in detecting and identifying abnormal pelvic masses remains, however, somewhat limited at present, owing largely to its lower power of both axial and lateral resolution and the inability to perform compound scanning with it.

In this chapter I demonstrate the various kinds of abnormal pelvic masses that can occur with pregnancy and determine the reliability of ultrasound in accurately diagnosing such masses.

TECHNIQUE AND BASIC PRINCIPLES

The technique of ultrasonic scanning of a pregnant patient with a suspected pelvic mass is basically the same as that described in previous chapters, that is, serial cross-sectional scans are obtained at 2 to 4-cm intervals both saggitally and transversely, and a three-dimensional image is then mentally created.

In dealing with pelvic masses, however, several points that may not be important in routine obstetric sonography should be stressed, as follows:

1. A full urinary bladder is absolutely essential for a proper study, especially if the suspected mass is deep in the pelvis or in the cul-de-sac.

2. Multiple additional sections at closer intervals (½–1.0 cm) should also be obtained in the region of the pelvic mass. On certain occasions oblique sections might also be necessary.

3. At certain specific sections through the mass several photographic prints must be obtained at varying gain or sensitivity settings to determine the true nature of the mass (i.e., cystic, solid, or mixed). Two specific characteristics in a mass are looked for in such a determination. The first is the so-called "fill in" pattern of the mass, where, on gradually increasing the gain setting, all purely cystic structures, including the bladder, remain echo free, in contrast to solid or mixed masses, which invariably fill in with echos (8) (Fig. 20–1). The second characteristic is the so-called "through transmission" or the ability to visualize the posterior wall of the mass. Cystic masses have clearly defined, thin posterior walls, whereas solid masses have a rather poorly defined one. Inflammatory masses, on the other hand, even though they are mostly cystic, have a clear but rather thick and irregular posterior wall owing to inflammation, edema, and adhesions.

4. A thorough review of the patient's history and symptoms is also mandatory, since on many occasions multiple different pathologic entities produce similar sonographic features, and knowledge of the patient's medical background coupled with an abdominal and pelvic examination whenever feasible may help in defining the location of planes that must be carefully scanned and assist the sonographer in interpreting some of the echograms.

GENERAL CONSIDERATIONS

When a pelvic mass is sonographically discovered in pregnancy, a careful evaluation of both the pregnancy and the mass must be made. The sonographic appearance of a gravid uterus at various stages of gestation is discussed elsewhere. As for the mass, it must be evaluated with regard to its size, consistency (solid or cystic), location, and origin.

The size of the mass can easily be measured by means of an electronic centimeter marker superimposed directly on the mass (see Fig. 20–7). Its consistency can be determined by varying the gain settings and by using transducers with different frequencies.

With the recent introduction of the newer gray-scale instrumentation, the resolution of most systems has markedly improved. For most pelvic sonograms a 3.5-MHz-long internal focus transducer is optimal. But when deep penetra-

FIG. 20–1. Schematic differentiation among a cystic, solid, and inflammatory mass by ultrasound. b, bladder, m, mass.

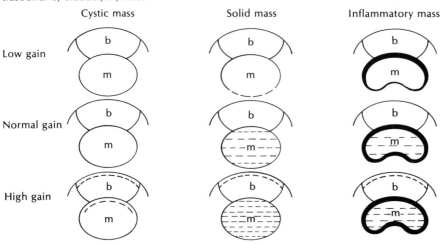

tion into the posterior wall of the pelvis or the abdomen, especially in the absence of a full urinary bladder, is needed, a 2.5-MHz transducer may be more helpful (11).

The location and origin of the mass are best determined by initially localizing and identifying the gravid uterus. The relationship of the mass to the uterus, that is, whether it is uterine or extrauterine, then becomes easier to determine. Table 20–1 outlines the various types of pelvic masses that may be associated with a pregnant uterus. Note that the major differential point is whether the mass is uterine or extrauterine in origin.

To evaluate the reliability of sonography in the diagnosis of pelvic pathology in pregnancy, we reviewed all the cases that had such a sonographic diagnosis for the past 4 years at the University of Miami Medical School and Jackson Memorial Hospital. Of 143 such cases encountered, 21 were either lost to follow-up or had an inadequate postpartum evaluation and thus were deleted from the study. In the remaining 122 cases the ultrasonic diagnosis was verified by pathologic or clinical means (Table 20–2). The correct diagnosis was made by ultrasound in 117 of 122 patients (95%).

FALSE PELVIC MASSES

Some gravidas present with a uterus that is "large for dates," and this leads the clinician to believe that the excessive uterine enlargement is due to an abnormal pelvic mass. In such cases ultrasound is useful in ruling out a pelvic mass that may be difficult to delineate by examination alone. Conditions leading to increased intrauterine enlargement are the following:

Inaccurate menstrual dates.

Fetal macrosomia and/or large placenta (diabetes mellitus, hydrops fetalis, postterm pregnancy.

Large abnormal fetal masses (abdominal and CNS masses) (Fig. 20–2).

Multiple pregnancy (Fig. 20–2).

Polyhydramnios (Fig. 20–2).

Occasionally, normal structures within a gravid uterus can also be mistaken for abnormal masses. The most common error made here is the occasional collection of amniotic fluid in the lower portion of the uterine cavity mimicking a cyst in that region (Fig. 20–3). With proper scanning techniques, however, this fluid collec-

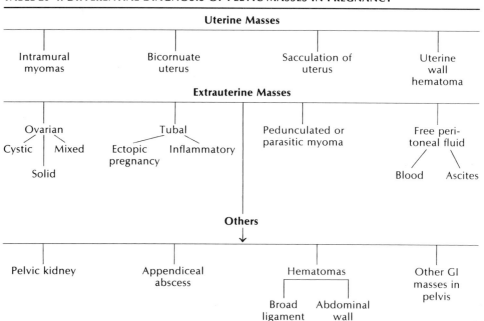

TABLE 20–1. DIFFERENTIAL DIAGNOSIS OF PELVIC MASSES IN PREGNANCY

Uterine Masses

| Intramural myomas | Bicornuate uterus | Sacculation of uterus | Uterine wall hematoma |

Extrauterine Masses

| Ovarian (Cystic / Mixed / Solid) | Tubal (Ectopic pregnancy / Inflammatory) | Pedunculated or parasitic myoma | Free peritoneal fluid (Blood / Ascites) |

Others

| Pelvic kidney | Appendiceal abscess | Hematomas (Broad ligament / Abdominal wall) | Other GI masses in pelvis |

TABLE 20-2. VARIOUS TYPES OF PELVIC MASSES IN PREGNANCY DIAGNOSED BY SONOGRAPHY

Condition	Correct diagnosis Proven pathologically	Proven clinically	Incorrect diagnosis Proven pathologically	Total
Uterine myoma	23	31	2*	56
Ovarian tumor	12	37	1†	50
Theca-lutein cysts associated with hydatidiform mole	1	5	1‡	7
Uterine wall hematoma	3	—	1§	4
Abdominal wall hematoma	2	—	—	2
Bicornuate uterus	—	2	—	2
Appendiceal abscess	1	—	—	1
Total	42	75	5	122

* In two patients marked degeneration of fibroids was incorrectly diagnosed as ovarian cysts
† Ovarian fibroma in the posterior cul-de-sac was incorrectly diagnosed as a uterine myoma
‡ Diagnosed as a missed abortion with a uterine myoma
§ Diagnosed as uterine myoma

tion can be shown to be leading to the cervical os inferiorly and to the remainder of the amniotic cavity superiorly. The normally existing thickened lower anterior uterine wall in the first trimester of pregnancy has also been occasionally confused with a myoma in that region (Fig. 20–3).

Certain normal extrauterine pelvic structures and echo patterns have also been occasionally mistaken for abnormal pelvic masses. These include the following:

1. Lateral pelvic wings (Fig. 20–4). These are the bilateral iliac bones extending medially toward the pelvis. The ileopsoas muscles are frequently seen lying medial to them. The iliac bones can easily be recognized by their winglike shape and by their location immediately underneath and medial to the iliac crests.
2. Ischial spines. These can be seen indenting the full bladder on vertical scans in the area of the lateral pelvic walls (Fig. 20–4).
3. Bowel artifacts. Air within loops of bowel is a poor sound transmitter and can occasionally create a false mass effect posterior to the loops of bowel. This can be readily recognized by

noting the absence of sound transmission through the area in question as well as by identifying the multiple thick and bright bowel echoes overlying it (Fig. 20–4).

Finally, the increased sensitivity of the newer gray-scale systems and the increasing use of compound scanning techniques have led to increased creation of artifactual reverberation, mostly along the proximal border of fluid-filled cavities. They are commonly seen along the anterior bladder wall and can extend to any adjacent cystic pelvic structures. These echoes can be confused with true echoes representing solid components in an otherwise cystic mass. Their true nature can be determined by comparing them to any existing echoes within the urinary bladder (see Fig. 20–14).

UTERINE MYOMAS

The most common pelvic mass associated with pregnancy is a uterine leiomyoma (56 of 122 cases of pelvic masses). They occur generally in 1 of 200 pregnancies, and most are small and have no clinical bearing on the outcome of the

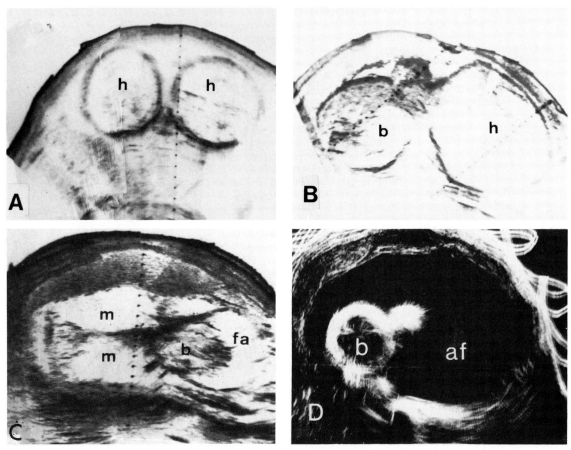

FIG. 20–2. Causes of increased intrauterine enlargement. **A.** Twins. **B.** Hydrocephalus. **C.** Fetal meningomyelocele and fetal ascites. **D.** Hydramnios; a, fetal ascites; af, amniotic fluid; b, fetal body; h, fetal head; m, meningomyelocele.

FIG. 20–3. False intrauterine masses. **A.** Collection of amniotic fluid in lower uterine region resembling a cyst. **B.** Thick lower anterior uterine wall resembling a myoma; af, amniotic fluid; b, bladder; h, fetal head; w, uterine wall.

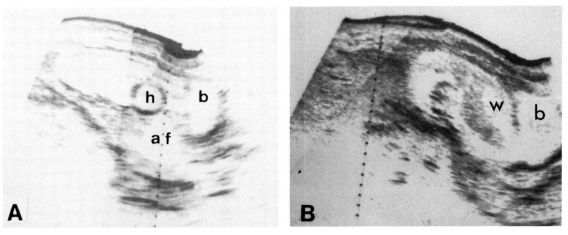

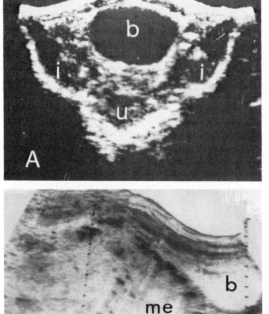

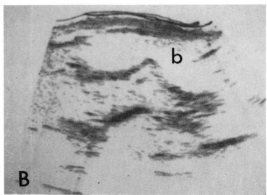

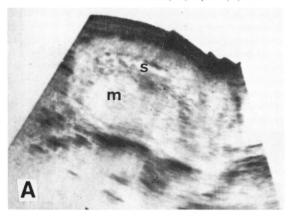

FIG. 20–4. False pelvic masses. **A.** Intrauterine pregnancy at 7 weeks with bilateral iliac bones. **B.** Ischial spine indenting the urinary bladder. **C.** False mass effect created by overlying loops of bowel; b, bladder; i, iliac bones; me, mass effect; u, uterus.

FIG. 20–5. Two large myomas compressing an 8 weeks' size gestational sac. **A.** Vertical scan **B.** Transverse scan; m, myoma; s, sac.

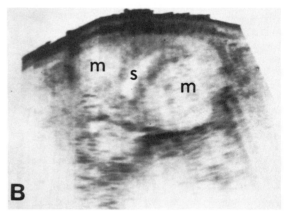

pregnancy. Large submucous myomas may, however, be associated with an increased rate of spontaneous abortions, owing to compression of the gestational sac (Fig. 20–5). In the second and third trimesters of pregnancy myomas are also known to be associated with premature labor, premature rupture of membranes, placental abruption, fetal malpresentation, and soft-tissue dystocia during labor. In the nonpregnant state most myomas are intramural, homogeneously solid and irregular, and therefore present with the following distinct sonographic features:

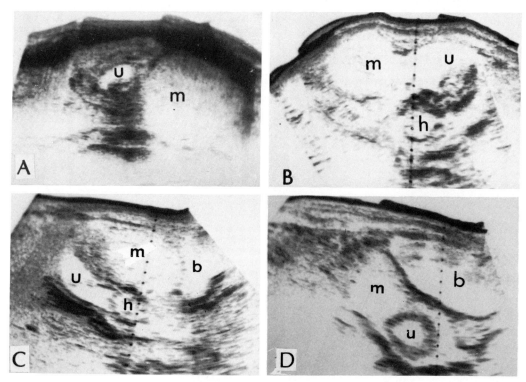

FIG. 20-6. Uterine myomas occupying varying positions within the pregnant uterus. **A.** Left-sided myoma. **B.** Right-sided myoma. **C.** Low anterior myoma. **D.** Fundal myoma; b, bladder; h, fetal head; m, myoma; u, pregnant uterus.

1. The uterus is usually irregularly shaped (Fig. 20–6).
2. No clear interface exists between the myoma and the uterus (Fig. 20–7).
3. The posterior wall of the uterus is poorly visualized, and its internal structure may exhibit a finely speckled appearance on gray-scale sonography (Fig. 20–7).

In pregnancy, however, myomas increase in size and undergo varying degrees of softening and degeneration. Thus, they become more transonic, and their internal texture changes to a more variable, coarse and complex echo pattern. With the introduction of gray-scale imaging (4) some other interesting ultrasonic features have become better recognized, as follows:

1. The degree of degeneration within a myoma is better appreciated and can therefore be more reliably quantitated and more closely observed in the symptomatic patients in whom surgery is contemplated (Fig. 20–8).

2. Calcifications within a myoma are more clearly seen and appear as bright, sonolucent areas, sometimes even resembling a fetal head (Fig. 20–9).
3. The interface between tissue is more clearly identified and the borders of myomas are more distinctly seen. As a result, the pressure exerted on a pregnant uterus by the myoma may be better appreciated (Fig. 20–10).

In occasional cases fibroids remain difficult to diagnose. This occurs when the degree of degeneration of the myoma during pregnancy is so severe that it mimics sonographically a semi-solid adnexal tumor (6). The two patients in whom ovarian masses were incorrectly diagnosed (Table 20–2) were found at laparotomy to have markedly degenerated soft fibroids (see Fig. 20–8). Both pregnancies were allowed to continue with the myomas, and healthy term infants were delivered. It is extremely difficult at present, even with improved instrumentation, to differentiate with certainty such atypical myomas in pregnancy from mixed ovarian tumors or possibly ovarian carcinomas. Since the risk of leaving a possible ovarian carcinoma in the pelvis throughout pregnancy is greater than the risk of exploratory laparotomy, the author recommends surgical exploration for diagnostic purposes (Table 20–3).

Occasionally with progression of pregnancy a myoma has been sonographically observed to

change its position in relation to the uterus. (Fig. 20–11). This phenomenon is probably due to the following two factors: 1) development of the lower uterine segment, causing the low uterine myoma to retract upwards; 2) gradual rotation of the uterus, usually toward the right side, and secondary rotation of the myoma attached to the uterine wall.

Two other groups of pregnant women with

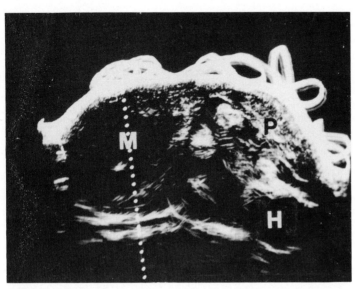

FIG. 20–7. Large uterine myoma with intrauterine pregnancy at 32 weeks. Note centimeter marker within myoma and the absence of line of separation between the myoma and the uterine cavity; H, fetal head; P, placenta.

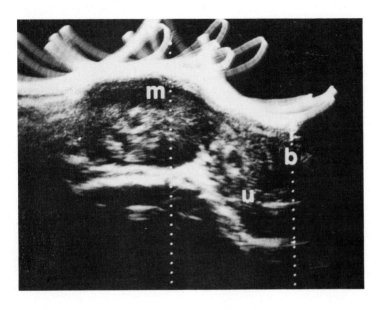

FIG. 20–8. Intrauterine pregnancy at 8 weeks with severely degenerated large fundal myoma. Note bright posterior wall and the line of separation between myoma and uterine fundus; b, bladder; m, myoma; u, uterus containing gestational sac.

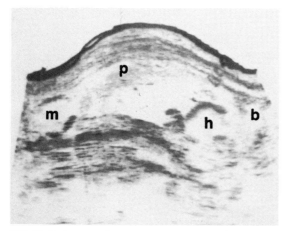

FIG. 20-9. Intrauterine pregnancy at 20 weeks with calcified myoma resembling fetal head; b, bladder; h, fetal head; m, calcified myoma; p, placenta.

fibroids also deserve further discussion. The first constitutes 12 patients who were refused a suction curettage because uterine size was greater than 12 weeks' gestation (Table 20–4). On sonographic evaluation, however, they were found to have uterine myomas associated with pregnancy of less than 12 weeks' duration (Fig. 20–12). Their pregnancies were all terminated uneventfully by suction curettage.

In the second group of two patients (Table 20–4) amniocentesis for second-trimester abortion was unsuccessful at presumably 15–16 weeks' gestation. On sonographic examination the pregnancies were found to be only 12–13 weeks in duration but were associated with uterine myomas. Amniocentesis was successful 3 weeks later. Thus, ultrasound is useful in the management of some women seeking termination of pregnancy (2), and should be accessible to all outpatient abortion clinics.

Finally it is noteworthy that about 50% of the gravidas with myomas were referred for a sonogram with no clinical suspicion of a pelvic mass (Tables 20–3 and 20–4). This is not surprising, since soft intramural myomas are often clinically indistinguishable from the normal myometrial wall. Posterior myomas in the second and third trimesters can also be easily missed, for they are beyond the reach of the examining hand. The sonographic diagnosis of uterine myomas associated with pregnancy in such unsuspected cases can play a major role in the subsequent management of these gravidas.

OVARIAN TUMORS

THE NORMAL OVARIES

With the development of gray-scale sonography, normal ovaries can often be well visualized in the first trimester of pregnancy. They measure approximately 2 × 3 cm and are located lateral to the uterus (Fig. 20–13). However, with the gradual enlargement of the gravid uterus, the normal ovaries become almost impossible to visualize.

FIG. 20-10. Large uterine myoma with degeneration compressing fetal thorax; M, myoma; T, fetal thorax.

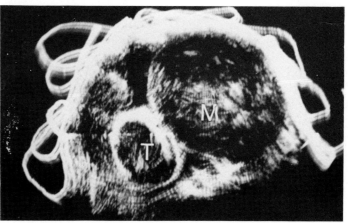

TABLE 20-3. UTERINE MYOMAS IN PREGNANCY WITH POSITIVE SONOGRAPHIC AND PATHOLOGIC CORRELATION

No. of cases	Clinical diagnosis	Sonographic diagnosis	Operation
2	IUP 8–10 weeks with myomas	IUP 8–10 weeks with myomas	Abortion hysterectomy
5	IUP with pelvic mass	IUP 14, 15, & 16 weeks with myomas	Abortion hysterectomy
3	IUP with pelvic mass	IUP with lower uterine myomas	Cesarian section
3	IUP large for dates	IUP 8–12 weeks with myomas	Abortion hysterectomy
4	IUP large for dates	IUP with large myomas	Myomectomy post suction curetage
1	Hydatidiform mole	IUP 11 weeks with 16-cm myoma	Abortion hysterectomy
1	IUP 16 weeks. Failed amniocentesis	Missed abortion with multiple myomas	Hysterectomy
1*	IUP with pelvic mass	IUP 17 weeks with 8 cm cul-de-sac mass. Probably myoma	Myoma found at exploratory laparotomy

* Patients had exploratory laparotomy because of uncertain clinical and sonographic diagnosis.

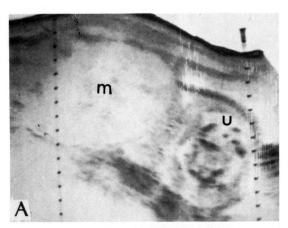

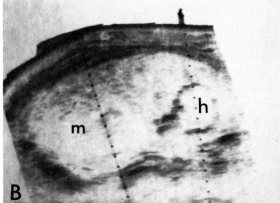

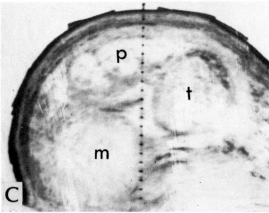

FIG. 20-11. A large myoma at variable positions in relation to the pregnant uterus at different stages of gestation. **A.** Vertical scan showing fundal myoma at 13 weeks' gestation. **B.** Transverse scan showing the same myoma occupying the right lateral side of the uterus at 18 weeks' gestation. **C.** Transverse scan showing myoma along right posterior uterine wall at 35 weeks' gestation; h, fetal head; m, myoma; p, placenta; t, fetal thorax; u, uterus.

TABLE 20-4. UTERINE MYOMAS IN PREGNANCY WITH POSITIVE SONOGRAPHIC AND CLINICAL FOLLOW-UP CORRELATION

No. of gases	Initial diagnosis	Sonographic diagnosis	Outcome
3	Routine obstetric scan	IUP + myomas	Vaginal delivery. Myomas felt postpartum
3	Large for dates	IUP + myomas	Vaginal delivery. Myomas felt postpartum
6	IUP + myomas	IUP + myomas	Vaginal delivery. Myoma felt postpartum
5	IUP + pelvic mass	IUP + myomas	Vaginal delivery. Myoma felt postpartum
2	IUP 15–16 weeks with failed amniocentesis	IUP at 12–13 weeks with myomas	Successful amniocentesis at 15–16 weeks under guidance of ultrasound. Myomas felt at postpartum examination
12	Large for dates	IUP + myomas	Suction curettage. Myomas felt at 4 weeks postoperative examination

FIG. 20-12. A 15-week-size myomatous uterus containing an 8-week gestational sac in its fundal region; three distinct myomas can be identified. The position of the gestational sac is important to determine for a safe and adequate suction curettage; m, myoma; s, gestational sac.

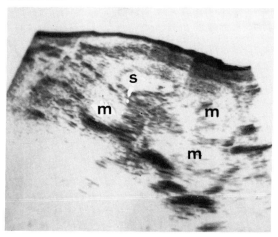

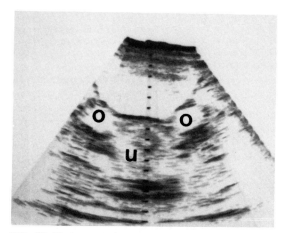

FIG. 20-13. Intrauterine pregnancy at 6 weeks with minimal enlargement of the ovaries bilaterally; b, bladder; o, ovaries; u, uterus.

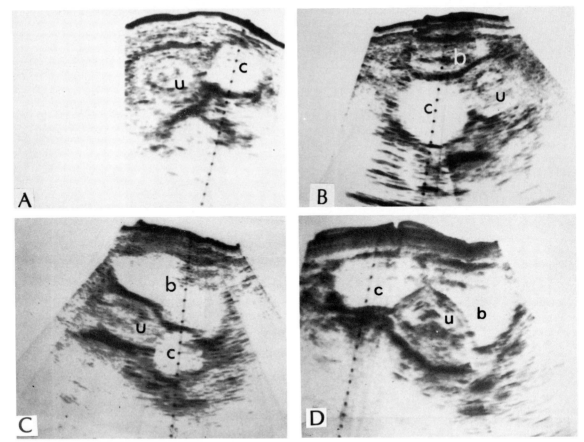

FIG. 20–14. Corpus luteum cyst occupying varying positions in relation to the pregnant uterus. **A.** Right side. **B.** Left side. **C.** Posterior cul-de-sac. **D.** Fundal. Note reverberation echoes within fundal cyst and bladder; b, bladder; c, cyst; u, uterus.

It is estimated that 1 in 1000 pregnancies is complicated by an ovarian tumor (3). These tumors can be sonographically classified into the following:

A. Simple unilocular cysts
  1. Corpus luteum cyst
  2. Paraovarian cyst
  3. Cystadenoma
B. Simple multilocular cysts
  1. Mucinous cysts adenoma
  2. Theca lutein cyst
  3. Polycystic ovaries
C. Complex masses
  1. Dermoid
  2. Hemorrhage and/or necrosis within cystic or solid mass
  3. Malignant tumor

D. Solid masses
  1. Benign (fibroma, thecoma, Brenner)
  2. Malignant

SIMPLE UNILOCULAR CYSTS

These cysts are easily detectable by ultrasound (9). They are regular in shape and usually well separated from the pregnant uterus and can occupy variable positions in the pelvis (Fig. 20–14). Frequent reverberation artifacts are seen in the anteriorly located ones (Fig. 20–15). They are echo free and have a well-defined, smooth posterior wall.

By far the most common ovarian tumor in pregnancy is the corpus luteum cyst (Tables 20–5 and 20–6). They occur in the first trimester of pregnancy and disappear by the 16th week of gestation. They can occupy any position within

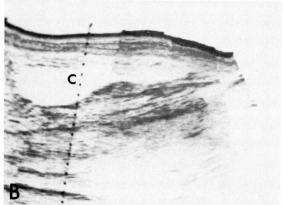

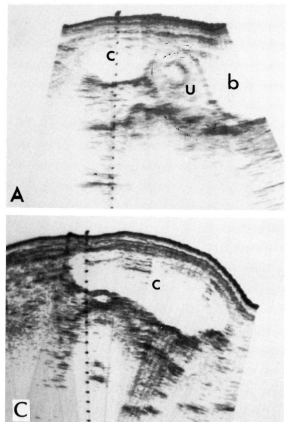

FIG. 20-15. Large paraovarian cyst discovered accidentally during a routine sonogram. Despite its size the soft cyst could not be adequately felt by physical examination. **A.** Vertical scan at mid line. **B.** Vertical scan at 3 cm left of midline. **C.** Transverse scan at level of umbilicus; b, bladder; c, cyst; u, uterus.

the pelvis (Fig. 20–14). Although it is estimated that about 10% of ovarian masses in pregnancy represent normal corpus luteum cysts that may be as large as 10 cm in diameter (3), in the author's series, 80% of ovarian masses diagnosed by ultrasound were corpus luteum cysts (Tables 20–5 and 20–6). The discrepancy may be attributed to two factors, as follows:

1. With the liberalization of abortion laws more patients are being examined in the first trimester and hence more corpora lutea are being discovered.
2. With the introduction of ultrasound more ovarian cysts previously unrecognized are being detected.

A large number of corpus luteum cysts are sonographically diagnosed in patients referred with a suspected diagnosis of an ectopic pregnancy.

The signs and symptoms of a patient with early intrauterine pregnancy with vaginal spotting and a corpus luteum cyst can be similar to that of an ectopic pregnancy, and the demonstration of a normal intrauterine pregnancy with an ovarian cyst can be of great assistance to the clinician (see Ch. 21).

Paraovarian and serous cyst adenomas, though purely cystic, can reach sizes much greater than corpus luteum cysts, and they persist after the 16th week of gestation (Fig. 20–15).

SIMPLE MULTILOCULAR CYSTS

These cysts are sonographically similar to the simple unilocular cysts but contain linear septations that vary in number and complexity (Fig. 20–16). They are commonly seen in mucinous cyst-adenomas and theca lutein cysts associated with ovarian hyperstimulation syndrome and hydatidiform moles.

TABLE 20-5. OVARIAN CYSTS IN PREGNANCY WITH POSITIVE SONOGRAPHIC AND PATHOLOGY CORRELATION

Initial diagnosis	Sonographic diagnosis	Surgery	Pathologic diagnosis	Correlation sonogram and pathology
IUP + post cul-de-sac mass	IUP 10 weeks + benign mass post cul-de-sac	Suction curettage Right S & O	Corpus luteum	+
IUP + right ovarian cyst	IUP 6 weeks + right adnexal cyst	D&C right S & O	Corpus luteum	+
IUP + right ovarian cyst	IUP 8 weeks + 10 cm right adnexal cyst	Suction curettage cystectomy	Corpus luteum	+
IUP 12 weeks + spotting	IUP 12 weeks + 12 × 14 cm left ovarian cyst	Cystectomy	Paraovarian cyst	+
IUP + mass	IUP 35 weeks + semi-solid mass	Ovarian cystectomy post-partum	Dermoid cyst	+
IUP large for dates	IUP 6 weeks + ovarian cyst, mixed in nature	Cystectomy	Dermoid cyst	+
IUP + ovarian cyst	IUP + dermoid	Suction curettage left ovarian cystectomy	Dermoid cyst	+
IUP large for dates	IUP 10 weeks with 6 cm left dermoid cyst	Suction curettage cystectomy	Dermoid cyst	+
IUP + ovarian cyst	12 weeks IUP and adnexal cyst with septations	Right oophorectomy	Mucinous cyst adenoma	+
IUP + ovarian cyst	IUP 10 weeks + left ovarian cyst with septations	Left S & O at 17 weeks gestation	Mucinous cyst adenoma	+
IUP with hydramnios and fetal demise	IUP 8 weeks + with 30 × 10 cm mucinous cyst adenoma	Ovarian cystectomy and suction curettege	Mucinous cyst adeno with small focus of early carcinoma	+
IUP + post cul-de-sac mass	IUP 37 weeks + post cul-de-sac cystic mass	Cesarean section and cystectomy	Cystic adenofibroma of ovary	+

TABLE 20-6. OVARIAN CYSTS IN PREGNANCY WITH POSITIVE SONOGRAPHIC AND CLINICAL FOLLOW-UP CORRELATION

No. of cases	Sonographic diagnosis	Outcome
12	Intrauterine pregnancy with benign adnexal cyst	Suction Curettage. No cyst at 6 weeks' follow-up
23	Intrauterine pregnancy with benign adnexal cyst	Cyst disappeared with progression of pregnancy
2	Intrauterine pregnancy with multiple gestation at 8 weeks with bilateral theca-lutein cysts. Ovarian hyper-stimulation syndrome	Cysts disappeared with progression of pregnancy

Mucinous cyst-adenomas (Fig. 20–16) are rare in pregnancy and are usually unilateral. They can assume large sizes and if ruptured can cause pseudomyoxoma peritonii, which can sonographically mimic ascites. Besides the septations, they can occasionally contain some solid elements.

Theca lutein cysts, though seen in normal pregnancy, are most commonly associated with either trophoblastic disease of pregnancy (30%) or ovarian hyperstimulation syndrome (20%–40%). They are often bilateral and can assume gigantic sizes (Fig. 20–17). Clinically such cysts must be recognized and their surgical removal avoided. When associated with trophoblastic disease, they regress spontaneously within several weeks following the evacuation of the

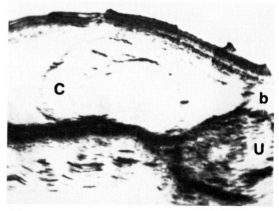

FIG. 20-16. Large mucinous cyst-adenoma and 8 weeks' pregnant uterus. Note septations within cyst. A small focus of early carcinoma was found histologically within the cyst; b, bladder; c, multiloculated cyst; u, uterus.

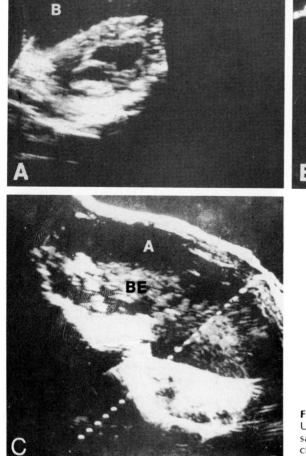

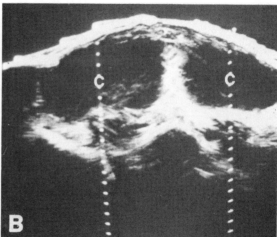

FIG. 20-17. Ovarian hyperstimulation syndrome. **A.** Uterus at 7 weeks' gestation showing two gestational sacs. **B.** Bilateral large theca-lutein cysts. **C.** Massive ascitic fluid; B, bladder; BE, bowel echoes; C, cysts; S, gestational sacs.

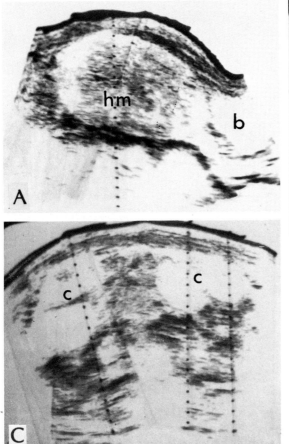

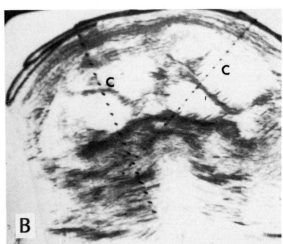

FIG. 20-18. Bilateral theca-lutein cysts in a molar pregnancy with regression following evacuation of the mole. **A.** A 15 weeks' size uterus containing the hydatidiform mole. **B.** Bilateral theca-lutein cysts prior to evacuation of the mole. **C.** Same cysts 2 weeks following evaucation; b, bladder; c, cysts; hm, hydatidiform mole.

hydatidiform mole (Fig. 20–18). The misdiagnosed case in Table 20–2 had a hydatidiform mole with theca lutein cysts. She was erroneously diagnosed by sonogram as having a missed abortion with uterine myomas, but this patient had the procedure performed with the old bistable technique; with improved instrumentation today, this kind of error should not occur.

The theca lutein cysts secondary to ovarian hyperstimulation syndrome are often associated with ascites (Fig. 20–17). The author encountered two such cases in his series (Table 20–6), one of whom developed massive hemorrhage within the cyst. These cysts also regress with progression of the pregnancy. The author recommends a diagnostic sonogram in all cases of ovarian hyperstimulation syndrome following induction of ovulation to detect the theca lutein cysts and the existence of multifetal gestations, which are often associated with this condition. It has been recommended (7) that all patients carrying three or more fetuses be kept on complete bed rest as soon as the diagnosis of multiple gestation is made.

COMPLEX MASSES

These ovarian masses contain variable echos but have no unique sonographic pattern. Dermoid cysts are the most common in this group (Table 20–5), and though these may show distinct areas of sonolucency within the cyst typical of a dermoid (5) (Fig. 20–19), we have at times seen dermoids with the most bizarre sonographic patterns. As previously mentioned, myomas with marked degeneration can also mimic complex ovarian tumors.

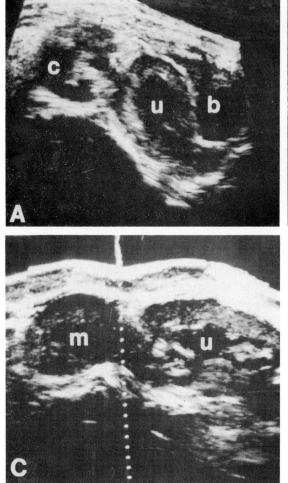
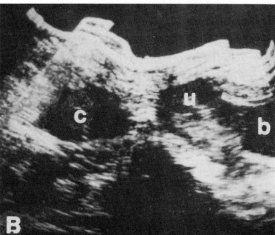

FIG. 20-19. Dermoid cyst adherent to fundus of 10 weeks' pregnant uterus. **B.** Same cyst separated from uterine fundus by pressure. **C.** Fundal myoma inseparable from uterine fundus by pressure; b, bladder; c, dermoid cyst; m, myoma; u, pregnant uterus.

SOLID MASSES

These masses, similar to solid myomas, are acoustically homogeneous, and their posterior wall is poorly visualized. In the author's series an ovarian mass in the posterior cul-de-sac was incorrectly diagnosed as a uterine myoma (Table 20–2).

In distinguishing uterine from adnexal masses, we have found it helpful in certain cases to apply pressure in the area of contact between the mass and the uterus in an effort to separate the two (Fig. 20–19). If the mass can be separated from the uterus, it is most likely extra-uterine. Obviously a pedunculated myoma cannot be ruled out with this maneuver.

Mixed and solid ovarian tumors associated with pregnancy are of great concern to the obstetrician because of fear of malignancy and possible torsion, hemorrhage, and/or rupture. The incidence of malignancy in ovarian tumors associated with pregnancy is approximately 2.5%–5% (3). In our series we encountered only one such case (incidence 2%) in which a small focus of carcinoma was found in the wall of a large 10×30 cm mucinous cyst-adenoma in a 17-year-old primigravida (Table 20–5).

Our approach regarding the management of patients with ovarian cysts in pregnancy is as follows:

1. If the ovarian mass is found in the first trimester and appears unequivocally cystic, we

recommend close clinical and sonographic follow-up. Corpus luteum cysts disappear in the second trimester.

2. If the ovarian mass is found to be either mixed or solid, or if a simple large cyst persists in the second trimester, surgical removal of the mass is recommended. The timing of the surgical procedure is left to the referring physician.

OTHER MASSES ASSOCIATED WITH PREGNANCY

Several rare but interesting conditions must also be considered in the differential diagnosis of pelvic masses in pregnancy, as follows:

1. Uterine wall hematomas. These must be considered any time a patient is found to have a pelvic mass following termination of pregnancy either by suction curettage or by amniocentesis. These hematomas are sonographically inseparable from the uterine wall and often contain variable echos, especially if clotting has occurred within them (Fig. 20–20). Since the liberalization of the abortion laws we have encountered four cases of broad ligament hematomas and correctly diagnosed three of them (Table 20–2).

2. Abdominal wall hematomas. These are cystic and echo free unless clotting has occurred within them. This diagnosis is made by ob-

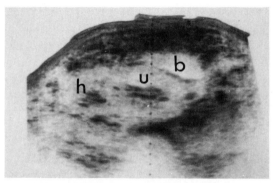

FIG. 20-20. Right uterine wall hematoma in an empty uterus following suction curettage; b, bladder; h, hematoma; u, uterus.

serving the mass above the peritoneal lining. Occasionally a well-encapsulated subserous myoma can be confused with an abdominal wall hematoma (Fig. 20–21).

3. Bicornuate uteri. These are very difficult to differentiate from a uterine myoma. We encountered two such cases (Table 20–2). Obtaining an accurate history from the patients helped in the diagnosis.

4. Inflammatory masses. These must be considered if the patient's history is suggestive of it. Acute pelvic inflammatory disease is extremely rare in pregnancy, and we did not encounter any such cases in our series. However we correctly diagnosed an appendiceal abcess in a patient at 16 weeks' gestation by consid-

FIG. 20-21. A. Abdominal wall hematoma at 28 weeks' gestation with a breech presentation. Note hematoma exterior to the linear peritoneal lining. **B.** Subserous myoma at 36 weeks' gestation. Note curved capsule of myoma continuous with myometrial wall; b, bladder; h, hematoma; FH, fetal head; M, myoma.

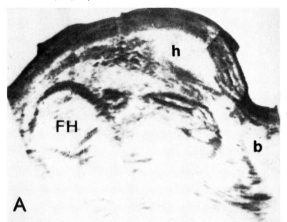

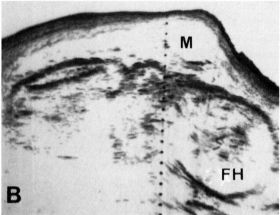

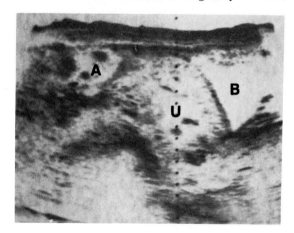

FIG. 20-22. Appendiceal abscess at 12 weeks' gestation. Note the irregularly shaped abscess with bright and thick posterior wall surrounding bright bowel echoes; A, abscess; B, bladder; U, uterus.

ering the sonographic findings (Fig. 20–22) in conjunction with her clinical symptoms (which may be misleading in pregnancy). The patient was successfully operated upon.

CONCLUSION

The rate of accuracy of ultrasound in the diagnosis of pelvic masses associated with pregnancy is better than 95%. Sonography is useful in the following: 1) confirming the presence of a pelvic mass, 2) detecting a hitherto unsuspected pelvic mass, 3) following the progress of a pelvic mass, 4) differentiating myomas from adnexal masses, and 5) solving difficult clinical situations encountered in patients being evaluated for procedures such as therapeutic abortions and amniocentesis.

REFERENCES

1. ACOG Newsletter, July 2, 1975
2. ATIENZA MF, BURKMAN RT, WIGHT DJ, KING TM: Ultrasonography in the management of induced abortion. In Sanders RC, James AE (eds): Ultrasonography in Obstetrics and Gynecology. New York, Appleton-Century-Crofts, 1977, pp 123–133
3. BARBER HR: Diagnosing and managing the unilateral mass. Contemp Obstet Gynecol 7:99, 1976
4. CARLSEN EN: Gray-scale ultrasound. J Clin Ultrasound 1:190, 1973
5. COCHRANE WJ: Ultrasonics in obstetrics and gynecology. Br J Radiol 40:604–611, 1967
6. HASSANI N: Ultrasonic appearance of pedunculated uterine fibroids and ovarian cysts. J Natl Med Assoc 66:432, 1974
7. JEWELEWICZ R, VANDE WEILE RL: Management of multifetal gestation. Contemp Obstet Gynecol 6:59, 1975
8. KOBAYASHI M: Illustrated Manual of Ultrasonography in Obstetrics and Gynecology. Philadelphia, JB Lippincott, 1974
9. QUEENAN JT, KUBARYCH SF, DOUGLAS DL: Evaluation of diagnostic ultrasound in gynecology. Am J Obstet Gynecol 123:453–65, 1975
10. SABBAGHA RE(ed): Ultrasound in obstetrics. Clin Obstet Gynecol 20:229, 1977
11. SAMPLE F: Pelvic inflammatory disease. In Sanders RC, James AE (eds): Ultrasonography in Obstetrics and Gynecology. New York, Appleton-Century-Crofts, 1977, pp 357–385
12. THOMPSON HE, TAYLOR ES, HOLMES JH et al: Ultrasound diagnostic techniques in obstetrics and gynecology. Am J Obstet Gynecol 90:472, 1964

21

Ectopic pregnancy

ALAN V. CADKIN, ALEX A. BEZJIAN,
RUDY E. SABBAGHA

The early recognition of ectopic pregnancy prior to the stage of rupture is a challenging diagnostic problem for the obstetrician. The use of ultrasound in women suspected of having an ectopic pregnancy is mandatory because differentiation between intrauterine and ectopic implantation is possible in the majority.

Clinically the patient with an unruptured ectopic pregnancy usually presents with amenorrhea, nausea, breast tenderness, vaginal bleeding, and/or lower abdominal pain. In many gravidas a history of previous ectopic pregnancy, pelvic inflammatory disease, tubal surgery, or use of an intrauterine device (IUD) may be elicited—data that may alert the physician to the possibility of ectopic gestation.

The diagnosis of ectopic pregnancy cannot be definitively made by physical findings such as vaginal bleeding, abdominal tenderness, and an adnexal mass. Further, laboratory tests used for detection of urinary chorionic gonadotropins (HCG) are positive in only 30–40% of gravidas with ectopic pregnancies. However, beta subunit HCG assays are almost always positive; although this indicates the presence of a pregnancy, the distinction between intrauterine and extrauterine implantation is not possible.

On the other hand sonography is particularly useful in differentiating normal from ectopic pregnancy especially in the presence of other physical findings, including the following: 1) uterine myomas, 2) retroverted uterus, 3) uterine anomalies, and 4) adnexal mass.

The diagnosis of a normal intrauterine pregnancy by ultrasound will spare the mother and fetus possible hazards pertaining to anesthesia and surgery. In addition, it will direct the physician to search for other possible intraabdominal pathology, including appendicitis, twisted adnexal tumor, pelvic infectious process, and ureterolithiasis—all of which may mimic ectopic pregnancy.

In the study of gravidas with suspected ectopic pregnancy the sonographer should consider unusual ectopic locations such as cornual implantations because their sonographic appearance may be similar to that of normal pregnancy. In these patients the clinical findings should not be ignored (1). By contrast, abdominal pregnancies, though rare, can be readily diagnosed by ultrasound. Additionally, in gravidas seeking pregnancy termination and from whom only decidual tissue is obtained by suction curettage, the use of diagnostic ultrasound may indicate whether the pregnancy is intrauterine or ectopic.

Bezjian followed the outcome of 102 women who were referred to ultrasound because of the possibility of ectopic pregnancy. In 73 patients (71.6%) the diagnosis of ectopic pregnancy was ruled out by ultrasound and the underlying pathology or absence of it was clarified, Table 21–1. In 29 women (28.4%) ectopic pregnancy could not be ruled out, and of these only 14 patients had an ectopic gestation. The pathology in the remaining 15 women is shown in the follow-

TABLE 21-1. DIAGNOSIS OF PATIENTS REFERRED FOR ULTRASOUND TO "RULE-OUT" ECTOPIC PREGNANCY (TOTAL 102)

Ultrasound diagnosis	No. of cases	Correct diagnosis
Ectopic	16	10
Cannot rule out ectopic	13	4†
Intrauterine pregnancy	12	12
IUP with cyst	17	17
IUP with myoma	1	1
IUP with inflammatory mass	1*	0*
Tuboovarian abscess	15	12‡
Cyst	10	10
Missed abortion	7	6
Retained POC with myoma	1	1
Normal findings	9	9

* Patient had an ectopic pregnancy.
† Four patients had ectopic pregnancies.
‡ Three patients with incorrect diagnosis all had simple ovarian cysts.

ing lists. In 1 patient the diagnosis of ectopic pregnancy was missed—a false-negative rate of 0.98%.

Patients with ectopic pregnancy:

Ultrasound consistent with ectopic pregnancy	10
Ultrasound cannot rule out ectopic pregnancy	4
IUP with inflammatory mass (missed diagnosis)	1

Clinical findings in patients who had an ultrasound that was consistent with ectopic pregnancy (total, 16):

Ectopic pregnancy	10
Tuboovarian abscess	2
Normal findings	2
Well-differentiated carcinoma of ovary	1
Fibroid uterus	1

Clinical findings in patients who had an ultrasound that could not "rule out" ectopic pregnancy:

Ectopic	4
Tuboovarian abscess	2
Corpus luteum cyst	2
Normal findings	2
Bicornate uterus with IUP	2
Dermoid cyst	1

UTERINE FINDINGS

In ectopic pregnancy the uterus may be normal to slightly enlarged. The internal echo pattern may consist of weak echoes, scattered strong and weak echoes, or a central thick linear band of echoes of moderate strength that represents decidual reaction, Figure 21–1. The presence of a positive pregnancy test without ultrasonic evidence of intrauterine pregnancy or extrauterine findings may be seen in the following conditions:

1. Ectopic pregnancy.
2. An early intrauterine pregnancy prior to the depiction of the gestational sac (less than 5 weeks).
3. Abnormal pregnancy such as blighted ovum or recent spontaneous abortion.

The demonstration of a normal centrally located or slightly eccentric intrauterine pregnancy virtually excludes an ectopic pregnancy except in the rare circumstance when an ectopic and intrauterine pregnancy coexist.

A pregnancy that appears normal but is not centrally located within the uterus may be seen in association with the following conditions:

1. An overdistended bladder.
2. Uterine myomas.
3. Bicornuate uterus.
4. Cornual pregnancy.
5. Ectopic pregnancy (discussed further under Ectopic Gestational Sac).

We have seen several cases where intrauterine blood clots presented as a small echo-free space in the center of the uterus surrounded by strong marginal echoes. This simulated a blighted ovum or early normal pregnancy, when in fact, the patient had an ectopic pregnancy (1).

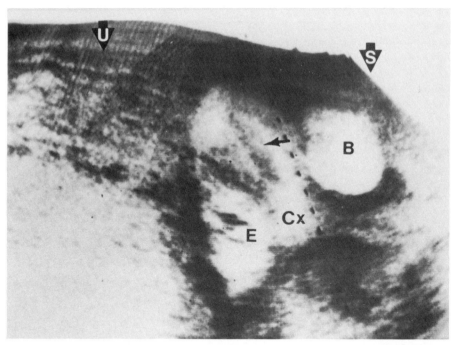

FIG. 21-1. Ruptured ectopic pregnancy in a patient who had 7½ weeks of amenorrhea with spotting for 1 week and diffuse abdominal pain. HCG level was positive. Longitudinal scan shows an enlarged uterus containing a thick central linear collection of moderate-strength echoes (**arrow**), which represents decidual reaction.There is a 6- × 3-cm complex mass (E) just posterior to the uterus that contains a few strong internal echoes. The strong echoes in the mass are due to interfaces within the clotted blood and are not fetal echoes; Cx, cervix; S, symphysis; U, umbilicus; B, bladder. (Cadkin AV, Motew M: Clinical Atlas of Gray-Scale Ultrasonography in Obstetrics. Courtesy of Charles C Thomas, Springfield, IL, 1979)

EXTRAUTERINE FINDINGS

ECTOPIC GESTATIONAL SAC

The demonstration of an intact ectopic gestational sac is difficult. However, since the advent of gray-scale ultrasound and with the use of a 3.5-MHz focused transducer it may be possible to depict the ectopic gestational sac and thus establish a positive diagnosis of ectopic pregnancy (4). Nonetheless, meticulous scanning technique is required to demonstrate the sac and to permit optimal differentiation of intrauterine from extrauterine pregnancy, Figure 21-2. Transverse scans angled perpendicular to the long axis of the uterus are often helpful. The sonographer should try to demonstrate the trophoblastic shell of dense echoes characteristic of the gestational sac outside the uterus, Figures 21-2 and 21-3. The demonstration of a live fetus or definite fetal

echoes within the sac is helpful in differentiating an ectopic pregnancy from a hemorrhagic cyst, abscess, or dermoid.

When trying to demonstrate whether a pregnancy is intrauterine or extrauterine, the sonographer should try to demonstrate uterine musculature surrounding the gestational sac. On rare occasion an intact ectopic sac may have a pseudointrauterine appearance (2); this may be due to hypertrophy of the musculature of the fallopian tube around the sac or to the echo pattern of an organized hematoma surrounding the sac simulating uterine echoes, Figure 21-4. In these cases, *careful analysis of the scan findings* is mandatory.

An ectopic sac may not be seen because of its small size, because it is obscured by overlying bowel or incorporated into a hemorrhagic mass, or because there has been a tubal abortion.

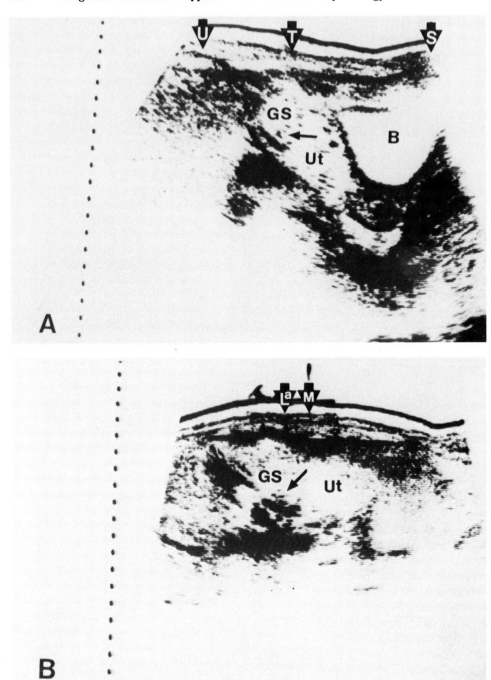

FIG. 21-2. Intact ectopic gestational sac in a patient who had 7 weeks of amenorrhea, a positive pregnancy test, and a possible right adnexal mass. **A.** Longitudinal scan shows a slightly enlarged uterus (Ut) with an intact gestational sac (GS) just superior to the uterine fundus. Notice the small fetal echo within the sac (**arrow**). **B.** Transverse scan at T shows a poorly defined gestational sac (GS) containing a small fetal echo (**arrow**) just to the right of the uterine fundus (Ut). The relatively echo-free appearance of the uterus is technical and with current gray-scale equipment, the sonographic detection of the ectopic sac is easier; S, symphysis; U, umbilicus; B, bladder; T, point at which transverse scan is obtained.

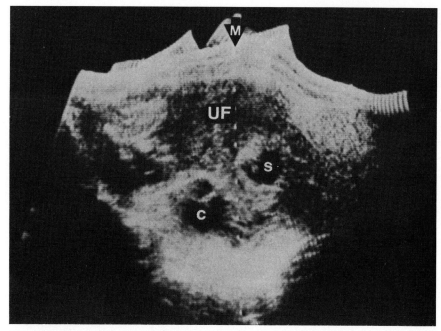

FIG. 21-3. Ruptured left ectopic pregnancy in a patient who had 9 weeks of amenorrhea, abdominal pain, and a pelvic mass. Transverse scan through the pelvis shows a cross section of the enlarged uterine fundus (UF). There is an intact sac (s) containing a small fetal echo in the left adnexal area outside the uterus. Note the collection of strong echoes outlining the sac owing to trophoblastic tissue. There is a small complex cystic mass (c) just posterior to the uterus due to blood clots. At surgery, there was an intact sac in the left tube and blood clots in the cul-de-sac. (Cadkin AV, Motew M: Clinical Atlas of Gray-Scale Ultrasonography in Obstetrics. Courtesy of Charles C Thomas, Springfield, IL, 1979)

EXTRAUTERINE MASS

When an ectopic pregnancy ruptures, a complex mass due to blood clots or an admixture of blood clots and products of conception usually forms. The outline of the mass is usually irregular and the internal echo pattern is complex (weak or strong echoes coupled with cystic areas), Figure 21-1 and 21-3. The mass may be located adjacent to the uterine fundus or in the cul-de-sac. In the presence of a "chronic ruptured ectopic" the uterus may be incorporated into the mass and may not be identifiable as a separate structure, Figure 21-5 (5). The sonographic differential diagnosis includes primarily pelvic inflammatory disease and endometriosis, see Chapter 22.

HEMOPERITONEUM

When there is intraperitoneal hemorrhage, blood may appear as a crescentic echo-free area in the cul-de-sac, Figure 21-6. This finding indicates the presence of free fluid and may also be seen with a ruptured cyst, minimal ascites, or pus. If bleeding is massive, an ascites-like picture may be seen (3).

ABDOMINAL PREGNANCY

A rare type of pregnancy is an abdominal pregnancy. Demonstration of fetal or placental echoes or both outside the uterus is daignostic. The placenta is usually mixed with bowel echoes and there is no well-defined amniotic space or chorionic plate, Figure 21-7. The fetal head must be at least 2 cm before it can be seen outside the uterus (3).

The figures in this chapter are reproduced from: Cadkin, AV and Motew, M, *Clinical Atlas of*

(*Text continues on p. 257*)

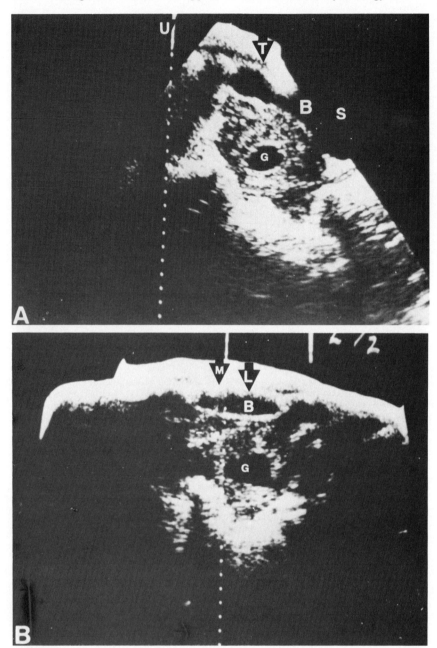

FIG. 21-4. Ruptured ectopic pregnancy with pseudointrauterine appearance. Pregnancy test was positive at 7 weeks of amenorrhea. **A.** Longitudinal scan at L shows a gestational sac (G) that appears to be in the uterus. There is irregularity of the uterine contour. **B.** Transverse scan at T shows the gestational sac (G) and a small uterine outline in cross section to the right. The ultrasonic diagnosis was an intrauterine pregnancy probably in the left horn of a bicornuate uterus. At surgery, there was a ruptured ectopic pregnancy in the isthmus of the left tube, and the sac was surrounded by organized hematoma. The uterus was anterior and just to the right of the midline; S, symphysis; U, umbilicus; B, bladder; T, point at which transverse scan is obtained; L, point at which longitudinal scan is obtained. (Cadkin AV, Motew M: Clinical Atlas of Gray-Scale Ultrasonography in Obstetrics. Courtesy of Charles C Thomas, Springfield, IL, 1979)

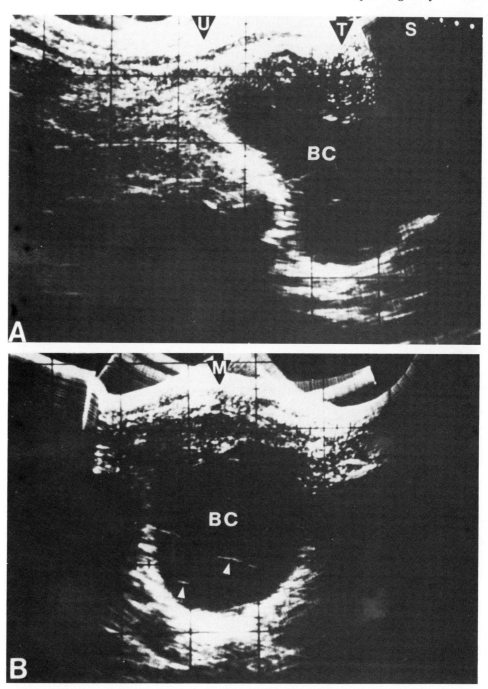

FIG. 21–5. Chronic ruptured ectopic pregnancy in a patient who had a normal period 10 weeks prior to this scan. At 6 weeks of amenorrhea, the patient had heavy vaginal bleeding and was diagnosed clinically as a complete abortion. She presented at the time of this scan with lower abdominal pain for 3 weeks, a large pelvic mass, and tenderness in the right lower quadrant. An IVP showed a large pelvic mass compressing the ureters with bilateral hydronephrosis. Longitudinal scan (A) and transverse scan (B) show a large predominantly cystic pelvic mass (BC) that contains a few small, weak internal echoes (**arrowheads**). The urinary bladder is empty and the uterus cannot be identified. At survey, there were organized blood clots filling the entire pelvis secondary to a ruptured tubal pregnancy; S, symphysis; U, umbilicus; T, point at which transverse scan is obtained.

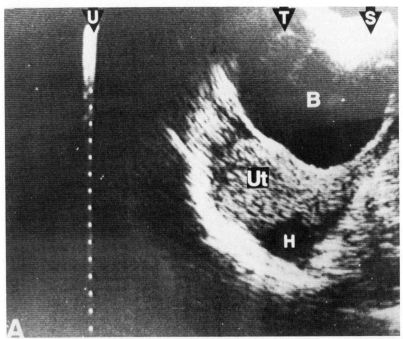

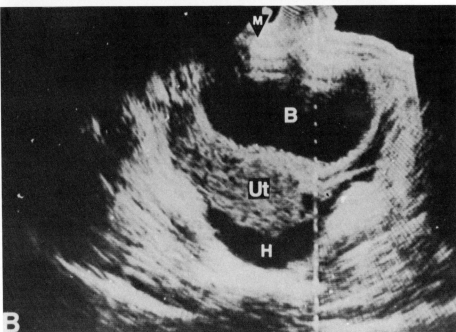

FIG. 21–6. Hemoperitoneum in a patient who had 13 weeks of amenorrhea with spotting for 2 weeks and a positive pregnancy test. **A.** Longitudinal midline scan shows a slightly enlarged uterus (Ut). There is no evidence of an intrauterine pregnancy. Just posterior to the uterus is a small collection of fluid due to hemorrhage (H) in the cul-de-sac. **B.** Transverse scan at T shows a cross section of the uterine fundus (Ut) and the crescentic echo-free area (H) due to blood in the cul-de-sac; U, umbilicus; T, point at which transverse scan is obtained; S, symphysis; B, bladder. (Cadkin AV, Motew M: Clinical Atlas of Gray-Scale Ultrasonography in Obstetrics. Courtesy of Charles C Thomas, Springfield, IL, 1979).

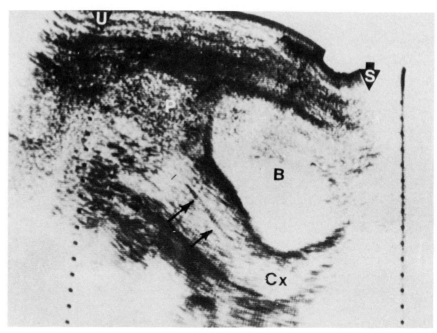

FIG. 21-7. Abdominal pregnancy in a patient who had a 15-week-size uterus on clinical examination and no products of conception were found by dilatation and curettage. Longitudinal scan shows a uterus of normal size containing a thin central linear echo (**arrows**). Adjacent to the uterine fundus is a collection of strong echoes (P) with a texture and echo density similar to placental tissue. At surgery, this was confirmed to represent placenta and there was a mummified fetus, 7.5 cm in crown-rump length (not seen on the ultrasound scan); Cx, cervix; U, umbilicus; B, bladder. (Cadkin AV, Motew M: Clinical Atlas of Gray-Scale Ultrasonography in Obstetrics. Courtesy of Charles C Thomas, Springfield, IL, 1979).

Gray-Scale Ultrasonography in Obstetrics. Courtesy of Charles C Thomas, Publisher, Springfield, Illinois, 1979.

REFERENCES

1. CADKIN A, MOTEW M: Clinical Atlas of Gray Scale Ultrasonography in Obstetrics. Springfield, IL, CC Thomas, 1979

2. CONRAD MR, JOHNSON J, JAMES AE: Sonography in ectopic pregnancy. In Sanders RC, James AE (eds): Ultrasonography in Obstetrics and Gynecology. New York, Appleton-Century-Crofts, 1977, p 113

3. KOBAYASHI M: Illustrated Manual of Ultrasonography in Obstetrics and Gynecology. Philadelphia, JB Lippincott, 1974

4. MAKLAD NF, WRIGHT CH: Gray-scale ultrasonography in the diagnosis of ectopic pregnancy. Radiology 126:221, 1978

5. ROGERS WF, SCHAUB M, WILSON R: Chronic ectopic pregnancy: ultrasonic diagnosis. J Clin Ultrasound 5:257, 1977

22

Ultrasound in gynecology

JAMES D. BOWIE

This chapter, a review of the applications of ultrasound to gynecology, is divided into two parts. The first deals with indications, technique, normal anatomy, and basic interpretation. The second covers the sonographic appearances of the more important diseases and their differential diagnoses.

INDICATIONS, TECHNIQUE, NORMAL ANATOMY, AND BASIC INTERPRETATION

INDICATIONS

Specific lists of indications are available for gynecologic sonography (4). Generally, conflicting or equivocal results from the history, physical examination, or laboratory test are indications of the need for sonography. In planning further evaluation or a specific surgical procedure, sonography provides information about the size, extent, and anatomic relationships of tumors and diseased and normal pelvic organs. This examination provides an objective way to follow a disease when therapeutic response may not be obvious, when several physicians may be involved in the patient's care, or when return visits to the physician are infrequent. When the patient or others may hold contrary opinions, a positive sonogram is objective evidence of disease. To go beyond these general indications to more specific ones requires an understanding of the diagnostic potential of the sonogram, which

is in part the subject of the remainder of this chapter.

TECHNIQUE
PRINCIPLES OF EXAMINATION

Each gynecologic sonogram requires three steps as follows: 1) formulate the problem, 2) do the study, and 3) make a diagnosis. Each step is limited by the previous one. In our laboratory, examinations consist of these two parts: a survey portion, which is essentially the same for every patient, and a special portion, which is unique for each patient.

SURVEY SECTIONS

The bladder should usually be maximally distended for an adequate sonographic study. Complete filling of the bladder may not be possible when a large pelvic mass is present, and the combination of an incompletely filled bladder and a large mass often makes it difficult to identify the uterus. Occasionally a very distended bladder causes diagnostic error. This occurs when the bladder displaces an ovarian mass to an unusual position or distorts the uterus, making the distinction between an intrauterine or a uterine wall abnormality difficult.

After the patient's bladder is distended, a series of parallel longitudinal sections and two series of parallel transverse sections cover the entire pelvis at 1-cm intervals to produce the survey. One of the sets of transverse sections is angled cephalad to be perpendicular to the usual position of the uterus; the other is angled caudad to be perpendicular to the vagina (2). The image format is chosen to use as much as possible of the scanconverter or digital matrix and still display the area of interest. Generally the 2–1 or 3–1 scales are used. The time gain compensation (TGC), or slope, should include the entire pelvic soft tissues. The equipment settings often need to be set to give appropriate amplification of superficial structures when the bladder is not interposed and reset, to prevent overamplification of structures posterior to the bladder. Transducers are selected from a variety of frequencies (2.25, 3.5, and 5 MHz) with different focal zones to provide optimal resolution and penetration. A 3.5-MHz, 19-mm face, long-focal-length transducer has proved useful for general purposes. Good scanning technique should fit the situation: small objects, structures with parallel sides, and internal textures are best appreciated with a linear, single-pass scan technique, structures with irregular outlines or interfaces between objects are often better shown by a modified compounding technique. The principles of good scanning technique follow:

1. Set the scan plane perpendicular to the surface of structures to be scanned.
2. Use at least two complete sets of parallel sections at right angles to each other.
3. Demonstrate all lines of closure and separation.
4. Avoid artifacts or direct them away from important structures.
5. Account mentally for every structure seen.

SPECIAL SECTIONS

Planning special sections requires experience and skill. Most frequently operators choose a unique oblique-scan plane to show the relationships of an abnormality to normal anatomy, or they use higher frequency transducers, lower gain settings, or higher gain settings to demonstrate the internal detail or transmission properties of an abnormality. Usually this part of the

examination requires an alteration of conditions related to the patient, equipment, or technique (see list that follows).

Conditions That Can Be Altered for Special Section

1. Patient parameters
   a. Preparation (bladder distention, cathartics, etc)
   b. Position (decubitus, Trendelenburg, upright, etc)
   c. Activities (breath holding, coughing, etc)
2. Equipment parameters
   a. Instrument (B-scan, real time)
   b. Mode (A-mode, B-mode, M-mode)
   c. Transducer
   d. Time gain compensation, gain, output
   e. Scan converter postprocessing
   f. Field size and magnification
3. Technique parameters
   a. Scan planes, intervals
   b. Transducer movement
   c. Pressure to displace objects

NORMAL ANATOMY

BLADDER

The bladder is limited anteriorly by the abdominal wall, laterally by the sides of the pelvis, posteriorly by the uterus and bowel, caudad by the symphysis or superior public ramus, and cephalad by bowel. When the bladder is distended, it assumes the shape permitted by surrounding structures. When it is not distended and the patient is supine, its most cephalad portion is posterior. Because of the ease with which this organ is distorted, lateral and posterior protuberances are found, which may appear separate from the bladder in some scanning planes. These should not be mistaken for cysts, and oblique scans will show their connection with the bladder.

UTERUS AND VAGINA

The uterus lies immediately posterior to the bladder and may be tilted anteriorly, posteriorly, or to either side. The size and shape of the normal uterus varies throughout life and from woman to woman. In the infantile uterus the cervix may be twice the diameter of the corpus and represent about two-thirds the total length of the uterus. The infantile uterus ranges from 2.0 to 3.3 cm in length and 0.5 to 1.0 cm in anteroposterior (AP) diameter (22) (Fig. 22–1). After puberty the total size of the uterus and the ratio of corpus to cervix increase until the diameter of the corpus is about twice that of the cervix. During the child-bearing years the size of the normal uterus varies greatly. Sample's in vivo measurements correspond to those made of resected specimens from nulliparous patients, indicating the length to range from 7.5 to 8.1 cm, the AP diameter from 1.8 to 2.0 cm, and the width from 2.4 to 5.0 cm (10, 23). The multiparous uterus measured about 1.2 cm more in each dimension. With occasional exceptions a uterus longer than 9.5 cm is abnormally enlarged. After menopause the uterus may become as small as in infancy (16), but this involution is variable.

In the sonogram the uterus is filled with moderate-intensity echoes of medium texture, which originate in the myometrium (Fig. 22–2). These echoes become more intense and numerous during early pregnancy and some ectopic pregnancies. A dark line, usually seen centrally within the uterus, is sometimes referred to as the "endometrial line" or as "endometrial echoes," though this line is more likely produced by a reflection from the interface between the endometrium and the secretions within the endometrial cavity and glands. A zone of slightly less intense echoes may be seen between this line and the myometrial echoes. It is unclear what this zone represents, but it may be in part the deeper layers of the endometrium.

The vagina has a characteristic appearance in both longitudinal and transverse scans (Figs. 22–2 and 22–3). There is a zone of low-intensity echoes surrounding a single—in a few cases double—thin stripe of more intense echoes. The low-intensity echo zone, which corresponds to the muscular and erectile tissue of the vagina, blends with the uterine wall, and the central stripe may be continuous with the endocervix. After a complete hysterectomy the upper end of the vagina has a characteristic tapered appearance.

FALLOPIAN TUBES, ADNEXA, AND OVARIES

The fallopian tubes and adnexa extend laterally from the cornua of the uterus, initially lying along the posterior surface of the bladder. The fallopian tube is divided into a short interstitial portion in the uterine cornua; an isthmic portion, 2–3 cm long, distal to the uterine cornua; and an ampullary portion, 5–8 cm long. The isthmic portion is most often seen in the normal patient, and when the ampullary portion is dilated, it may be seen along the lateral and posterior pelvis. The broad ligament and other supportive structures have not been distinguished as separate structures.

In the nulliparous the ovaries are usually in the ovarian fossa, which lies posterior to the psoas muscle and the external iliac vessels and anterior to the piriformis muscle (23). At the time of ovulation the uteroovarian ligament is shortened and the ovary is seen nearer the uterus. In some women, the ovary may be fixed in this position and in contact with the uterus presumably as a result of an abnormality of the uteroovarian ligament (6). The ovarian volume determined by ultrasound is 0–0.7 cm^2 for 1–2 years, 0.13–0.9 cm^2 for 2–12 years, and 1.8–5.7 cm^2 for 13–20 years (23). The normal ovary is approximately $1 \times 2 \times 3$ cm, or about one-fourth to one-third of the normal uterine diameter; if it exceeds one-half the uterine diameter, it is porbably enlarged (28). These sonographic measurements are slightly smaller than those obtained from resected specimens. Size as measured by sonography varies during the menstrual cycle, reaching normal maximums at ovulation and in the premenstrual phase (1). After menopause the ovaries atrophy and become smaller.

COLON AND RECTUM

The appearance of the rectum varies, but usually there is some gas present, which produces strong echoes and an acoustic shadow. Fecal material or retained enemas in the rectum may simulate a pelvic mass. Reexamination after a cathartic may be required if the location of the mass or evidence of anteriorly placed gas suggests this

(*Text continues on p. 264*)

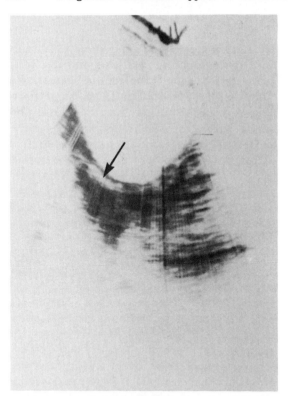

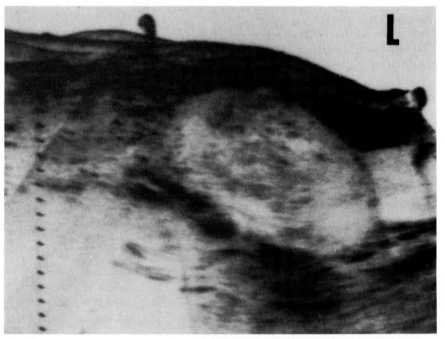

FIG. 22-1. Longitudinal section of an infantile uterus **(arrow).** The corpus is small in relation to the cervix, which represents most of the volume of the infantile uterus.

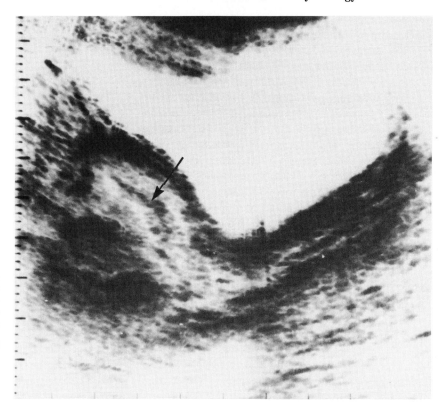

FIG. 22–2. Longitudinal section of the normal adult uterus. A central line of echoes **(arrow)** identifies the endometrial cavity. This is surrounded by a zone of low-intensity echoes, which is surrounded by moderate-intensity echoes. The parallel lines of low intensity echoes separated by a dark line represent the vagina, which is continuous with the uterus.

FIG. 22–3. Transverse section of the normal vagina. Usually a single central line of echoes is seen.

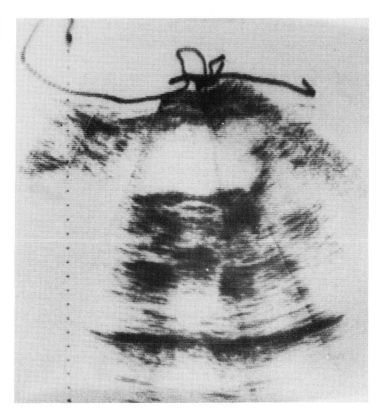

possibility. A water enema is useful in identifying the rectum and localizing the cul-de-sac (21). The rectosigmoid can sometimes be identified as an acoustic shadow between the uterus and ovary (22) (Fig. 22–4). A loop of sigmoid is often seen superior and anterior to the uterine fundus on longitudinal scans. The distended bladder displaces the remainder of the bowel from the true pelvis, but occasionally portions of small bowel or colon remain, often because of previous surgery, and give a false appearance of a pelvic mass. When the examiner cannot define all the borders of a mass or the mass changes shape, this problem should be suspected. If additional filling of the bladder or repeating the examination does not help, it may be necessary to perform additional studies, for example, computed tomography of the pelvis with dilute oral contrast material in the small bowel.

PELVIC MUSCLES

The iliopsoas, piriformis, and internal obturator muscles are important landmarks. These muscles usually produce weak echoes except for the strong central zone of echoes seen in the iliopsoas. The lower margin of this muscle defines the usual location of the ovaries (Fig. 22–4), which are anterior to the piriformis at the same level and best seen in a transverse scan with cephalic angulation. The external iliac artery, vein, and lymph nodes are located medial to the iliopsoas. These structures are not frequently seen, and a mass in this region is usually the result of lymph node enlargement (Fig. 22–5). The internal iliac artery, vein, and sciatic nerve lie posterior to the ovary and anterior to the piriformis muscle. One of these structures may be shown to branch on longitudinal sections (23). The ureter is at about the same level as these structures but slightly more medial and anterior. The internal obturator and levator ani muscles, which are better seen when the transverse sections are angled caudad (Fig. 22–6), help to define the limits of the pelvis. The sacrum and iliac wings are usually seen, and the iliacus muscle can be shown anterior to the ilium. In scans of poor quality the acoustic shadow of the iliac wing is sometimes mistaken for a mass. Visualization of structures posterior to the anterior surface of the sacrum can also be misleading.

BASIC INTERPRETATION

The ultrasonographer should develop a systematic way of approaching each case. One approach is to begin by identifying the bladder and uterus in each section. This is an important step, and failure to accomplish successfully it often leads to error. Next, identify as much as possible of the normal anatomy, ovaries, adnexa, bowel, and muscle groups. If an abnormality seems to be present, try to decide whether the abnormality is within the uterine cavity, a part of the uterus, or outside the uterus. If special sections seem to be required for this decision but have not been done, the patient should be restudied before an opinion is given.

After the anatomic relationships have been decided, each abnormality should be classified by its ultrasound characteristics. Generally, four characteristics are looked for as follows: outline, substructure, texture, and sound transmission properties. Each category may be subdivided. For example, outline includes shape, distinctness of margin, width of margin, and others. Substructure refers to recognizable structures within a mass, such as septa, blood vessels, calcifications, and collections of fluid. Texture refers to the background echoes, other than artifacts, that fill in an area, which have no known specific anatomic correlate. Sound transmission is judged in comparison to adjacent normal structures (often the bladder and uterus) and by a subjective familiarity with certain combinations of transducers and settings on each machine.

Finally, secondary or additional findings are evaluated. These include the apparent mobility of a mass, its effects on adjacent structures, and the presence of additional abnormalities such as ascites, uterine enlargement, and fluid in the cul-de-sac. When all these steps have been taken, the disease process may often be easily recognized, but in some cases the solution is not apparent. In these cases a single diagnosis cannot be made, but a list of diagnositc possibilities with some estimate of their relative probabilities can be offered.

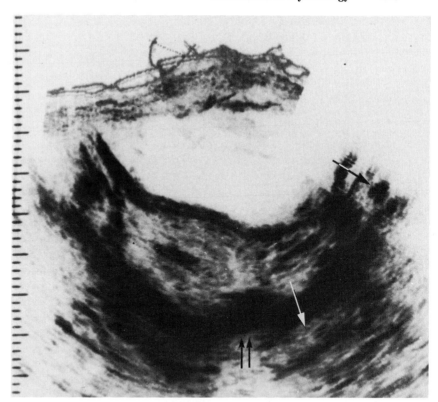

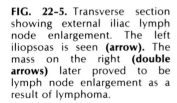

FIG. 22-4. Transverse section of the normal uterus. The iliopsoas and piriformis muscles are seen on the left **(arrows).** A dark group of echoes **(double arrows)** and an acoustic shadow between the ovary and uterus is produced by the sigmoid colon.

FIG. 22-5. Transverse section showing external iliac lymph node enlargement. The left iliopsoas is seen **(arrow).** The mass on the right **(double arrows)** later proved to be lymph node enlargement as a result of lymphoma.

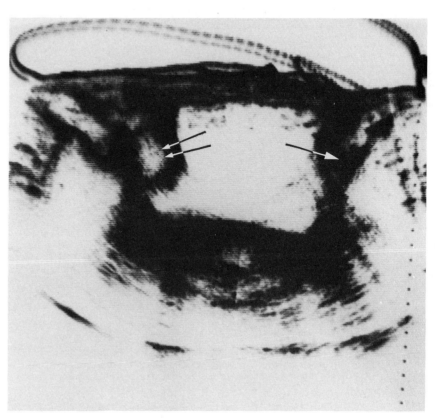

SONOGRAPHIC APPEARANCE OF COMMON CONDITIONS

The most common diseases, unrelated to pregnancy, seen in our case material are uterine myomas, pelvic inflammatory disease (PID), ovarian and parovarian cysts, dermoid cysts, cystadenoma and cystadenocarcinoma of the ovary, and endometriosis. The first two, uterine myomas and PID, are by far the most frequent. Although not strictly a disease, location of an intrauterine contraceptive device (IUCD) is a common problem. Endometrial carcinoma, adenomyosis, and carcinoma of the cervix are important diseases, but they are not frequently seen in our laboratory, because sonography does not add useful clinical information except under unusual circumstances. Solid ovarian tumors and carcinoma of the vagina or fallopian tube are also rarely encountered.

SONOGRAPHIC APPEARANCE OF COMMON CONDITIONS

UTERINE LEIOMYOMAS, MYOMAS, FIBROMYOMAS, OR FIBROIDS

It may not be an exaggeration to say that a complete understanding of the sonographic appearances of uterine leiomyomas and their differential diagnoses implies a working knowledge of ultrasound applied to gynecology. These common tumors are found in one-fifth of women over age 30 and may occur from the second decade through old age, though they are by far more common in the reproductive years. They are usually multiple; in only 2% of cases are they singular (26). Leiomyomas may be located anywhere in the uterus but are less often found in the cervix. These tumors may be intramural, subserous, or submucous; they may extend into the broad ligament or may even detach from the uterus.

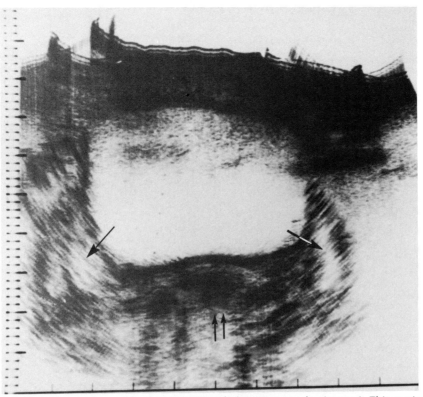

FIG. 22–6. Transverse section showing internal obturator muscles **(arrows).** This section was made with 15 degrees of caudal angulation. The rectum **(double arrows)** produces an acoustic shadow posterior to the vagina.

There are generally four sonographic appearances of uterine fibroids, as follows: a small, localized mass in the uterine wall; an enlarged but almost normally shaped uterus; replacement of the uterus by a distorted mass; and a solid mass associated with a normal uterus (Fig. 22–7). These appearances seem to offer opportunities for confusion, but in practice this seldom happens. Two observations are appropriate. The first is that a large portion of the mass in most fibroids is inseparable from the uterus. Whereas in many sections a separation may be seen, careful study usually shows large reproducible areas where the two are joined. This is usually true even of pedunculated fibroids. Other conditions that may simulate the appearance of a mass inseparable from the uterus are adhesions, inflammatory masses, ectopic pregnancies, and broad ligament hematomas. When the continuity with the uterine wall does not provide a clue to the true nature of a fibroid, the second observation usually does. Although these tumors vary in the amount of fibrous tissue relative to muscle, the attenuation of higher frequency sound in these is greater than in other solid masses. This phenomenon is less pronounced in rapidly growing fibroids (Fig. 22–8), but even those with areas of cystic degeneration usually show some regions with the characteristic attenuation properties (Fig. 22–9). Calcified solid ovarian tumors and dense ovarian fibromas may show similar preferential attenuation. This appearance is dependent on proper technique. With use of a 3.5- or 5-MHz transducer, the machine must be adjusted so that the posterior of a normal uterus will be completely demonstrated, but an increase of attenuation or decrease in gain will lose this definition (2). In practice, after a little experience, the appropriate settings are easily found and very useful.

Leiomyomas have a well-defined, smooth or lobulated border. The internal texture, which is homogeneous and coarse, may not be apparent at lower gain settings (Fig. 22–10). The degree of coarseness and ease of demonstration of the texture vary for unknown reasons, perhaps related to the age, growth rate, and composition of the tumor. A characteristic circular pattern of the internal texture, which probably depends on the relationship of the scan plane to the tumor architecture, may be seen in some cases. Fi-

broids in the cul-e-sac are reported to lack internal echoes (26). In our experience fibroids in that location have the same appearance as fibroids elsewhere (Fig. 22–11). This apparent lack of internal echoes is the result of insufficient amplification because the fibroid is too far from the transducer (i.e., beyond the "knee" of the TGC curve) or because there are intervening fibroids present that excessively attenuate the sound. The most common substructures seen are calcifications, which may appear as localized, diffuse, or ring-like echoes (9) (Fig. 22–7C). Some investigators (5), including the author, have been unable to associate a sonographic appearance with any specific type of degeneration except cystic degeneration, which appears as a localized area of fluid that may be easier to identify with higher frequency transducers. Often an area of degeneration is associated with strong internal echoes (Fig. 22–12), but we have also observed this echo pattern when the pathologist found no evidence of degeneration.

Leimyosarcoma. It is uncertain whether leiomyosarcoma arises most often de novo from the uterine wall or from preexisting uterine leiomyomas (24). These tumors are seen from the fourth decade throughout life. Although they are rare, they represent from one-half to three-fourths of all uterine sarcomas. These are typically large tumors, which have better sound transmission than most fibroids and may contain areas of liquefaction. This sonographic appearance is indistinguishable from rapidly growing or degenerating fibroids except when there is evidence of distant metastasis or local invasion.

PELVIC INFLAMMATORY DISEASE (PID)

This group of diseases is estimated to affect from one-tenth to one-third of the adult female population and includes gonococcal, pyogenic, and tubercular infections of the genital system. Although any portion of the genital tract may be infected, it is the 1 patient in 10 with involvement of the upper tract, primarily the fallopian tubes, that is of interest to the ultrasonographer.

Early in the disease sonography may detect no abnormality. The initial sonographic findings

(*Text continues on p. 274*)

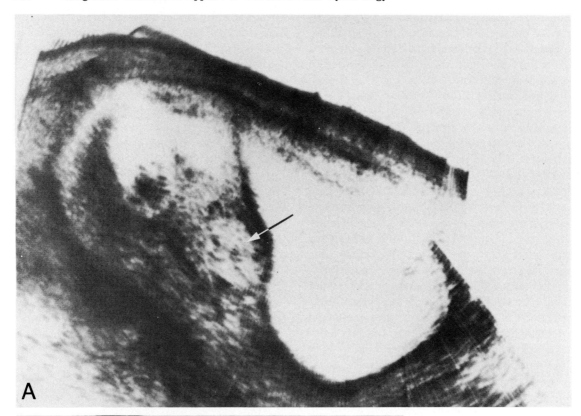

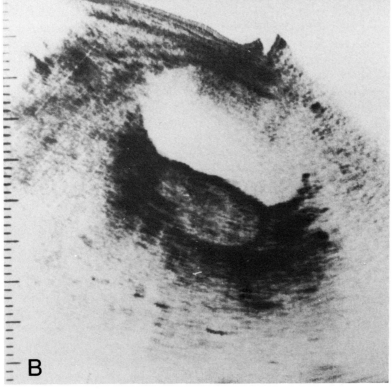

FIG. 22–7. A. Longitudinal section showing a small intramural fibroid **(arrow).** If the patient is pregnant, as in this case, intramural fibroids must not be confused with transient thickenings of the uterine wall. **B.** Longitudinal section of a uterus that is enlarged because of fibroids. There is a slight lobulation at the superior surface and some distortion of the normal shape, which help distinguish this appearance from other causes of uterine enlargement.

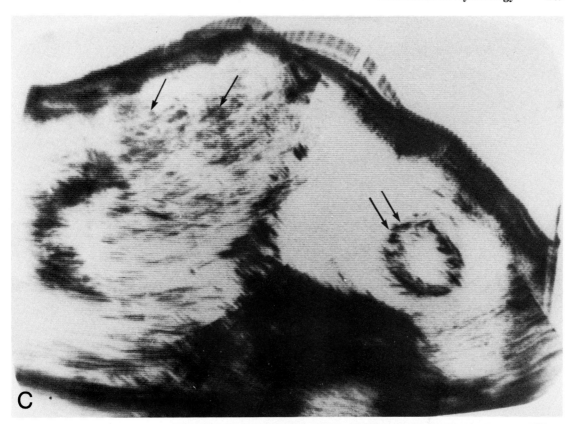

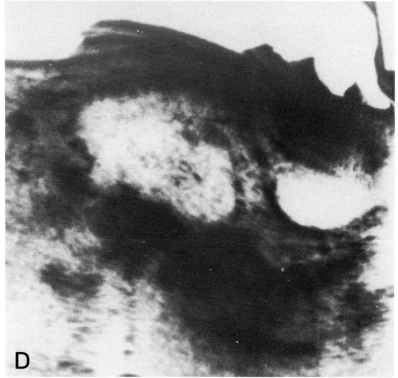

FIG. 22-7C. Longitudinal section of a large fibroid. Three types of calcifications are seen. The diffuse scattered and amorphous localized calcification **(arrows)** are similar. The ring-like calcification **(double arrow)** is seen here in a large region of degeneration characterized by a different internal texture and increased sound transmission. **D.** Longitudinal section of a fibroid adjacent to a normal portion of the uterus. Usually this appearance is limited to a few sections.

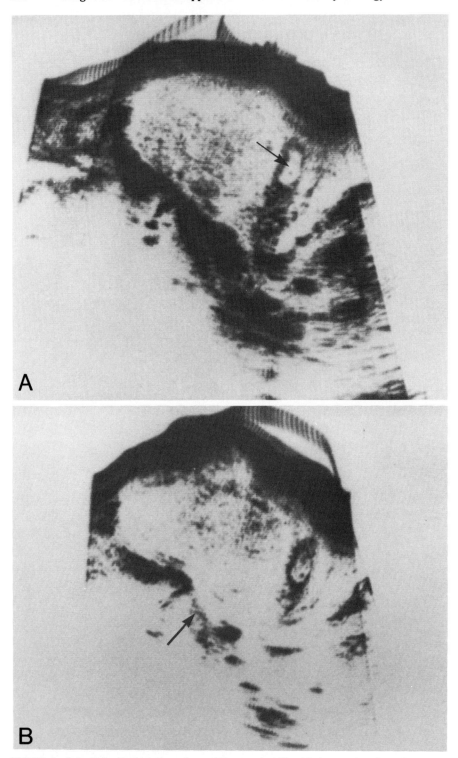

FIG. 22-8. A. Longitudinal section of a rapidly growing fibroid. A gestational sac **(arrow)** is seen. **B.** High-frequency section similar to Fig. 22–8B. The poor definition of the posterior wall **(arrow)** indicates greater than average attenuation of the sound for soft tissue.

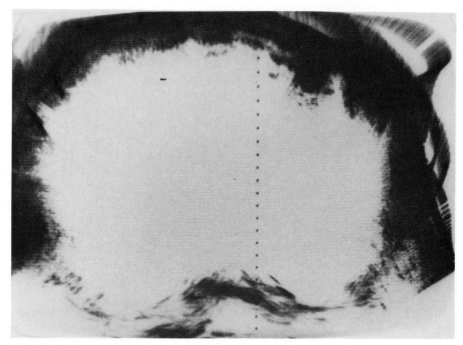

FIG. 22–9. A transverse section of the cephalad portion of the large fibroid with degeneration seen in Fig. 22–7C. The posterior wall and intensity of echoes beyond it indicate poor transmission of sound.

FIG. 22-10. A. A transverse section showing the internal texture of a fibroid. Often this circular pattern can be identified. **(Continued)**

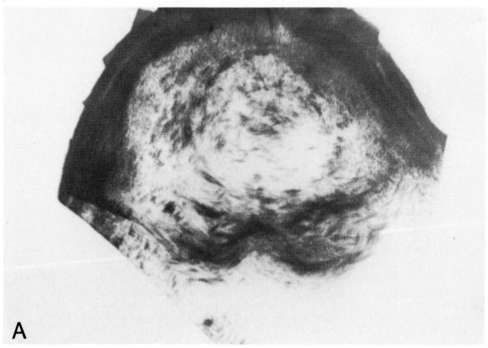

A

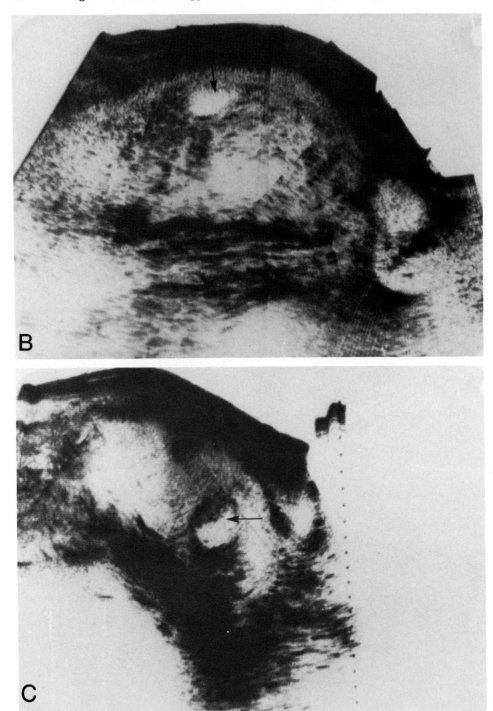

FIG. 22-10. (*Continued*) B. A longitudinal section showing the internal texture of a fibroid. In this section the circular pattern is not seen, but an area of cystic degeneration is shown **(arrow). C.** A longitudinal section of an early intrauterine pregnancy **(arrow)** within a fibroid uterus. This appearance should be distinguished from Fig. 22-10B.

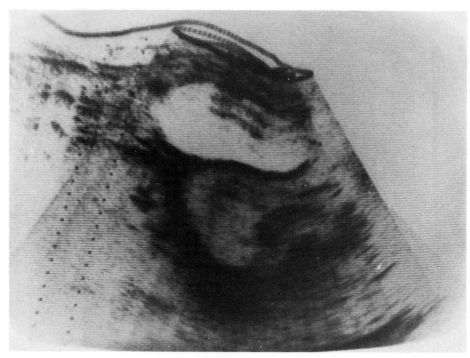

FIG. 22-11. Longitudinal section of a small fibroid in the cul-de-sac. The internal texture may be more difficult to demonstrate in these cases.

FIG. 22-12. Longitudinal section of a degenerating fibroid. These internal echoes are often seen when degeneration occurs but are not always an indication of degeneration.

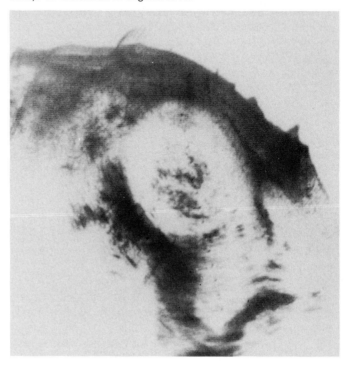

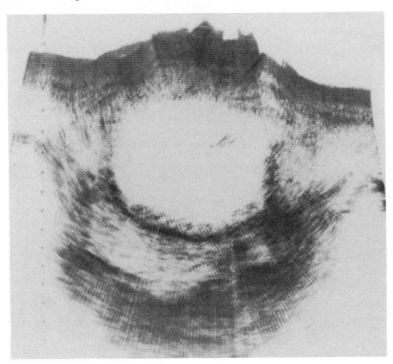

FIG. 22-13. Transverse section from a patient with acute pelvic inflammatory disease (PID). The right adnexa is enlarged, and the interface between the ovary and uterus are indistinct.

are a slight increase in the visibility of the fallopian tube and a small number of fluid-containing areas either within the tube or around it. When the infection is more severe, there is enlargement of the fallopian tube, ovaries, and ligaments with a decrease in intensity of internal echoes (Fig. 22–13). The uterus may also show a similar loss of echo intensity, and all the pelvic structures, including the surrounding muscles, may appear to blend together. Superficially, this produces a confusing picture because the uterus cannot be identified. In transverse scans these inflammatory masses conform to the shape of the pelvis, and on longitudinal scans they often have an irregular cephalad extent, which may contain portions of entrapped bowel (Fig. 22–14). This appearance may be deceptive. In some cases PID has a smooth cephalad extent, and sometimes fibroids have the irregular appearance of PID. If a large fluid area is seen within the mass, a tuboovarian abscess is often present. The use of focused higher frequency transducers and careful technique frequently permits the identification of the uterus in cases where it cannot otherwise be identified.

In the chronic active stages of the disease, a dilated fallopian tube is often seen. This elongated structure lies along the side of the pelvis and extends posteriorly. It may appear as a single, sausage-shaped, fluid-filled structure (Fig. 22–15), but in many cases because of adhesions, fibrosis, and folding of the fallopian tube there is a "chain of lakes" appearance (Fig. 22–16). Involvement of the fallopian tubes by PID is usually but not invariably bilateral. Depending on the activity of the disease, additional fluid-filled pockets of infection may be seen, and there may be some loss of definition of surrounding structures as a result of either adhesions or inflammatory changes.

Frequently the sonogram cannot distinguish the appearance of the chronic active disease from the chronic quiescent, particularly when the fallopian tubes are enlarged. When the clinical information is not helpful, serial studies are of value in demonstrating the static nature of quiescent disease. Often the only result of previous infections may be an alteration of the pelvic anatomy by thickening of the adnexa and formation of adhesions, which draw the uterus and ovary together (Fig. 22–17).

In the appropriate clinical setting the diag-

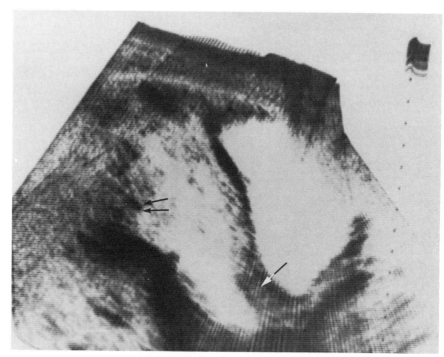

FIG. 22-14. Longitudinal section of acute PID. A portion of the uterus **(arrow)** can still be identified, though sometimes this is not possible. The cephalad border is irregular, and groups of echoes, which probably represent bowel **(double arrow)**, protrude into the mass.

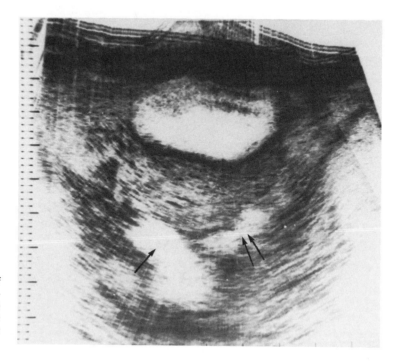

FIG. 22-15. Transverse section of chronic active PID. The larger dilated right fallopian tube **(arrow)** extends more posteriorly than the dilated left fallopian tube **(double arrow).**

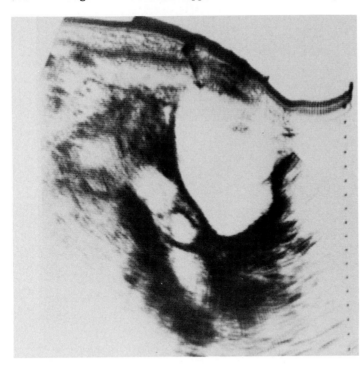

FIG. 22–16. Longitudinal section of chronic active PID. The folding of the enlarged fallopian tube gives the appearance of several oval-shaped fluid collections because of the two dimensional nature of the scanning plane.

FIG. 22–17. Transverse section of chronic quiescent PID. The right adnexa lacks detail and appears thick. A small hydrosalpinx is seen on the left **(arrow).**

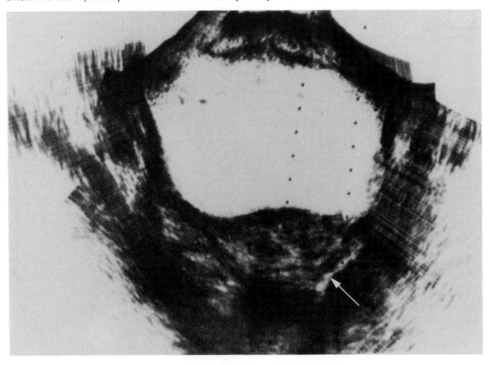

nosis of PID is easily confirmed by ultrasound. When, however, PID coexists with other pelvic pathology, in particular ovarian cyst or ectopic pregnancy, the diagnostic problems are greater. These latter two conditions usually go unrecognized, and the state of activity of the PID is often overestimated. On some occasions pedunculated fibroids have been mistaken for pelvic abscesses (14, 25). The differential diagnosis of these conditions is discussed in more detail later.

OVARIAN CYSTS

These common extrauterine masses are often of no significance. The difficulty arises in distinguishing the ovarian, parovarian, and fimbrial cyst from the true ovarian neoplasm and other conditions that contain fluid, such as ectopic pregnancy, endometrial cyst, or infection. The types of "ovarian" cysts are follicular, corpus luteum, fimbrial (hydatid of Morgagni), and parovarian (mesonephric).

The normal follicle may be as large as 3 cm, and only larger masses are considered "cysts." Follicular cysts are usually less than 6 cm but may become as large as 10 cm. A smooth, echo-producing border surrounds many small cystic masses of ovarian origin and is a common finding with follicular cysts (Fig. 22–18). They are unilocular, but the presence of several cysts in a single ovary may give a multilocular appearance. Hemorrhage may be present and give the appearance of a soft-tissue area within the mass (Fig. 22–19). These cysts are often associated with endometrial hyperplasia, fibroids, and hormone therapy.

Corpus luteum cysts are luteinized follicles that have accumulated fluid or blood (Fig. 22–20). The sonographic picture is indistinguishable from follicular cysts. Theca lutein cysts result from luteinization of theca cells, not granulosa cells (Fig. 22–21). These are usually large and multiple when chorionic gonadotrophin titers are increased, as in hydatidiform mole, multiple pregnancy, erythroblastosis fetalis, gonadotrophin administration, or with hyperreactio luteinalis. These are covered in more detail in other chapters.

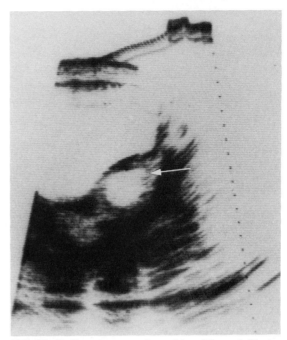

FIG. 22-18. Transverse section with a 3.5-cm follicular cyst on the left. There is an echo-producing zone **(arrow)** around the fluid-containing central portion of the mass.

FIG. 22-19. Transverse section of a hemorrhagic follicular cyst on the right. The appearance is the same for a hemorrhagic corpus lutein cyst.

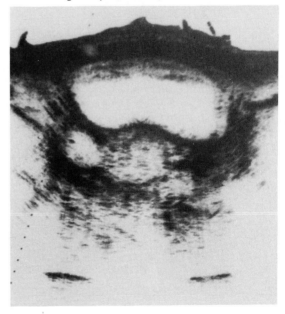

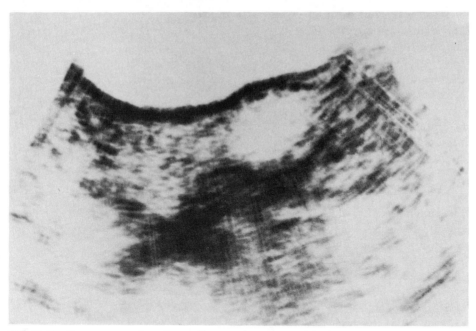

FIG. 22–20. Transverse section of a small corpus lutein cyst of the left ovary. The appearance is similar if not indistinguishable from that of a follicular cyst.

FIG. 22–21. Transverse section of a theca lutein cyst seen to the right of the uterus, which contains a gestational sac **(arrow)**. Several thin septa **(double arrow)** are seen within the cyst.

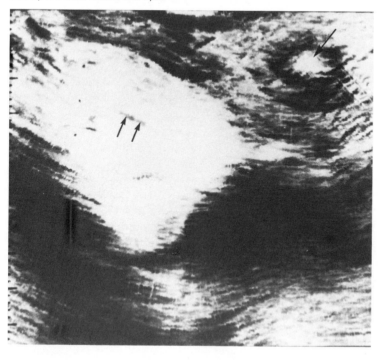

Fimbrial and parovarian cysts may be as large as 18 cm and are thin walled and usually unilocular, though occasionally thin septa are seen (Fig. 22–22).

The ovarian and parovarian cysts must be distinguished from the ovarian neoplastic cysts, endometrioma, and ectopic pregnancy. Although this cannot always be done with certainty, the small size and typical simple unilocular appearance should indicate the possibility of benign disease. Because most of these regress spontaneously, following them at intervals of 2–3 weeks, over several menstrual cycles if necessary, is important to show both the failure to grow and the eventual regression. When a mass fails to regress, invasive diagnostic techniques are usually indicated.

OVARIAN NEOPLASMS

True neoplasms of the ovary may be largely fluid-containing, of a mixed appearance, or solid. The pathologic types of these tumors are numerous, but the majority are either serous or mucinous cystadenomas and cystadenocarcinomas. This discussion is limited to these more common lesions and a few of the solid ovarian tumors because of their importance in differential diagnoses.

Cystic ovarian neoplasms, mucinous and serous cystadenoma and cystadenocarcinoma, comprise about half of all ovarian neoplasms. These tumors are more commonly benign than malignant, and the serous and mucinous forms are about equally common. Both types are bilateral in one-fifth to one-third of cases. Although the size varies greatly, they usually exceed 8 cm in diameter when clinically apparent.

The typical ultrasound appearance is a spheroid mass with well-defined borders. Both the serous and mucinous varieties are usually unilocular but may be multiocular (Fig. 22–23). The internal texture is more readily apparent when the mass contains large amounts of mucin, but at 5 MHz a fine uniform internal texture can also be shown in some serous tumors (Fig. 22–24). This texture is not specific for these neoplasms but may be seen in ovarian metastasis as well. These tumors have good transmission properties, which can be shown by the use of either low-gain studies or high-frequency transducers.

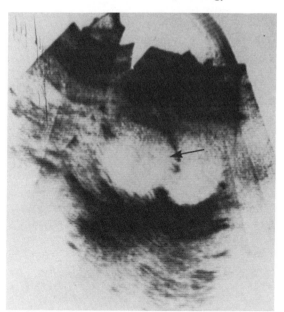

FIG. 22-22. Longitudinal section of a 6-cm fimbrial cyst **(arrow).** The anterior echoes and apparent irregularity of the posterior wall are artifacts.

The two problems in the diagnosis of these tumors are to distinguish them from simple cysts and to separate the benign and malignant tumors. Neither of these problems can be solved entirely by the use of ultrasound. A larger size, the presence of septation, and internal demonstrable structures and textures assist in distinguishing the neoplasms from simple cysts. Thickening and irregularity or nodularity of walls or septa are seen more in malignant tumors, but exceptions are common (Fig. 22–25). The presence of ascites is a strong indication of malignancy (8), though ascites may be present with benign tumors or even fibroids. Kobayashi (12) described four appearances that are suspicious for malignancy, as follows: 1) a large mass with scattered internal echoes, 2) focal septal thickening, 3) fine echoes distributed along the inner wall, 4) irregular mass with mixed linear and scattered echoes. There are enough exceptions to these rules that exact tissue diagnosis is always required.

Metastatic neoplasms to the ovaries are not rare and may account for one-fourth of malignant ovarian neoplasms (27). These are usually the result of metastasis from the gastrointestinal tract (especially the colon) or breast, though

(*Text continues on p. 283*)

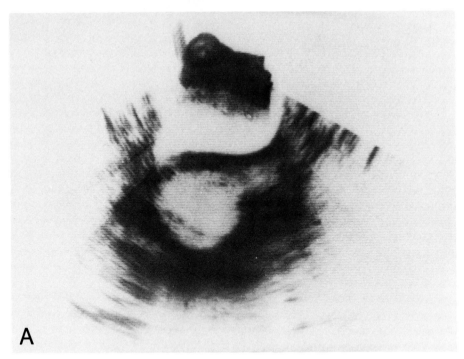

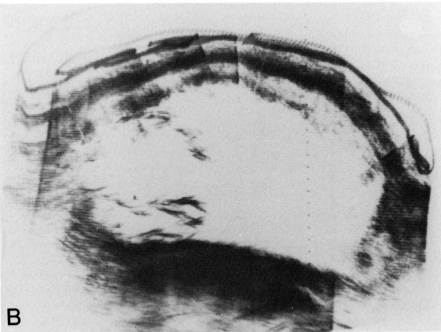

FIG. 22-23. A. Section of a 7.5-cm serous cystadenoma of the right ovary. A posterior septum can be seen within the mass. **B.** Longitudinal section of a very large mucinous cystadenoma. Thick, irregular septa were present throughout the mass. **(Continued)**

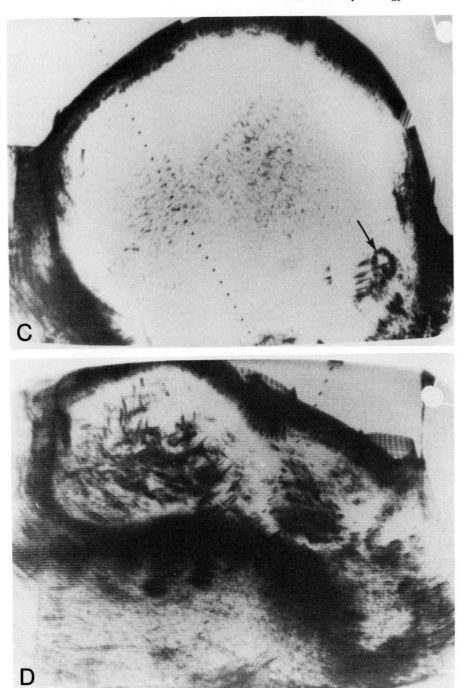

FIG. 22-23C. (*Continued*) Section of a large mucinous cystadenocarcinoma, which shows few internal structures. The distribution of the internal texture is probably a result of an improper TGC setting. One localized substructure can be seen **(arrow),** and a single septum was identified. **D.** Section of a large papillary mucinous cystadenocarcinoma. Compare this malignant tumor to Fig 22–23B.

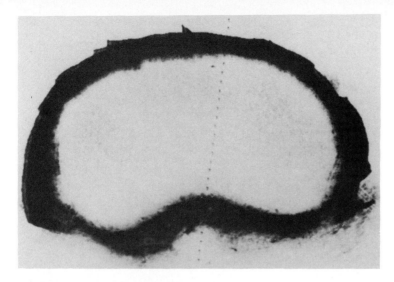

FIG. 22-24. Transverse section of a large serous cystadenoma. This unilocular unseptated tumor has a fine internal texture, which was demonstrated with a 5-MHz transducer.

FIG. 22-25. A. Transverse section of a papillary serous cystadenocarcinoma. A single septum **(arrow)** and a few irregular echoes are seen in this tumor. Compare this with the benign tumor in Fig. 22-23A. **B.** Longitudinal section showing solid mesenteric metastasis **(arrow)** from the tumor seen in Fig. 22-25A.

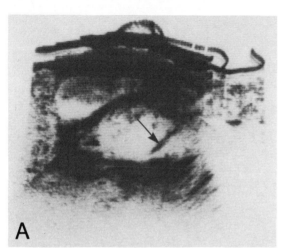

A

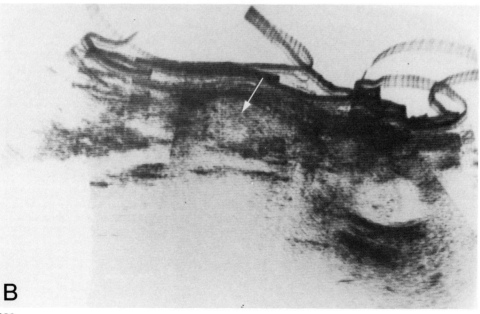

B

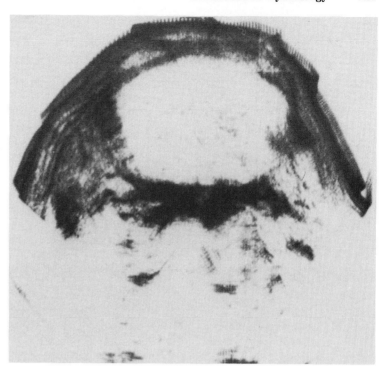

FIG. 22–26. Transverse section of a large Krukenberg tumor resulting from metastasic colon carcinoma. The scattered internal echoes and good penetration are similar to those of many other ovarian tumors.

other tumors (from the genital organs) are included in the broad classification of Krukenberg tumors (Fig. 22–26). These neoplasms have an appearance of homogeneous echoes within a mass with good sound transmission, similar to that found in the mucinous cystadenoma (20). They are usually bilateral but may appear on sonograms as either a single mass or a bilobulated mass.

Two other tumors of surface epithelium are endometrial tumors and clear-cell tumors, both of which are predominantly solid with small fluid-containing areas. Pathologically the Brenner tumors belong to this group of epithelial tumors and are usually solid, though the proliferating variety may form large cysts.

Solid ovarian tumors are less common than the cystic tumors. A wide range of pathologic diagnoses is associated with these masses. The more common ones are ovarian fibromas, thecomas, and Brenner tumors. Solid ovarian carcinomas are also found occasionally. The benign tumors have margins that are frequently smooth or lobulated with an overall spherical shape; however, slower growing masses may develop a shape that conforms to surrounding structures.

These tumors usually have a homogeneous internal structure with medium internal echo texture (Fig. 22–27). Similar to other soft-tissue areas such as the uterus, solid ovarian tumors usually transmit sound without preferential attenuation at higher frequencies but in some cases may have increased attenuation of sound in comparison to fibroids (17). Although the benign solid ovarian tumors may have areas of degeneration and calcification, these are not a prominent feature. Malignant solid ovarian tumors, on the other hand, not only have a more irregular border but also typically have a heterogeneous internal structure with areas containing fluid and uneven sound transmission (Fig. 22–28). Most of the smaller solid tumors are diagnostic problems and either are not recognized during the ultrasound examination or are thought to be uterine fibroids. Occasionally they are overdiagnosed when small ovarian cysts are mistaken for solid tumors.

BENIGN CYSTIC TERATOMAS

Benign cystic teratomas account for about one-fifth of ovarian neoplasms and are most often

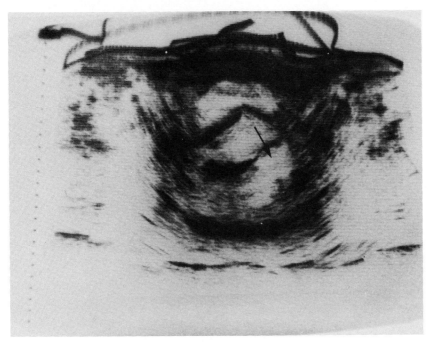

FIG. 22–27. Section of a solid thecoma **(arrow)** showing the uniform internal texture.

FIG. 22–28. Section of a malignant solid ovarian tumor **(arrow)** showing a heterogeneous internal structure with fluid-containing areas **(double arrow).** This was a poorly differentiated malignant granulosa cell tumor.

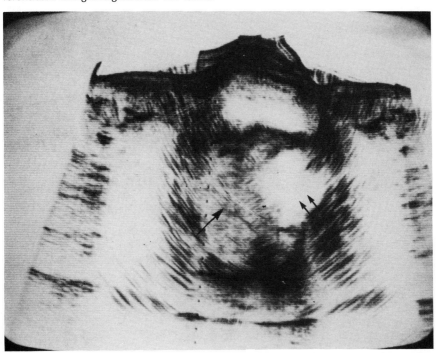

seen in children and in young adults. Solid teratomas are usually found in children. About 20% of dermoid cysts are said to be bilateral and less than 1% are malignant.

These tumors are usually spheroid but may be multilobular or very bizarre in shape. Three-fourths of these tumors are less than 10 cm in diameter, and they are rarely very large unless malignant. The margins of this type of mass are well defined unless solid elements are contiguous with it. Characteristically, this tumor appears as a fluid-filled mass with a localized, echo-producing internal portion (Fig. 22–29). This latter area is frequently eccentric in location and often casts an acoustic shadow that obscures part of the remainder of the tumor. The echogenic area need not contain calcification, teeth, or bone to produce sound attenuation and has generally been shown to represent a conglomerate of hair and sebum (7). When a fluid-fluid level is seen, the more echogenic fluid on the top represents a layer of fat and other materials (Fig. 22–30). When similar fluid-fluid levels are seen in infected or hemorrhagic cysts, the echo-producing fluid seeks the dependent position (Fig. 22–31).

Occasionally dermoid cysts may appear entirely cystic, but more often this is a false appearance resulting from incomplete scanning of the mass (Fig. 22–32). Entirely solid tumors in the prepubertal age group are often hard to recognize because of the difficulty of distinguishing these from surrounding bowel (Fig. 22–33). It is particularly important in these cases to have a distended bladder. Solid dermoids usually have higher intensity internal echoes, which are coarser than other solid ovarian tumors.

ENDOMETRIOSIS

Endometriosis is a common disease of menstruating women, producing pelvic pain, dysmenorrhea, and infertility. Like the pathologic findings, the ultrasound appearances range widely from predominantly solid to entirely cystic masses. This condition represents a problem in differential diagnosis and in most cases cannot be distinguished from PID. Most often the ovaries are involved, but the fallopian tube, broad ligament, and cul-de-sac may also be affected.

(*Text continued on p. 288*)

FIG. 22-29. Transverse section of a 12-cm dermoid cyst, which has a characteristic fluid-fluid level. The strongly reflective substructure **(arrow)** casts an acoustic shadow. (Courtesy of Dr. David Rochester, Evanston Hospital.)

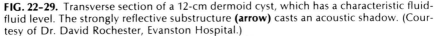
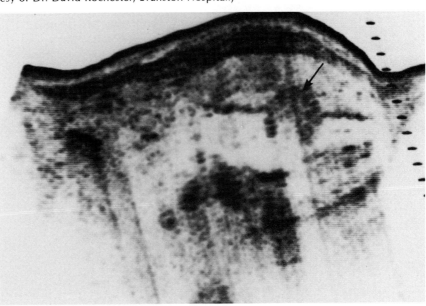

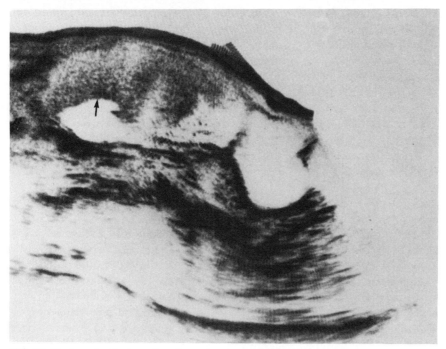

FIG. 22–30. Longitudinal section through a large dermoid cyst with a fluid-fluid level **(arrow)**.

FIG. 22–31. A. A longitudinal section of a cystic granulosa cell tumor that contains a fluid-fluid level **(arrow)** as a result of hemorrhage. The echo-producing mass was thought to result from blood clots **(double arrow). (Continued)**

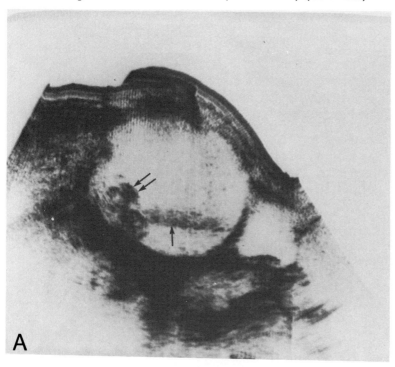

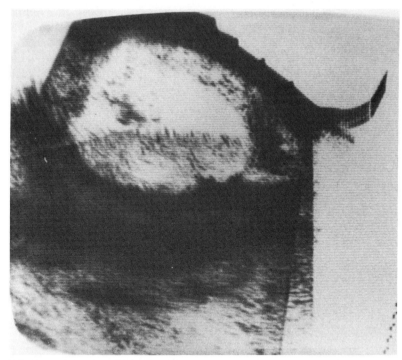

FIG. 22–31. (Continued) B. A longitudinal section of an infected renal cyst with a fluid-fluid level. The more echo-producing fluid is in a dependent position.

FIG. 22–32. Section of a predominantly cystic terotoma, in which the characteristic echo-producing mass **(arrow)** was seen in only a few of the sections.

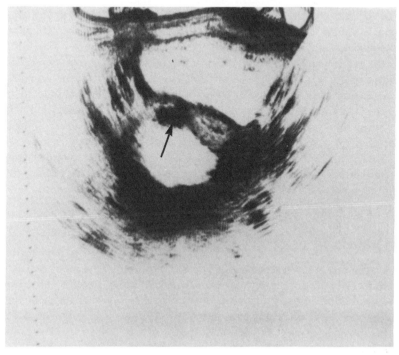

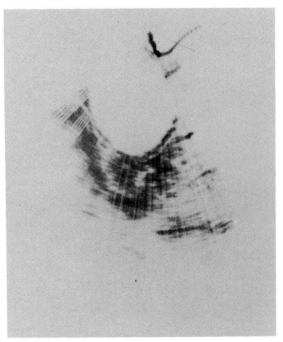

FIG. 22-33. Section of an entirely solid dermoid tumor of the right ovary. Because of the strong internal echoes this tumor may be mistaken for bowel or artifacts in some cases.

The two common ultrasound appearances of endometriosis are a solid thickening of the adnexal region (Fig. 22-34) and a unilocular thick-walled cystic mass corresponding to a "chocolate" cyst (Fig. 22-35). These cystic masses are usually less than 5 cm but may be as large as 15 cm. They are occasionally multiple, appearing as a multilocular mass or "chain of lakes" similar to that in hydrosalpinx. Blood within the cyst may produce internal echoes. Clearly the problem is to distinguish endometriosis from PID, which cannot be done from the sonogram alone. Endometriosis is also in the differential diagnoses of ovarian cyst and cystic neoplasms of the ovary.

ADENOMYOSIS

Adenomyosis is endometriosis of the myometrium. Because the sonogram usually reveals no abnormalities, this condition has received little attention in the ultrasound literature (13, 26). In three-fourths of cases of adenomyosis, the uterus is seen to be enlarged. Unlike the typical presentation of fibroids, adenomyosis often pro-

duces a symmetric enlargement of the uterus, but smooth, localized areas of enlargement may also be identified. A confusing factor is that fibroids and adenomyosis frequently occur together. Typically the adenomyosis involves the inner two-thirds of the myometrium and produces a slight decrease in the echo content of the involved areas, and sometimes echo-producing interfaces, resulting from hemorrhage or secretions, are found within an area of adenomyosis (Fig. 22-36). These findings may be indistinguishable from either normal endometrial echoes or fibroids. In up to 40% of cases adenomyosis is seen in association with external endometriosis, which is a combination that may be particularly difficult to distinguish from pelvic inflammatory disease.

INTRAUTERINE CONTRACEPTIVE DEVICES (IUCD)

During reexamination after insertion of an IUCD about 1 in 10 patients have no visible string. This finding may be caused by spontaneous expulsion of the IUCD, the string having been cut too short; retraction of the IUCD itself; enlargement of the uterus from either pregnancy or fibroid tumor growth; or perforation of the uterus by the IUCD. Perforation is thought to occur at the time of insertion of the IUCD (18), but the rate of migration from the uterine cavity varies. The clinician may investigate the problem of a missing string by sonography; radiography, including hysterosalpingography; and uterine sounds or probes, which may be used in combination with radiography. Sonography is the most appropriate study in a patient whose uterus has grown in size, is possibly pregnant, has symptoms of perforation, or has an associated pelvic mass. In general, when the IUCD is seen by sonographic examination, it has been accurately localized, but if sonography does not find the IUCD, it may still be present in the pelvis. In these cases plain film radiography is a useful and important supplement. On longitudinal section the Lippes loop consists of two to five dots or short lines (Fig. 22-37). To show these characteristic lines, do not scan the area too rapidly or with excessive gain, either of which may cause the characteristic dots to appear as a continuous line. The Copper-"7" has a long limb, which can be seen on longitudinal section, and a

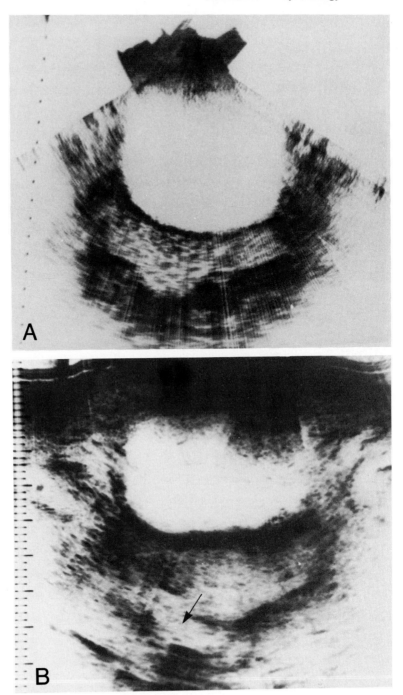

FIG. 22-34. A. Transverse section of the pelvis in a patient with endometriosis. The ovaries and other adnexal structures are inseparable from the uterus. **B.** Transverse section of treated endometriosis with adnexal thickening. The right tube is slightly enlarged **(arrow).** Compare this appearance with Fig. 22-15.

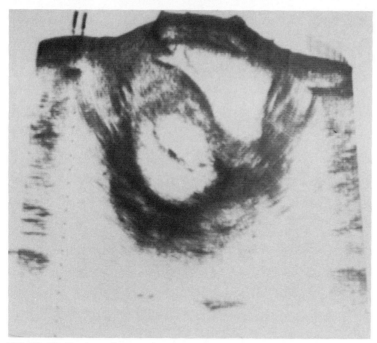

FIG. 22–35. Section of a 7-cm endometrioma of the right ovary. The mass was located in the cul-de-sac and associated with dense adhesions.

FIG. 22–36. Longitudinal section of a uterus that is enlarged because of adenomyosis. A few scattered strong echoes **(arrow)** can be seen within the area of adenomyosis.

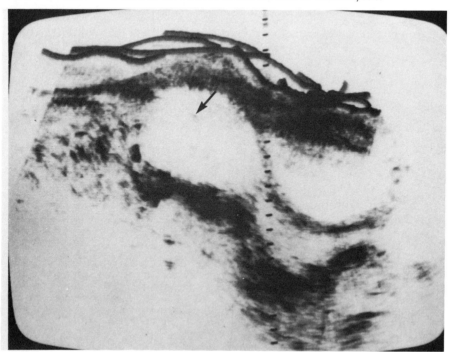

short limb seen on transverse (Fig. 22–38). Oblique sections often show two distinct echoes. The Copper-T is similar to the "7" except that the short upper limb can be demonstrated to cross in a typical "T" shape. The Saf-T-Coil produces a series of echoes along the coil portion and a linear echo along its central part. The Dalkon Shield, often difficult to recognize, appears as a small line of strong echoes seen in the uterus both on longitudinal and transverse sections.

The IUCD can be hidden by coexisting intrauterine abnormalities such as blood clots or an incomplete abortion (Fig. 22–39). An IUCD outside the uterine cavity is difficult to identify but can be seen when it is partially within the uterus (11). When an IUCD is present in the uterus along with an intrauterine pregnancy, the IUCD can reliably be seen only early in the pregnancy (Fig. 22–40). We have rarely identified an IUCD after the first trimester, and the sixth through the ninth weeks are ideal for confirming the presence of an IUCD with a pregnancy.

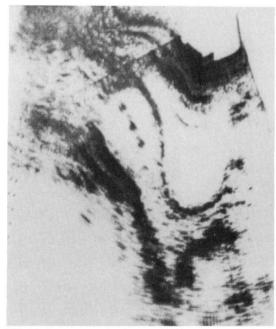

FIG. 22-37. Longitudinal section through a Lippes loop showing the characteristic line of dots.

FIG. 22-38. Longitudinal section of a copper "7" IUCD **(arrow).** The mass **(double arrow)** seen above the uterus was an ovarian cyst displaced by the distended bladder.

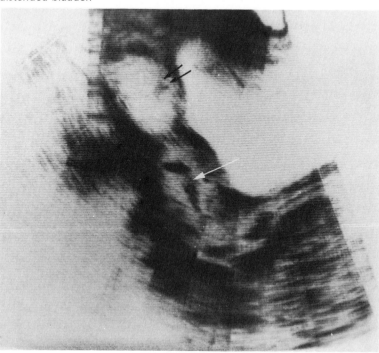

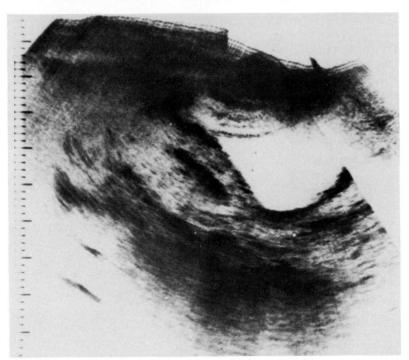

FIG. 22–39. Longitudinal section of a patient with both a Lippes loop and an incomplete abortion. The IUCD could not be satisfactorily distinguished from the echoes resulting from the incomplete abortion.

FIG. 22–40. A. Longitudinal section showing the upper limb **(arrow)** of a copper "7" IUCD and an intrauterine gestation of 6 weeks.**(Continued)**

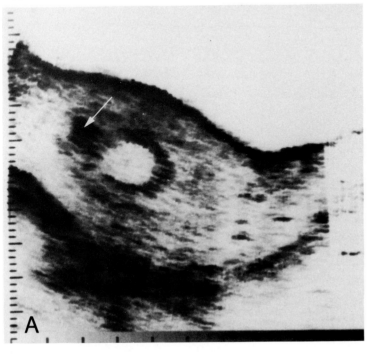

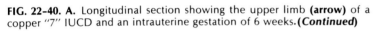

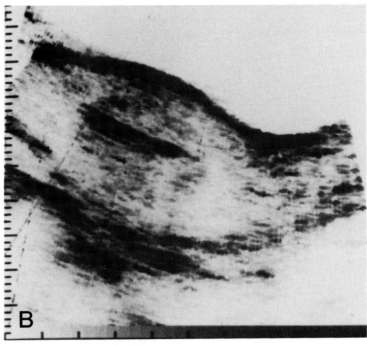

FIG. 22–40. (*Continued*) B. The long limb of the copper "7" IUCD can be seen in a section immediately to the right of Fig. 22–40A.

NONGYNECOLOGIC PELVIC MASSES

The ultrasonographer should be familiar with the sonographic appearance of important nongynecologic conditions, including pelvic kidney, rectal or sigmoid carcinoma, and metastasis to the pelvis. The sonographic distinction of pelvic kidneys from ovarian tumors is not always easy; with improved resolution the substructure of the kidney can be recognized and the nature of the mass suspected. Nevertheless the expediency of examining the patient prone and confirming that one kidney is not in its normal location should not be ignored. Infrequently the sonographer is asked to diagnose rectal or sigmoid carcinoma. When bulky enough to be seen by sonography, this tumor is an irregular, solid mass with a nonhomogeneous internal texture, which varies from moderately strong echoes to very strong echoes (Fig. 22–41). Because of the internal pattern it is difficult to identify lumph nodes or to find evidence of local spread of colon or rectal tumors. Krukenberg tumors have been discussed elsewhere and must be distinguished from primary ovarian neoplasms. Drop metastases from intestinal malignancies often form a platelike thickening in the cul-de-sac. Although these metastases may occasionally resemble slow-growing ovarian tumors, the patient's history provides the important information for the differential diagnosis. When presacral masses and other pelvic masses are closely associated with the limits of the pelvis or radiography shows bony changes, computed tomography often provides important information (3) for their evaluation.

In pediatric patients sonography gives a noninvasive way to confirm the presence or absence of a uterus or ovaries, but its value in complex urogenital anomalies remains uncertain. Hydrometrocolpos can be demonstrated by sonography as an elongated, fluid-filled mass replacing the uterus. Although this is usually a condition of infants and adolescents, it may also be an acquired condition in older women who have cervical obstruction following surgery or radiation. In many patients various forms of bicornuate uterus can be confirmed by ultrasound (Fig. 22–42), but usually hysterosalpingography provides the important details if reconstructive surgery is planned.

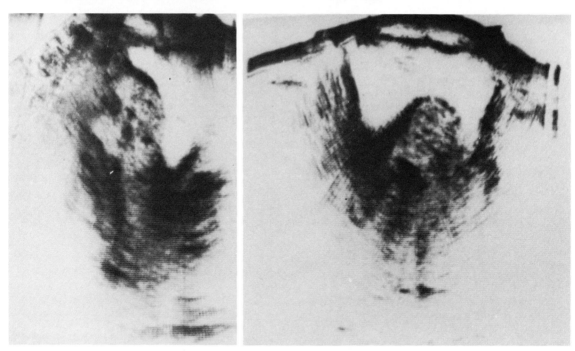

FIG. 22-41. A. A longitudinal section of a large rectal carcinoma in a male patient. **B.** A transverse section showing the impression of the rectal carcinoma in Fig. 22–41A on the bladder. The heterogeneous internal texture is typical of these tumors.

FIG. 22-42. Transverse section of a bicornuate uterus. This appearance may be difficult to distinguish from uterine fibroids.

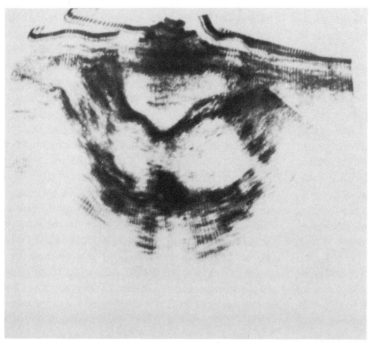

DIFFERENTIAL DIAGNOSIS

INTRAUTERINE ABNORMALITIES

Intrauterine abnormalities have two important patterns. The first is one of strong echoes within the uterine cavity, which may be the result of missed abortion, incomplete abortion, retained products of conception, hydatidiform mole, or IUCD. The second is a fluid mass with the uterine cavity, which may be a normal intrauterine pregnancy, a blighted ovum, or a hematocolpos. Because most intrauterine problems are related to pregnancy and covered in other chapters, these are not discussed at length.

UTERINE MASSES

The other group of patterns present as uterine masses. The three variations of these patterns are an enlarged uterus, a mass apparently replacing the uterus, and a mass inseparable from the uterus.

When the uterus appears enlarged but retains a recognizable uterine shape, the differential diagnosis includes the following: 1) normal variant, 2) fibroids, 3) adenomyosis, 4) endometrial carcinoma. An unusually large but otherwise normal uterus is most often seen in the multiparous patient during the child-bearing years. Not only is the normal shape retained but also the normal proportion of fundus to cervix, as well as the proportions of length to width to AP diameter. In those patients in whom the enlargement is a result of fibroids, some disproportion of width to length to AP diameter is frequently seen. After careful scanning with higher frequency transducers, texture differences corresponding to large fibroids can often be identified in the uterus. In many cases adenomyosis is difficult to recognize and cannot be reliably distinguished from normal variants. Sometimes the involvement is extensive enough to show areas within the myometrium characteristic of adenomyosis. Enlargement of the uterus associated with endometrial carcinoma cannot often be distinguished from enlargement due to other causes, and its appearance is similar to adenomyosis, though the age and clinical presentation are usually different.

In the next pattern to be described the uterus appears to be replaced by a mass. Because this may be an incorrect assumption, the differential diagnosis includes fibroids, PID, solid ovarian tumors, mixed fluid and solid ovarian tumors, and some nongynecologic pelvic malignancies. When large fluid-filled masses are seen and the uterus cannot be identified, these masses are almost always nonuterine in origin, and it is likely that the uterus must either be displaced or obscured by the mass. When the mass is solid, the correct diagnosis is usually uterine fibroids. Demonstration of their characteristic features is enough to establish this diagnosis. Poor transmission of sound at higher frequency is a particularly helpful feature. Calcified ovarian tumors may give the appearance of fibroids, but these are rare. The other common pathology to present with this appearance is pelvic inflammatory disease, which is most often seen when the clinical setting is such that there is no difficulty in the differential diagnosis. The shape of the mass caused by PID is more irregular, particularly at its junction with the bowel; on transverse sections the mass tends to fit the shape of surrounding structures (Fig. 22–43). Surrounding pelvic musculature remains unaffected by fibroids but may lose definition in PID. When higher frequency transducers are used, small fluid-filled areas are often seen in PID and transmission of sound is much greater than in fibroids. Both a degenerating fibroid and a fibroid on a twisted pedicle have been reported to have the appearance of PID. We have not encountered this problem using special sections at high frequency and low gain. At 3.5 and 5 MHz even complicated fibroids have large areas of poor penetration. An ectopic pregnancy may form a mass of blood clots adherent to and surrounding part of the uterus. This appearance may be difficult to distinguish from fibroids, though, as in PID, the transmission properties are different.

Large solid ovarian tumors may rarely present with this appearance. When the patient is scanned carefully, the uterus can often be identified as a separate structure. Although fibroids tend to be more lobulated in outline, in some cases we have been unable to correctly distinguish large solid ovarian tumors from fibroids (Fig. 22–44). Solid ovarian tumors have in general produced a pattern that is difficult to distinguish from other possibilities.

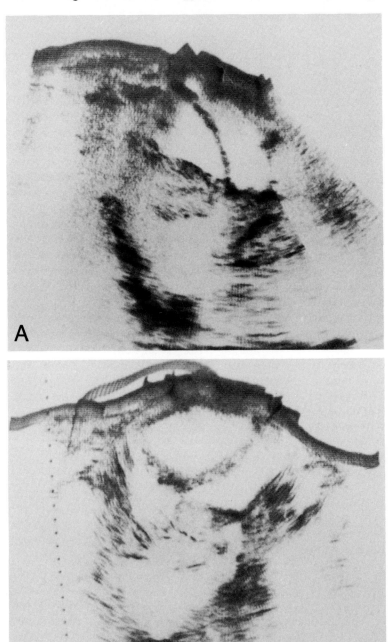

FIG. 22–43A. Longitudinal section of a patient with PID showing fluid anterior and posterior to the uterus. **B.** Transverse section of a patient with advanced PID. The inflammatory masses tend to fit the surrounding pelvic structures.

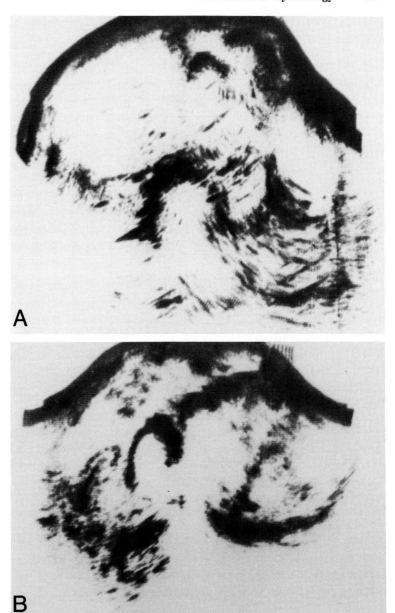

FIG. 22–44. A. Longitudinal section of a large solid calcified ovarian tumor (fibrothecoma cell). The uterus cannot be distinguished from this mass, which has a heterogeneous appearance and some areas of good sound transmission. **B.** Transverse section of the same tumor as in Fig. 22–44A showing the acoustic shadow produced by large areas of calcification.

Mixed fluid and solid ovarian masses may be difficult to tell from degenerating fibroids when the uterus has not been identified. These ovarian masses are rapidly growing tumors and tend to be more spheroid and not as lobulated or asymmetrical as fibroids. The solid elements that separate the fluid areas do not attenuate sound at higher frequencies as strongly as those in fibroids. Frequently ascites is seen in the cul-de-sac; this finding may occur rarely with benign tumors and fibroids. Occasionally carcinoma of the rectum, colon, or cervix may have so completely invaded surrounding pelvic structures that the uterus cannot be identified, but clinical information or findings easily distinguish these conditions.

Although the final pattern of uterine masses to be described is a common one, arriving at a correct diagnosis is frequently difficult. In this pattern a normal uterus or part of a normal uterus is seen, but a mass is also present that cannot be entirely separated from the uterus. Usually this appearance is caused by fibroids, but the differential diagnosis includes PID, ectopic pregnancy, endometriosis, broad ligament hematoma, and solid ovarian tumors.

As previously stated, fibroids are rarely singular, and the apparent connection to the uterus is usually broad. In addition, the texture of the adjacent uterine wall is usually similar to that of the fibroid and unlike that of the normal myometrium. These observations and the sound transmission properties of fibroids are generally enough to give the correct diagnosis.

Pelvic inflammatory disease may have a similar appearance in both acute and chronic cases. When the uterine wall texture is normal, PID is not often mistaken for fibroids. When, however, inflammatory changes affect the appearance of the uterus, the attenuation differences between PID and fibroids give very important diagnostic clues. In addition, PID tends to be bilateral in distribution and more readily conforms to the shape of surrounding structures. An ectopic pregnancy can produce a similar appearance, and in some cases hemorrhage and subsequent blood clots either fill the tube or are adherent to the uterus and give the appearance of a homogeneous mass inseparable from the uterus. A fluid-containing structure corresponding to the gestation may or may not be identified within this mass. Although such masses do not have the attenuation properties of fibroids, they may easily be mistaken for PID. An ectopic pregnancy may appear similar to a pregnancy occurring within a uterus containing fibroids. The distinguishing features are better transmission of sound through blood clots and better definition of the gestational sac when it is intrauterine. In many cases we have not discovered a reliable finding to distinguish ectopic pregnancy from the other possibilities, particularly from PID. The pregnancy test is helpful, being positive in half to three-fourths of ectopic pregnancies, and with the availability of more sensitive hormone assays this difficulty in diagnosis will be further decreased.

Benign solid ovarian tumors tend to have regular outlines. The clue to distinguishing these tumors from the others is the completely normal appearance of the adjacent uterus; both its shape and myometrial texture are unaltered by a nearby solid tumor. A difficulty arises, however, if the patient has both fibroids and solid ovarian tumors. In these cases, just as when PID coexists with ovarian cysts or ectopic pregnancy, we have no reliable way of establishing the correct diagnosis. Endometriosis can mimic PID, and when it presents with this ultrasound pattern, it should be included in the PID-ectopic pregnancy differential diagnosis. Hematoma of the broad ligament may also appear as a mass inseparable from the uterus. The history of a recent curettage is a valuable clue. Hematomas in the pelvis have a variety of appearances, and although they vary from solid to entirely fluid, they have uniformly good transmission. These masses become gradually smaller, but they can become infected and enlarge as pelvic abscesses.

EXTRAUTERINE MASSES

The final group of patterns, the extrauterine masses, have traditionally been categorized as cystic, mixed, and solid. The almost purely fluid-containing (or cystic) masses are usually ovarian or parovarian cysts. Ovarian neoplasms, dermoids, PID, and endometriosis should be included in the differential diagnosis. When the mass is spheroid, sharply defined, and small (less than 5cm), it is probably an ovarian cyst. Some ovarian neoplasms may have this appearance but are generally larger and show growth on subsequent examinations. Dermoids may have this appearance. Chronic PID may have the appearance of a fluid-containing extrauterine mass, but the shape of this mass is more typically elongated and its margins are less well defined. In addition, other changes associated with PID may be found. A rare ovarian pregnancy may take the appearance of an extrauterine mass (Fig. 22–45).

The group of fluid-filled masses with either substructure or solid elements are usually ovarian tumors; metastatic tumors to the ovary may have this appearance, and pedunculated fibroids have been reported to be indistinguishable from other conditions in this group. When the distinctive features of each of these diseases, as discussed earlier, are used in the differential diag-

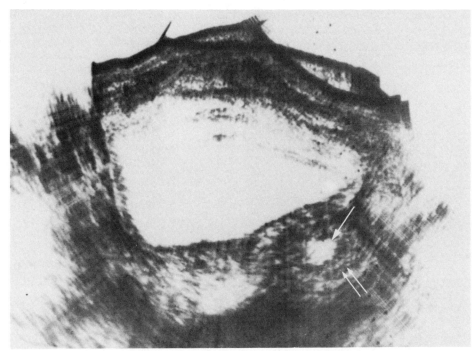

FIG. 22–45. Transverse section showing an ovarian pregnancy **(arrow)** to the left of the uterus. The fluid-containing portion of the mass was entirely surrounded by a solid outer ring **(double arrow).**

nosis, there are usually few problems in establishing a correct diagnosis. PID (abscess), endometriosis, and ectopic pregnancy are often difficult to distinguish, and when one is considered, the others should not be excluded. Most of the problems in this group arise when several conditions are found in the same patient.

The solid extrauterine masses are usually solid ovarian tumors, fibromas, thecomas, Brenner tumors, solid adenocarcinomas, or dermoids. Occasionally hematomas, endometriosis, and colon carcinoma are included in this group. The features of these last three have been discussed. The former conditions are encountered infrequently, and the spectrum of sonographic presentation for each pathologic entity is not sufficiently well described to speculate on possible ways of distinguishing among these.

CONCLUSION

That sonographic examination of the female pelvic organs is a useful diagnostic test has been established. Cochrane reported an 82% accuracy (5) regarding size, location, and structure using biphasic equipment. A later report by Queenan (19) indicates 21% of examinations were diagnostic, 74% confirmatory, and 5% misleading. Levi compared sonographic diagnoses with clinical findings and concluded this combination would reduce false-negative results considerably (15). This report also found that the sensitivity of sonography to the presence of disease was 98% for masses larger than 2 cm. Our review of gray-scale examinations indicated an equally high sensitivity and an accuracy of 85% (2). A more recent review by Lawson found an accuracy of 91% (14).

Since each author defines the correctness of a diagnosis somewhat differently, these figures cause some confusion. What represents a reasonable diagnostic goal for the sonogram is uncertain. To expect an exact tissue diagnosis is unrealistic, but merely to determine the presence or absence of normality is a failure to use the full potential of sonography. The appropriate goal is the maximum utility of sonography in patient management as measured by alteration and improvement of care given to the patient. It is hoped that this standard will be used when the information in this chapter is applied.

Acknowledgment

I would like to give special thanks to Ms. Elizabeth Blake for her help in preparing this manuscript and to Dr. Axel Kunzmann for his advice and comments.

REFERENCES

1. ANDERSON CF, JASSO L, GILES HR, HEINE MW: Cyclic variations in ultrasonographic evaluation of the female pelvis. Presentation No. 515. Twenty-second Annual Meeting of the American Institute of Ultrasound in Medicine (AIUM), Dallas, November, 1977

2. BOWIE JD: Ultrasound of gynecologic pelvic masses: the indefinite uterus and other patterns associated with diagnostic error. J Clin Ultrasound 5:323–328, 1977

3. CARTER BL, KAHN PC, WOLPERT SM, HAMMERSCHLAG SB, SCHWARTZ AM, SCOTT M: Unusual pelvic masses: a comparison of computed tomographic scanning and ultrasonography. Radiology 121:383–390, 1976

4. COCHRANE WJ: Ultrasound in gynecology. Radiol Clin North Am 13:457–467, 1975

5. COCHRANE WJ, THOMAS MA: Ultrasound diagnosis of gynecologic pelvic masses. Radiology 110:649–654, 1974

6. DECKER A: Culdoscopy. Philadelphia, FA Davis, 1967, p 143

7. GUTTMAN PH JR: In search of the elusive benign cystic ovarian teratoma: applications of the ultrasound "tip of the iceberg" sign. J Clin Ultrasound 5:403–406, 1977

8. HANEY AF: Estimation of malignant risk of pelvic disease by acoustic appearance. Presentation No. 333. Twenty-first Annual Meeting of the American Institute of Ultrasound in Medicine (AIUM), San Francisco, August, 1976

9. HASSANI N: Ultrasonic evaluation of uterine fibroids: the sonic shadow sign. J Natl Med Assoc 67:307–310, 1975

10. HERTIG AT, GORE H: Female genitalia. In Anderson WAD (ed): Pathology, 6th ed. St. Louis, CV Mosby, 1971, p 1489

11. IANNIRUBERTO A, MASTROBERODINO A: Ultrasonic localization of the Lippes loop. Am J Obstet Gynecol 114:78–82, 1972

12. KOBAYASHI M: Illustrated Manual of Obstetrics and Gynecology. Philadelphia, JB Lippincott, 1974, p 90

13. KOBAYASHI S, SEKIBA K, NIWA K, AKAMATSU N: Fundamental and clinical study of the ultrasonic classification of uterine myomas. Presentation No. 314. First Annual Meeting of the World Federation of Ultrasound in Medicine and Biology, San Francisco, August, 1976

14. LAWSON TL, ALBARELLI JN: Diagnosis of gynecologic pelvic masses by gray-scale ultrasonography: analysis of specificity and accuracy. Am J Roentgenol 128:1003–1006, 1977

15. LEVI S, DELVAL R: Value of ultrasonic diagnosis of gynecological tumors in 370 surgical cases. Acta Obstet Gynecol Scand 55:261–266, 1976

16. MILLER EI, THOMAS RH, LINES P: The atrophic postmenopausal uterus. J Clin Ultrasound 5:261–263, 1977

17. MORLEY P, BARNETT E: The use of ultrasound in the diagnosis of pelvic masses. Br J Radiol 43:602–616, 1970

18. PIIROINEN O: Ultrasonic localization of intrauterine contraceptive devices. Acta Obstet Gynecol Scand 51:203–207, 1972

19. QUEENAN JT, KUBARYCH SF, DOUGLAS DL: Evaluation of diagnostic ultrasound in gynecology. Am J Obstet Gynecol 123:453–465, 1975

20. ROCHESTER D, LEVIN B, BOWIE JD, KUNZMANN A: Ultrasonic appearance of the Krukenberg tumor. Am J Roentgenol 129:919–920, 1977

21. RUBIN C, KURTZ AB, GOLDBERG BB: Water enema: a new ultrasound technique in defining pelvic anatomy. J Clin Ultrasound 6:28–33, 1978

22. SAMPLE F: Pelvic inflammatory disease. In Sanders RC, James AE Jr (eds): Ultrasonography in Obstetrics and Gynecology. New York, Appleton-Century-Crofts, 1977

23. SAMPLE WF, LIPPE BM, GYEPES MT: Gray-scale ultrasonography of the normal female pelvis. Radiology 125:477–483, 1977

24. SILVERBERG SG: Leiomyosarcoma of the uterus. Obstet Gynecol 38:613–628, 1971

25. UHRICH PC, SANDERS RC: Ultrasonic characteristics of pelvic inflammatory masses. J Clin Ultrasound 4:199–204,1976

26. VON MICSKY LI: Sonographic study of uterine fibromyomata in the non-pregnant state and during gestation. In Sanders RC, James AE Jr (eds): Ultrasonography in Obstetrics and Gynecology. New York, Appleton-Centruy-Crofts, 1977

27. WEBB MJ, PECKER DG, MUSSEY E: Cancer metastatic to the ovary: factors influencing survival. Obstet Gynecol 45:391–396, 1975

28. ZEMLYN S: Comparison of pelvic ultrasonography and pneumography for ovarian size. J Clin Ultrasound 2:331–339, 1974

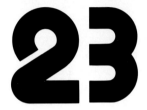

23

Ultrasound in gynecologic oncology

INTRODUCTION

The use of diagnostic ultrasound in the evaluation and management of patients with suspected or proved pelvic malignancy is extremely valuable. Although sonography is not diagnostic of malignancy, when correlated with the history and physical examination, it can assist in the differential diagnosis of pelvic disease and provide information that may influence management decisions. In some cases the ultrasound study simply confirms the pelvic examination findings, while in others additional information is revealed that alters the differential diagnosis.

Sonography is a safe, simple, noninvasive examination that should be the first procedure in the workup of a patient with a definite or suspected pelvic mass (8, 19, 21, 26). Since ultrasound gives a true spatial relationship of the pelvic structures, it is usually possible to determine where a mass arises. Confirmation of the exact origin of a pelvic mass can considerably alter the management of the patient. In addition to information about the origin of the mass, it is possible to measure the size and determine the character of a mass and make important observations regarding extension to other structures in malignant disease. For these reasons abdominal-pelvic sonography is valuable in the preoperative assessment of patients with suspected pelvic masses. After surgery it can be used to evaluate complications and recurrence of malignant tumors. In patients receiving radiation therapy ultrasound plays a very important role in establishing radiation fields and obtaining anatomic information for radiation dosimetry measurements. It is useful for following response to radiation or chemotherapy and for detecting or confirming recurrence of disease. The application of sonography in patients with pelvic malignancy is described and illustrated in this chapter.

APPLICATIONS

DETECTION OF PELVIC DISEASE

Ultrasound examination provides a new dimension in the study of the soft-tissue structures within the pelvis. When the sonographic findings are correlated with the bimanual examination, a clearer picture of the anatomy and pathologic condition within the pelvis is obtained. The main indication for sonography of the pelvis in the nonpregnant female is the presence or suspicion of a pelvic mass on pelvic examination. If the palpable mass is a normal structure, such as the uterus or ovary, the three-dimensional sonographic study will illustrate this. On the other hand, demonstration of an extraorganal space-occupying structure is confirmation that a pathologic situation exists, and further evaluation is indicated.

Abnormal variations in the size, configuration, or echographic characteristics of pelvic organs may be the earliest indication of disease, and these findings also require evaluation. In these situations the main contribution of ultrasound examination is the detection or confirmation of pelvic abnormality. This very important contribution in the clinical management of patients should not be overlooked by gynecologists.

CHARACTERIZATION OF PELVIC MASSES

Once the existence of a pelvic mass has been confirmed by ultrasound, it is important that it be characterized as much as possible to assist in the differential diagnosis. Although the test is not specific for the histopathology of a pelvic disease state, it is of considerable value in assessing the malignant potential.

Although there is no ultrasonic pattern that indicates malignancy of a mass lesion, a complex, or mixed solid and cystic appearance, is more likely to be found in a malignant tumor. A solid echogenic pattern can be seen in malignant or benign tumors. Benign cysts, which usually arise in the ovaries, are typically sonolucent with thin, well-defined walls. Septations or localized thickening of the wall of a cyst should raise the suspicion of malignancy. The finding of ascites in a patient with a solid or complex mass strongly suggests pelvic malignancy.

The sonographic characterization of a mass, when correlated with the patient's history, age, and bimanual examination, as well as related findings, such as ascites or evidence of liver metastasis, greatly assists in establishing the potential for malignancy. The total information facilitates the decisions necessary in the management of the patient, in particular, whether surgical exploration or conservative management is indicated. Findings indicating a high potential for malignancy require surgical intervention for confirmation of histology.

PREOPERATIVE ASSESSMENT

Diagnostic ultrasound examination can provide extremely valuable information about the origin and textension of tumors in the pelvis and should be considered as part of the routine preoperative work-up for these patients. Although the examination does not usually give a specific diagnosis, it has been shown to be 82%–91% accurate in documenting the presence, size, and location of a mass in the pelvis (17, 18).

ORIGIN

The determination of the origin of a mass in the pelvis will assist in the preoperative differential diagnosis and may influence what other diagnostic studies are done before surgical intervention. The single most helpful finding that the ultrasonography can provide the clinician is whether the mass is uterine or extrauterine. Uterine masses may be approached directly by cervical and uterine biopsy before exploratory surgery. This procedure is not likely to be informative for an extrauterine mass, but intravenous pyelography and barium enema may be. In some cases ultrasound will reveal that an extrauterine mass is of abdominal origin, rather than pelvic. Further work-up for gastrointestinal malignancy is indicated in this situation, and the findings may alter the surgical approach.

Uterine Masses. Ultrasound is most useful in determining whether there is a tumor of the uterus when the physical examination is equivocal. The uterus is easily outlined on routine sonography by scanning through a distended bladder (23). Uterine size is accurately determined by using the centimeter markers that can be displayed on the image. An assessment can be made of uterine position—whether it is anteverted or retroverted or displaced to one side of the pelvis. This finding may explain a mass palpable on bimanual examination.

The sonographic finding of uterine enlargement raises suspicion of disease within the uterine cavity or a benign or malignant tumor of the uterine wall. Cervical biopsy and endometrial curettement would distinguish these two possibilities. On the other hand, if the uterus is of normal size and the endometrial tissues are normal, the pelvic disease is not likely to be of uterine origin.

The most common tumor-causing uterine enlargement is leiomyoma. Uterine enlargement may be diffuse, or a mural mass may be outlined. These benign, solid tumors characteristically produce diffuse, low-intensity echoes and poor sound transmission on gray-scale sonography. If calcification is present, strong clusters of dense echoes with poor transmission will be identified. Central areas of lucency due to necrosis may also be demonstrated.

In most cases it is not possible to distinguish leiomyoma from malignant sarcoma of the uterus. Sarcoma also produces uterine enlargement because of the growing mass within the uterine cavity or wall. The echoes produced by the sarcoma are usually very intense, and often there are relative cystic areas within the tumor. Since sarcomas often involve the uterine cavity, a relatively lucent band produced by the normal uterine wall may be seen surrounding the dense, irregular echoes from the sarcoma (Fig. 23–1).

Trophoblastic disease of the uterus also presents as an enlarged uterus. Suspicion is aroused clinically when the uterine size exceeds that expected for the stage of gestation. This is usually associated with marked elevation in the gonadotropin levels. The characteristic internal appearance of hydatidiform mole on gray-scale sonography is a low-level echo mass with multiple small cysts filling the entire uterus (11, 20). The cystic spaces within a mole represent areas of hemorrhage and necrosis. In approximately 30% of cases of mole, bilateral multiloculated cystic ovarian masses are present. These represent theca-lutean cysts. The differential diagnosis of hydatidiform mole includes fibroid tumor with degeneration, retained placenta, missed abortion, endometritis, and sarcoma. By correlating the sonographic findings with the patient's age, history, gonadotropin levels, and findings on endometrial curettement, the diagnosis can be established.

A malignant tumor of the cervix or uterine fundus can also cause a mass of uterine origin. Ultrasound examination has not been of signifi-

cant value in diagnosing lesions confined to the cervix, since these are readily visualized and palpated by pelvic examination. It has been noted, however, that exophytic lesions confined to the cervix or lower uterine segment characteristically produce a mass with very dense internal echoes (Fig. 23–2).

Carcinoma of the uterine fundus cannot be identified in its early stages but may produce uterine enlargement as the tumor grows. This enlargement is usually symmetrical. Thickening of the endometrial cavity may occur with endometrial carcinoma. This cannot, however, be distinguished from other causes of this finding, which include cystic glandular hyperplasia, incomplete abortion, ectopic pregnancy, and retained blood clots. Clinical correlation and endometrial biopsy are necessary to distinguish these disease states.

Extrauterine masses. The most common origin of an extrauterine mass is the ovary. These lesions may be benign or malignant. Specific distinction is not possible with ultrasound, but the finding of well-defined, thin-walled, bilateral cystic lesions is usually indicative of benign disease. Malignancy within a cyst is suggested by the identification of thickening of the cyst wall, areas of solid echogenic tissue within the cyst, or grossly thickened septa. Clotted blood or thick mucus can produce echoes within the cyst that may mimic solid tissue and lead to misinterpretation of the nature of the mass. Ovarian malignancy should be suspected when there is a solid tumor with internal echoes located laterally in the pelvis. Benign tumors of the ovary, such as fibroma, can also give a solid appearance (Fig. 23–3).

Complex tumors, with both solid and cystic components, are usually malignant (6, 9, 10, 16, 24). Large dermoid cysts are usually complex, however, and may have septations. In some cases standard radiography will demonstrate fat or tooth structure in the tumor to help in the differential diagnosis of dermoid or teratoma. Although the appearance of most ovarian masses does not permit a specific histologic diagnosis, a mass separate from the uterus and containing disorganized internal echoes and a complex ap-

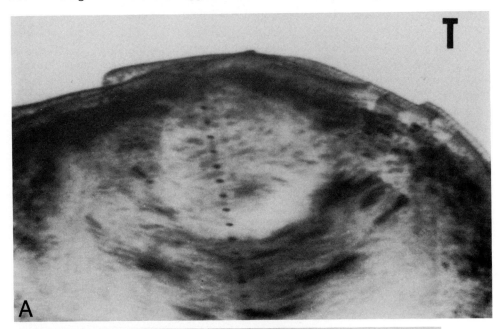

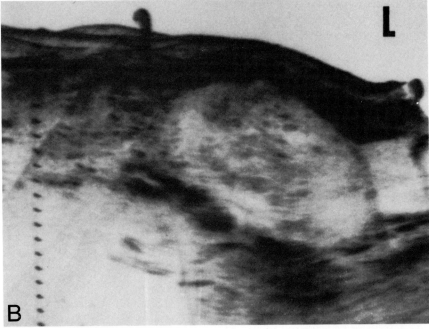

FIG. 23–1. Sarcoma of the uterus. **A.** Transverse scan. **B.** Longitudinal scan. The uterus is enlarged and there are clusters of dense echoes from the centrally located tumor. The surrounding uterine wall is less echogenic. **C.** Gross specimen showing the convoluted solid tumor filling the uterine cavity.

FIG. 23-1. (*Continued*)

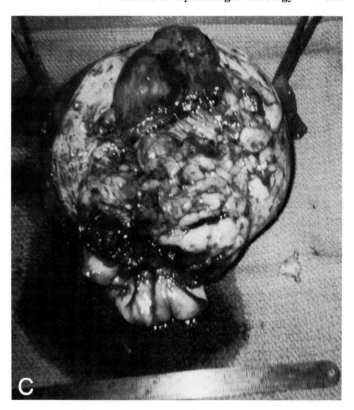

pearance suggests ovarian carcinoma. The finding of ascites in a patient who has a solid or complex pelvic mass strongly suggests neoplastic disease (Fig. 23–4).

Malignant tumors of the colon can also present as an extrauterine pelvic mass. These tumors are echogenic, and the margins are usually somewhat irregular. The barium enema will distinguish a mass of colon origin from other extrauterine masses.

Another malignant condition that can present as a mass in the pelvis is lymphoma. Large lymphomatous nodes in the external or internal iliac chain may present as extrauterine pelvic masses. Characteristically they are sonolucent, well marginated, and laterally located. Often they are multiple or bilateral. Ultrasound findings are not specific, but the diagnosis is suspected when the ultrasound scan of the retroperitoneal and abdominal region shows other areas of involvement, or the patient presents with peripheral nodal disease and has an established diagnosis of lymphoma. The sonar findings indicate involvement of the pelvic lymph nodes with disease and thus assist in staging of disease.

Krugenberg tumor of the ovary cannot be distinguished from primary ovarian carcinoma. These metastatic lesions also usually present as a complex mass, with homogeneous, low-level internal echoes, possibly imbedded in a fluid matrix (22). The history of a breast, gynecologic, orgastrointestinal malignancy in a patient with this sonographic finding should raise the suspicion that this is a metastatic tumor. If the colon is the primary lesion, the carcinoembryonic antigen level may be elevated.

There are many benign conditions that should be included in the differential diagnosis of extrauterine masses. These include abscess, hematoma, and endometrioma. They have a similar

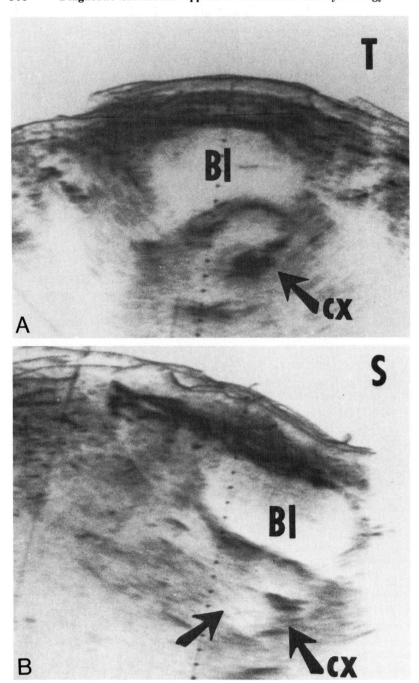

FIG. 23-2. Carcinoma of the cervix. **A.** Transverse scan. **B.** Sagittal scan. Exophytic, echogenic mass involving the lower uterine segment and cervix (CX); BI, bladder.

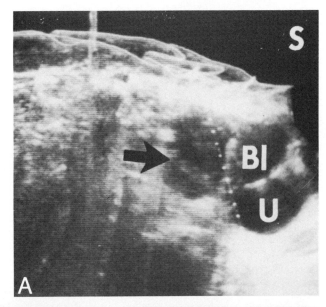

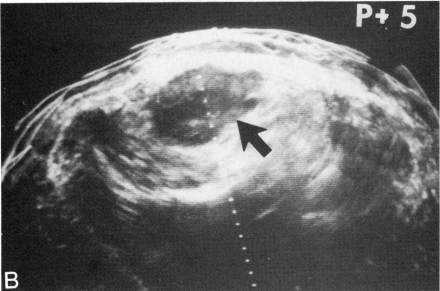

FIG. 23–3. Carcinoma of the ovary. **A.** Sagittal scan. There is a 5- × 6-cm echogenic mass (**arrow**) compressing the bladder (Bl); U, uterus. **B.** transverse scan, 5 cm above the pubis. The solid mass with irregular margins measures 6 × 9 cm in this plane.

sonographic appearance. They are usually well-defined mass lesions and may be either faintly echogenic or cystic in appearance. Tuboovarian abscess is often multiloculated. Ectopic gestation has a characteristic appearance, and the history and clinical course is usually diagnostic. Patients with lymphocele usually have a history of trauma or surgery, and the diagnosis can be suspected clinically. They are typically sonolu-

cent and thin walled. Hydrosalpinx presents as an extrauterine mass that is usually sonolucent. The unilateral appearance and clinical history are usually helpful in establishing this diagnosis. Generally, the diagnosis of these benign conditions can be suspected when the ultrasound finding is correlated with the history and clinical findings.

Rarely, a patient may present with a pelvic

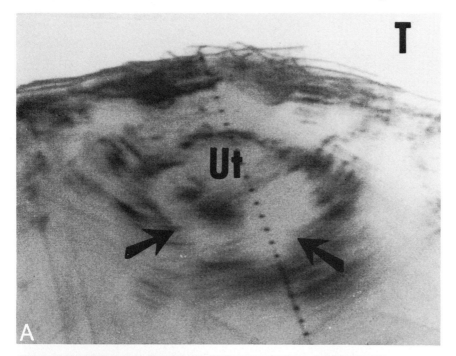

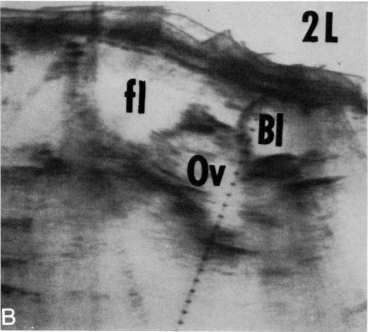

FIG. 23-4. Bilateral carcinoma of the ovary with ascites. **A.** Transverse scan showing bilateral complex masses (**arrows**) lateral to the uterus (Ut). The echo-free area anterior to the uterus is ascitic fluid. **B.** Sagittal scan 2 cm to the left of midline shows the left ovarian mass (Ov) and ascites (fl); Bl, bladder.

mass that is extrauterine in origin and has the typical sonographic appearance of a kidney, with demonstration of the pelvocalyceal system. This is diagnostic of a pelvic kidney and would not be an indication for surgery.

EXTENSION

In addition to documenting the presence, size, and location of a pelvic mass, ultrasonography can detect findings that not only are suggestive of malignancy but also assist in the clinical staging of the disease. These findings include evidence of direct extension to other pelvic structures, such as the bladder or lateral pelvic sidewall, lymph node metastasis in the pelvis or periaortic region, hematogenous spread to the liver, ascites, and peritoneal implants. Documentation and verification of these situations will significantly influence the management of the patient with pelvic malignancy and is a major reason for routine sonographic examination in patients with pelvic malignancy prior to treatment.

Direct Extension

LATERAL PELVIS. The extension of central pelvic tumors to the lateral pelvis advances the stage of disease and influences the treatment and prognosis. In some patients it may be difficult to document lateral extension by bimanual pelvic examination because of obesity, scarring from previous surgery, or anatomic distortion due to the primary tumor. In these situations sonography can assist the clinician in determining lateral extension from carcinoma of the cervix and uterus. Whereas minimal infiltration cannot be detected, mass-like thickening in the parametrial or paracervical regions usually indicates tumor. Inflammatory changes do not usually produce the bandlike echogenic soft tissue prominence seen with tumor. The documentation of extension to the pelvic side wall usually indicates unresectability (Fig. 23–5).

BLADDER. Ultrasonography can be of value in documenting extension of pelvic neoplasm to the bladder. The sonographic finding of mucosal thickening in the bladder near a pelvic tumor should raise suspicion of invasion of the bladder

FIG. 23-5. Carcinoma of the cervix. Transverse scan. The tumor extends to the left lateral pelvic side wall (**arrows**) and produces marked parametrial thickening; Bl bladder.

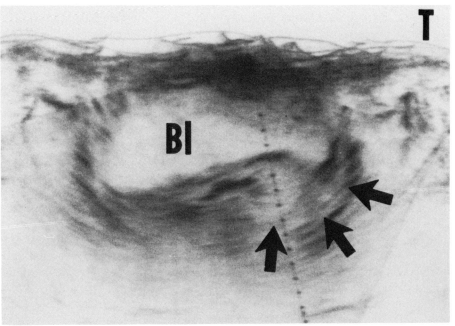

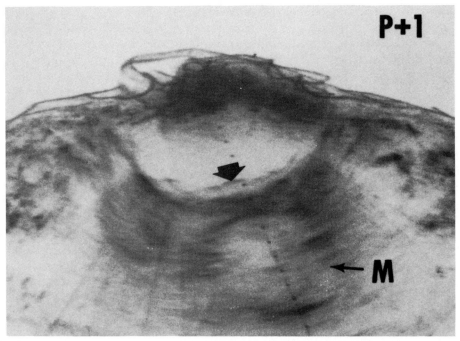

FIG. 23-6. Tumor extension to the bladder with mucosal edema (**arrow**). Recurrent carcinoma of the ovary producing an irregular solid mass (M). Transverse scan, 1 cm above the pubis.

(Fig. 23-6). Cystoscopy and biopsy of the bladder in the area of sonographic abnormality are indicated for complete staging.

Lymphatic Extension. Lymph nodes involved with tumor characteristically enlarge to produce mass lesions. Depending on the location of the enlarged nodes and the resolution of the sonographic system, these nodes are detectable when they become a certain size. In the pelvis, nodes 3 cm or more in diameter can be outlined. In the paraaortic region those 2 cm or greater can be demonstrated (5). Although documentation of enlarged nodes in the pelvic and paraaortic regions in patients with pelvic malignancy is not specific for tumor, this finding usually indicates metastatic disease. The absence of enlarged nodes by sonography does not rule out lymphatic involvement, since node enlargement may not occur with early microscopic involvement.

Enlarged lymph nodes in the pelvis appear as sonolucent, well-defined, concentric masses located laterally. Involvement of specific node chains, such as the external iliac, internal iliac, or inguinal nodes can often be determined (Fig. 23-7).

Paraaortic lymph node enlargement produces a characteristic appearance. The nodes lie anterior and lateral to the vertebral body, and as they enlarge, they may displace the vena cava and aorta from their normal location along the spine. Multiple sonolucent, lobulated masses in the paraaortic region, with or without displacement of the major vessels, is diagnostic of retroperitoneal lymph node enlargement (Fig. 23-8).

In our experience sonography has been 94% accurate in detecting enlarged lymph nodes in the retroperitoneum in patients with Hodgkin's disease and lymphoma (5). No one has yet documented the accuracy in gynecologic malignancy. In a number of cases of cervical and ovarian carcinoma in our series sonography has demonstrated enlarged nodes in the paraaortic region that were subsequently confirmed by exploratory laparotomy and biopsy to be malignant metastasis. Since a negative study cannot exclude microscopic disease involvement in the

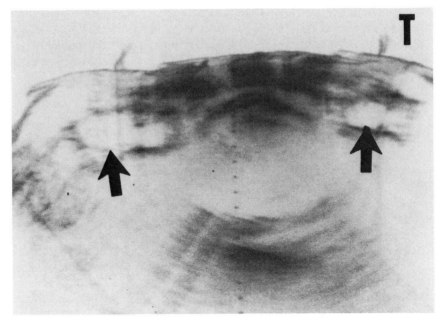

FIG. 23-7. Enlarged external iliac lymph nodes (**arrows**). Carcinoma of the vulva. Transverse scan.

FIG. 23-8. Enlarged paraaortic lymph nodes (**arrows**). Carcinoma of the cervix. Transverse scan. The lobulated, echogenic, enlarged nodes have displaced the aorta (a) away from the spine (s).

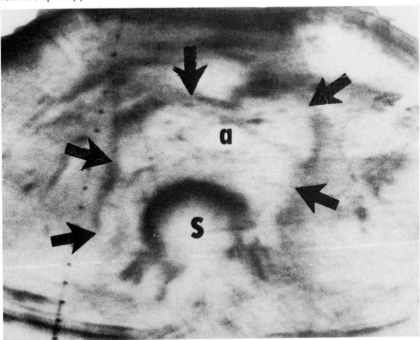

nodes, this technique will not replace staging laparotomy in patients with negative scans. However, the demonstration of enlarged nodes by sonography with confirmation by lymphangiography would indicate disease spread outside of the pelvis and may negate the need for exploratory laparotomy for staging.

Hematogenous Spread. The most frequent site of hematogenous metastasis from pelvic malignancy is the liver. Sonography is an effective method of documenting metastatic foci in the liver. The liver should, therefore, be scanned as part of the sonographic study of patients with suspected or proved gynecologic neoplasm.

The sonographic appearance of liver metastasis is quite variable. Four different patterns have been reported (13, 25). These are as follows: dense, lucent, bullseye, and mixed. The most common pattern is that of single or multiple echodense foci within the liver parenchyma. These lesions may coalesce into lobular masses. Metastatic adenocarcinoma usually has this dense appearance. A second common manifestation of hepatic metastasis is that of a well-defined sonolucent area surrounded by normal liver parenchyma. Fine, low-level echoes can be recorded within these lesions, indicating that they are solid (Fig. 23–9).

The third type is the bullseye lesion, with a dense, central focus surrounded by a more lucent periphery. The fourth type presents as a mixed pattern, with diffuse inhomogeneity. These usually display multiple coarse, dense and/or lucent areas, but without a dominant pattern of focal lesions. The pattern of hepatic metastasis from gynecologic malignancies is not specific.

If liver sonography reveals one of the patterns of metastasis, the findings should be confirmed by abnormal liver function study. The single most valuable function test is the alkaline phosphatase. If the clinical and laboratory picture is not consistent with liver abnormality, documentation by biopsy is preferable, if the result will significantly modify patient management. Biopsy can be performed at laparoscopy with direct visualization or percutaneously by use of a special ultrasound biopsy transducer.

Ascites. The presence of ascites in a patient with a solid or complex pelvic mass usually in-

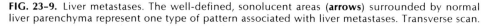

FIG. 23–9. Liver metastases. The well-defined, sonolucent areas (**arrows**) surrounded by normal liver parenchyma represent one type of pattern associated with liver metastases. Transverse scan.

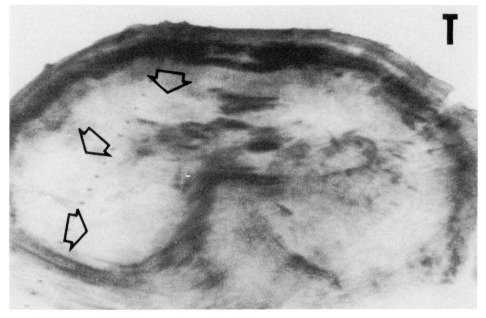

dicates malignancy. Fluid in the pelvis and abdominal cavity is easily demonstrated (14). It has been estimated that as little as 100 mm can be detected (12). Fluid accumulates in the most dependent portions of the abdominal cavity. Therefore, with the patient in the supine position for examination, small amounts of fluid will be seen in the pelvis and upper abdomen behind the liver. This fluid is sonolucent and provides excellent echo-free contrast around the solid, echo-producing organs such as liver, uterus, and bladder wall (Fig. 23–10).

Some have tried to make a distinction between benign and malignant ascites (16, 17, 24). In benign ascites due to cirrhosis or heart failure, loops of bowel float freely in the fluid centrally in the peritoneal cavity, and the flanks bulge with the fluid. In malignant ascites the loops are often adherent to each other or the peritoneal surface. However, adhesions from previous surgery or infection can also cause this loculated appearance.

Free fluid is distinguished from cystic masses and loculated fluid collections by reexamining the patient in lateral decubitus position. Free fluid will shift to the dependent region; loculated fluid or cyst will not change in appearance with a change in position.

Sonography can be used to determine the best location for paracentesis. The needle is placed away from the identifiable loops of bowel and mesentery. Reexamination after fluid removal determines the amount of residual fluid. The examination is repeated at the time of reevaluation of the patient to determine if repeat paracentesis is needed for reaccumulation of fluid.

Peritoneal Implants. The documentation of ascitic fluid in patients with gynecologic malignancy usually indicates advanced disease, with extrapelvic spread and serosal implants. If the amount of fluid is sufficient to displace bowel from the serosal surface of the abdominal wall, it may be possible to document peritoneal implants. The side of the implant demonstrable will depend on the resolution of the sonographic system. We have visualized peritoneal implants 1 cm in diameter (Fig. 23–11). The documentation of peritoneal implants and ascites would indicate advanced neoplastic disease and a nonsurgical management problem.

RADIATION THERAPY PLANNING

Ultrasound is a very valuable tool for obtaining anatomic information for radiation treatment planning (2, 3, 4). In many situations this information cannot be obtained by any other noninvasive method. Use of this technique can idealize therapy plans for patients receiving either external or internal radiation for pelvic malignancy.

EXTERNAL RADIATION

External irradiation is commonly used to treat pelvic malignancy, either initially or for postoperative surgical recurrence. If a mass is present, sonography is indicated to determine the location and size of the mass prior to the establishment of the radiation field. The ultrasound information and other available information about the extent of tumor are used to place the field on the patient's external surface. Sonography allows direct visualization of the margins of the deep tumor as the fields are being marked. Scanning in both the transverse and longitudinal planes gives three-dimensional information about the tumor position and shape, and the hand-held transducer is used to determine at which point on the skin surface the radiation field margins should be located to encompass all of the mass and a suitable margin of normal tissue (Fig. 23–12).

This dynamic method of establishing radiation fields has been shown to be more accurate than clinical palpation (7). Use of sonography for external irradiation field setup for pelvic tumors decreases the chance of underdosage to the tumor because of anatomic miss.

In addition the scan produces an accurate contour of the patient in the region of treatment and shows the relative position of the tumor to the body surface. This information is used in the radiation dose calculations to further improve the radiation technique. Moreover, the relative position of the bladder and rectum in the treatment volume can be documented by ultrasound.

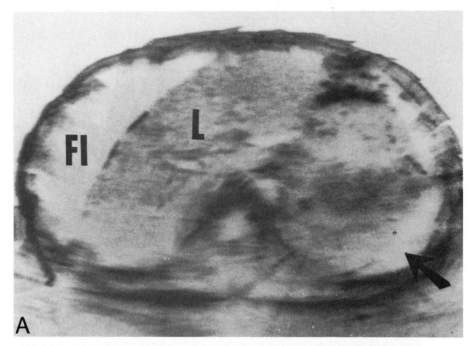

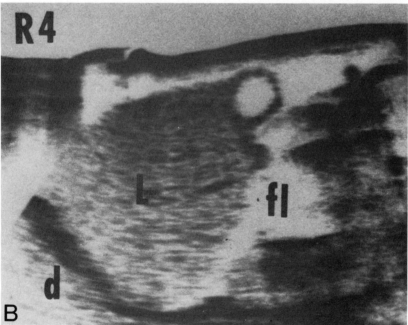

FIG. 23–10. A. Fluid (Fl) surrounding the liver (L) and in the left flank (**arrow**). **B.** Longitudinal scan, 4 cm to the right of midline. Fluid (fl) surrounds the liver (L). Note the gallbladder at the anterior tip of the liver; d, diaphragm.

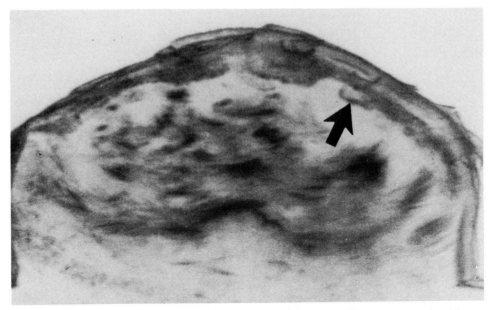

FIG. 23-11. Peritoneal implant (**arrow**) from carcinoma of the cervix. The tumor is outlined by ascitic fluid, which displaces the loops of bowel from the serosal surface. Transverse scan.

This information can assist in the development of plans that minimize the dose to these radiosensitive normal structures. Sonography can, therefore, theoretically improve the quality of external irradiation therapy for patients with pelvic malignancy by providing anatomic information that will decrease the risk of tumor miss and help prevent overdosage of normal organs.

INTRACAVITARY RADIATION

Intracavitary radiotherapy is frequently used in the treatment of carcinoma of the endometrium. It can be used preoperatively or in combination with external irradiation with an intent to cure. In using intrauterine irradiation it is imperative that the size and shape of the uterus be known so that adequate doses can be given to the myometrium, but maximum tolerable doses to the surrounding radiosensitive structures such as bladder, rectum, and small bowel will not be exceeded. The size of the uterus and the anatomy within the pelvis can easily and accurately be determined by sonography prior to insertion of intracavitary applicators (Fig. 23–13). Determining the uterine size and configuration prior

to insertion allows proper selection of an appropriate applicator. In some cases ultrasound may reveal abnormal pelvic masses that would alter the treatment plan (Fig. 23–14).

Scanning the pelvis following insertion of an afterloading applicator is safe and easily performed. Individualized dosimetry can be devised, depending on the position of the applicator, the uterine size and configuration, and the relative position of the bladder (Fig. 23–15). The afterloading technique allows selection of radioactive sources to fit the clinical problem and permits consistent radiation doses to be delivered to critical points within the pelvis.

Ultrasound examination is also indicated after any intrauterine application when there is a possibility of uterine perforation by the applicator. The tandem position can easily be localized by the strong echoes from its surface and the relative position of the tandem to the uterus documented. If it is not within the uterine cavity, perforation has occurred (Fig. 23–16). This is the only noninvasive, direct method of detecting this serious situation. Confirmation of perforation by sonography requires removal of the applicator.

Whereas the uses of sonography in gyneco-
(*Text continues on p. 319*)

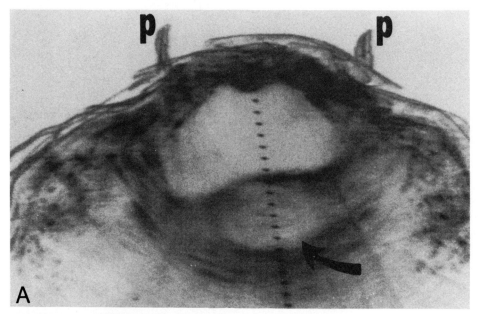

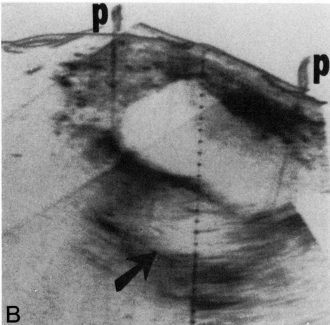

FIG. 23–12. External irradiation fields for recurrent carcinoma of the ovary, posthysterectomy. **A.** Transverse scan. **B.** Longitudinal scan. The solid tumor (**arrow**) is outlined behind the bladder. The radiation field margins (p) are marked on the display by lifting the transducer. The patient's skin is also marked at these points to locate the radiation field on the body surface. The depth, shape, and size of the tumor can be determined from the display for dosimetry calculations.

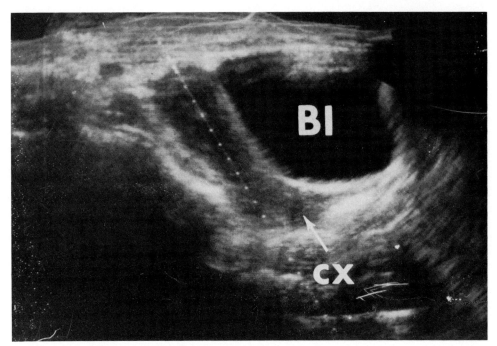

FIG. 23–13. Longitudinal scan of the uterus before intracavitary treatment. The uterus is long and narrow (11 × 3.5 cm) and is anteverted; cx, cervix, Bl, bladder. A single tandem applicator rather than the multiple capsule technique was used because of the shape of the uterus. The dose to the bladder was monitored to prevent overdosage.

FIG. 23–14. Transverse pelvic scan before intracavity treatment for adenocarcinoma of the uterine cavity. A 2.5-cm mass (M) is present in the right pelvis. Radiation therapy was aborted, and exploratory laparotomy revealed carcinoma of the right ovary with metastasis to the endometrial cavity. The patient was treated surgically; Ut, uterus, Bl, bladder.

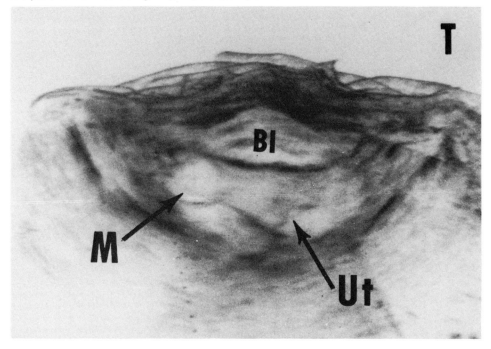

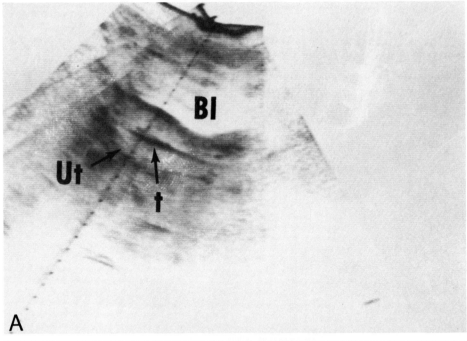

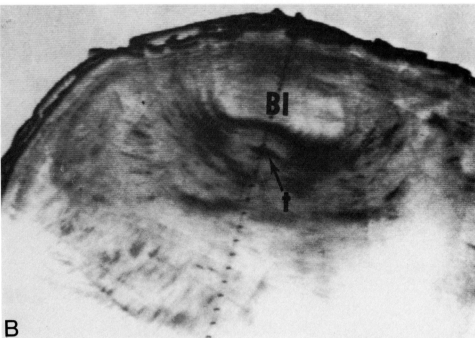

FIG. 23–15. Intracavitary applicator in the uterus. **A.** Sagittal scan. **B.** Transverse scan. The intra-uterine tandem (t) can be outlined within the uterus (Ut), and the uterine wall thickness measured for dosimetry calculations; Bl, bladder.

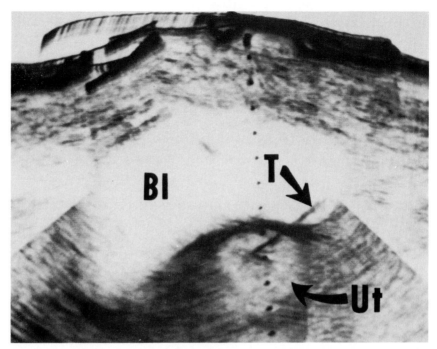

FIG. 23–16. Uterine perforation by an intracavitary applicator in a patient with carcinoma of the cervix. Transverse scan. The tandem (t) can be seen within the bladder (Bl). Ut, lower uterine segment.

logic diagnosis are well documented, the application of this modality in radiation therapy for gynecologic malignancy has been limited to a few treatment centers. With the current availability of diagnostic ultrasound equipment in most modern hospitals this important application should be more widely used by radiation therapists. Sonography is a simple and reliable method of obtaining precise anatomic information that allows individualized external and internal radiation treatment programs to be developed. This should result in improved cure rates and reduced complications in the treatment of patients with pelvic malignancy.

FOLLOW-UP
SURGERY

In the immediate postoperative period sonography can be helpful in evaluating the deep pelvic anatomy when abscess, hematoma, or fluid collections are suspected clinically. The occurrence of a drop in hematocrit or tempera-ture elevation in a postoperative patient is an indication for sonography. If there are no suprapubic dressings, the pelvis can usually be adequately examined by compound scanning through a slightly distended bladder. If there is postoperative ileus, bowel gas may prevent satisfactory examination. The sonographic finding of a mass in the pelvis in these clinical situations indicates that one of these complications has occurred.

By use of sonographic criteria alone, hematoma and abscess cannot be distinguished. Both appear cystic early, and with clotting or necrosis, internal echoes may be demonstrated (Fig. 23–17). Fluid collections, such as lymphocele, are typically cystic. After initial documentation of a mass, sonography is used to follow response in patients treated conservatively (15). If surgical drainage is performed, ultrasound examination is used to record the completeness of resolution or to detect further recurrence.

Sonography can play a valuable role in the late follow-up of patients treated initially by

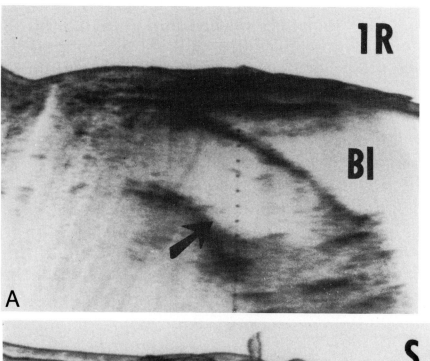

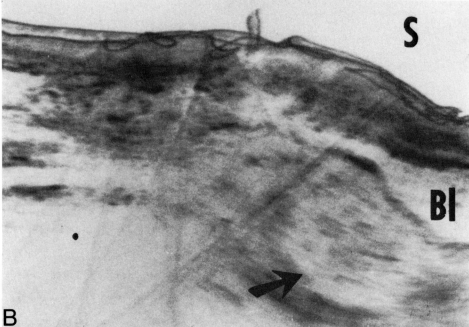

FIG. 23–17. Postoperative complications following hysterectomy. **A.** Abscess. There is a sonolucent mass (**arrow**) behind the bladder (Bl). Sagittal scan, 1 cm to the right of midline. **B.** Hematoma. There is an echogenic mass (**arrow**) behind the bladder (Bl). Sagittal scan, midline. The echo pattern is not characteristic, and the lesions cannot be distinguished by ultrasound characteristics alone.

surgery. If the bimanual pelvic examination is equivocal or suspicious for a mass in the pelvis, sonography is performed to rule out or document recurrence (Fig. 23–18). The scan can be done with no special patient preparation and can usually be completed in 15 min with no patient discomfort. A negative scan usually indicates that it is safe to defer further evaluation until the next routine follow-up. Confirmation of a pelvic mass by ultrasound examination indicates, however, the need for immediate workup for recurrent malignancy.

Since central pelvic masses as small as 2 cm can be detected with sonography, this test may demonstrate lesions not palpable in the postoperative patient. In some cases disease reactivation can be detected before it is clinically evident by routine examination by ultrasound. This early detection of occult disease may improve the salvage rates in patients with recurrence after surgery.

RADIATION AND CHEMOTHERAPY

Sonography is a safe, simple, and inexpensive method of following response of pelvic tumors to radiation or drug therapy. A base-line scan is performed at the beginning of therapy. For radiation therapy patients serial scans are performed at appropriate intervals during the treatment program and compared to the initial pretherapy scan. Monitoring in this manner allows modification of radiation fields as tumor size changes.

Similarly, ultrasound is used to follow patients on prolonged chemotherapy for pelvic malignancy. The ultrasound examination can be performed on the day of follow-up examination and compared with the previous scans. The tumor size is graded as "no change, increased or decreased." This assessment is used in correlation with the other clinical information by the clinician to make decisions in chemotherapeutic management (Fig. 23–19). In patients who have responded completely to radiation or chemotherapy, ultrasound is an added parameter that can be used to detect reactivation of disease. Previously irradiated patients are often difficult to evaluate by pelvic examination because of radiation adhesions in the vagina. Sonography

can show the status of the uterus and other pelvic structures beyond the scar tissue. Recurrence usually presents as a mass and is detectable by ultrasound study. Whether the tumor is confined to the uterus or extends to the lateral pelvis or to the pelvic or paraaortic lymph nodes can be documented (Fig. 23–20). The information obtained by this noninvasive technique greatly assists in initial restaging of the recurrence and facilitates appropriate treatment decisions. If there is documentation of extension out of the pelvis or to the pelvic side wall, the patient is not controllable by surgery, and radiation or chemotherapy must be considered for management.

LIMITATIONS OF SONOGRAPHY

The major limitation of sonography in pelvic malignancy is the lack of specificity of the findings. This prevents distinction between benign and malignant pelvic masses. Biopsy is still necessary to make the histologic diagnosis, after a mass is documented by sonography.

The other major limitations regard technical problems in examination. Gas or barium in the bowel may interfere with transmission of the sound waves and prevent adequate evaluation of the pelvic structures. This is especially true in the patient with adynamic ileus secondary to pain or surgery. One of the most common interpretation errors is mistaking loops of fluid-filled bowel for mass lesions (17).

Surgical dressings may prevent the contact application of the ultrasound transducer to the skin surface and must be removed if the study is to be performed. Careful cleansing of the transducer surface with antiseptics will usually prevent the introduction of infection at the surgical site. Postoperative patients may have tenderness in the surgical wound that will prevent adequate skin contact of the transducer. These problems are rare, however, and satisfactory examination can be performed in the majority of cases.

PROSPECTS

It is inevitable that technical improvements will be made in diagnostic ultrasound systems that

(*Text continues on p. 324*)

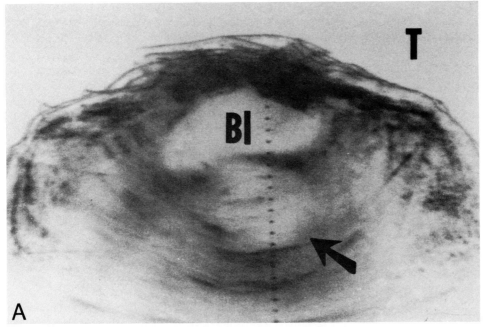

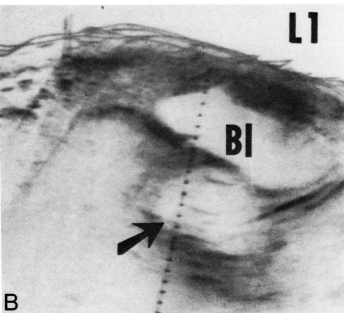

FIG. 23-18. Tumor recurrence after surgery. Carcinoma of the ovary. **A.** Transverse scan. **B.** Sagittal scan, 1 cm to the left of midline. A 7.5 × 9 × 10-cm solid mass (**arrow**) posterior to the bladder (Bl) is documented by sonography.

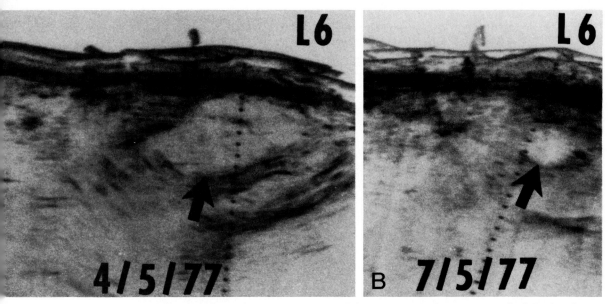

FIG. 23-19. Response to therapy. Carcinoma of the ovary. Sagittal scan 6 cm to the left of midline. **A.** An 8-cm solid metastasis (**arrow**) is demonstrated in the lower abdomen before treatment. **B.** The same mass (**arrow**) measures 3 cm in diameter after 3 months of chemotherapy. It was not palpable at the time of this examination.

FIG. 23-20. Recurrent carcinoma of the ovary after hysterectomy. Sagittal scan 1 cm to the left of midline. There is a 3.5-cm solid mass (M) posterior to the bladder (Bl). This represents midpelvic recurrence. Also demonstrated is a 3-cm presacral node (N), indicating lymphatic metastasis away from the central pelvis and nonresectability.

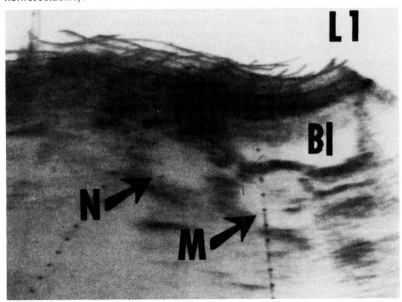

will greatly enhance resolution and definition. These developments should increase the contributions of ultrasound in the management of patients with pelvic malignancy. More specific diagnosis should be possible. Computer analysis of subtle differences in echo patterns from within solid tumors has the potential of allowing noninvasive tumor identification (1). Refinement in equipment design has already occurred and allows supplemental transrectal and transvaginal scanning. This technique may significantly improve the diagnostic potential of ultrasonography in patients with pelvic tumors.

There has been some speculation that computerized axial tomography will replace sonography in the evaluation and management of patients with malignancy. Although large masses can be detected, both the character of the mass or the extension to surrounding tissues have not been determined with great accuracy by axial tomography. Early investigators have shown that ultrasound and computerized tomography reveal the same information, and do not complement one another in the detection of pelvic diseases. The safety, simplicity, and relative low cost of ultrasound examination delegate this study to be first choice for initial study of pelvic masses and for the majority of applications discussed in this chapter.

CONCLUSION

Although sonography is not diagnostic of the histopathology of pelvic masses, important information about the origin, characterization, size, and extension of mass lesions can be obtained quickly and safely. In some cases the ultrasound study simply confirms the pelvic examination findings, while in others, additional information is revealed that is helpful in the differential diagnosis. The examination is indicated when there is suspected or definite pelvic mass of undetermined origin, since the information it can provide may be extremely valuable in the management of the patient.

In patients with confirmed pelvic malignancy, ultrasound is valuable in the pretreatment assessment, particularly regarding extension of tumor beyond the primary site. It assists in radiation therapy planning for external and intracavitary techniques. It can be used to follow response of mass lesions to radiation or chemotherapy and, after surgery, can be used to evaluate suspected complications or recurrent malignancy.

Since this noninvasive examination is safe for the patient, easy to perform, and relatively inexpensive, it should play an increasingly important role in the field of gynecologic malignancy, especially as more clinicians become aware of the possible contributions it can make in the management of their individual cases.

REFERENCES

1. BIRNHOLZ J: (Letter): Ultrasonography of ovarian masses. N Engl J Med 294:906, 1976
2. BRASCHO D: Radiation therapy planning with ultrasound. Radiol Clin North Am 13:505–521, 1975
3. BRASCHO D: Tumor localization and treatment planning with ultrasound. Cancer 39:697–705, 1977
4. BRASCHO D, BRYAN J, WILSON E: Diagnostic ultrasound to determine renal size and position for renal blocking in radiation therapy. Int J Radiat Oncl Biol Phys 2:1217–1220, 1977
5. BRASCHO D, DURANT J, GREEN L: The accuracy of retroperitoneal ultrasonography in Hodgkin's disease and non-Hodgkin's lymphoma. Radiology 125:485–487, 1977
6. CAROVALE R, SAMUELS B: (Letter): Complex ovarian mass on ultrasound: primary or metastatic tumor? N Engl J Med 294:446–447, 1976
7. CARTER S, DENNY I, TISH D, MARTY R, DAVIS M: Ultrasonic evaluation of radiation therapy ports. J Clin Ultrasound 5:103–106, 1977
8. COCHRANE W: Ultrasound in gynecology. Radiol Clin North Am 13:457–466, 1975
9. COCHRANE W, THOMAS M: Ultrasound diagnosis of gynecologic pelvic masses. Radiology 110:649–654, 1974
10. DONALD I, ABDULLA U: Ultrasonics in obstetrics and gynecology. Br J Radiol 40:604–611, 1967
11. FLEISCHER A, JAMES A, KRAUSE D, MILLIS J: Sonographic patterns in trophoblastic diseases. Radiology 126:215–220, 1978
12. GOLDBERG B, GOODMAN G, CLEARFIELD H: Evaluation of ascites by ultrasound. Radiology 96:15–22, 1970
13. GREEN B, BREE R, GOLDSTEIN H, STANLEY C: Grayscale ultrasound evaluation of hepatic neoplasms: patterns and correlations. Radiology 124:203–208, 1977

14. HIINING R, KINSER J: The diagnosis of ascites by ultrasonic tomography (B-scan). Br J Radiol 46:325–328, 1973

15. KAPLAN G, SANDERS R: B-scan ultrasound in the management of patients with occult abdominal hematomas. J Clin Ultrasound 1:5–13,1973

16. KRATOCHWIL A: Ultrasonic diagnosis in pelvic malignancy. Clin Obstet Gynecol 13:898–909, 1970

17. LAWSON T, ALBARELLI J: Diagnosis of gynecologic pelvic masses by gray-scale ultrasonography: analysis of specificity and accuracy. Am J Roentgenol 128:1003–1006, 1977

18. LEVI S, DELVAL R: Value of ultrasonic diagnosis of gynecologic tumors in 370 surgical cases. Obstet Gynecol Scand 55:261–266, 1976

19. MORLEY P, BARNETT E: The use of ultrasound in the diagnosis of pelvic masses. Br J Radiol 43:602–616, 1970

20. PERLMUTTER G, GOLDBERG B: Ultrasound in obstetrics and gynecology. J Reprod Med 20:1–21, 1978

21. QUEENAN J, JUBARYCH E, DOUGLAS D: Evaluation of diagnostic ultrasound in gynecology. Am J Obstet Gynecol 123:453–465, 1975

22. ROCHESTER D, LEVIN B, BOWIE J, KUNZMANN A: Ultrasonic appearance of the Kurkenberg tumor. Am J Roentgenol 129:919–920, 1977

23. SAMPLE W, LIPPE B, GYEPES M: Gray-scale ultrasonography of the normal female pelvis. Radiology 125:477–483, 1977

24. SAMUELS B: Usefulness of ultrasound in patients with ovarian cancer. Semin Oncol 2:229–233, 1975

25. SCHEIBLE W, GOSINK B, LEOPOLD G: Gray-scale echographic patterns of hepatic metastatic disease. Am J Roentgenol 129:983–987, 1977

26. THOMPSON H, TAYLOR E, HOLMES J et al: Ultrasound diagnostic techniques in obstetrics and gynecology. Am J Obstet Gynecol 472, 1964

24

Breast imaging

ELIZABETH KELLY-FRY

In the past decade ultrasound visualization techniques have been widely used as a routine clinical tool for examination of various soft-tissue regions of the body and in the past 5 years significant advances have been made in this instrumentation. In the Western world, however, application of ultrasonic instrumentation for breast examination has, by comparison, been quite limited. Considering the present critical need for improved accuracy of detection of breast cancer by noninvasive methods, in terms of the current capability of ultrasound techniques, ultrasound breast examination programs should give first priority to the goal of applying ultrasound at its current level of relative sophistication to assist the physician in the differential diagnosis of breast pathologies. Additionally, in view of the nonionizing character of ultrasonic energy, emphasis should be placed on repeated examination of subjects with a previous diagnosis of "benign breast pathology" to accomplish early detection of the malignant changes that may take place, after a period of time, in benign conditions. In designing instrumentation to achieve these specific goals, particular attention should be devoted to using present knowledge of the structural characteristics of both benign and malignant breast masses, as revealed by other examination techniques and, in particular, mammography and histology.

There are a number of other aspects of ultrasound technology, such as computerized tomography, computer image enhancement, and so forth, Doppler techniques, that have relevance to detection of breast cancer, but these are not the subject of this paper. The primary purpose of this paper is to provide background knowledge of the development of currently standard ultrasound visualization techniques for breast examination and to relate this past history to clinical needs at the time of this writing (1978).

BACKGROUND

During an approximate 10-year period, starting in the early 1950s, John Wild and associates and Douglas Howry and his coinvestigators performed the studies that are the foundation for present investigation on the use of ultrasound for breast examination (32–35, 95–100). In 1951 John Wild and Donald Neal published results on the application, for breast examination, of a military ultrasound instrument. The unit consisted of a hand-held, 15-MHz quartz crystal transceiver mounted at one end of a water-filled chamber, with the other end sealed by a rubber membrane that was placed directly over the area of the tumor (95). Standard electronic equipment was used for energizing the crystal, amplifying the returned echo signals, and displaying the A-mode responses on a cathode ray tube (98, 100). By 1951, 19 breast patients, in addition to the first 2 examined with the original instrument, were diagnosed with newly constructed A-mode ultrasound instrumentation (97). In making their diagnoses, Wild and Reid analyzed three possibly significant aspects of the A-mode echograms, but the only data that appeared significant were the ratio of the area beneath the vertical deflection (ie, the A-scope trace, which represents the average returned sound) for a tumor, and that of normal breast tissue. The normal breast, or control, in most cases was the opposite breast of the same subject. On the basis of these and later results, Wild and Reid concluded: "In general, cancer tissue returned more sound than normal control tissue and that nonmalignant tissue returned less sound than normal control tissue" (99). This finding influenced the course of future studies in this field.

Wild and Reid also developed a two-dimensional breast-imaging technique by pivoting the crystal through a 45 angle and electronically synchronizing the scanning motion to the trace of the cathode ray tube (96, 97). The instrumentation was in a very early stage of development at that time, however, and only a single case of use of the instrument was reported; but by 1956 Wild and Reid published results on the examination of 77 patients by B-scan visualization (98, 99). By this time the scanning equipment had been modified to the extent that, instead of the crystal's pivoting through an angle, it moved in a linear mode in the water chamber. The detector unit was hand held, with an unfocused, 9-mm-diameter, 15-MHz quartz transceiver crystal mounted on one end of a 2-cm-long water-filled tube sealed with a thin rubber membrane. Coupling of the sound to the skin was made by pressure contact of the rubber membrane to the wet skin surface. The linear motion of the transducer in the water-filled tube and, thus, length of tissue examined for each scan, was 6.5 cm. The depth of penetration in the tissue was 4 cm. The detector unit was applied only to breast areas that were known to harbor an abnormal structure. No attempts were made to use the ultrasound technique to detect unsuspected pathologies (98).

There are a number of important aspects to Wild and Reid's investigations of the use of ultrasound to examine breast, but particularly significant were their clear differentiation of cysts, successful detection of malignant tumors, and

their attempts to set criteria for differentiating benign from malignant tumors (99).

Howry's instrumentation differed in a number of ways from that of Wild and Reid. The most significant differences were the use of a much lower frequency, a focused sound beam, lower intensity of sound, and direct water coupling between the transducer and skin surface (34). The unique aspect of a varable focus of the quartz transducer was provided by two lenses and a concave reflector. The type of scan was B-mode linear at a frequency of 2 MHz (32). The coupling technique consisted essentially of immersion of the scanning equipment and subject in a large tank of water. Although scanning of the breast, with a patient sitting in the water tank, is possible, it is not practical from a clinical point of view. This coupling technique was a limiting factor in Howry's early studies.

Howry and associates' first published results on the breast were concerned with excised rather than intact specimens (35). B-mode echograms were shown for a normal breast and breasts with intact malignant tumors. For the normal breast a sharp reflection was demonstrated from the skin line, but there were essentially no echoes from the interior aspects of the breast. Malignant tumors located within the normally nonecho interior regions were recognizable by the echoes received from anterior surfaces of the tumors. An important aspect of Howry's early work was the attempt to accomplish a precise comparison between the tissue information provided by the echogram and the tissue structures known to be present in the cross section of tissue scanned. Scanning the breast in serial fashion, followed by slicing of the breast tissue at the cross-sectional regions that were traversed by the sound beam and photographing the sliced surfaces, provided the comparison data. Unfortunately, however, since so few sound reflections were received from the interior regions of the breast (except for the limited echoes from the tumor surface), few definitive correlations could be made.

In a 1957 publication Howry explained the basis of a newly developed compound circular scanning system, which was designed so that the transducer moved horizontally and simultaneously traveled around the structure under study (32). The coupling system used with the new scanner remained essentially the same, namely, direct immersion of the patient. Although the design of the water tank had been improved, the necessity of immersing the greater part of the patient's body in water during the scan remained a clinically difficult technique. In his final publication, concerned with studies of ultrasound visualization of breast tissue, Howry indicates, in an illustration, that the breasts of the subject were supported by a gauze mesh brassiere during scanning (33). It can be assumed, therefore, that the patients sat in the scanning tank with the breasts supported by a relatively sound-transparent covering. Some subjects were examined by the same technique except that the breasts were uncovered.*

The breast echograms shown by Howry in the above-mentioned 1965 publication include successful detection of benign pathologies, such as cysts, fibroadenomas, and lipomas. Further, the individual echogram characteristics of these three types of tumors are relatively distinct. A number of types of malignant tumors are shown, including an adenocarcinoma, a stellar breast carcinoma, a far-advanced carcinoma with the "orange peel" skin symptom, and a medullary carcinoma. With the exception of the adenocarcinoma (which may have been of small dimension), and the medullary carcinoma (which contained cystic degenerative processes), reflections are shown not only from the tumor surface but also from internal areas of the malignant mass.

From the viewpoint of present knowledge regarding attenuation or shadowing of ultrasound in the path of malignant tumors and Howry's earlier demonstrations of the acoustic shadowing effect of inanimate targets, it might be expected that Howry would have detected shadowing in the region of malignant tumors. Two of the factors which might explain this failure are: 1) Howry did not obtain echoes from deeply located, normal breast tissue regions (using his early instrumentation) and, thus, attenuation shadows would not have been detectable under such circumstances; and 2) the compound scan

* Personal communication.

equipment applied in the later studies would have masked the shadowing phenomena.

As early as 1956 Kikuchi, Uchida, Tanaka, and Wagai reported research in Japan on cancer diagnosis by ultrasonic techniques that included an application of the method for breast tumor detection (64). The technique outlined for the breast involved B-scanning, using small-diameter, unfocused transducers (5 to 10 MHz), immersed in a rubber water bag resting on the surface of the breast. Echograms of a normal breast and breasts containing a benign and malignant tumor were displayed, but since the research was at a very preliminary stage, the results obtained were primarily significant in regard to the potential of the method. Additionally, this work was the starting point of detailed clinical studies done by a number of investigators in Japan (14, 16, 30, 36, 42, 62–64, 66–74, 82, 86, 89–92, 101–103). Much of the early work published in Japanese journals did not come to the attention of investigators in other parts of the world, but it should be recognized that the early Japanese clinical studies were the sequential progression of the work of Drs. Wild and Howry and are significant to current clinical studies in this field (16, 30, 42, 62).

Although the details of all of the work done by Japanese scientists cannot be discussed here, a brief outline of some of the significant developments is presented below. T. Kobayashi's 1974 review of investigations performed in Japan and in other parts of the world provides concise information on the studies of the many Japanese scientists who contributed to this field (66, 67). With the permission of the author, the summarized data on the echogram parameters studied by Japanese investigators and the results obtained are shown here in Tables 24–1 and 24–2 (66).

Fukuda and Wagai's 1964 report outlines results obtained by examination of 170 breast patients with B-scan instrumentation using sector scanning and a 5-MHz frequency transducer (16). The overall accuracy of differentiating between a benign and malignant tumor was 92%; 77 malignant cases were identified ultrasonically, and 8 of these in an early stage of develop-

TABLE 24–1. DIFFERENTIAL DIAGNOSTIC CRITERIA PROPOSED BY JAPANESE INVESTIGATORS FOR BREAST CANCER*

Investigator	Year Reported	Differential Points
Wagai	1969	Type a: strong irregular pattern; Type b: relative homogeneous pattern; Type c: malignant homogeneous pattern.
Hirose et al	1970	1) Disappearance of the back echo of the tumor; 2) irregular boundary echo of the tumor
Shima	1973	1) Irregular boundary echo of the tumor; 2) inhomogeneity of internal echoes of the tumor; 3) disappearance of back echo of the tumor.
Takahara et al	1972	1) Shape; 2) irregularity; 3) internal echoes; 4) back echo; 5) STC rate measurement by combined use of A-mode.
Tsutsumi et al	1972	Measurement of decibel difference at two points when internal echoes disappear and when back echo completely disappears, as an attenuation increases. Malignant—decibel difference 0–15 dB; benign—decibel difference over 16 dB.
Yokomori et al	1972	Measurement of ultrasonic absorption by the tumor in decibels at two points when back echo of the tumor starts to disappear and when back echo completely disappears, as an attenuation increases. Absorption strength is greater by malignant tumor than by benign tumor.
Nobuoka et al	1972	Measurement of decibel difference at two points when surrounding breast tissue echoes disappear and when back echo completely disappears as an attenuation increases. Malignant—decibel difference approximately 6 dB.
Sato	1972	Malignant; first pattern (echo-poor shadow). Benign; second pattern (echo-rich shadow) (lateral gutter).
Kobayashi et al	1972	1) Complete disappearance of distal limit of the tumor echo (malignant); 2) acoustic middle shadow sign (malignant); 3) bilateral disappearance of distal limit of tumor echo (benign); 4) tadpole-tail sign (benign); 5) lateral shadow sign (benign).
Fujii et al	1973	Type A: conglomerated echo pattern; Type B: irregular transparent pattern; Type C: transparent pattern with attenuation.

* Kobayashi T: Jpn J Clin Oncol 4(2):149, 1974 (with permission of the author).

TABLE 24–2. ACCURACY OF DIFFERENTIAL DIAGNOSIS OF BREAST TUMORS BY JAPANESE INVESTIGATORS USING ULTRASONIC DETECTION TECHNIQUES*

Author Year		Fujii 1970	Hirose 1970	Tsutsumi 1970	Furuki 1971	Kobayashi 1973	Total or Average
Total cases examined Diagnostic accuracy rate		296	—	452	1000	618	2366
Cases histologically proved	Malignant	103	430	141	165	57	896
	Benign	141	—	311	234	43	729
Overall accuracy	Malignant	82%	84%	90%	90%	89%	87%
	Benign	80%	80%	88%	—	70%	80%
Scirrhous carcinoma		—	—	—	93%	100%	97%
Papillary carcinoma		—	—	—	68%	88%	78%
Medullary carcinoma		—	—	—	89%	84%	87%
T_0—less than 1.0 cm		—	60%	—	56%	—	58%
T_1—less than 2.0 cm		70%	—	74%	89%	80%	81%
T_2—more than 2.1 cm to below 5.0 cm		86%	—	94%	—	93%	93%
T_3—more than 5.0 cm		86%	—	100%	—	100%	100%

* Adapted from Kobayashi T: Jpn J Clin Oncol 4(2):155, 1974 (with permission of the author).

ment (presumably a T_1 classification or a tumor less than 2 cm in diameter). The most important aspect of the report is an attempt to define the characteristics of the echogram pattern of malignant tumors. It is indicated that, when localized, irregular, intense reflections are found in the area of a mass, this is a sign of the presence of a cancerous tumor. It is also mentioned, however, that, if a cancer is relatively large, the interior (rather than highly reflecting) is echo free, with essentially no reflections received from within or from the distal border of the tumor. As the authors point out, attenuation of the ultrasound must be taking place in the latter case to an extent that insufficient sound penetrates the tumor to allow reflections from the distal border. Therefore, two distinctly different echo patterns for malignant tumors were found, namely (1) intense, localized reflections from the surface with some echoes from within the tumor; and (2) an echogram pattern showing essentially no echoes from the interior regions of the malignancy but, in fact, attenuation of the sound beam by the malignant tumor.

In the Kaketa and Wagai 1970 report, three categories of echogram patterns for malignant breast tumors are discussed, namely, the two described in the 1964 report and a third type that resembles the pattern of benign tumors to the extent that few echoes are found within the tumor and the inferior border of the tumor can be imaged (42). The differentiating characteristic of this type of malignant tumor, in comparison to benign masses, is its irregular border in contrast to the smooth boundaries of benign tumors.

Gradually, in Japan, ultrasound visualization, generally using a frequency of 5-MHz, became an accepted clinical technique for breast examination (71–74, 86, 89). As shown in Table 24–1, during this period of evolving clinical application, a number of image pattern characteristics were investigated. Dr. Wagai's differentiation of three distinct image patterns for malignant tumors is significant in this regard. However, the image pattern for malignant tumors found by Wild, Reid, and Howry (namely, intense reflection of the sound energy by the cancerous tumor) did not prove to be a readily detectable characteristic. Rather, the attenuation properties of malignant masses (as judged by "acoustic shadowing") appeared to be the most significant clue for differential diagnosis. Further, the unique image pattern found for benign masses, namely, an enhancement of the reflected sound by the posterior wall of the tumor, accompanied by two narrow shadows on either side of this enhanced image (designated as the "tadpole" sign), was easily distinguishable from that of attenuating masses.

The concepts of time gain control (TGC) of the amplifier system and sensitivity graded tomography (SGT) had been introduced rather early in the breast studies done by Japanese investigators, and, generally, these continued in use (42, 62). Gray-scale techniques were added to clinical breast-scanning equipment, and increasing attention was given to the smooth or jagged character of the walls of tumors and to the homogeneous or heterogeneous character of the echo from within the tumor (68, 69, 91, 92). Kobayashi found that fat necrosis produced an attenuation shadow that was comparable to the shadow produced by a malignant mass, as judged by visual image inspection (72). Recent studies in Japan confirmed earlier findings of other investigators that medullary carcinoma is not highly attenuating and that it has an image pattern similar to that of a benign tumor (68, 91). The success of Japanese physicians, in terms of percentage of correct diagnoses, may be judged from Wagai and Tsutsumi's (91) results, namely, for patients scanned during the period 1966 to 1975, correct diagnoses of malignant masses (no tumor size specified) was accomplished in 89.4% of the cases. The application of gray-scale techniques gave essentially the same level of overall diagnostic success, but the diagnostic accuracy for tumors less than 2 cm in diameter (T_1) was improved (to 80%) over earlier efforts. The smallest tumor detected was 5 mm in size. These results are in general agreement with those outlined by Kobayashi in his summary of the work of Japanese investigators (67). The primary current diagnostic criteria used by many Japanese clinicians in diagnosing breast pathologies by means of currently standard ultrasonic visualization techniques are summarized in Table 24–3 (67, 70, 91).

Yokoi, Ito, and associates have studied the use

**TABLE 24-3. VISUALIZATION PATTERNS OF
VARIOUS PARAMETERS OF BREAST MASSES**

	Benign	Malignant
1. Surrounding wall structure	Smooth	Irregular
2. Internal echo pattern	Homogeneous or echo-free (cyst)	Nonuniform
3. Posterior wall visibility (in reference to entrance of sound beam)	Intense (enhanced) reflection and two narrow, adjacent shadows (tadpole sign)	Not visible (or poorly visible); presence of acoustic shadow in this region

of color display for ultrasound breast examination (36, 101–103). Their approach is to digitize the ultrasound echo signals via application of an A/D converter and store the digitized signals on cassette or videotape, with color display used to correspond to an intensity range of echo levels. This stored data can then be presented in color B-scan images. The image patterns in these color displays are, however, extremely complex, since the breast tissue structures that are the source of the signals are multistructured. To deal with this problem, computer techniques simplify the color presentation by emphasizing tissue data such as contour of structures and, additionally, improve resolution. Included as part of this instrumentation system is C-mode scanning, allowing a cross-sectional image of a coronal plane of the breast at any selected depth. Apparently, imaging this plane provides a distinct advantage for analysis of breast masses, especially in regard to their wall structure (101).

Finally, Japanese investigators were the first to attempt the use of ultrasound as a screening agent (90, 91). Their screening program has been underway since 1975 in Toyama Prefecture in Japan and has been subsequently expanded to provide screening in several other prefectures in Japan.* For these programs an ultrasound unit is installed in a relatively small van that tours the countryside to permit examining as many subjects as possible with one instrument. Since it is generally known that the majority of breast

tumors are found in the upper, outer quadrant of the breast, only this region is ultrasonically examined (at 5-mm spacing intervals) for the specific purpose of keeping examination time to a minimum.* (Manual examination of the entire breast precedes the ultrasound examination and if any abnormal area is detected by that procedure then that region is also scanned.) A 5-MHz small diameter, single-focus transducer, linear scanning, water bag coupling, combined with 35-mm film recording are standard features of the instrumentation. In terms of mass screening for early detection of tumors, the 5-mm spacing between scans and the restriction of the scanning to the upper, outer quadrant are limiting compromises, but, nonetheless, this program is yielding valuable data.

In the decade of the sixties relatively few scientists outside of those in Japan carried out detailed studies on the use of ultrasound techniques for examination of the breast. A 1966 paper by Evans et al discusses a new commercial ultrasound B-mode instrument designed for examination of liver, kidney, and breast (13). A quite large water bag was used as a coupling medium, and scans were done at a frequency of 2.5 MHz with an unfocused transducer. Cysts were well demonstrated, but the authors questioned the capabilities of this technique in distinguishing between solid benign and malignant masses. Holmes' 1967 publication demonstrates a highly reflecting scirrhous carcinoma and a clearly defined cyst by use of a compound scan technique (31). (The precise frequency was not specified.) For this study the patients were in a sitting position with the breast pressed against a soft plastic window coupled to a large water tank containing the scanning unit.

The ultrasound scanner described by Wells and Evans in a 1968 publication was specifically designed for breast examination and included direct water coupling between breast surface and transducer (93). Coupling was accomplished by placing the patient in a prone position and immersing both breasts in a water bath built into an examination couch. The transducer was an unfocused, 2.5–cm–diameter, 2–MHz lead titanate zirconate unit. There were a number of

---

* Personal communication.

* Personal communication.

interesting features to this instrument, including swept gain, compound sector scanning, and the ability to scan both breasts simultaneously. Only preliminary results are shown in this paper, and, unfortunately, the instrument was not extensively used in subsequent clinical investigations.

The breast studies of DeLand are of interest from the viewpoint that, as early as 1969, he applied a system that included a single sending transducer, combined with an array of four receiving transducers (11). Using a direct water coupling technique, with the subject in a supine position, this investigator found that malignant tumors classified as scirrhous gave echogram patterns showing irregular borders and echoes from within the tumor, while malignant tumors classified as medullary had regular margins with no echoes from within the tumor. Of considerable interest is the fact that some scans were made on surgically removed breasts and the results compared to presurgery scans of the same breast.

E. Kelly-Fry, as chief investigator under a program sponsored by the Department of Health, Education and Welfare (HEW), Cancer Control Program, was apparently the first to recognize the potential of ultrasound visualization for breast screening, and to attempt to obtain the data that would allow screening for very early breast cancer by means of pattern recognition techniques (45). Additionally, the early studies of this investigator and associates, initiated in 1968, represent the first application of an on-line computer control system for ultrasound breast examination of human subjects (43–46, 49, 52–54, 57–59). The long range objectives of this program as outlined in a 1969 report to HEW are significant to current diagnostic problems, namely:

1) to develop knowledge of the correlation between acoustic echo patterns and normal and abnormal breast tissue structure; and 2) to develop and demonstrate the feasibility of applying ultrasonic visualization techniques to mass screening methods. It was recognized from the beginning that the chances for successful development of these objectives in a reasonable period of time would be advanced if sophisticated scanning techniques were coupled with the latest development in data processing and presentation. It was also recognized that meaningful

results are fundamentally dependent upon the design and construction of the transducer array and the method of coupling the sound energy to the breast tissue (45).

In pursuing these aims a sophisticated sector mode, B-scanning visualization system was used which featured a sending-receiving transducer system (applied in the pulse-echo mode) designed to provide both good lateral and range resolution (15). The improved lateral resolution was associated with a unique feature of this system, namely, a wide aperture parabolic mirror, fabricated of a hardened resin with embedded micro-sized tungsten particles. The highly polished front surface of this unit provided an excellent mirror and any sound energy that penetrated this front surface was effectively absorbed and scattered by the particle embedded resin. The sending transducer was a 3-MHz frequency unit with a front face plastic focusing lens; the 4-mm diameter receiving transducer had a frequency response of 15 MHz. With the aid of the on-line digital computer, this visualization system was used in 1968–1969 to automatically scan millimeter by millimeter, breasts of normal subjects and of patients with various pathologies, including cancer. In later studies, wide aperture single focus, lower frequency (1.7 and 2.4 MHz) transceiver type transducers were applied (58).

The improved resolution was not confined to a depth of tissue in the immediate area of the focus of the transducer but could be made available for essentially the entire depth of the breast. This was accomplished as follows: gating circuitry permitted only echoes emanating from a certain linear distance on either side of the focus (a preselected region of best focus), to be processed for final imaging display; the computer provided automatic control of the transducer motion in depth so that the chosen focal region was placed in a stepwise, sequential fashion, through the full depth of the tissue (15). The computer also provided program control of receiver gain as a function of range and echo amplitude. Each of the focal band segments could be recorded at different amplifier gain settings. The completed image of each breast cross section was presented in a single picture constructed from the single-focus segments. This system was, in essence, a multiple-focus, wide dynamic range system that eliminated the problems of time variable gain and allowed SGT to be displayed on a single picture. An additional feature of this instrumentation system was the choice of either the normal, two-dimensional, "flat" B-mode imaging or a presentation designated as "relief display," which gave an impression of three dimensions and provided more structural information than the usual flat presentation (15, 44, 59).

This instrumentation system was used in conjunction with a direct water coupling technique, with the subject in a supine position and with no body regions other than the breasts being subjected to the water bath (43, 58). The coupling technique, which involved the use of a seal around the borders of each breast, permitted the completely exposed breasts to float in an open water bath and the scanning transducer to freely move over both breasts in almost any chosen direction; thus, no limitations were imposed in regard to the size of breasts acceptable for complete scanning.

Initially, in this investigative program, primary emphasis was placed on attempts to delineate echogram patterns of the normal breast (over the age range of young to old) by scanning each subject under known and precisely comparable conditions of instrumentation sensitivity (45, 58, 59). This approach was based on the premise that, if such characterization could be accomplished, then recognition of deviations from normal could form the basis of an early breast cancer detection method (45). Subject selection was based on specific experimental goals with subjects classified as normal after a clinical examination and a radiologist's interpretation of mammographic findings (45). In pursuit of the above aims it was demonstrated that certain standard classifications of breast tissue types, such as glandular or fatty, can be recognized by their echogram patterns and that specific benign breast diseases such as fibrosing adenosis can also be identified by this approach (58). Additionally, E. Kelly-Fry and G. Kossoff (using a hand-held, direct contact, transducer unit devised by G. Kossoff) determined average acoustic velocity values of breasts in vivo and corre-

lated their findings with breast structure as interpreted by age and mammogram information (45, 58). The subsequent Kossoff, Kelly-Fry, and Jellins studies, confirming and expanding these results, clearly identified breasts that were largely composed of fat (by their low acoustic velocity values) and differentiated them from denser breasts, such as those of normal, young subjects (which have higher acoustic velocity values) (78).

The patient examinations carried out under the E. Kelly-Fry et al program were primarily devoted to scanning the specific regions of "palpable" solid and cystic masses. However, attempts were also made to locate "nonpalpable" breast masses by detailed (millimeter-by-millimeter) scanning of the whole breast. Biopsy data of the detected tumor masses were correlated with the visualization results, and, to a limited degree, postoperative scanning was done on some of the surgically removed masses (45, 46). Ultrasound studies were also done on fresh, whole breasts just after their surgical removal. These investigations showed that the excised breast can provide good experimental data that are applicable to breasts in vivo (46).

Subsequent to these studies of fresh excised breasts, E. Kelly-Fry and H. S. Gallager carried out precise studies on formalin-fixed excised breasts containing known, intact malignant tumors that had not been subjected to any prior biopsy procedures (47–49, 52). These special preparations were scanned in precise detail using the previously mentioned computer-based instrumentation. After the ultrasound scans these specimens were subjected to whole-breast sectioning and histologic staining. It was possible with this approach to compare (on a one-to-one basis) the tissue structures portrayed on the echogram as a cross section through the breast and the histologic cross section that showed the actual tissue structures in the path of the sound beam. Included in the findings of this study were the following: 1) ultrasonic scanning of formalin-fixed breast tissue is a valid research method that provides diagnostic information applicable to ultrasound scanning of the breasts of patients in vivo; 2) malignant masses classified under the broad histology category of "breast carcinoma of no special type," examined at scanning frequencies as low as 1.7 MHz; attenuated the incoming sound beam to the extent of producing an acoustic shadow; and 3) the attenuation of the sound was associated with the complete cellular malignant mass but was increased in regions of necrosis or fibrosis. (Recently Kelly-Fry and associates carried out an additional study with this same type of unique breast preparation in which computer signal processing of ultrasound transmission data [Fast Fourier Transform] was used to determine precise information on frequency-dependent attenuation values of the malignant mass and normal tissue regions (60). This data was correlated with x-ray, ultrasound visualization and histologic information (48).)

In summary, the early studies of E. Kelly-Fry et al demonstrated both the advantages of applying advanced, computer-based ultrasound instrumentation for diagnosis of breast pathologies, and the potential of this technique for early breast cancer detection. In that regard, the studies directed at identification of overt breast masses in patients' breasts demonstrated, first, the ability of ultrasound to locate precisely a tumor both in terms of distance in depth (from the skin line) and in terms of its geometric placement in respect to other breast demarcation areas (such as nipple). (In essence, complete contour of nonattenuating masses could be determined in a relatively short time with the aid of a computer-based, automatic scanning system. Highly attenuating masses could also be precisely located, but their total contour could not always be determined, since the posterior walls were not always visualized due to the attenuation.) Second, these studies demonstrated identification of cystic structures by their characteristic smooth walls and non-echo interiors and detection of multiple cysts of varying sizes widely distributed throughout the breasts. The in vivo and the excised-tissue studies clearly demonstrated the presence of an "attenuation shadow" associated with the most commonly occurring type of malignant breast tumors (for the limited number of cases studied). The complexities involved in detecting a malignant tumor in its early stages of development were recognized in these initial investigations, and research approaches to their solution were suggested (48). Subsequent studies of E. Kelly-Fry and associates are discussed later in this paper.

In the late 1960s some European investigators initiated studies on ultrasonic detection of breast tumors. The work of Kratchowil and Kaiser is of interest from the viewpoint that, using a simple B-mode contact scanner, these investigators examined breast tumors at two different frequencies and attempted to make diagnostic decisions on the basis of comparison of echogram patterns obtained at the different frequencies (79). Ossoinig and Kaiser et al were generally successful in differentiating between cysts, fibroadenomas, and carcinomas (using an A-mode technique at a frequency of 8 MHz), but malignant tumors less than 2.5 cm were not found by this method (83). Relatively recently, Pluygers attained (for a small patient population) a diagnostic accuracy of 100% for cysts, 85% for fibroadenomas, and 75.8% for malignant tumors with the use of Japanese instrumentation (water bag coupling, automatic mechanical scanning, 5-MHz frequency) (84). However, the resolution of the system limited the detection of deeply located malignant tumors to those of 1 cm in size or larger.

Apparently, the most extensive ultrasound studies in Europe have been carried out by Gros and associates (22–28). An important aspect of the instrumentation (direct contact, A-mode/B-mode scanner) is the availability of interchangeable transducers of 2, 4, and 6 MHz frequencies (27). These authors used the frequency response characteristics of tissue to differentiate between solid and liquid-filled masses and attempted to differentiate between benign and malignant masses by this technique (27). Their efforts to correlate thermography and ultrasound visualization (and to obtain quantitative data on the attenuation characteristics of normal breast tissue and of various types of breast tumors) are of particular interest (22, 23). In summarizing their ultrasound studies of more than 8000 breast patients (including 1000 cases of breast cancer), Gros et al indicate that they found seven distinct B-mode echographic patterns for breast carcinoma; that the echo pattern for malignant tumors is more homogeneous than that of normal tissues of the breast; and that, in general, the edges of malignant tumors are extremely smooth. Both of these findings (i.e., a homogeneous echo pattern and smooth edges) are in contrast to the finding of most Japanese clinicians for malignant tumors. The attenuation values found for breast carcinoma by these investigators range from 2 to 4 dB/cm, with an upper limit of 10 dB/cm (24). It was also found that tumors 2 to 5 cm in diameter do not greatly attenuate ultrasound. Histologic studies made by these investigators showed that fibrous tissue, adipofibrous interfaces, microcysts, microcalcifications, and spicules are the significant structures that define echogram patterns and, in particular, attenuation patterns. These authors also found the following: fibrous tissue is the predominant factor in echogram patterns, considerable variability is common in regard to the attenuation characteristics of fibrous tissue (i.e., such tissue may be highly attenuating or lightly attenuating), and cellular density is not significant to echogram pattern images.

Starting with a 1971 publication by Jellins et al, scientists from the Commonwealth Acoustics Laboratory in Australia reported results of applying ultrasound compound scanning to study of the breast (17, 18, 37–41, 75–78, 85). The transducer used in most of these studies was a 4-cm-diameter, 2-MHz unit with a 10-cm radius of curvature that moved in a lateral plane across the breast, while oscillating ±30° about its axis, to provide a compound scan (simple sector and linear scans were also available) (40, 85). The method of transducer–breast coupling used was that mentioned in the E. Kelly-Fry et al studies. Jellins et al indicated that application of this instrumentation system on patients showed the following: scirrhous carcinoma tumors less than 2 cm in diameter have a low level of echoes from internal regions, jagged boundaries, and they exhibit significant attenuation of ultrasound; large tumors of this type are less characteristic and the boundaries may not be jagged; single cases of mucoid and anaplastic carcinoma tumors were found not to attenuate the sound beam (40). Multiple cysts (including those less than 1 mm in diameter), benign tumors, and the normal tissues of the breast were well displayed with this instrumentation system (the smallest scirrhous carcinoma detected was 0.5 cm in diameter). A comparatively recent ultrasound instrument developed by this same group of Australian scientists (17, 18, 77) features eight motor-driven, large-aperture (7.0 cm), focused transducers for the purpose of providing either rapid, compound, or simple sector scanning. This instrument is designed as a multipurpose scanner (abdomen, thyroid, breast). Relatively low-frequency transducers were used in the early units (less than 2.5 MHz); more recent models have frequencies of 3 MHz. During breast scanning procedures the patient is prone with breasts directly immersed in a water bath. Good penetration of the sound beam for noncompressed breasts, the ability to automatically scan both breasts in a relatively short time, in either the transverse or longitudinal direction, good resolution and gray scale display are the advantages of this instrument.

Baum developed an ultrasound visualization system, specifically designed for examination of the breast, in which the subject is in a sitting position, with the undraped breasts suspended in a water-filled tank (1–5). For each examination approximately 60 sector scans are done at 3-mm vertical steps, with a focused, 2.25-MHz transducer. One unique feature of Baum's studies is the use of a color-coded, isodensitometric printout of the breast with a specific color assigned to each 3-dB change in gray scale (6). The goal of these studies is to improve the capability of the examiner to visually characterize the echo patterns of various benign and malignant pathologies.

Although, at this writing, the use of ultrasound for breast examination in the United States still remains in a relatively inactive state (in comparison to other areas of medical ultrasound), physicians have, in the past several years, shown an increased interest in ultrasonic breast examination. In view of the lack of readily available commercial ultrasound breast scanning instruments, some physicians have used commercial scanners (designed for other purposes) for examination of the breast (9, 65, 80, 81, 87). For example, Laing (applying a standard commercial medical ultrasound unit) scanned approximately 50 patients with palpable breast masses and compared the results with information obtained by mammography (80, 81). Direct-contact transducers of 2.25 and 5.0

MHz were used, and the breasts were taped to keep them as stationary as possible during the scan. Despite the limitations of the instrumentation system in respect to ultrasonically differentiating benign and malignant solid tumors, it was found that inclusion of the ultrasound technique in the clinical protocol improves clinical diagnostic accuracy when used in conjunction with mammography. More recently Teixidor and Kazam, using a B-mode contact scanner (5-MHz transducer) examined 200 breast patients by ultrasound visualization and mammography (87). The results obtained by these authors are significant, namely, only 38.6% of cysts were correctly diagnosed by mammography, while 100% were correctly identified by ultrasound examination. However, only 78.8% of the carcinomas were correctly diagnosed with ultrasound alone, while 94% were correctly identified by mammogram examination. When mammography and ultrasound were combined, the successful diagnostic rate for carcinomas increased to 97%. In the case of fibroadenomas, 53% were identified by mammography alone, 70.6% by ultrasound, and 88% by the two methods combined. Cole-Beugelet and Beique not only applied conventional B-mode and A-mode scanning techniques but also used two separate commercial "rapid scanners" in their studies, namely, a system that provided a continuous (16 times per second) B-scan by means of two rotating, 2.5-MHz transducers and a parabolic mirror in an enclosed water path and a water-enclosed, oscillating 7-MHz transducer unit that produced a continuous, sector B-scan repeated 10 times per second (9). With the high-frequency transducer head assembly applied directly to the breast surface, a penetration depth of 4.5 cm was attained. As in the Laing and Teixidor and Kazam studies, Cole-Beugelet and Beique found that, when used in conjunction with mammography, ultrasound improves the diagnostic accuracy obtained by application of mammography alone and aids in the differentiation of certain unique masses that could not be delineated on mammograms. Unfortunately, it was not possible, while using these adaptations of commercial instruments for breast examination, to identify small solid tumors. Laing experienced difficulty in identifying

tumors less than 2 cm in diameter, whereas Cole-Beugelet found a 20% failure rate for detection of tumors less than 2 cm in diameter, using the 2.5-MHz continuous scanner (9). Nonetheless, if it is recognized that these commercial instruments included serious limitations in design (insofar as breast examination is concerned), then the findings of these investigators are encouraging in regard to future clinical applications of standard ultrasound instrumentation for detection of breast pathologies.

Comparatively recent studies of a number of investigators on the development of ultrasonic computerized tomographic imaging techniques for breast examination can be expected to have a significant influence on future ultrasonic breast cancer detection methods (8, 10, 12, 19–21). Discussions of these investigations, however, as well as those of Calderon et al on attenuation values of excised malignant and benign tumors (7), by E. Kelly–Fry et al on the use of FFT (Fast Fourier Transform) techniques for studies of frequency dependent attenuation values of malignant tumors (60) and alterations of phase angles of ultrasound transmitted through a malignant tumor (61), and by Wells et al on the use of Doppler ultrasound for detection of breast carcinoma (94) are not included in this paper. Recent extensive studies by many investigators on tissue scattering phenomena may also be expected to play a significant role in ultrasonic breast examination.

DISCUSSION

Although, except in Japan, there has been (to date) a general lack of commercial equipment specifically designed for ultrasonic breast examination, it can be expected that many types of ultrasound breast scanning instruments will become available in the immediate future. As is evident from the work discussed here, there are a number of unknown factors in regard to interactions between sound waves and breast tumors, and there are discrepancies between the results obtained by different investigators who have studied these interactions. It is also clear, however, that, despite these difficulties, clinically successful results have been obtained by a number of investigators (for reasonably large patient population) in ultrasonically diagnosing breast tumors 2 cm and more in diameter. There is a serious need, however, to detect and diagnose small malignant tumors (i.e., those less than 0.5 cm in diameter). Problems associated with ultrasonic detection and diagnosis of such small masses, on a routine clinical basis, should be solvable in a relatively short time period if interdisciplinary terms of bioacoustic scientists, clinicians, and pathologists, working with adequate instrumentation, perform detailed studies for this specific purpose. Although increased numbers of these interdisciplinary programs will probably emerge in the near future, clinicians now entering the field of ultrasonic breast diagnosis have to be acutely aware not only of the limitations of present knowledge but also of the significant contributions they can make to this much-neglected field. The following is a brief summary of some aspects of recent interdisciplinary laboratory based but clinically oriented studies of the author and associates (50, 51, 56).

A laboratory designed linear-scan, B-mode visualization system that allows easy interchange of transducers, precise placement of the focus of the transducer at any depth within the breast, a choice of water bag or direct fluid coupling, and the ability to scan the breasts in steps as small as 1 mm (in either the transverse or longitudinal direction) has been applied by E. Kelly-Fry and associates to examine breasts in vivo. The ability to scan in both the longitudinal (sagittal) and transverse plane is helpful because, for some malignant tumors, there seems to be a "best" scanning plane orientation in respect to obtaining good diagnostic images. Figure 24–1 shows an artist's rendering of these two planes as examined by a scanning transducer. The subjects are examined in a supine position.

Single-focus transducers ranging in frequency from 2.25 to 5.0 MHz were designed by the present author for the studies carried out with this instrument. In designing these transducers, emphasis was placed on obtaining good lateral and range resolution, over the full depth of the breast, for the specific technique of coupling the sound to the tissue. Until such time that more advanced transducers (including phased array)

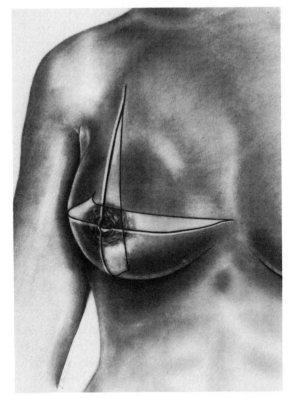

FIG. 24–1. Artist's view of transverse and longitudinal planes of the breast.

are specifically designed for breast examination, such simple focused transducers (either of the lens or disc type), when appropriately designed, can be used in clinical programs to obtain much-needed data on breast structure. The importance of various design factors (which may have a specific influence on successful detection of discrete structures in the breast) was experimentally verified by breast phantom target testing, followed by scanning of patients with the various experimental units. Since resolution capability of a transducer and its associated electronic systems are related to a number of design factors and to the specific tissue structures under examination, this type of investigation is important to early detection of breast carcinoma. It was determined by use of these specially designed but relatively simple transducers that cysts 1 to 3 mm in diameter and attenuating masses of the order of 3 mm in size can be readily detected; additionally, normal components of breast, such as subcutaneous fat, Cooper's ligaments, primary ducts, and pectoralis muscle, can be definitively imaged (47) (see Figs. 24–5 through 24–10).

The most appropriate type of ultrasound–breast surface coupling technique, for noncontact type scanners, was considered in terms of its function as one unit of a clinical system that, ideally, should be capable of 1) displaying the normal tissues of the breast in their natural relations to each other, including the fine tissue structures (such as ductal structures); and 2) detecting an overt mass located deep within a large breast. For item 1, direct fluid coupling between breast and transducer was found to be the best technique. In regard to item 2, the water bag technique, because of its compression of the breast, has two definite advantages; it considerably decreases the length of the tissue path that the sound field must traverse and thus allows transducers with higher frequencies to be used; the problem of loss of sound at a sharp angle of entrance is eliminated by the flattening of the tissues. Disadvantages of the water bag method are possible wrinkling that air can be trapped between skin and bag, forming a barrier to the entering sound. This is particularly difficult to avoid in the areolar region where the surface structure is uneven. If a water bag is used, it should be light translucent to allow viewing of the breast through the bag.

Insofar as the position of the patient is concerned, it was found, on the basis of comparing the prone and supine positions, that the supine orientation has many advantages for breast scanning. By starting from the supine position, the patient's position can be adjusted, just prior to scanning, to provide the best angle of sound entrance between the transducer and tumor region. In the current clinical program, the tumor region, as found by palpation or x-ray examination, is marked on the skin prior to scanning and this region (as directly viewed through the water bag) placed in its best orientation in respect to the position of the transducer. Normally, depending on the location of the breast mass, the patient can either be resting on her back or can be slightly turned to rest partially on one shoulder. During the scanning procedure the breast may be repalpated if there is any uncertainty

regarding the precise location of the tumor in reference to the scanning plane, and the position of the patient may then be adjusted, if necessary. A further significant advantage of the supine orientation is that it is possible to easily scan the outermost regions of the breast and axilla from this position.

A particularly significant result of these laboratory based studies (insofar as differential diagnosis of breast tumors by pulse-echo techniques is concerned) is the finding that the attenuation (as judged by acoustic shadowing) of some densely fibrous benign tumors (scanned at frequencies of 4.4 MHz and more) is such that their echogram patterns are visually indistinguishable from those of malignant masses. A small percentage of subjects whose breasts contained highly attenuating masses (as judged by intense acoustic shadowing) were conclusively diagnosed, on the basis of biopsy examination, as having fibrocystic disease (60). In addition, all of these subjects had specific breast tissue alterations: epithelial hyperplasia, inflammation, collagen deposits, fibrosis, or calcification. However, fat necrosis, known to be sound attenuating (72), was not detected by the pathologist in any of these cases. Apparently the frequency-dependent attenuation coefficient for these specific benign masses had a value which, although less than that of the attenuation coefficient of malignant tumors, was sufficiently high to result in a dark shadow when examined by a pulse-echo system (which involves two passes of the sound beam through the tissue) at frequencies of the order of 4.5 MHz. However, until more quantitative clinical techniques are available, it appears possible to qualitatively differentiate these "highly attenuating benign tumors" from attenuating malignant tumors by reexamining, at lower frequencies (of the order of 2 MHz or less), all masses found to be highly attenuating when scanned at the higher frequencies. Although a shadowing phenomenon may still be present in the image pattern of benign tumors examined at lower frequencies this light shadow should be distinguishable from the dark shadow shown by most malignant tumors for this same low frequency range. The author and associates have performed preliminary clinical studies that seem to confirm the value of this interim approach (56). The tissue studies of Vucicevic et al are also of interest in regard to this approach (88). Clearly, there is a serious need for further quantitative studies on the attenuation characteristics of benign and malignant tumors, including investigations on the relationship of these characteristics to basic tumor structure and to individual structural components of the mass (7, 60).

Normal structures of the breast that also cause acoustic shadowing are the nipple and, to a lesser degree, the surrounding areola (47, 60). The extent of this shadowing is dependent on a number of factors, including the beam width, the depth of placement of the focus, the frequency of the transducer, and the tissue structure of the nipple itself, which, in fact, can vary from subject to subject. A completely opaque shadow imaged in the region below the nipple is a common finding for simple linear or sector scanning systems. Although, as shown in Figures 24–9 and 24–10, it is possible to image nipple structure and tissue structures located deep to the nipple by scanning directly over this area with a simple linear scan system, it is recommended that, when attempts are being made to detect a tumor so located, reliance *not* be placed on transmission of the sound directly through the nipple. Depending on the design of the instrument, transmission via the lateral aspect of the breast to the region deep to the nipple can usually be accomplished by angling the scanning head and carefully positioning the patient. It is also recommended that, in addition to examination at the higher frequencies, lower frequencies (of the order of 2 MHz) be applied when this area is scanned.

A clinical ultrasound breast examination program based on application of the knowledge gained in these laboratory studies and, in particular, information on the significance of transducer characteristics, is now underway at Indiana University Medical Center.* Patients who have a palpable mass within their breast or some other indication of the presence of a breast pathology are the primary subjects in this program.

---

* These studies are being done in association with Patricia M. Harper, M.D., Indiana University School of Medicine, who directs the clinical aspects of this program.

In view of the fact that, as discussed above, ultrasound breast examination techniques have not been as extensively used as other ultrasound methods, this program has been designed to make use of both mammography and ultrasound for a certain period of time. This approach, at this point in time, gives the patient the maximum advantage.

The current program has been specifically designed to accomplish the above aims with the use of simple but relatively fast scanning, clinically practical ultrasound instrumentation. This was accomplished by modifying a commercial ultrasound unit (designed in Japan for breast examination) to allow substitution of the original transducer with specially designed transducers and to provide for a number of other changes. As finally modified the ultrasound instrument is a linear scan, B-mode visualization system with an analogue scan converter, TV image display, step-variable attenuation control, time gain compensation, and translucent water bag coupling with the patient in a supine position. Breast images are recorded in a multiple format on 8^-10 x-ray film. The linear travel of the transducer covers a tissue viewing distance of 12 cm; nine sweeps are automatically taken in a 30-sec interval, with a choice of 5-mm or 1-mm spacing distance between each scan interval. Automatic scanning at 1-mm spacing distances is also provided. The scanning plane can be oriented in almost any direction (i.e., transverse, longitudinal, or oblique). Four specially designed, single-focus, interchangeable transducers ranging in frequency from 2.25 to 5.0 MHz are being used in this program in order to study the effects of frequency and transducer design characteristics.

An x-ray unit with low radiation dosage (400 mRad) and microfocal spot imaging is used for mammography.

Figures 24-2 through 24-10, obtained with the previously clinical ultrasound visualization system, illustrate the definitive imaging of both normal breast structures and of commonly found breast pathologies that can be accomplished with comparatively simple visualization systems. The transducer applied for these specific cases was designed by the present author to provide good (1- to 2-mm in tissue) range and

(*Text continues on p. 344*)

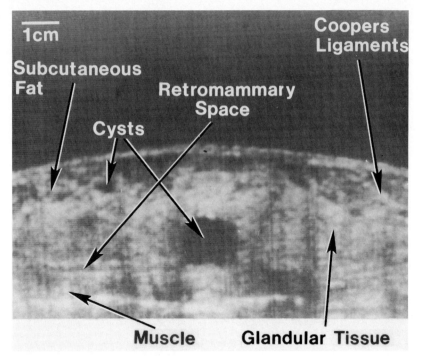

FIG. 24-2. Echogram of breast of 45-year-old subject with fibrocystic disease. A large component of glandular tissue is evident in this image, but scans of other areas of this same breast showed menopausal changes. The large cyst seen in this figure was located inferior to the areola; the structural image pattern to the right of this cyst represents tissue deep to the nipple (water bag coupling and a 3.7 MHz focused transducer).

FIG. 24-3. Echogram of 17-year-old subject with a subcutaneous fibroadenoma. Note homogeneous echoes from within mass (water bag coupling and 3.7 MHz focused transducer).

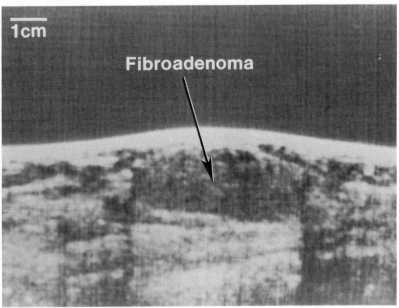

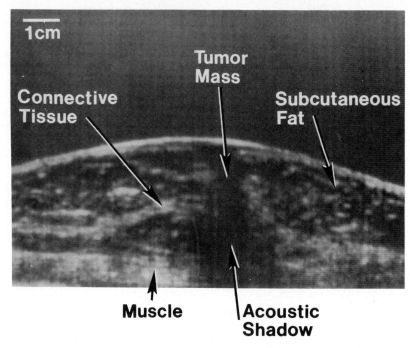

FIG. 24-4. Echogram of 58-year-old subject with an infiltrating ductal, 1 cm diameter, carcinoma. Note the well-displayed postmenopausal breast tissue changes and the presence of an acoustic shadow deep to the tumor (water bag coupling and 3.7 MHz focused transducer).

FIG. 24-5. Echogram of breast of 58-year-old subject with fibrocystic disease. Note, in addition to display of cystic mass, clear imaging of both subcutaneous structures, such as Cooper's ligaments, and the deeply located pectoralis muscle (water bag sound coupling and 3.7-MHz frequency transducer).

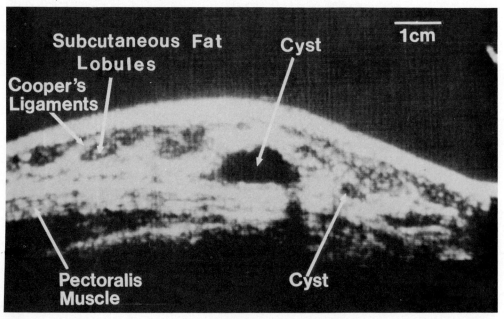

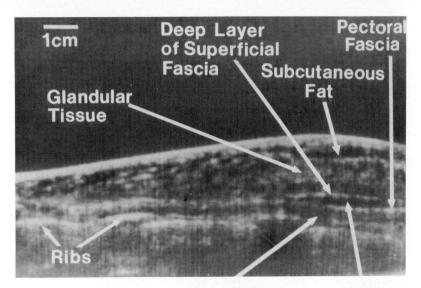

FIG. 24–6. Echogram of breast of normal young (age 25) subject demonstrating precise imaging of individual breast structures (water bag sound coupling and 3.7-MHz frequency transducer).

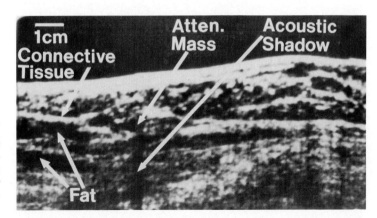

FIG. 24–7. Echogram of breast of a 75-year-old subject with a 3-mm attenuating tumor. Note excellent imaging of structural components of the older breast, namely, layers of fat interspersed by fine connective tissue strands (water bag sound coupling and 3.7 MHz frequency transducer).

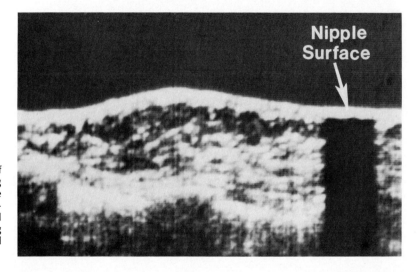

FIG. 24–8. Echogram of breast of 58-year-old subject, illustrating complete obscuration of tissue structures deep to the nipple because of attenuation of the sound beam by the nipple (water bag coupling and a 3.7 MHz focused transducer). See text.

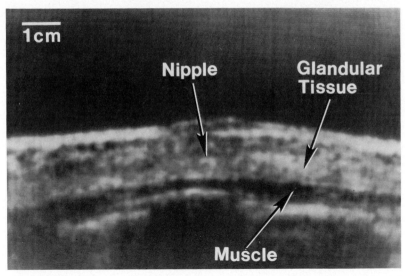

FIG. 24–9. Echogram of 22-year-old subject illustrating imaging of the nipple and structures deep to the nipple (water bag coupling and a 3.7 MHz focused transducer). See text.

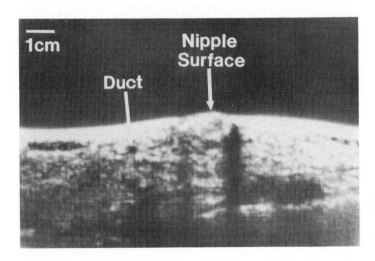

FIG. 24-10. Echogram of breast of 3-week post-partum subject. Note excellent imaging of ductal structures deep to nipple surface (water bag sound coupling and 3.7 MHz frequency transducer).

lateral resolution, and to meet the requirement of penetration of the sound beam from skin to pectoral muscles for large-breasted individuals. The transducer is a single focus, small f/number unit with a midband frequency of 3.7 MHz, a beam width (i.e., the distance across the focal region perpendicular to the direction of propagation of the beam) with a diameter of 0.8 mm at 3 dB down, 1.2 mm at 6 dB down, and 1.9 mm at 10 dB down. The range resolution of this unit is less than 1 mm for test targets and of the order of

1 mm for tissue. Its average intensity output is 23 mWcm^{-2}. An echogram of a middle-aged subject with fibrocystic disease is shown in Figure 24-2. The complete lack of internal echoes, and the smooth wall structure, are the primary diagnostic indicators of this pathology. Note the presence of the small cysts in addition to the primary fluid mass. Figure 24-3 demonstrates the type of image obtained in the case of a fibroadenoma in the breast of a 17-year-old subject. The fine echoes from within the mass, combined

with a smooth wall structure, are clear indicators of a fibroadenoma. In both Figures 24-2 and 24-3, an enhancement of the echoes in the posterior regions of the masses is present. Although not a necessary component, this characteristic is commonly observed in the case of cysts and fibroadenomas. The image pattern received from a highly attenuating malignant mass in the breast of a 58-year-old subject is shown in Figure 24-4. In addition to the sharp outlining of the superior borders of the mass and the acoustic shadowing in the region deep to the tumor mass, note the precise detailing in this image of the commonly found features for postmenopausal breasts, namely, a prominent layer of subcutaneous fat, an almost total absence of glandular tissue, and a large component of fat and connective tissue located in the deep layers. Additionally, the pectoralis major muscle of this subject is well displayed. The subcutaneous fat lobules and suspensory ligaments are exceptionally well displayed in the echogram of the breast of a 58-year-old subject with fibrocystic disease shown in Figure 24-5. The characteristic structure of a healthy young breast, namely, a subcutaneous fat layer which is small in comparison to the well-defined, ordered pattern of glandular tissue is well illustrated in Figure 24-6. The echogram of a 75-year-old subject (Figure 24-7) with a 3-mm attenuating mass in her breast evidences, in addition to normal postmenopausal changes, a random image pattern. Figure 24-8 illustrates an opaque nipple shadow which obscures all structures deep to the nipple, while Figures 24-9 and 24-10 (which were obtained by scanning the nipple regions of young subjects—one a normal 21-year-old (Fig. 24-9), the other a 3-week postpartum (nonbreast-feeding) subject demonstrate that structures deep to the nipple can be visualized (see earler discussion). The precise detailing in Figure 24-9 of the circular structures of the nipple should be noted.

Since the above described clinical program has been underway for a relatively brief time, statistical and other detailed data on diagnostic findings will not be presented here, but preliminary results will be reported elsewhere (29, 55, 56).

In regard to general results, it has been found that scanning in small (1- to 2-mm) step intervals in regions of a presumed mass is an essential requirement for correct diagnoses of tumor masses. Malignant tumors are usually not homogeneous, and they may include a variety of types of tissue components ranging from jagged- to smooth-walled, and from highly attenuating to cystic. Therefore, ultrasound examinations based on scanning a mass with large step intervals, such as 5 mm, may lead to an erroneous diagnosis. In the current program each patient is scanned in 1-mm step intervals in the region of a palpable mass (or the area designated as suspicious by mammography).

The overall clinical results to date indicate that for malignant masses the combined approach of mammography and ultrasound visualization can provide very high percentages of correct diagnostic diagnoses, and that this is more effective in differential diagnosis than either technique used exclusively, while for benign breast pathologies, ultrasound apparently can achieve a higher diagnostic accuracy than mammography. In that regard, fibroadenomas can be accurately diagnosed by either mammography or ultrasound if the subject is middle-aged or older, but for young subjects with dense breasts, ultrasound is a more accurate technique. In the case of cysts, ultrasound is the diagnostic method of choice for individuals of all ages, and is of particular value for young subjects. It was found, for example, that ultrasound definitively imaged cystic structures in dense young breasts of subjects whose mammograms had not revealed any abnormalities. Additionally, in many cases masses that were indeterminate in appearance on mammograms (even after thorough examination with x-ray magnification techniques) were shown, by ultrasound visualization, to be cystic. It was also found that even in those cases where cystic structures could be diagnosed by mammography, many more cystic lesions can be detected with acoustic imaging than with the radiographic imaging (including very small cystic structures revealed by the 1-mm step scanning). It is recommended, therefore, that in any clinical program in which x-ray and ultrasound are used as a combined technique, ultrasound imaging should be the initial examination performed, since this may eliminate the necessity of mammography. This is particularly true in the case of young subjects.

SUMMARY

The work of a number of investigators in many parts of the world has demonstrated the clinical usefulness of ultrasonic visualization techniques for diagnosis of both benign and malignant breast masses. To date, however, worldwide application of this method has been limited and, as a result, the potential of this method for differential diagnoses of breast pathologies and for breast cancer detection has been only partially realized. At present there is a serious need for additional, readily available, commercial ultrasound instrumentation that has been designed to meet the specific requirements associated with breast examination. As a minimum goal, such instrumentation should be capable of clearly imaging overt masses with dimensions of the order of 3 mm and of definitively diagnosing the malignant or benign nature of such small masses. Cooperative efforts between commercial companies, ultrasound scientists, engineers, and physicians in pursuing such goals would considerably decrease the time required to attain this level of success. During this imminent period of evolvement of improved ultrasound breast scanning instruments, physicians can have a major influence on further development of this field by applying, to as many patients as possible, presently available ultrasonic units for detection and diagnosis of breast pathologies. This approach on the part of physicians would stimulate the development of more sophisticated ultrasound breast examination instruments including those designed for mass screening.

ACKNOWLEDGEMENTS

The author gratefully acknowleges the financial support of research on ultrasound examination of the breast by the Showalter Residuary Trust, the Grant County Cancer Society, and the Indianapolis Center for Advanced Research, Inc. Special thanks and acknowledgment is given to the assistance of George Gardner in the ultrasound research, and to the various staff members of the Fortune-Fry Research Laboratory who contributed to many aspects of the instrumentation development and testing. Special thanks is also given to the secretarial assistance of JoAnne Drake.

REFERENCES

1. BAUM G: The detection of breast tumors by ultrasound methods. In Radiologic and Other Biophysical Methods in Tumor Diagnosis. Chicago, Year Book Medical, 1975, pp 405–414

2. BAUM G (ed): Ultrasonographic examination of the breast. In Fundamentals of Medical Ultrasonography. New York, GP Putnam Sons, 1975, pp 380–402

3. BAUM G: High resolution ultrasound mammography. In White D, Barnes R (eds): Ultrasound in Medicine, Vol 2. New York, Plenum, 1976, pp 469–470.

4. BAUM G: Ultrasound mammography. Radiology 122:199–205, 1977

5. BAUM G: Current status of ultrasound mammography. In White D, Lyons EA (eds): Ultrasound in Medicine, Vol 4. New York, Plenum, 1978, pp 299–311

6. BAUM G: The need for color coding in ultrasound mammography. J Clin Ultrasound 6:76–82, 1978

7. CALDERON C, VILKOMERSON D, MEZRICH R, ETZOLD KF, KINGSLEY B, HASKIN M: Differences in the attenuation of ultrasound by normal, benign, and malignant breast tissue. J Clin Ultrasound 4(4):249–254, 1976

8. CARSON PL, DICK DE, THIEME GA, DICK ML, BAYLY EJ, OUGHTON TV, DUBUQUE GL, BAY HP: Initial investigation of computed tomography for breast imaging with focused ultrasound beams. In White D, Lyons EA (eds): Ultrasound in Medicine, Vol 4. New York, Plenum, 1978, pp 319–322

9. COLE-BEUGELET C, BEIQUE RA: Continuous ultrasound B-scanning of palpable breast masses. Radiology 117:123–128, 1975

10. CRIBBS RW, ARNON S: High resolution synthetic aperture imaging. In White D, Brown RE (eds): Ultrasound in Medicine, Vol 3B. New York, Plenum, 1977, pp 1455–1462

11. DELAND FH: A modified technique of ultrasonography for the detection and differential diagnosis of breast lesions. Am J Roentgenol 105(2):446–452, 1969

12. DICK DE, BAY HP, CARSON PL: Hardware design of an ultrasound CT scanner. Proc Rocky Mountain Bioengineering Symposium 13:31–35, 1977

13. EVANS GC, LEHMAN JS, BRADY LW, SMYTH MG, HART DJ: Ultrasonic scanning of abdominal and pelvic organs using B-scan display. In Grossman CC, Holmes JH, Joyner C, Purnell EW (eds): Diagnostic Ultrasound. New York, Plenum, 1966, pp 369–415

14. FIJIMORI M, SAKAUCHI G, IZUO M, FUJII T, SARTO S, UEHARA C: Ultrasonic diagnosis of breast diseases. Med Ultrasonics 6(1):42–43, 1968 (Japan Society of Ultrasonics in Medicine)

15. FRY WJ, LEICHNER GH, OKUYAMA D, FRY FJ, KELLY-FRY E: Ultrasound visualization system employing new scanning and presentation methods. J Acoust Soc Am 44(5):1325–1338, 1968

16. FUKUDA T, WAGAI T (eds): Annual Report (1964) of the Medical Ultrasonics Research Center. Tokyo, Japan, Juntendo University School of Medicine, Mituba Printing, 1965, pp 1–33

17. GARRETT WJ, KOSSOFF G, CARPENTER D: Clinical studies with the Octoson. In White D, Brown R (eds): Ultrasound in Medicine, Vol 3A. New York, Plenum, 1977, pp 585–594

18. GARRETT WJ, KOSSOFF G, CARPENTER DA, RADOVANOVICH G: The Octoson in use. In White D, Barnes R (eds): Ultrasound in Medicine, Vol 2. New York, Plenum, 1976, pp 341–349

19. GLOVER GH: Computerized time-of-flight ultrasonic tomography for breast examination. Ultrasound Med Biol 3:117–127, 1977

20. GREENLEAF JF, JOHNSON SA, BAHN RC, RAJAGOPALAN R: Quantitative cross-sectional imaging of ultrasound parameters. In deKlerk J, McAvoy BR (eds): 1977 Ultrasonics Symposium Proceedings. New York, IEEE, 1977, pp 989–994

21. GREENLEAF JF, JOHNSON SA, BAHN RC, SAMAYOA WF, HANSEN CR: Images of acoustic refractive index and of attenuation: relation to tissue types within excised female breast. In White D, Brown RE (eds): Ultrasound in Medicine, Vol 3B. New York, Plenum, 1977, pp 2091–2093

22. GROS CM, DALE G: Interet de l'amplification logarithmique en echographie. J Radiol Electrol Med Nucl 56(6–7):487–490, 1975

23. GROS CM, DALE G, GAIRARD B, GAUTHERIE M: Correlations echothermographiques mammaires. J Radiol Electrol Med Nucl 56(6–7):481–486, 1975

24. GROS CM, DALE G, GAUTHERIE M, GAIRARD B, HAEHNEL P: Echography-radiography-histology correlation in breast cancer. In Proceedings of European Congress of Ultrasound in Medicine. New York, American Elsevier, 1975, pp 253–261

25. GROS CM, GAUTHERIE M, BOURJAT P, DALVIT G: Complimentarite des methodes physiques. Ann Radiol (Paris) 17(8):775–784, 1974

26. GROS CM, HAEHNEL P, DALE G, GAIRARD B: Echographie mammaire. J Radiol Electrol Med Nucl 55(8–9):611–614, 1974

27. GROS CM, JACOB M: Echographie mammaire et thyroidienne. J Radiol Med Nucl 52(3–4):222–228, 1971

28. GROS CM, JACOB M: Echographic mammaire: un cas clinique. J Radiol Med Nucl 53(10):680–681, 1972

29. HARPER P, KELLY-FRY E: Combined use of mammography and ultrasound visualization using a laboratory-modified commercial breast scanner to improve differential diagnosis. Proceedings of the 23rd Annual Meeting of AIUM, 1978, San Diego, p 131

30. HAYASHI S, WAGAI T, MIYAZAWA R, ITO K, ISHIKAWA S, UEMATSU K, KIKUCHI Y, UCHIDA R: Ultrasonic diagnosis of the breast tumor and cholelithiasis. J Surg Obstet Gynecol 70:34–40, 1962

31. HOLMES JH: Diagnosis of tumor by ultrasound. In Avel DM (ed): Progress in Clinical Cancer. New York, Grune & Stratton, 1967, pp 135–150

32. HOWRY DH: Techniques used in ultrasonic visualization of soft tissue. In Kelly E (ed): Ultrasound in Biology & Medicine. Washington DC, American Institute of Biological Sciences, 1957, pp 49–65

33. HOWRY DH: A brief atlas of diagnostic ultrasonic radiologic results. Radiol Clin North Am 3:433–452, 1965

34. HOWRY DH, BLISS WR: Visualization of soft tissue structures of the body. J Lab Clin Med 40:579–592, 1952

35. HOWRY DH, SCOTT DA, BLISS WR: The ultrasonic visualization of carcinoma of the breast and other soft tissue structures. Cancer 7:354–358, 1954

36. ITO K, YOKOI H, TATSUMI T: Quantitative color ultrasonography. Computer aided simultaneous tomogram method. In deVlieger M, White DN, McCready VR (eds): Proceedings, 2nd World Congress on Ultrasonics in Medicine, 4–8 June 1973, New York, American Elsevier, 1974, pp 366–372

37. JELLINS J, KOSSOFF G: Velocity compensation in water coupled breast echography. Ultrasonics 11:223–226, 1973

38. JELLINS J, KOSSOFF G, BUDDEE FW, REEVE TS: Ultrasonic visualization of the breast. Med J Aust 1:305–307, 1971

39. JELLINS J, KOSSOFF G, REEVE TS: Detection and classification of liquid filled masses in the breast by grey scale echography. Radiology 125:205–212, 1977

40. JELLINS J, KOSSOFF G, REEVE TS, BARRACLOUGH BN: Ultrasonic grey scale visualization of breast disease. Ultrasound Med Biol 1:393–404, 1975

41. JELLINS J, REEVE TS: Breast echography compared with xerography. In White D, Lyons EA (eds): Ultrasound in Medicine, Vol 4. New York, Plenum, 1978, pp 313–318

42. KAKETA K, WAGAI T (eds): Annual Report (1970) of the Medical Ultrasonics Research Center. Tokyo,

Japan, Juntendo University School of Medicine, Mituba Printing, 1971, pp 1–39

43. KELLY-FRY E: A study of ultrasonic detection of breast disease. First Quarterly Report, USPHS Cancer Control Program, PH86–68–193, 1968, pp 1–4

44. KELLY-FRY E: A study of ultrasonic detection of breast disease. Second Quarterly Report, USPHS Cancer Control Program, PH86–68–193, 1968, pp 1–14

45. KELLY-FRY E: A study of ultrasonic detection of breast disease. Third Quarterly Report, USPHS Cancer Control Program, PH86–68–193, 1969, pp, 1–18

46. KELLY-FRY E: A study of ultrasonic detection of breast disease. Progress Report, USPHS Cancer Control Program, PH86–68–193, 1970, pp 1–12

47. KELLY-FRY E: The use of ultrasound methods to detect changes in breast tissue which precede the formation of a malignant tumor. In Kessler LW (ed): Acoustical Holography, Vol 7. New York, Plenum, 1977, pp 1–20

48. KELLY-FRY E: Research approaches to breast tissue visualization by ultrasound methods. In Fry FJ (ed): Ultrasound: Its Applications in Medicine and Biology. Amsterdam, Elsevier Scientific, 1978, pp 637–672

49. KELLY-FRY E, FRANKLIN TD JR, GALLAGER HS: Ultrasound visualization of excised breast tissue: an experimental approach to the problem of precise identification of structure from echogram data. Proceedings of Acoustical Society of America, Washington DC, April, 1971

50. KELLY-FRY E, FRY FJ, GARDNER GW: Recommendations for widespread application of ultrasound visualization techniques for examination of the female breast. In White D, Brown RE (eds): Ultrasound in Medicine, Vol 3A. New York, Plenum, 1977, pp 1085–1088

51. KELLY-FRY E, FRY FJ, SANGHVI NT, HEIMBURGER RF: A combined clinical and research approach to the problem of ultrasound visualization of breast. In White D (ed): Ultrasound in Medicine, Vol 1. New York, Plenum, 1975, pp 309–320

52. KELLY-FRY E, GALLAGER HS, FRANKLIN TD JR: In vivo and in vitro studies of application of ultrasonic visualization techniques for detection of breast cancer. Proceedings of IEEE Sonics-Ultrasonics Symposium, Miami, December, 1971

53. KELLY-FRY E, GIBBONS LV: Application of ultrasonic visualization methods for study of the normal female breast and for demonstration of breast pathologies. Proceedings of 10th International Cancer Congress, Houston, May, 1970

54. KELLY-FRY E, GIBBONS LV, KOSSOFF G: Characterization of breast tissue by ultrasonic visualization methods. Proceedings of Acoustical Society of America, San Diego, November, 1969

55. KELLY-FRY E, HARPER P: Indications and comparative diagnostic value of combined echography and x-ray mammography for breast diseases—a preliminary report. In Proceedings of 3rd European Congress on Ultrasonics in Medicine, Bologna, October, 1978

56. KELLY-FRY E, HARPER P, GARDNER GW: Possible misdiagnosis of sound attenuating breast masses as detected by ultrasound visualization techniques and solutions to this problem. In Proceedings of the 23rd Annual Meeting of AIUM, San Diego, October, 1978, p 129

57. KELLY-FRY E, HINDMAN HA JR, TOWNSEND C, FRANKLIN TD JR., COLBERT JR: Application of ultrasonic methods for the characterization of breast tissue and for demonstration of the presence of breast pathologies. Proceedings of IEEE Sonics-Ultrasonics Symposium, San Francisco, November, 1970

58. KELLY-FRY E, KOSSOFF G, HINDMAN HA JR: The potential of ultrasound visualization for detecting the presence of abnormal structures within the female breast. Proceedings of IEEE Ultrasonics Symposium, 1972, pp 25–30

59. KELLY-FRY E, OKUYAMA D, FRY FJ: The influence of biological and instrumentation variables on the characteristics of echosonograms. In Bock J, Ossoinig K (eds): Ultrasono Graphia Medica. Vienna, Austria, Verlag der Wiener Medizinischen Akademie, 1969, pp 387–393

60. KELLY-FRY E, SANGHVI NT, FRY FJ, GALLAGER HS: Frequency dependent attenuation of malignant breast tumors studied by the Fast Fourier Transform technique. In Linzer M (ed): Ultrasonic Tissue Characterization II. NBS Special Publication 525. Washington DC, US Govt Printing Office, 1979, pp 85–91

61. KELLY-FRY E, SANGHVI NT, FRY FJ, GARDNER GW, GALLAGER HS: Determination of alterations of phase angle of ultrasound transmitted through a malignant breast tumor: a preliminary investigation. In White D, Lyons EA (eds): Ultrasound in Medicine, Vol 4. New York, Plenum, 1978, pp 493–501

62. KIKUCHI Y: Way to quantitative examination in ultrasonic diagnosis. Med Ultrasonics 6(1):1–8, 1968 (Japan Society of Ultrasonics in Medicine)

63. KIKUCHI Y: Present aspects of ultrasonotomography for medical diagnosis. In Stroke GW, Kock WE, Kikuchi Y, Tsujuichi J (eds): Ultrasonic Imaging and Holography: Medical, Sonar, and Optical Applications. New York, Plenum, 1974, pp 229–286

64. KIKUCHI Y, UCHIDA R, TANAKA K, WAGAI T: Early cancer diagnosis through ultrasonics. J Acoust Soc Am 29:824–833, 1957

65. KLEIN RI, DUMOND S: Ultrasonic evaluation of poorly circumscribed benign masses. In White D,

Brown RE (eds): Ultrasound in Medicine, Vol 3A. New York, Plenum, 1977, pp 1149–1150

66. KOBAYASHI T: Present status of differential diagnosis of breast cancer by ultrasound. Jpn J Clin Oncol 4(2):145–157, 1974

67. KOBAYASHI T: Review: Ultrasonic diagnosis of breast cancer. Ultrasound Med Biol 1:383–391, 1975

68. KOBAYASHI T: Gray-scale echography for breast cancer. Radiology 122(1):207–214, 1977

69. KOBAYASHI T: Grey scale echography for early breast cancer. In White D, Brown RE (eds): Ultrasound in Medicine, Vol 3A. New York, Plenum, 1977, pp 1089–1099

70. KOBAYASHI T: Clinical Ultrasound of the Breast. New York, Plenum, 1978

71. KOBAYASHI T, TAKATANI O, HATTORI N, KIMURA K: Clinical investigation for the differential diagnosis of breast tumor by means of the degraded sensitivity method of ultrasonotomogram (II). Med Ultrasonics 10(1):81–86, 1972 (Japan Society of Ultrasonics in Medicine)

72. KOBAYASHI T, TAKATANI O, HATTORI N, KIMURA K: Study of sensitivity-graded ultrasonotomography of breast tumor (preliminary report). Med Ultrasonics 10(1):38–40, 1972 (Japan Society of Ultrasonics in Medicine)

73. KOBAYASHI T, TAKATANI O, HATTORI N, KIMURA K: Clinical investigation for the differential diagnosis of breast tumor by means of the sensitivity graded method of ultrasonotomography (III). Med Ultrasonics 11(1):1–4, 1973 (Japan Society of Ultrasonics in Medicine)

74. KOBAYASHI T, TAKATANI O, HATTORI N, KIMURA K: Differential diagnosis of breast tumors. Cancer 33(4):940–951, 1974

75. KOSSOFF G: Improved techniques in ultrasonic cross-sectional echography. Ultrasonics 10:221–228, 1972

76. KOSSOFF G: Display techniques in ultrasound pulse echo investigations: a review. J Clin Ultrasound 2(1):61–72, 1974

77. KOSSOFF G, CARPENTER DA, ROBINSON DE, RADOVANOVICH G, GARRETT WJ: Octoson—a new rapid general purpose echoscope. In White D, Barnes R (eds): Ultrasound in Medicine, Vol 2. New York, Plenum, 1976, pp 333–339

78. KOSSOFF G, KELLY-FRY E, JELLINS J: Average velocity of ultrasound in the human female breast. J Acoust Soc Am 53(6):1730–1736, 1973

79. KRATCHOWIL A, KAISER P: Die darstellung der erkrankungen der weiblichen brust im Ultraschallschnittbildverfahren. In Bock J, Ossoinig K (eds): Ultrasono Graphia Medica, Vol III. Vienna, Austria, Verlag der Wiener Medizinischen Akademie, 1969, pp 119–126

80. LAING FC: Ultrasonographic evaluation of breast

masses. J Association Canadienne Radiologistes 27(4):278–282, 1976

81. LAING FC, HERZOG KA: Ultrasonic evaluation of breast masses. In White D (ed): Ultrasound in Medicine, Vol 1. New York, Plenum, 1975, p 331

82. NAKAO J, MASADE A, TUSDA H: Ultrasonic examination of breast tumors. Med Ultrasonics 6(1):44–45, 1968 (Japan Society of Ultrasonics in Medicine)

83. OSSOINIG K, KAISER P, KOLB R, LECHNER G: Echographische und rontgenologische befunde bei erkrankungen der mamma. In Bock J, Ossoinig K (eds): Ultrasono Graphia Medica, Vol III. Vienna, Austria, Verlag der Wiener Medizinischen Akademie, 1969, pp 127–133

84. PLUYGERS E: Diagnostic ultrasonore, par echographie A et B, des affections mammaires. J Belge Radiol 58(1):15–29, 1975

85. REEVE TS: Ultrasonic display of breast cancer. In White D, Brown RE (eds): Ultrasound in Medicine, Vol 3A. New York, Plenum, 1977, pp 1141–1142

86. SHIMA F, FUTAGAWA S: Ultrasonic examination of breast tumor. Med Ultrasonics 10(1):40, 1972 (Japan Society of Ultrasonics in Medicine)

87. TEIXIDOR HS, KAZAM E: Combined mammographic-sonographic evaluation of breast masses. Am J Roentgenol 128:409–417, 1977

88. VUCICEVIC ZM, WEN L-Y, WEBB R, MITCHELL G: Ultrasonic tissue differentiation. Bibl Ophthalmol 83:190–197, 1975

89. WAGAI T: Present state of the clinical application of ultrasonography. In Stroke GW, Kock WE, Kikuchi Y, Tsujuichi J (eds): Ultrasonic Imaging and Holography: Medical, Sonar, and Optical Applications. New York, Plenum, 1974, pp 553–566

90. WAGAI T, TSUTSUMI M: Mass screening of breast cancer by grey scale serial echography. In White D, Brown RE (eds): Ultrasound in Medicine, Vol 3A. New York, Plenum, 1977, pp 1147–1148

91. WAGAI T, TSUTSUMI M: Ultrasound examination of the breast. In Logan WW (ed): Breast Carcinoma: The Radiologists Expanded Role. New York, John Wiley & Sons, 1977, pp 325–342

92. WAGAI T, TSUTSUMI M, ISHIHARA A: Detection of breast cancer by grey-scale serial echography. In White D, Brown RE (eds): Ultrasound in Medicine, Vol 3A. New York, Plenum, 1977, pp 1143–1145

93. WELLS PNT, EVANS KT: An immersion scanner for two-dimensional ultrasonic examination of the human breast. Ultrasonics 6:220–228, 1968

94. WELLS PNT, HALLIWELL M, SKIDMORE R, WEBB AJ, WOODCOCK JP: Tumour detection by ultrasonic Doppler blood-flow signals. Ultrasonics 15(5):231–232, 1977

95. WILD JJ, NEAL D: Use of high-frequency ultrasonic waves for detecting changes of texture in living tissues. Lancet 1:655–657, 1951

96. WILD JJ, REID JM: Application of echo-ranging tech-

niques to the determination of structure of biological tissues. Science 115:226–230, 1952

97. WILD JJ, REID JM: Further pilot echographic studies on the histologic structure of tumors of the living intact human breast. Am J Pathol 28:839–861, 1952

98. WILD JJ, REID JM: Echographic visualization of lesions of the living intact human breast. Cancer Res 14(4):277–283, 1954

99. WILD JJ, REID JM: Diagnostic use of ultrasound. Br J Phys med, 1956, pp 1–11

100. WILD JJ, REID JM: Progress in the techniques of soft tissue examination by 15 mc pulsed ultrasound. In Kelly E (ed): Ultrasound in Biology and Medicine. Washington DC, American Institute of Biological Sciences, 1957, pp 30–48

101. YOKOI H, ITO K, INQUE T: C- and T-mode ultrasonic diagnosis equipment. Toshiba Rev 95:34–46, 1975

102. YOKOI H, ITO K, ITOH M, YUTA S, MATSUMOTO M: Clinical applications of real time color C-mode scanning of ultrasound tomogram by digital techniques. In White D, Brown RE (eds): Ultrasound in Medicine, Vol 3B. New York, Plenum, 1977, pp 1725–1737

103. YOKOI H, TATSUMI T, ITO K: Quantitative colour-ultrasonography by means of a computer aided simultaneous tomogram. Ultrasonics 13(5):219–224, 1975

25

Office real-time imaging

CHARLES W. HOHLER

The recent development of portable, relatively inexpensive real-time ultrasound scanners (with gray-scale capabilities) has not only enhanced the use of ultrasound in university hospital-based departments (of obstetrics and gynecology and radiology) but has also led to the use of this diagnostic modality by obstetricians in their private offices.

The author has collected data to show how cost effective this real-time equipment is and how it is incorporated into overall patient care in offices of specialists in obstetrics and gynecology (1).

To find out what use patterns are evolving, a survey of 25 ob-gyn practices using real-time ultrasound was conducted in November 1978. These practices were in geographic areas distributed all over the United States and were randomly selected from a list of physicians supplied by a manufacturer of real-time ultrasound equipment.*

SURVEY RESULTS AND COMMENTS

All 25 practices responded to the survey questionnaire. The results are discussed under eight broad categories, as follows:

* ADR Corporation, Tempe, Arizona.

1. Office setting
2. Personnel
3. Referral patterns and alternate resources
4. Economics and use
5. Third-party reimbursement
6. Medicolegal considerations
7. Education
8. The future of office-based real-time ultrasound

OFFICE SETTING

Of the physicians surveyed two-thirds are in single- or multispecialty groups and the remainder are in solo ob-gyn practice; 42% have had real-time equipment for less than 6 months, whereas 58% have been using this ultrasound modality for at least 1 year.

Of those surveyed 53% allot less than 15 min per scan for each patient, and the remainder set aside 15–30 min for the examination; 58% use ultrasound as the need arises, that is, during regular patient appointments. But 42% designate slots of time especially for scanning.

COMMENT

The relative speed with which a complete examination by real-time apparatus can be performed depends on the amount of teaching and patient instruction one wishes to do at the time of the scan.

PERSONNEL

Of the physicians surveyed 70% perform the sonar examination personally; however, 26% use nonphysician "assistants" for obtaining most of the scans. In 4% of practices all scanning is performed by "assistants."

The majority of the assistants performing these office-based scans are either nurses or office personnel trained by the physician specifically to do obstetric and gynecologic imaging. Only two practices employ a diagnostic medical sonographer registered in the American Society of Ultrasound Technical Specialists (ASUTS).

COMMENT

Whereas real-time ultrasound may appear to be relatively easy, the scan and its interpretation may be quite difficult, particularly in the hands of the poorly trained individual. It is the author's position that real-time office ultrasound examinations should be a "do-it-yourself project" performed by the physician. The reasons are the following: first, very few obstetricians are presently experienced or skillful sonographers—traits that can be acquired only by actual scanning and continuing education; the combination of inexperienced sonologists (physician sonographers) and inadequately trained assistants can only increase the possibility of diagnostic errors and, in turn, the physician's medicolegal liability. Second, because of his grasp of pelvic anatomy and pathophysiology the trained obstetrician-gynecologist is in a position to place ultrasound views of the pelvis and developing fetus in better clinical perspective than a nurse or technologist. Third, relying on an assistant takes away the opportunity for close contact between the obstetrician and the patients in a setting ideal for teaching and exchange of information. Such interaction with the patient and, perhaps, other members of her family may lead to better compliance with physician instructions, especially in high-risk pregnancies.

REFERRAL PATTERNS AND ALTERNATE COMMUNITY ULTRASOUND RESOURCES

Whereas 53% of respondents scan only their own patients, 42% of practices surveyed accept referrals for sonar imaging from other physicians in their community. Approximately 95% of office scans are done for obstetric indications. Very few physicians accept patient self-referrals.

Of those practices surveyed 58% have access to other ultrasound equipment in their community, usually located within a hospital-based department of radiology; 5% are able to use the services of other private practices in their community; 37% have no other diagnostic ultrasound resource in their community.

COMMENT

These results are remarkable. As little as 5 years ago, fewer than 30% of practitioners had diagnostic ultrasound services available in their community; until 4 years ago this meant a contact B-scanner and a university-based procedure not even universally accepted as useful or necessary for good obstetric and gynecologic care.

For many practitioners availability of sonar equipment is not the same as clinical utility. Although more than half of the respondents do have a nearby ultrasound facility available to them, they still elect to purchase their own equipment in an attempt to provide fast, reliable, and low-cost service to their patients.

In the long run each practitioner should judge for oneself the economic, political, professional, and community influences that bear upon the decision to acquire real-time office equipment. Before acquiring such equipment, physicians in any community should discuss the best means of providing ultrasound services. At the very least this mode of communication among physicians will lead to improvement in patient care by creating appropriate referral patterns for sonar examination.

ECONOMICS AND USE

Of the total respondents 68% purchased their equipment directly, and 27% either arranged for 5-year leases or took private bank loans.

In the average practice a mean of 13 initial and 8 repeat real-time examinations are performed per week. The number of patients scanned in different practices is shown in the following list.

Number of Gravidas Scanned in Different Obstetric (Ob) Practices

Ob Practices (%)	Gravidas Scanned (%)
15	<25
10	26–50
10	51–75
25	76–100
40	100

Note that, in 40% of surveyed practices, all obstetric patients are being scanned, at least once, between 20 and 30 weeks of gestation.

The mean fees for initial and repeat scans are $47.00 and $23.00 respectively. The mean monthly overhead expense averaged $258.00 (range $35.00–$700.00, depending on purchase arrangements of the equipment). The "hidden" costs of ultrasound scans include filing, postage, secretarial time, supplies, coupling agent, and physician time spent not only in performing scans but also in continuing education.

THIRD-PARTY REIMBURSEMENT

Of the respondents 56% were refused payment by at least one insurance carrier; 78% of such refusals were by the "Blues."

COMMENT

Since diagnostic ultrasound is not a routine screening examination reimbursement for indicated tests should not be refused. Furthermore, denial of insurance coverage based on the belief that diagnostic ultrasound as a radiologic procedure is not justifiable. The reason: ultrasound is neither an x-ray-related procedure nor one which falls exclusively within the province of the radiologist. To remedy this situation it is essential for obstetricians to exercise patience, maintain a spirit of active cooperation, and remain willing to communicate with officials of insurance companies to educate them regarding the multidisciplinary approach of diagnostic ultrasound. In the meantime patients should be informed that some insurance companies deny coverage for sonar examinations.

MEDICOLEGAL CONSIDERATIONS

The importance of proper records cannot be overemphasized. In view of the fact that 43% of respondents scan up to 25% of their patients more than once, a means of retrieving information from previous examinations is important.

Figure 25–1 shows the form the author uses to keep a record of the indications for each sonar examination. The sonar results are typed on another form. Records such as these are important documents of the patient's history and correlate clinical and ultrasound data. In addition, if, at some future date, questions arise regarding the reason for the ultrasound examination or the interpretation of the echograms, good records will form the basis for communication between physician and concerned party.

It would seem prudent, at present, to limit diagnostic B-scan ultrasound examinations to definite medical indications that are readily identifiable. Mothers who simply want to see the fetus or find out the sex should, in the author's opinion, be discouraged from such examinations. Nonetheless, maternal anxiety may in certain instances be construed as a reason for an ultrasound examination.

In today's litigious climate a poor reproductive outcome may be related to improper use of diagnostic ultrasound, especially if the test was performed in early pregnancy. In this event the obstetrician who cannot produce clear records of the indication for sonar may become vulnerable to medicolegal action. The obstetrician-sonologist who accepts the responsibility of performing office real-time imaging should continually review and analyze the number of scans performed, indications, results, and so forth, and should document continuing education credits in this field.

On the other hand, ultrasound is a well-established diagnostic entity, essential to patient care and widely accepted as the method of choice for the examination of the pregnant uterus (2). Thus, physicians and hospital ad-

ULTRASOUND OBSTETRIC EXAMINATION RECORD

Name _____ Date _____

Address _____ Exam No.QB— _____

_____

Phone _____ [ ] NEW   [ ] REPEAT

Indication: *Medical Complications:*

[ ] Gestational Age   [ ] Diabetes—Class
[ ] Multiple Gestation   [ ] Rh-Negative sensitized
[ ] Bleeding (1, 2, 3 trimester)   [ ] Hypertension
[ ] Mole   [ ] IUD in situ (Type _____)
[ ] IUGR   [ ] Toxemia
[ ] FDIU   [ ] Renal Disease
[ ] C-section   [ ] Anemia
[ ] PROM   [ ] Heart Disease
[ ] Dating for Ab   [ ] Drug Abuse
[ ] Amniocentesis   [ ] Other _____
_____ Genetic
_____ Fetal Maturity   Smoker [ ] No [ ] Yes
_____ Fetal Distress   Last Delivery Date _____
[ ] Research

Comments:

Patient Data:

Age _____ G _____ P _____
Ht _____ ft _____ in.   PP wt _____ lb   Present Wt _____ lb
LMP _____ Normal [ ] Yes [ ] No
Cycle length _____ days
EDC by LMP _____   Dates "Firm" [ ] Yes [ ] No
Fundal ht: _____ cm   GA(by LMP) _____ Wk
                                  GA(by U/S)   Wk (50th %)

FIG. 25–1. Example of a form used to keep a record of the indications for each sonar examination.

ministrators involved in the delivery of obstetric care may find themselves at increased risk for medicolegal action if they fail to provide diagnostic ultrasound services for their gravid patients.

EDUCATION

In comparison to contact scanners, real-time ultrasound apparatus are somewhat easier to handle. Nonetheless, competence in scanning and interpretation of images can be acquired only by experience, correlation of sonar diagnosis with clinical outcome, and continuing education. This last should include periodic reviews of the literature and attendance of meetings at both local and national levels. Anything less may not only lead to medicolegal liability but also be harmful to patients.

THE FUTURE

Since 90% of respondents expect to do more scans in their office next year and since 40% are already scanning all their patients between 20–30 weeks' gestation, it is apparent that an ever-increasing reliance on diagnostic ultrasound is truly a national trend.

The economics of office ultrasound seem very sound. Office use is becoming practical even on a limited budget. Ownership or lease of real-time equipment must be an individual decision, based on tax investment credit, depreciation and other personal financial considerations. However, it would be well to remember that with rapidly changing technology, 5 years can see considerable change in available equipment and prices; 5 years ago, for instance, real-time grayscale B-scanners were not even commercially available.

In summary the results of the survey conducted by the author indicate that the incorporation of real-time ultrasound into private practice has been found to be affordable, even for the solo practitioner, and useful in the clinical management of pregnant women. Furthermore, the use of this modality in an office setup may restructure antenatal care in the United States. The long term implications of these changes in the overall obstetric health care system remain to be critically assessed.

REFERENCES

1. HOHLER CW: Private practice use of real-time B-scan ultrasound in obstetrics and gynecology. J Clin Ultrasound 6:241–243, 1978
2. LELE PP: Application of ultrasound in medicine. N Engl J Med 286(24):1317–1318, 1972

26

Maternal organ imaging

HARVEY L. NEIMAN

Diagnostic ultrasound has advanced rapidly in the past several years owing to significant improvements in instrumentation. In particular, refinements in gray-scale image-processing techniques have accounted for much of this growth. Obstetric ultrasound is one area where the usefulness of this imaging modality has been most dramatic. However, the use of ultrasound in diagnosis of abdominal pathology has paralleled that of obstetrics. A more limited use has been found for diagnostic ultrasound in the evaluation of multiple abnormalities of the head and neck, chest, and extremities. These indications are now well established and are in daily clinical usage. The types of disease processes that can be diagnosed and in particular those that may be seen in the obstetric patient are discussed in this chapter.

The same basic concepts of interpretation are of value whether referring to an obstetric case or a nonobstetric problem. A fluid-filled space appears anechoic (echo free) whether it be the amniotic fluid or the serous fluid of a benign renal cyst. Solid structures appear echogenic whether they be the placenta or the normal hepatic parenchyma. Gray-scale ultrasound has progressed, however, to the point where further tissue characterization can be done. Slight differences in echogenicity within the liver can be noted and may be of utmost importance. Solid metastatic deposits to the liver may have an echo architecture only minimally different from the surrounding normal hepatic parenchyma (Fig. 26–1). Intrahepatic biliary radicals as small as 3 mm can be appreciated and differentiated from hepatic and portal veins.

Fluid-filled structures are sharply marginated, anechoic at various gain settings and have acoustic enhancement or strong transonicity (Fig. 26–2). Fluid-filled masses have the additional characteristic of generally being rounded or ovoid. An abscess with internal debris or a homogeneous cellular solid tumor may appear similar to a cyst at lower gain settings. But these lesions develop internal echoes at higher gain settings and have no evidence of acoustic enhancement. Appreciation of tissue texture is therefore most important in ultrasound and is a critical factor in diagnosis.

ANATOMY

Familiarity with normal upper abdominal vascular landmarks is essential for interpretation of cross-sectional images. Routinely, scans are obtained in transverse and longitudinal planes. Prone, oblique, and decubitus sections are also obtained, depending on the clinical problem. Compound, linear, and sector scanning techniques are used to maximize the diagnostic information.

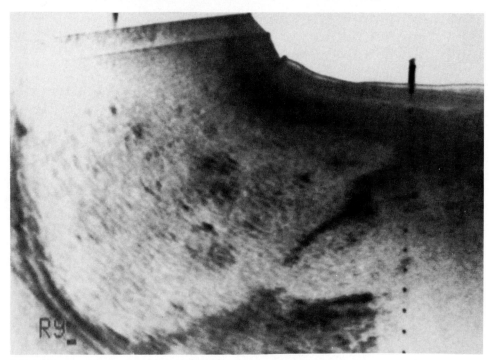

FIG. 26–1. Note the multiple echogenic, rounded mass lesions throughout the right lobe of the liver. Longitutinal section, 9 cm to the right of the midlength.

FIG. 26–2. Rounded, anechoic, sharply marginated mass with acoustic enhancement (**arrowhead**). This is a characteristic appearance for a simple renal cyst. The anechoic tubular structure within the liver is a hepatic vein.

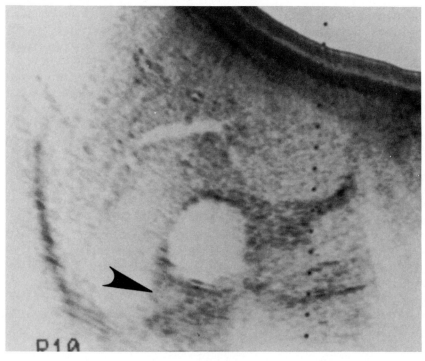

Identification of the abdominal vasculature may be important for diagnosis of intrinsic disease within these vessels. More commonly, however, these vessels serve as key landmarks for identification of parenchymal organs.

Routinely, the aorta, inferior vena cava, and superior mesenteric artery can be identified. The celiac artery and its major branches can be seen on a good-quality study (Fig. 26–3). The right renal artery and occasionally the left renal artery may also be imaged (35). On the venous side the left renal vein is constantly seen, whereas the right renal vein is more variable in its ability to be imaged (38) (Fig. 26–4). The hepatic veins within the liver are also invariably imaged. The portal venous system also serves as an important anatomic landmark, the splenic, superior mesenteric, and portal veins being consistently seen (7, 24). With appropriate scanning techniques the common bile duct can also be generally imaged (23).

The liver is easily identified and presents as a homogeneously echogenic structure with a characteristic architecture. Normal hepatic vein and portal vein radicals can be seen throughout. (Fig. 26–2) The right lobe of the liver is optimally studied with single-pass, longitudinal, sector scans of the right upper quadrant. The left lobe is best seen on transverse, single-pass, sector scans. The gallbladder is seen as a rounded or ovoid anechoic structure in the right upper quadrant (Fig. 26–5A and B).

The pancreatic bed or the pancreas itself can be identified by use of significant vascular landmarks. The pancreas lies ventral to the easily identifiable superior mesenteric artery. The splenic vein courses from the splenic hilum to the porta hepatis and lies on the dorsal and cephalic surface of the pancreas. The first and second portions of the duodenum cradle the head of the pancreas and can frequently be seen on a good-quality ultrasound examination. The uncinate process of the pancreas can also be identified encircling the superior mesenteric artery and vein. The pancreas itself appears as a homogeneously echogenic structure slightly more dense than the adjacent liver. (13).

In longitudinal sections the renal outline is ovoid, the parenchyma having low-level echogenicity. In transverse sections the kidney outline is rounded (Fig. 26–5B) The more centrally located collecting structures are quite echogenic

FIG. 26–3. Normal upper abdomen, 12 cm above the level of the umbilicus. The lower arrowhead points to the left renal vein as it courses to the left and ventral to the abdominal aorta. The gastroduodenal artery is seen (**arrowhead**). To the right of this structure is the common bile duct. Note the homogeneous appearance to the right and left lobes of the liver.

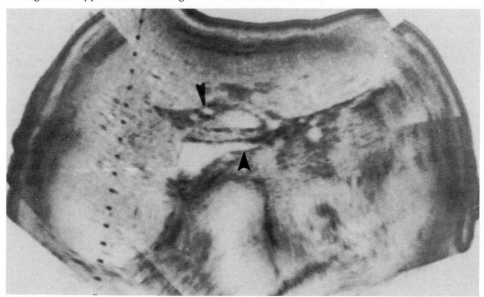

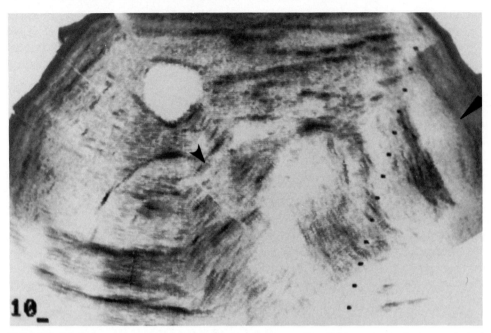

FIG. 26–4. Digital scan convertor image of upper abdomen; the right renal vein is demonstrated (**small arrowhead**) extending from the inferior vena cava to the right kidney. The rounded anechoic structure to the right of the midline is the gallbladder. The left side of the scan demonstrates the spleen (**large arrowhead**).

and densely packed. This central echo complex actually consists of the collecting system, hilar vessels, and sinus fat. On supine scans the right kidney is seen in close apposition to the liver, and the left kidney may be seen in close relationship to the spleen. With appropriate scanning techniques and newer instrumentation differentiation between the renal cortex and medulla can be obtained and the corticomedually junction identified (33).

It is essential to visualize the aorta, inferior vena cava, and right kidney on abdominal studies, for their structures serve as key criteria for identifying a diagnostic quality scan. Obesity and large volumes of intestinal gas are impediments to the passage of sound. An examination of the upper abdomen may be suboptimal or uninterpretable if these latter factors are excessive. Ultrasound remains an operator-dependent technique and requires close cooperation between the physician in charge, the technologist, the instrumentation, and the referring physician. There can be great variation in quality, depending on these independent factors.

Medical and surgical diseases in pregnancy may be caused by the following: 1) conditions arising in pregnancy, 2) intercurrent disease, 3) extrinsic factors, 4) preexisting disease. Numerous diseases and syndromes exist that fit these criteria. Ultrasound has proved to be of value in many conditions that affect the nonpregnant as well as the pregnant patient. This chapter primarily concerns itself with abnormalities that have been identified as being related to pregnancy and diagnosable by ultrasound.

GALLBLADDER AND PANCREAS

One of the most accurate uses of ultrasound is in the study of the gallbladder (21). Indications for gallbladder ultrasound are the following: 1) the nonvisualizing gallbladder by oral cholecystography, 2) the equivocal oral cholecystogram in which it is difficult to differentiate overlying bowel gas from gallstones, 3) the patient in whom it is desirous to avoid radiation, 4) the patient with an allergy to contrast material. Ultrasound has, therefore, a significant role in the

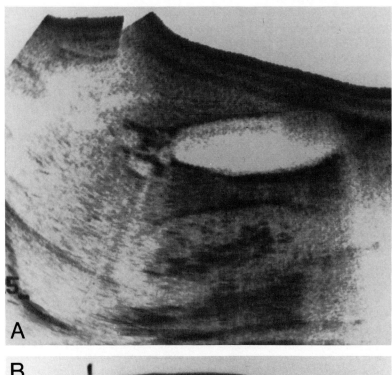

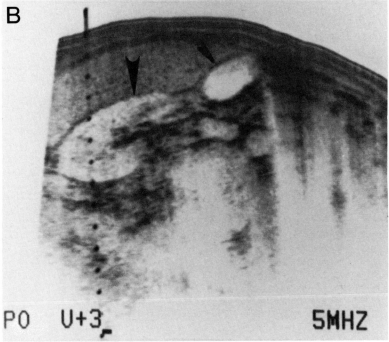

FIG. 26–5. A. Longitudinal section 5 cm to the right of the midline demonstrating the well-marginated, ovoid-shaped gallbladder. The right kidney is immediately dorsal to the gallbladder. **B.** Transverse scan demonstrating the relationship of the gallbladder (**small arrowhead**) and the right kidney (**large arrowhead**). Note the centrally located, dense echos within the right kidney from the collecting structures.

pregnant patient who presents with right upper quadrant pain.

Gallstones appear as dense echogenic complexes within the fluid-filled gallbladder (Fig. 26–6). The size of this echogenic area varies with the size of the gallstone. The prominent acoustic interface between the surrounding bile and the gallstone serves as an excellent reflector of sound waves with resultant acoustic shadowing behind the gallbladder. This dropping out of the echo pattern behind gallstones is seen in 60%–70% of cases and adds certainty to the diagnosis. Many studies have shown that gallbladder ultrasound is approximately 91% accurate in the detection of gallstones (125). Multiple views, including decubitus and upright sections of the gallbladder, are essential for this degree of accuracy, for gas in the hepatic flexure of the colon and duodenal bulb may simulate gallstones. Fine particulate matter in the gallbladder from gravel and sludge can also be diagnosed. Chronic cholecystitis may be demonstrated as a small, contracted, thick-walled gallbladder. Ultrasonic nonvisualization in a fasting patient is good circumstantial evidence of a chronically diseased gallbladder. Progression of disease with subsequent formation of a pericholecystic abscess can also be detected (3).

Cholodocholithiasis can be diagnosed by ultrasound with accuracy. In fact, ultrasound is 96% accurate in detecting dilation of the common bile duct (2). Obstructive jaundice can be differentiated in approximately 91% of cases. The diagnosis is based on detecting not only the dilated common bile duct but also the dilated intrahepatic biliary radicals (28, 29, 43).

Ultrasound has become the primary imaging technique for diseases of the pancreas. The pancreas or the pancreatic bed can be visualized in most patients. Occasionally, as previously noted, gas in the stomach and intestines obscures detail. Changing the patient's position (i.e., prone position for tail of pancreas) and filling the stomach with water may improve visualization in this latter group.

In acute edematous pancreatitis (Fig. 26–7)

FIG. 26–6. High-level echogenic complex within the gallbladder, with characteristic acoustic shadowing from a gallstone. Patient presented with right upper quadrant pain and is at 31 weeks' gestation.

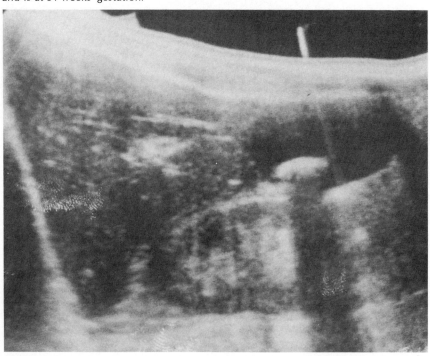

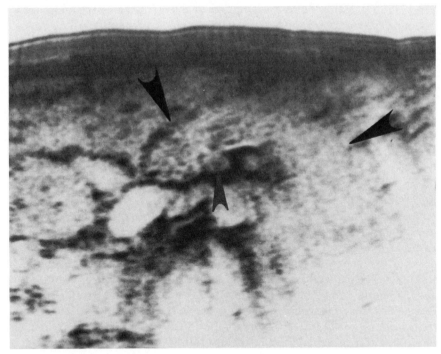

FIG. 26–7. Generalized enlargements of the pancreas secondary to acute edematous pancreatitis. The pancreas has slightly diminished echogenicity. The smaller arrowhead points to the superior mesenteric vein, the superior mesenteric artery being immediately to the left.

the gland usually enlarges uniformly and has decreased echogenicity. Multiple techniques exist for estimating an enlarged pancreas. Whereas no method is entirely accurate, in general the head of the pancreas should not exceed 3 cm in ventral–dorsal dimension, the body 2.5 cm, and the tail 2.0 cm. In acute pancreatitis there may also be a "silhouetting" of the margin between the pancreas and splenic vein (44). Occasionally, the disease processes may be focal, in which case the ultrasound appearance simulates that of a mass lesion. In the age group relating to pregnancy, however, the incidence of carcinoma is exceedingly uncommon. If the acute pancreatitis is secondary to an impacted common duct stone, then this latter abnormality may also be identified. Recently, dilatation of the pancreatic duct has been described with carcinoma and presumably may be seen in patients with obstruction from a stone and secondary pancreatitis (15).

Chronic pancreatitis is difficult to diagnose by ultrasound, for the atrophic gland cannot be differentiated from the surrounding peripancreatic tissues. But in chronic relapsing pancreatitis the edematous portion may be diagnosed. Calcification within the pancreas in individuals with chronic pancreatitis has also been described. Computed body tomography is more accurate than ultrasound in the evaluation of chronic pancreatic disease (40), but the radiation levels from this imaging technique make it relatively contraindicated in pregnancy.

In a large series pancreatic ultrasonography was correct 87% of the time in separating patients with a normal pancreas from those with abnormality (22).

KIDNEY AND ADRENAL

Evaluation of the poorly functioning or nonfunctioning kidney is of particular importance in the pregnant patient. Ultrasound has proved to be of great value in this clinical setting.

Several patterns of hydronephrosis have been

identified (37). Early, there is separation of the collecting system complex of echoes with development of a central echo-free area (Fig. 26–8). This is surrounded by well-defined echoes from the wall of the renal pelvis. With newer instrumentation dilated infundibula and calices can be identified (Fig. 26–9). Later, the collecting system echoes contain multiple centrally located echo-free areas, the so-called "O" sign and "C" sign. Finally, with advanced hydronephrosis, renal tissue may no longer be identified, and the kidney has the appearance of a multilobulated, fluid-filled sac (Fig. 26–10).

Hydronephrosis, particularly of the right kidney, occurs frequently during pregnancy. Ultrasound is an ideal technique for evaluating and continually monitoring the degree of hydronephrosis. The patient can be scanned supine or supine oblique, and therefore the study is easy to obtain. Possible concurrent disease in the left kidney can be evaluated at the same time. This may allow for an explanation of deteriorating renal function in the pregnant patient.

Renal calculi can also be detected with gray-scale ultrasonography (6). Renal stones are generally strong reflectors and have associated acoustic shadowing. Chronic renal parenchymal disease has recently been described as demonstrating characteristic changes on the ultrasound study. With increasing severity of disease there is progressively greater loss of the renal margin, increasing echogenicity of the renal parenchyma, and dispersal of the central collecting complex of echoes (19). Cortical scarring of chronic pyelonephritis can be identified. Differentiation of chronic glomerulonephritis, collagen–vascular disease, and nephrosclerosis can be made with less certainty. Little work has been done on the ultrasound changes in the kidney in toxemia of pregnancy, but identification of chronic renal parenchymal disease and differentiation from obstructive uropathy are of obvious clinical importance in the pregnant patient. With recent demonstration of intrarenal anatomy, including cortex, medulla, and arcuate vessels, there should be further advancements in defining the changes of medical renal diseases (8).

FIG. 26–8. Minimal changes of hydronephrosis with slight separation of the collecting system echoes.

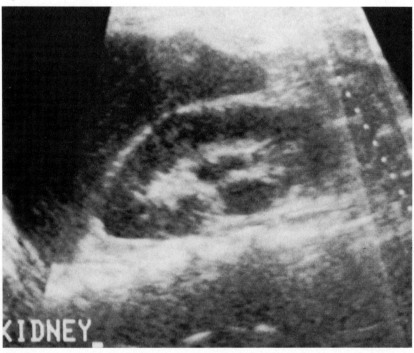

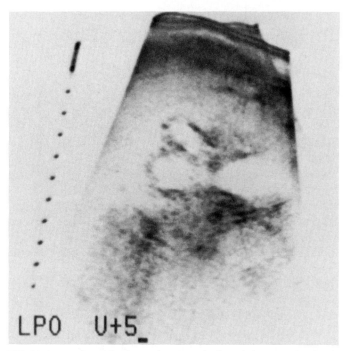

FIG. 26–9. Moderate hydronephrosis with clear definition of individual dilated major calices. Patient is at 34 weeks' gestation with progressively decreasing renal function. The right kidney demonstrates similar findings.

FIG. 26–10. Advanced hydronephrosis. There is loss of renal parenchyma and marked pyelocaliectasis of the right kidney. The left kidney is normal in this patient at 27 weeks' gestation.

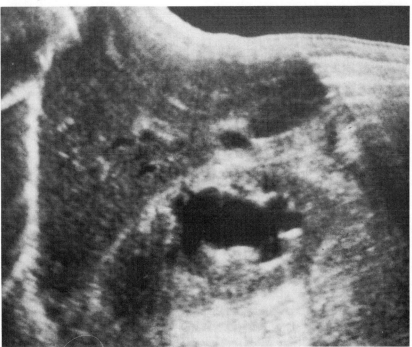

The adrenal gland can be imaged with ultrasound, but this is more easily done with CT (4).

THYROID AND SUPERFICIAL MASSES

Many aspects of thyroid metabolism are affected by pregnancy. The gland itself may enlarge in 25%–85% of patients. The diagnosis of hyperthyroidism may be difficult, for many of the values in thyroid function tests normally rise in pregnancy. Additionally, a solitary nodule may be difficult to differentiate from a generalized increase in thyroid size (41).

The standard imaging technique for the thyroid gland is the radionuclide scan. Ultrasound is an excellent adjunctive procedure that has the ability to determine thyroid volume (31), diagnose the presence of a nodule, and differentiate the cystic from the solid lesion.

The thyroid gland can be scanned by using either a water bath or a contact transducer. If a contact scan is done, a 5-MHz, 6-mm-diameter transducer should be used.

Ultrasound displays the glandular tissue of the thyroid as a homogeneous, low-level, echogenic structure lying in front of and on each side of the trachea. Posterior to the right and left lobes of the thyroid are seen the common carotid artery and internal jugular vein.

The cold nodule on a radionuclide scan presents a diagnostic dilemma, for this lesion may represent a cyst or a solid mass. Ultrasound clearly demonstrates a thyroid cyst as a rounded, anechoic, sharply marginated lesion (Fig. 26–11). A thyroid adenoma and carcinoma present a characteristic appearance of a solid mass lesion (Fig. 26–12) (34).

Other superficial masses (i.e., the parotid gland and breast) can be studied in a similar fashion (30).

VASCULAR

One of the earliest uses of ultrasound was in the detection of abdominal aortic aneurysms. Except for intercranial lesions, aneurysms anywhere within the body can be detected by ultrasound. Normal vessels demonstrate sharp margination with gentle tapering from proximal to distal, an anechoic center, and a diameter that is of expected size.

The normal abdominal aorta measures a maximum of 3.0 cm in diameter. The normal popliteal artery has been shown to be 0.8 cm ± 0.2 cm in diameter, irrespective of age (9).

The major advantage of ultrasound in the diagnosis of intraabdominal and peripheral aneurysms is the noninvasiveness of the study. Additionally, thrombus within an aneurysm can be visualized. Aneurysms of the visceral branches, such as a splenic artery aneurysm, are occasionally detected (14).

Differentiation of a baker's cyst from lower extremity deep-vein thrombosis can be important in the pregnant patient. Ultrasound demonstrates a baker's cyst as an anechoic, lentiform mass in the posterior calf. Depending on the amount of proliferative synovium, there is a variable amount of internal echoes.

Deep-vein thrombosis cannot be diagnosed by B-scan or real-time ultrasound. The latter diagnosis may be made noninvasively with the use of Doppler ultrasound and impedance plethysmography. With the present imaging techniques, thrombus in a peripheral vein cannot be seen, but thrombus within the inferior vena cava or an arterial aneurysm can be demonstrated.

ABSCESSES

Abscesses may occur secondary to operative procedures, hematagenous spread, or penetrating trauma. All these situations may be of moment in the pregnant and postpregnant patient. Ultrasound serves as a useful technique for detection of abscesses. No patient preparation is required, except that the patient's bladder should be distended for pelvic ultrasound examination.

Most abscesses are anechoic and have defined margins and acoustic enhancement. Abscesses that contain debris may, however, have internal echoes. The wall of an abscess is usually not as sharply defined as that of a cyst (Fig. 26–13). Abscesses generally are spherical or ellipsoidal, though they may be crescentic when in a con-

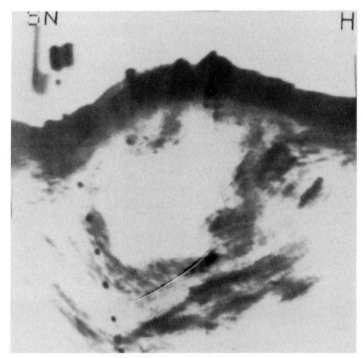

FIG. 26-11. Somewhat irregularly shaped anechoic mass in the right lobe of the thyroid. This palpable nodule presented as a photon-deficient area on the radionuclide scan. The ultrasound is characteristic of a cyst.

FIG. 26-12. Two echogenic mass lesions in the left lobe of the thyroid secondary to adenomata.

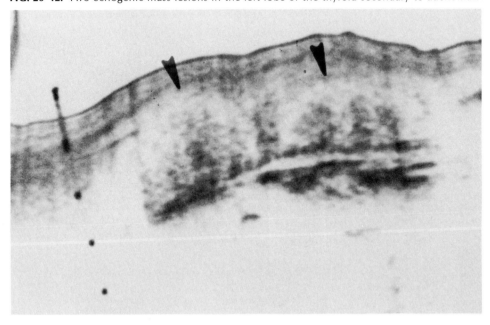

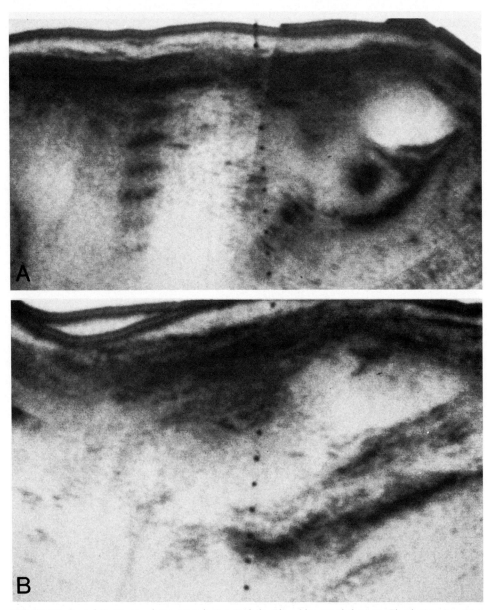

FIG. 26–13. A and **B.** Hypoechoic mass lesion in left side of lower abdomen. The lesion is somewhat poorly marginated and is compatible with the clinically suspected abscess. The patient is 2 weeks postcesarean section and presented with a picture suspicious for abscess. Note the electronic marker with which we are able to determine volume.

fined space. They also tend to displace adjacent structures (11).

Right subphrenic abscesses present little difficulty in diagnosis. The liver serves as an acoustic window, the right hemidiaphragm being easily imaged. Left subphrenic abscesses are more difficult to image, for the gas-filled stomach and splenic flexure of the colon obscure visualization. A single-pass, linear or sector scan in longitudinal plane with the patient in a left anterior oblique position has been found to facilitate greatly the visualization of the left upper quadrant.

Abscesses in the general peritoneal cavity usually present little difficulty in detection. However, whereas ultrasonography detects fluid collections readily, it is nonspecific in terms of the type of fluid. Pus, blood, or fluid in a distended loop of bowel may appear similar. The presence of a recent incision or a surgical drain complicates the performance of the procedure. In spite of these drawbacks ultrasound has been shown to be efficacious in abscess detection, having been shown in one series to have been 93% accurate (12).

An appendiceal abscess is a particular consideration in the patient of childbearing age. This lesion has an identical appearance to abscesses elsewhere, the specific diagnosis being made in correlation with the clinical picture. Regional enteritis of the terminal ilium with surrounding inflammatory reaction is in the differential diagnosis. The latter usually demonstrates, however, multiple thick-walled anechoic or hypoechoic areas in the right lower quadrant.

Pelvic abscesses also have the same ultrasonic properties as abscesses elsewhere. A fluid-filled bladder is, however, important for diagnosis. Postvoid scans should also be obtained for further confirmation (20).

PREGNANCY AND CANCER

Whether pregnancy exerts a specific effect on neoplastic disease continues to be a topic of interest. The older literature suggested a positive relationship. These observations have, however, been reappraised. Breast carcinoma in pregnancy is relatively rare. Carcinoma of the cervix

has an incidence of approximately 1 case/2000 pregnancies. Hodgkins disease has been reported to occur approximately once in 6000 pregnancies. Malignant melanoma, leukemia, and neoplasms of the stomach, colon, and pancreas occur in an incidence unrelated to gestation (18).

The obstetrician in the span of his practice is therefore likely to encounter a pregnant or recently pregnant patient with cancer. Ultrasound can play a significant role in the diagnosis and staging of neoplastic disease in this patient population.

The normal liver presents a homogeneous echo architecture interrupted only by the tubular anechoic hepatic veins and portal veins. Metastatic disease to the liver is of obvious clinical significance in the staging of neoplastic disease. Ultrasound has been shown to be an efficacious technique with respect to sensitivity as well as specificity (5). There are five basic patterns to the ultrasound appearance of metastatic disease to the liver (16, 39), as follows. 1) A metastatic deposit may appear more echogram than the surrounding liver (Fig. 26–1). The mass or masses are generally poorly marginated and range from being faintly more echogenic to intensely echo producing. 2) A deposit may be hypoechoic with respect to the surrounding liver. A variant of this is the Bull's Eye lesion that is frequently seen (Fig. 26–14). 3) Anechoic metastatic deposits have also been described as occurring primarily in sarcomatous lesions metastatic to the liver that have undergone necrosis. 4) The liver may be diffusely involved, areas containing all three of the previous types. 5) An area of abnormal echo architecture may exist within the liver. The echogenicity of the area is the same as the surrounding parenchyma, but the architectural pattern is different. This has been most commonly seen in our experience with primary tumors of the liver, though metastatic disease can occasionally cause this appearance. With present equipment the pattern of the metastasis is not specific for a primary tissue type.

Normal intrahepatic biliary radicals are not seen on standard sections through the liver. When these structures are dilated, they can, however, be appreciated on ultrasound sections.

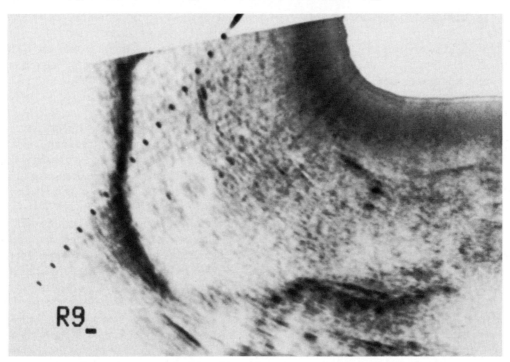

FIG. 26-14. Bull's Eye lesion in right lobe of liver secondary to metastatic ovarian carcinoma.

Dilated intrahepatic biliary radicals appear as single or multiple branching tubular structures that demonstrate acoustic enhancement (42). Mass lesions, such as lymphadenopathy, within the area of the porta hepatis can be detected, as well as the changes of biliary obstruction, with a high degree of accuracy (27, 36).

Periaortic adenopathy has also been determined by ultrasound with a high degree of accuracy (32). Those neoplasms that cause enlargement of lymph nodes, such as Hodgkin's disease and Non-Hodgkin's lymphoma can be imaged (Fig. 26-15). The adenopathy is seen as multiple masses or as a hypoechoic band adjacent to the abdominal aorta. These masses are of variable size and may silhouette the margin of the aorta. At first inspection the mass may simulate an abdominal aortic aneurysm, but it can be differentiated by careful scanning and evaluation of the margin between the abdominal aorta and suspected mass. With recent improvements in ultrasound instrumentation the adenopathy is increasingly seen as multiple discrete hypoechoic masses. Ultrasound can also be used as an effective means of monitoring patients to deter-

mine the effect of chemotherapy for change in tumor volume. Obviously, mass lesions in other portions of the peritoneal cavity and pelvis can also be studied, the ultrasound characteristics being dependent on the nature of the mass.

Ascites can be diagnosed easily with the use of ultrasound. Ascitic fluid is seen to collect in the lateral gutters and in the pelvis. If there is enough fluid, it is seen to involve much of the abdomen with bowel floating centrally (Fig. 26-16). Abdominal wall and peritoneal implants from tumors such as ovarian carcinoma can sometimes be visualized. Ascitic fluid can be differentiated from abscess, hematoma, cystic mass, and lymphocele (45).

Renal cystic disease is a common abnormality in the population. An incidental renal cyst may, therefore, be seen on a study of the pregnant patient. This is frequently seen during the work-up for gestational age. Renal cysts are sharply marginated, rounded, anechoic mass lesions at all gain settings with strong transonicity (17). A mass lesion that does not follow these criteria strictly must be considered solid until proved otherwise. While quite rare in the 20- to

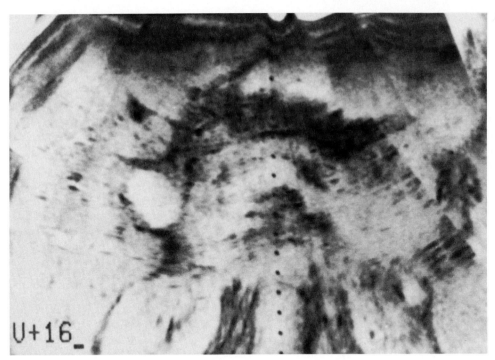

FIG. 26–15. Hypoechoic band in the periaortic region. Aorta is poorly visualized because of silhouetting by the large mass. Malignant melanoma.

FIG. 26–16. Large volume of ascitic fluid secondary to ovarian carcinoma. Individual loops of intestine are seen, for the wall is well visualized by fluid contained within the lumen as well as by the extraluminal ascites.

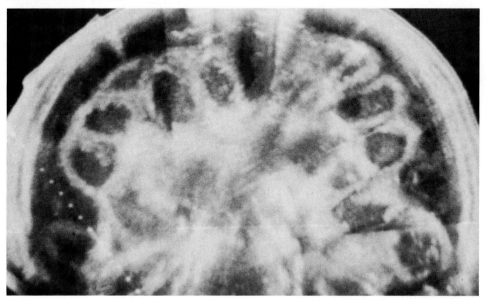

40-year-old group, renal cell carcinoma must be a consideration if the renal mass is not clearly a cyst (26).

Pleural effusion is another manifestation of metastatic malignancy. Ultrasonography provides an accurate means of differentiating pleural fluid from other entities that cause opacity of the chest x-ray. Ultrasound also localizes the fluid for thoracentesis, particularly in those cases with loculated effusion (10).

REFERENCES

1. ANDERSON JC, HARNED RK: Gray-scale ultrasonography of the gallbladder: an evaluation of accuracy and report of additional ultrasound signs. Am J Roentgenol 129:975–977, 1977

2. BEHAN M, KAZAM E: Sonography of the common bile duct: value of the right anterior oblique view. Am J Roentgenol 130:701–709, 1978

3. BERGMAN AB, NEIMAN HL, KRAUT B: Ultrasonic evaluation of pericholecystic abscesses. Am J Roentgenol (in press)

4. BERNARDINO ME, GOLDSTEIN HM, GREEN B: Gray-scale ultrasonography of adrenal neoplasms. Am J Roentgenol 130:741–744, 1978

5. BRYAN PJ, DINN WM, GROSSMAN ZD et al: Correlation of computed tomography, gray-scale ultrasonography and radionuclide imaging of the liver in detecting space-occupying processes. Radiology 124:387–393, 1977

6. CACCIARELLI AA, YOUNG N, LEVINE AJ: Gray-scale ultrasonic demonstration of nephrocalcinosis. Radiology 128:459–460, 1978

7. CARLSEN EN, FILLY RA: Newer ultrasonographic anatomy in the upper abdomen: in the portal and hepatic venous anatomy. J Clin Ultrasound 4:85–90, 1976

8. COOK JH, ROSENFIELD AT, TAYLOR KJ: Ultrasonic demonstration of intrarenal anatomy. Am J Roentgenol 129:831–835, 1977

9. DAVIS RP, NEIMAN HL, YAO JST et al: Ultrasound scan in diagnosis of peripheral aneurysms. Arch Surg 112:55–58, 1977

10. DOUST BD, BAUM JK, MAKALD MD et al: Ultrasonic evaluation of pleural opacities. Radiology 114:135–140, 1975

11. DOUST BD, QUIROZ F, STEWART JM: Ultrasonic distinction of abscesses from other intra-abdominal fluid collections. Radiology 125:213–218, 1977

12. FILLY RA, CALLEN PW: Ultrasonography in the evaluation of nontraumatic abdominopelvic emergencies. In The Radiologic Clinics Of North America. Philadelphia, WB Saunders, 1978, pp 159–173

13. FILLY RA, CARLSEN EN: Newer ultrasonographic anatomy in the upper abdomen. II. The major system veins and arteries with a special note on localization of the pancreas. J Clin Ultrasound 4:91–96, 1976

14. FILLY R, FREIMANIS AK: Thrombosed hepatic artery aneurysm. Radiology 97:629–630, 1970

15. GOSINK BB, LEOPOLD GR: The dilated pancreatic duct: ultrasonic evaluation. Radiology 126:475–478, 1978

16. GREEN G, BREE RL, GOLDSTEIN HM et al: Gray-scale ultrasound evaluation of hepatic neoplasms: patterns and correlations. Radiology 124:203–208, 1977

17. GREEN WM, KING DL, CASARELLA WJ: A reappraisal of sonolucent renal masses. Radiology 121:163–171, 1976

18. GREENSPAN EM, LESNICK GJ: Pregnancy and cancer. In Medical, Surgical, and Gynecologic Complications of Pregnancy. Baltimore, Williams & Wilkins, 1965, pp 290–300

19. KRUGLIK GD, NEIMAN HL, WOODRUFF A et al: Ultrasound correlations in non-obstructive chroinic renal disease. Radiology (in press)

20. LAING FC, JACOBS RP: Value of ultrasonography in the detection of retroperitoneal inflammatory masses. Radiology 123:169–172, 1977

21. LAWSON TL: Gray-scale cholecystosonography: diagnostic criteria and accuracy. Work In Progress 122:247–250, 1977

22. LAWSON TL: Sensitivity of pancreatic ultrasonography in the detection of pancreatic disease. Radiology 128:733–736, 1978

23. LEE TG, HENDERSON SC, EHRLICH R: Ultrasound diagnosis of common bile duct dilatation. Radiology 124:793–797, 1977

24. LEOPOLD GR: Gray-scale ultrasonic angiography of the upper abdomen. Radiology 117:665–671, 1975

25. LEOPOLD GR, AMBERG J, GOSINK BB et al: Gray-scale ultrasonic cholecystography: a comparison with conventional radiographic techniques. Radiology 121:445–448, 1976

26. MAKLAD NF, CHUANG VP, DOUST BD et al: Ultrasonic characterization of solid renal lesions: echographic, angiographic, and pathologic correlation. Radiology 123:733–739, 1977

27. MALINI S, SABEL J: Ultrasonography in obstructive jaundice. Radiology 123:429–433, 1977

28. NEIMAN HL, MINTZER RA: Accuracy of biliary duct ultrasound: comparison with cholangiography. Am J Roentgenol 129:979–982, 1977

29. NEIMAN HL, MINTZER RA: Gray-scale ultrasonography of the biliary duct system: comparison with percutaneous transhepatic cholangiography. In Ultrasound In Medicine, Vol 4. New York, Plenum Press, 1977, pp 121–123

30. NEIMAN HL, PHILLIPS JF, JACQUES DA et al: Ultrasound of the parotid gland. J Clin Ultrasound 4:11–14, 1976

31. RASMUSSEN SN, HJORTH L: Determination of thyroid volume by ultrasonic scanning. J Clin Ultrasound 2:143–147, 1975

32. ROCHESTER D, BOWIE J, KUNZMANN A et al: Ultrasound in the staging of lymphoma. Radiology 124:483–487, 1977

33. ROSENFIELD AT, TAYLOR KJW: Gray-scale ultrasound in the imaging of urinary tract disease. Yale Biol Med 50:335–353, 1977

34. SACKLER JP, PASSALAQUA AM, BLUM M et al: A spectrum of diseases of the thyroid gland as imaged by gray-scale water bath sonography. Radiology 125:467–472, 1977

35. SAMPLE WF: Techniques for improved delineation of normal anatomy of the upper abdomen and high retroperitoneum with gray-scale ultrasound. Radiology 124:197–202, 1977

36. SAMPLE WF, SARTI DA, GOLDSTEIN LI et al: Gray-scale ultrasonography of the jaundiced patient. Radiology 128:719–725, 1978

37. SANDERS RC: Renal ultrasound. Radiol Clin North Am 8:417–434, 1975

38. SANDERS RC, CONRAD MR, WHITE RI: Normal and abnormal upper abdominal venous structures as seen by ultrasound. Am J Roentgenol 128:657–662, 1977

39. SCHEIBLE W, GOSINK BB, LEOPOLD GR: Gray-scale echographic patterns of hepatic metastatic disease. Am J Roentgenol 129:983–987, 1977

40. STANLEY RJ, SAGEL SS, LEVITT RG: Computed tomographic evaluation of the pancreas. Radiology 124:715–722, 1977

41. STOWERS JM: Medical disorders, Sect 3, Alimentary and endocrine system. In Combined Textbook Of Obstetrics And Gynaecology. London, Churchill Livingstone, 1978, pp 210–219

42. TAYLOR KJW, CARPENTER DA, MCCREADY VR: Ultrasound and scintigraphy in the differential diagnosis of obstruction jaundice. J Clin Ultrasound 2:105–109, 1974

43. TAYLOR KJW, ROSENFIELD AT: Gray-scale ultrasonography in the differential diagnosis of jaundice. Arch Surg 112:820–825, 1977

44. WALLS WJ, GONZALEZ G, MARTIN NL et al: B-scan ultrasound evaluation of the pancreas: advantages and accuracy compared to other diagnostic techniques. Radiology 114:127–134, 1975

45. YEH HC, WOLF BS: Ultrasonography in ascites. Radiology 124:783–790, 1977

27

Echocardiography

SHERIDAN N. MEYERS, JAMES V. TALANO

Echocardiography is a noninvasive procedure, free from discomfort, that lends itself well to the study of pregnant women with possible cardiac disease. Because of its safety, ease of performance, and reproducibility, repeated studies and longitudinal evaluations are possible. Ultrasonic examination of the heart is performed, with almost equal ease, for evaluation of inpatients and outpatients—even at the bedside. In echocardiography the use of contrast media or catheters is not necessary; this is of particular advantage since introduction of such media may alter cardiac physiology (myocardial contractility, serum osmolality, vascular tone), and the placement of catheters may result in arrhythmias and intracardiac conduction disturbances. Ultrasound recording may be interfaced with other noninvasive techniques such as phonocardiography, electrocardiography, and apexcardiography, permitting better evaluation of a specific phenomenon. Because ultrasound transducers are pulsed at a rate of approximately 1000 times/sec, the time course of cardiac events can be very accurately followed; this is even better than clinical cineangiography, where angiograms are usually recorded at rates of 30–120 frames/sec. The rapidity of transducer pulsing is especially useful for observing moving structures as may be found in the heart. Thus, the size of the heart and its components can be accurately and reproducibly measured, cardiac structural anatomy can be evaluated, and good

estimates of alteration in cardiac physiology can be made.

The purpose of this chapter is to demonstrate the usefulness of echocardiography when applied to a patient population in which special care is desired to prevent iatrogenic injury and yet provide information necessary for evaluation of the heart. Accordingly, examples are provided of those cardiac disorders, both acquired and congenital, that may be expected to be encountered in an adult population. The salient features of each disorder are included, but those aspects that are presently considered to be controversial are either presented as such or have not been included. Further, consideration is given to two-dimensional cross-sectional echocardiography because this technique has enhanced ultrasonic evaluation of the heart. The reader is referred to standard textbooks for tables of normal values. The history of ultrasound in the evaluation of the heart is both interesting and dramatic but cannot be reviewed in this chapter, and the reader is also referred to standard references for this information.

M-Mode Echocardiography

Interpretation of echocardiograms is relatively easy. In marked contrast, however, the technical skills required for an adequate ultrasound examination of the heart are demanding. The sources of failure of an echocardiographic examination is more often related to the adequacy of the technical performance of the examination rather than to the skills required for interpretation. The sonologist should be careful about making inappropriate diagnoses as a result of 1) inadequate adjustment of equipment (gain, reject, control), 2) recording artifacts, and 3) failure to record important structures. Ultrasound does not conduct well through air, as in the lungs, and much of the sonic beam is reflected from bone. Therefore, certain approaches to the heart from the chest wall are more suitable than others. An echocardiographic examination is usually started with the transducer placed in the fourth intercostal space lateral to the left sternal border, with the ultrasound beam directed posteriorly. Slight angulation of the transducer cephalad or caudad may be necessary to obtain appropriate echoes from cardiac structures. Turning the patient slightly to his or her left side may be helpful. Depending on variations in body build and cardiac position relative to the thorax, a better echocardiogram may sometimes be obtained if the transducer is placed in the third or fifth intercostal space.

Another approach, useful in individuals with expanded lungs as in chronic obstructive pulmonary disease, is to place the transducer in the subxyphoid region and direct the ultrasound beam toward the left shoulder. The heart can then be scanned by moving the transducer in an arc from left to right. Other approaches such as supraclavicular, suprasternal, or esophageal (with a specially designed esophageal transducer) (36) may be of additional benefit in certain circumstances when the more common approaches are inadequate.

A longitudinal M-mode scan between the apex of the heart and the base, including the aorta and left atrium, is a necessary component of a complete echocardiographic examination (Fig. 27–1). Perhaps one of the more useful landmarks in the echocardiogram is the mitral valve with its characteristic M-shaped motion (Fig. 27–2) (33, 123). Early in diastole the anterior mitral leaflet opens into the left ventricle (toward the transducer positioned on the anterior chest wall) inscribing an upward movement

(D–E slope Fig. 27–2). As the rapid blood flow through the mitral valve decreases (and the left atrium empties) the anterior mitral leaflet starts to close toward the mitral orifice, moving posteriorly (away from the transducer) (E–F slope Fig. 27–2). When an effective mechanical atrial contraction is present, the increased movement of blood from the left atrium to the left ventricle causes the anterior mitral leaflet to again move into the left ventricular chamber, toward the transducer, resulting in the inscription of the "A" wave. With the onset of ventricular systole, as left ventricle pressure rises, the mitral valve again moves toward the closed position with the anterior leaflet moving posteriorly away from the transducer (A–C, Fig. 27–2). This characteristic M-shaped motion is readily identified and serves as a useful starting point in the orientation and identification of surrounding echoes. Motion of the posterior mitral leaflet is similar to the anterior valve. This motion is, however, directed toward the left ventricular posterior wall and away from the transducer positioned on the anterior chest wall. The echocardiographic inscription of the posterior mitral leaflet is of small magnitude because it is shorter than the anterior leaflet.

As one performs a longitudinal M-mode scan toward the base of the heart, one can see that 1) the anterior leaflet of the mitral valve becomes continuous with the posterior aortic wall (aortic–mitral continuity); 2) the posterior wall of the left ventricle becomes continuous with the posterior left atrial wall at the atrioventricular groove; 3) the interventricular septum becomes continuous with the anterior aortic wall. When one scans toward the apex of the left ventricle, the mitral valve leaflets become continuous with structures that have a similar position. These represent the chordae tendineae. More caudally (toward the apex) the chordae tendineae extend to the posterior papillary muscle.

In viewing the left ventricular posterior wall its endocardial and epicardial surfaces can be seen; during systole it moves toward the center of the left ventricular chamber (anterior and closer to the transducer) and becomes thicker. The endocardial surface of the posterior left ventricular wall is the most rapidly moving pos-

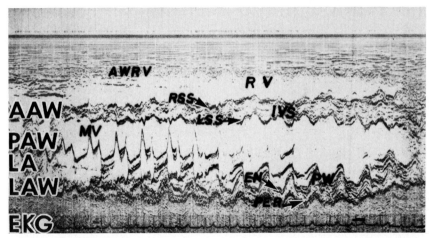

FIG. 27-1. Longitudinal M-mode scan of heart from base (**at left**) to apex (**at right**). The interventricular septum (IVS) is continuous with the anterior aortic wall (AAW). The mitral valve (MV) has the characteristic motion described in the text, and the anterior mitral leaflet is continuous with the posterior aortic wall (PAW). The left atrium (LA) is posterior to the aorta. The posterior left atrial wall (LAW) is continuous with the posterior wall of the left ventricle (PW), and the endocardium (EN) and pericardium (PER) can be identified. The right (RSS) and left (LSS) sides of the interventricular septum can be clearly seen. The excursion of the IVS and PW is greater near the apex of the left ventricle, as is often normally seen. The right ventricular cavity (RV) and anterior wall of the right ventricle (AWRV) can be seen.

FIG. 27-2. Normal mitral valve—E—point of maximum diastolic opening; F—point of closure in early diastole; A—atrial opening of mitral valve; C—point of closure of mitral valve in early systole; D—point of opening of mitral valve in early diastole; aml—anterior mitral leaflet; pml—posterior mitral leaflet; ivs—interventricular septum.

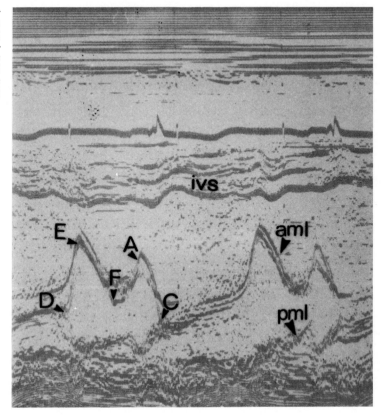

terior structure during systole. This feature can be used to help distinguish it from the chordae tendineae.

The interventricular septum normally and physiologically functions as part of the left ventricle. Thus, during systole its left side moves toward the center of the left ventricular chamber. Additionally, at the end of systole there is a notch in the left side of the interventricular septum thought to result from anterior movement of the entire heart (65).

The anterior and posterior aortic walls appear as two parallel undulating lines that move anteriorly (toward the chest wall) during systole and posteriorly during diastole; this is thought to be the result of movement of the heart and great vessels during the cardiac cycle. Within the aorta the normal aortic valve leaflets are represented by thin echoes that during systole have a boxlike appearance within the center of the aorta (Fig. 27–3A). The anterior echo is thought to represent the right coronary cusp and the pos-

terior echo the noncoronary cusp (33). The left coronary cusp (usually not visualized) may be represented by an echo moving through the center of the box. This cusp lacks anterior or posterior displacement because it moves perpendicular to the direction of the ultrasound beam. In diastole the cusps come into apposition and form a single, midline, somewhat more dense echo.

The first moving band of echoes seen behind the chest wall is thought to represent the anterior free wall of the right ventricle (Fig. 27–1). Usually only a small portion of the right ventricular chamber is seen with M-mode echocardiography and is often represented by a small echo-free space anterior to the right side of the interventricular septum. This space as it continues superior and anteriorly to the aortic root represents the right ventricular outflow tract.

If the transducer is angled more medially portions of the tricuspid valve which has a pattern of movement similar to that of the mitral

FIG. 27–3. A. Normal aortic valve. The right coronary leaflet (rcl) and the noncoronary leaflet (ncl) appear thin and open fully in systole and in diastole form a single echo that lies in the center of the aortic root; aaw—anterior aortic wall; paw—posterior aortic wall; LA—left atrium. **B.** Aortic valve in a patient with idiopathic hypertrophic subaortic stenosis. In midsystole there is midsystolic closure (msc) of the aortic valve.

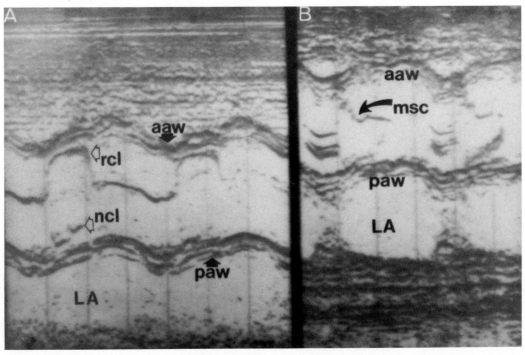

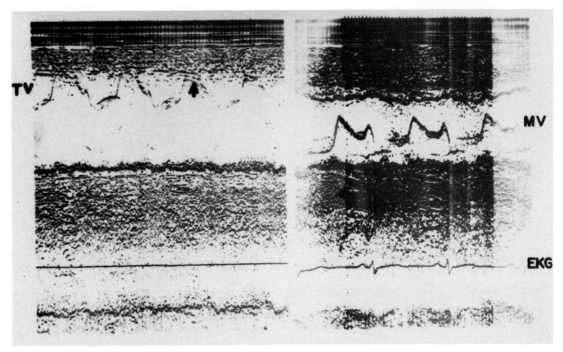

FIG. 27-4. Tricuspid valve. **A.** TV showing decreased E–F slope (**arrow**) suggesting tricuspid stenosis. **B.** Mitral valve (MV). At catheterization the patient had congenital tricuspid stenosis.

valve, can be seen (Fig. 27–4). If the transducer is directed superiorly and laterally (to the left of the aortic valve), a portion of the pulmonic valve can be recorded.

With M-mode echocardiography, usually only the posterior leaflet of the pulmonic valve is recorded. Its characteristic motion has been well described by Weyman et al (116) (Fig. 27–5). As a result of right atrial contraction and the effects of the transmitted pressure on the pulmonic valve an initial slight posterior movement is recorded ("a" wave). The leaflet then moves slightly anteriorly to the "b" point, the position of the pulmonic valve at the onset of ventricular ejection (Fig. 27–5). During ventricular systole the valve opens posteriorly to the fully opened position ("c" point) followed by a gradual anterior movement during systole to the "d" point (Fig. 27–5). With the onset of diastole there is rapid closure to the "e" point. The leaflet then gradually moves posteriorly, point "f."

In the presence of pulmonary hypertension the maximal amplitude of the "a" wave during the inspiratory phase of quiet respiration is generally equal to or less than 2 mm. The e–f slope is either reduced or negative (meaning that it moves anteriorly rather than posteriorly). There is also systolic fluttering and midsystolic closure of the pulmonic valve, the latter being the most specific finding in pulmonary hypertension (117) (Fig. 27–6). The opening slope (b–c) of the pulmonic valve is increased, and the right ventricular preejection period is prolonged (79).

In the presence of pulmonic valvular stenosis the "a" wave of the posterior pulmonic valve leaflet may have an increased amplitude. This may be the result of a normal or reduced pulmonary artery pressure, an increased right ventricular end-diastolic pressure, and an increased force of right atrial contraction (117).

On the other hand, with pulmonary infundibular stenosis the pulmonic valve exhibits high-frequency, coarse fluttering noted primarily during systole but which can extend into diastole (117). The fluttering may be the result of a turbulent stream of blood distal to the infundibular obstruction striking the pulmonary valve.

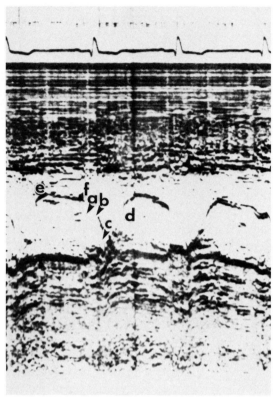

FIG. 27-5. Normal pulmonic valve. (See text for explanation of movement during various phases of the cardiac cycle.)

Evaluation of Left Ventricular Function

Measurements of the left ventricle can provide useful information. The left ventricular internal dimension in diastole (LVID$_d$) is measured as the distance between the endocardial echoes of the left side of the interventricular septum and the left ventricular posterior wall at end-diastole. This is often taken at the peak of the R-wave of the QRS complex (33). The left ventricular internal dimension in systole (LVID$_s$) is measured as the distance between the endocardial echoes of the left side of the interventricular septum and the posterior wall of the left ventricle at end-systole. This may be taken at the peak of posterior motion of the interventricular septum (33). However, since the peak posterior movement of the interventricular septum and the peak anterior movement of the posterior wall of the left ventricle often do not occur simultaneously, various points are used by different investigators to represent the end of systole. These dimensions alone provide a crude estimate of left ventricular chamber size and function. If the left ventricular internal dimension is increased, one may suspect a dilated left ventricle. If the difference between the left ventricular internal dimension in systole is much smaller

FIG. 27-6. Echocardiogram of a patient with pulmonary hypertension. Note the flat e–f slope (**open arrow**) and midsystolic notching of the pulmonic valve (PV) (**solid arrow**) in the right panel. The M-mode scan on the left side of the figure demonstrates the relationship between right ventricle (RV), left ventricle (LV), mitral valve (MV), tricuspid valve (TV), aortic valve (AV), and left atrium (LA); ivs—interventricular septum; pw—posterior wall left ventricle.

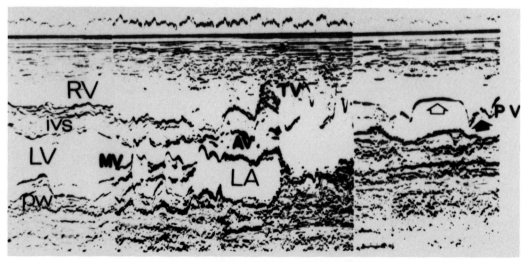

than that in diastole, one may expect a good ejection fraction, but if there is only a small difference between the two measurements, one may expect a decreased ejection fraction. Left ventricular dilatation associated with an exaggerated excursion of the interventricular septum (>8 mm) and left ventricular posterior wall suggests the presence of left ventricular volume overload; this is seen in significant aortic regurgitation, mitral regurgitation, and a large left-to-right shunt (ventricular septal defect or a patent ductus arteriosus).

One must remember that only two points on the left ventricle are being used to make complex assumptions in estimating left ventricular size and function. These assumptions are erroneous if 1) the two points used are not representative of the remainder of the left ventricle and 2) there are differences in beam angulation between measurements, 3) abnormalities in left ventricular geometry, and 4) segmental regions of differing function. Despite the many theoretical objections and practical problems, many of the measurements used to evaluate left ventricular function, though not always correct in absolute value, may provide a determination useful in evaluating left ventricular function and correlate well with the trend of measurements derived from other techniques.

Although a number of formulae and correction factors have been offered for calculation of left ventricular volume (35, 85, 110), stroke volume (88), and ejection fraction, a simple method is to cube the $LVID_d$ to calculate left ventricular end-diastolic volume (EDV) and cube $LVID_s$ to calculate left ventricular end-systolic volume (ESV) (85). Left ventricular ejection fraction is then calculated as:

$$\frac{(LVID_d)^3 - (LVID_s)^3}{(LVID_d)^3}$$

Another means of looking at this same information is to calculate the percent fractional shortening of the left ventricle:

$$\frac{LVID_d - LVID_s}{LVID_d} \times 100.$$

The mean rate of circumferential fiber shortening (mean Vcf) expressed as circumferences/sec is calculated (18):

$$\frac{LVID_d - LVID_s}{LVID_d \times LVET}$$

In other words the circumferential shortening of the left ventricle

$$\left(\frac{LVID_d - LVID_s}{LVID_d} \right)$$

is divided by the left ventricular ejection time (LVET). Left ventricular ejection time may be measured from the carotid pulse recording, the echocardiographic aortic valve opening during systole, or the time from the peak of the QRS to the point of maximal anterior movement of the left ventricular posterior wall less 50 msec (the preejection period) (18).

Analysis of the movement of the left ventricular posterior wall has been used in the past as a measure of left ventricular function but appears to be less useful than other measurements. In the presence of segmental myocardial disease the posterior wall if primarily involved may not move nearly as well as the remainder of the ventricle. To the contrary, if other segments of the left ventricle are functioning poorly, the posterior wall may be compensating for these other segments and have exaggerated motion.

Inspection of the various regions of the left ventricle can provide useful information. For example, if a portion of the interventricular septum or the posterior wall of the left ventricle is seen to contract less well than the remainder of the ventricle or possibly to become thin in systole with paradoxical motion (features seen in dyskinesia), segmental disease (ischemic heart disease, trauma, coronary artery embolism) is suspected. On the other hand, if one sees a dilated left ventricle contracting poorly and equally in all visible regions, a diffuse process such as a cardiomyopathy may be suspected.

Rosenblatt et al (95) noted that the left ventricular ejection phase indices (left ventricular minor diameter percentage shortening, the echocardiographic calculated ejection fraction, and the echocardiographic calculated mean velocity of circumferential fiber shortening [Vcf]) provided the best estimate of myocardial function. These were useful in assessing compensated or decompensated volume overload (aortic regurgitation, mitral regurgitation) and pressure overload (aortic stenosis). It was thought that the percentage change in minor diameter shortening appeared to be the easiest used measurement because 1) there was not much difference between the discriminating ability of these three indices, 2) left ventricular ejection time is more difficult to measure on the echocardiogram and varies between individuals and with different diseases, and 3) the ejection fraction offers no significant advantage over measurement of the minor diameter.

Motion of the mitral valve has been used by some to assess indirectly certain alterations in left ventricular performance (92). In addition, mitral valve movement has been used to assess blood flow indirectly from left atrium to left ventricle. The precise usefulness of mitral valve movement in the indirect evaluation of blood flow and cardiac function is uncertain at present. Vignola et al (113) noted that changes in E–F slope of the mitral valve appeared to be related to changes in left ventricular compliance (pressure-volume), particularly during the early part of diastole.

Konecke et al (59) studied the relationship between the pattern of mitral valve movement and left ventricular diastolic pressure. They reported that in patients with elevated left ventricular end-diastolic pressure and a prominent left ventricular A wave ("atrial kick") there was prolongation of mitral valve closure (A–C interval). Differences in atrioventricular conduction were corrected for by subtracting the A–C interval measured on the echocardiogram from the P–R interval measured from a simultaneously recorded electrocardiogram. Values ≦0.06 sec were associated with left ventricular end-diastolic pressures ≧20 mm Hg and a left ventricular "A" wave ≧8 mm Hg. Patients with elevated left ventricular early diastolic pressure had a decreased velocity of mitral valve opening (reduced D–E slope) and an accentuated A wave on the mitral echogram. Yow and Reichek (122) reported poor correlation between the A–C slope duration, and excursion and left ventricular end-diastolic pressure and found many false positives. More recently Lewis et al (63) found the PR minus AC interval to be a poor predictor of left ventricular end-diastolic pressure; when followed through a variety of maneuvers designed to change acutely the left ventricular

diastolic pressure in the same patient, the PR minus AC interval showed little change.

Katz, Karliner, and Resnik (54) followed 19 patients through pregnancy and evaluated changes in cardiac function using noninvasive techniques. Heart rate increased: left ventricular ejection time decreased, which was greater and more significant when the patient was in the supine position than when in the left lateral decubitus position. The left ventricular internal dimensions at end-diastole and end-systole increased during pregnancy when recorded with the patient in the left lateral decubitus position. The left atrial dimension was observed to increase while the aortic dimension remained unchanged. The E–F slope of the mitral valve was noted to decrease when recorded in the supine position but not in the left lateral decubitus position: this was thought to be due to interference on venous return by the enlarging uterus. Calculated left ventricular mass increased during pregnancy and decreased postpartum, suggesting the development and then regression of hypertrophy. The decreased ratio of posterior wall thickness to left ventricular wall radius was consistent with the development of eccentric hypertrophy. Ejection fraction, Vcf, and percent of fractional shortening did not appear to have changed significantly. Despite the development of volume overload, the shortening characteristics and other measured parameters of left ventricular function remained within normal limits.

Mitral Valvular Stenosis

In mitral valvular stenosis acquired as a result of rheumatic carditis the mitral valve leaflets often appear thickened. Because of the reduced mitral valve orifice size, blood flow through the mitral valve is impaired and emptying of the left atrium into the left ventricle is prolonged. As a result the diastolic closing velocity of the anterior mitral valve leaflet (E–F slope) is reduced (123). The "A" wave is often blunted or almost absent. The posterior mitral valve leaflet is usually seen to move parallel to the anterior mitral leaflet, as opposed to the normal opposite direction of these two leaflets in diastole (31). This latter feature when present appears to be diagnostic for mitral valvular stenosis (Fig. 27–7, 8). There

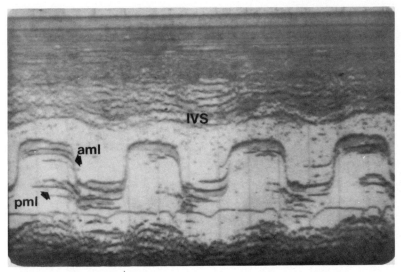

FIG. 27-7. Mitral valvular stenosis. The anterior mitral leaflet (aml) and the posterior mitral leaflet (pml) appear thickened and have a similar direction of movement characteristic of mitral valvular stenosis. The E–F slope is reduced; ivs—interventricular septum.

FIG. 27-8. Mitral stenosis with thickening of anterior mitral valve leaflet (AMVL) and posterior mitral valve leaflet (PMV). Note the posterior mitral leaflet moves in the same direction and parallel to the anterior mitral leaflet. There is a reduced mitral valve excursion in diastole, and the E–F slope is reduced. Calcification of the mitral annulus (MA) is seen as a dense band of echoes between the mitral valve and the posterior wall of the left ventricle (PW). The left atrium (LA) is enlarged. The aortic valve (AV) demonstrates a reduced opening and slightly thickened leaflets.

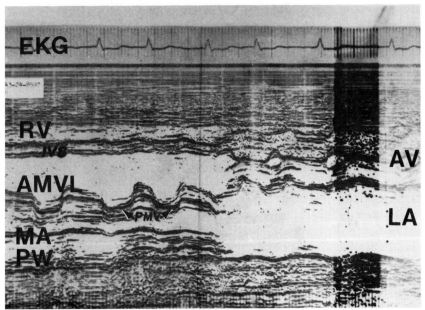

have been several reports of instances in which posterior mitral leaflet movement appeared normal in the presence of mitral stenosis documented by cardiac catheterization and surgery (7, 34, 62). Nevertheless, in these instances, other accompanying echocardiographic features of mitral stenosis may be sufficient to at least raise the suspicion of its presence.

Severity of Mitral Stenosis

Mitral valve excursion, commonly measured as the anterior–posterior distance between the D and E points, is reduced as the mitral valve leaflets become less pliable. Some cardiologists use the excursion of the mitral valve as a parameter in the decision-making process of whether a commissurotomy or valve replacement is necessary. Specifically, if mitral valve excursion is less than 1.5 to 2 cm, a successful commissurotomy is less likely. Others believe that mitral valve excursion is of limited usefulness for predicting the optimal surgical procedure (19). The severity of mitral stenosis may also be evaluated by other parameters. First, the persistence of thin mitral valve leaflet echoes suggests pliable leaflets with less fibrosis. Secondly, a slower diastolic mitral valve closing velocity (E–F slope) suggests a more severe mitral stenosis.Again, although this may be useful, several reports indicate that it is not entirely reliable (19).

Associated Cardiac Findings

Associated cardiac findings in the presence of mitral stenosis include decreased left ventricular dimension (especially in the presence of pure, isolated mitral valvular stenosis), increased left atrial dimension (Fig. 27–8), and at times increase in right ventricular dimension. With cardiac failure, pericardial effusion may appear. In the presence of pulmonary hypertension there may be alterations in the pulmonic "a" wave as well as other movements of the pulmonic valve discussed earlier. When tricuspid regurgitation is present (often functional and secondary to pulmonary hypertension with right ventricular failure), paradoxical motion of the interventricular septum and increase in right ventricular diastolic dimension may be seen. Motion of the posterior aortic wall has been used to evaluate left atrial emptying indirectly and relate this to obstruction to flow across a stenotic mitral valve (106). Left atrial thrombi are not readily visualized with M-mode echocardiography, though perhaps more information will be obtained with two-dimensional sector scanning.

Mitral Regurgitation

Mitral regurgitation may have a variety of etiologies; some of these result in specific abnormalities of the mitral valve that are apparent on the echocardiogram (14). In some types of mitral regurgitation, however, the abnormality of the mitral valve is not currently detected by echocardiography. Nonetheless, in these patients the pathophysiology may be suspected by the presence of features that are secondary to mitral regurgitation, namely, left ventricular volume overload, left atrial volume overload, and increased mitral excursion in diastole.

In the presence of known mitral regurgitation a left ventricle showing evidence of left ventricular volume overload in the face of a normal ejection fraction suggests the preservation of ventricular function. On the other hand, the association of a dilated ventricle with reduced ejection fraction suggests impaired ventricular function. When the latter findings are accompanied by a murmur of mitral regurgitation, papillary muscle dysfunction should be entertained as the etiology.

The presence of a large left atrium with other evidence for mitral regurgitation would be in keeping with a chronic process. However, when mitral regurgitation and left ventricular volume overload are associated with a normal left atrium, an acute process is likely. Thus, valuable information can be obtained from an echocardiogram regardless of whether a specific pattern of mitral regurgitation is present.

Mitral Valve Prolapse

The clinical syndrome of mitral valve prolapse is well known, with its classic midsystolic click and mid- to late systolic murmur, the frequently associated findings of cardiac arrhythmias, non-specific electrocardiographic abnormalities, and a complex of clinical symptoms, including chest pain (4). The echocardiographic picture of mitral valve prolapse is fairly characteristic (Figs. 27–9, 10) (26, 66). As mentioned previously, with the onset of systole the mitral leaflets normally come into apposition, and move slowly to a more anterior position throughout systole until the mitral valve leaflets open at the beginning of the following diastole. When mitral valve prolapse is present, the echoes representing either one or both mitral leaflets are seen to move posteriorly, usually in midsystole, and remain there until the end of systole, at which time they move anteriorly. In some instances the two leaflets may move either parallel to the anterior chest wall (flat C–D slope) or slightly posteriorly (negative C–D) before a more abrupt midsystolic posterior movement is seen. In other instances there may be holosystolic posterior prolapse of the mitral leaflets. Occasionally, the mitral leaflets are seen to move anteriorly in early systole and then move posteriorly in midsystole and late systole (86) (Fig. 27–10). This initial anterior movement should not be confused with the abnormal mitral valve movement seen in idiopathic hypertrophic subaortic stenosis. In the latter condition the abnormal anterior movement of the mitral valve begins after the onset of systole, and the valve remains anterior and adjacent to the interventricular septum throughout midsystole—returning to a more posterior position before the end of systole. In addition the other features of idiopathic hypertrophic subaortic stenosis are usually absent when the early anterior movement of the mitral valve is a result of mitral valve prolapse. In some instances of mitral valve prolapse, the mitral leaflets are seen to move into the left atrium and against the posterior left atrial wall. Further, during systole (especially during midsystole and late systole) multiple-layered echoes are seen.

In patients with myxomatpus degeneration of the mitral valve, frequent seem with prolapse,

FIG. 27–9. Mitral valve prolapse. In midsystole there is posterior prolapse **(arrow)** of the mitral valve (MV); ivs—interventricular septum.

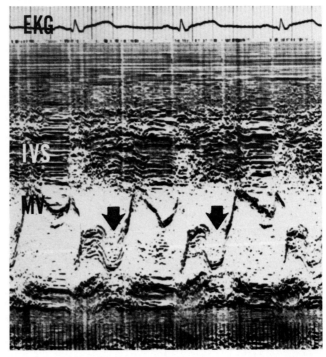

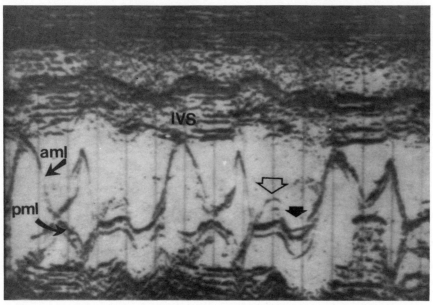

FIG. 27–10. Mitral valve prolapse. This shows the early systolic anterior movement (**open arrow**) that is sometimes seen preceding midsystolic posterior prolapse (**solid arrow**) of the mitral valve. This should not be confused with the systolic anterior movement of the mitral valve seen in idiopathic hypertrophic subaortic stenosis; ivs—interventricular septum; aml—anterior mitral leaflet; pml—posterior mitral leaflet.

the leaflets may appear thickened and multiple echoes may be seen. In the presence of pericardial effusion, valve motion may appear to be distorted and there may be the appearance of mitral valve prolapse when in actuality it is not present (76). Finally, excessive caudal angulation of the transducer may result in the false appearance of mitral valve prolapse (66). Systolic prolapse of the mitral valve has also been seen in the presence of primary pulmonary hypertension (42).

Flail Mitral Valve

In the presence of ruptured chordae tendineae, the mitral valve leaflets may become flail and a somewhat different echocardiographic pattern is seen. When the anterior mitral leaflet is flail, there is increased amplitude of movement of the anterior mitral leaflet so that it may touch the interventricular septum in diastole and the left atrial wall in systole. The leaflet itself is often thin with a coarse, irregular notching seen during diastole within the E–F slope; in systole there

are many layers of echoes and the anterior mitral leaflet assumes a position somewhat more posterior than normal (33, 107).

With a flail posterior mitral leaflet (Fig. 27–11), echoes representing the posterior mitral leaflet and chordae tendineae are seen in the left atrium during systole. The anterior and posterior mitral leaflets do not coapt during systole. Often in early diastole the posterior leaflet appears to come off the posterior left atrial wall or atrioventricular segment with a very rapid anterior movement staying in the so-called "neutral position" throughout most of diastole (33, 107).

Mitral Insufficiency (Rheumatic)

When mitral regurgitation is due to rheumatic involvement, the mitral valve echoes often appear wide and dense, suggesting either fibrous thickening or calcification (14). One method of qualitatively assessing the density of the structure is to relate the density of the mitral valve echoes to the density of the interventricular septum and the posterior left ventricular wall

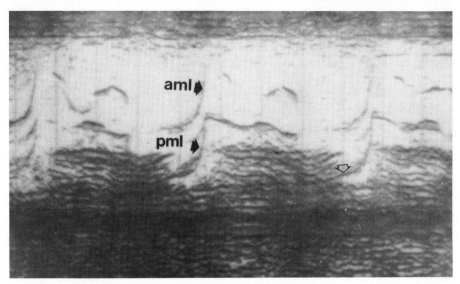

FIG. 27–11. Flail posterior mitral leaflet (pml) with abnormal motion described in the text. The open arrow points to the posterior mitral leaflet against the posterior wall in systole. The posterior mitral leaflet remains separated from the anterior mitral leaflet (aml) throughout systole and diastole.

(14). In the instance of a rheumatic mitral valve, as the gain of the echocardiography is reduced, the mitral valve leaflets continue to appear dense while the interventricular septal and left ventricular posterior wall echoes begin to disappear. It has also been noted that the mitral valve diastolic closing velocity is reduced in the presence of rheumatic mitral valvular disease.

Calcified Mitral Annulus

At times a heavily calcified mitral annulus has been associated with the murmur of mitral regurgitation. The echocardiogram may demonstrate a band of dense echoes between the mitral valve leaflet and the endocardial surface of the posterior wall of the left ventricle (Fig. 27–8). Because of problems with lateral resolution, these dense echoes at times may appear to be superimposed on the endocardium (25). With the transducer angulated cephalad these dense echoes usually end at the level of the atrioventricular junction, though at times they have appeared to end in the left atrium. With the transducer pointed caudally the dense echoes may extend toward or to the posterior papillary

muscle (37). These echoes may be seen to move anteriorly during systole and posteriorly in diastole, having the movement that has been described for the mitral valve annulus (14). The motion of these echoes may resemble that of the posterior wall of the left ventricle; at times, even an initial posterior movement during the isovolumic phase of systole may be seen (37). The similarity of movements of the calcified mitral annulus and the posterior ventricular wall may lead to the erroneous diagnosis of pericardial effusion. Thus, under these circumstances care should be exercised in obtaining and interpreting the echocardiogram (37).

Hypertrophic Cardiomyopathy

Hypertrophic obstructive cardiomyopathy is a disease that clinically presents with a wide spectrum of manifestations. At one extreme is the presence of only asymmetric septal hypertrophy (ASH) with the features of an interventricular septum disproportionately thickened in comparison to the left ventricular posterior wall (47, 49). In addition, during systole the percentage of thickening is less than normal and septal excursion is usually reduced. Rossen et al (97) found the interventricular septum to thicken during systole by 30%–64% in normal individuals and 0%–22% in patients with idiopathic hypertrophic subaortic stenosis. They also found interventricular septal excursions to average 5–10 mm in normals and 1–6 mm in patients with asymmetric septal hypertrophy. A more severe form of this disease is idiopathic hypertrophic subaortic stenosis (IHSS). In IHSS, during systole, the anterior mitral leaflet moves abnormally toward the interventricular septum, obstructing ventricular outflow and producing a measurable systolic pressure gradient within the left ventricle (Figs. 27–12, 13). This abnormal systolic anterior movement (SAM) of the anterior mitral leaflet begins after the onset of sys-

tole. The leaflet then approaches the interventricular septum or touches it throughout midsystole, finally returning posteriorly before the end of systole. The closeness and duration of approximation between the anterior mitral leaflet and the interventricular septum provide an estimate of the severity of obstruction to flow (Figs. 27–12, 13B) (48). After either ventriculoseptomyectomy, mitral valve replacement or the use of beta-blockade agents a decrease or disappearance of SAM may be noticed echocardiographically (9, 87, 104). Similarly, after therapy the dimension of the left ventricular outflow tract increases.

In IHSS left ventricular chamber size is usually reduced. Because the myocardium is thickened and less compliant (resulting in im-

FIG. 27-12. Idiopathic hypertrophic subaortic stenosis. The interventricular septum (IVS) is disproportionately thickened with respect to the left ventricular posterior wall (PW), has a reduced systolic excursion, and thickness less than normal during systole. The left ventricular chamber is small, a common finding in this condition. During systole there is abnormal anterior motion of the anterior mitral leaflet (**open arrow**), and it comes into close approximation with the interventricular septum; aml—anterior mitral leaflet; pml—posterior mitral leaflet.

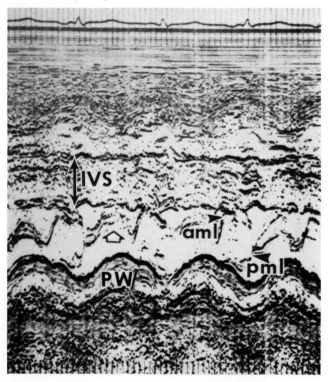

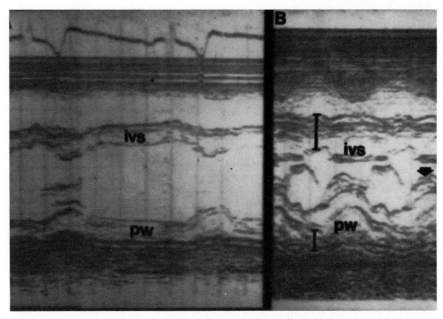

FIG. 27–13. A. Normal heart demonstrating normal systolic thickening and excursion of interventricular septum. **B.** Idiopathic hypertrophic subaortic stenosis. The interventricular septum (ivs) is disproportionately thickened with respect to the left ventricular posterior wall (pw). The interventricular septum appears to have diminished systolic thickening and excursion. Note the abnormal systolic anterior movement of the mitral valve (**solid arrow**).

pedance to inflow of left ventricle) the diastolic closing velocity of the anterior leaflet of the mitral valve (E–F slope) may be reduced.

Further, because of midsystolic obstruction within the ventricle, flow of blood from the left ventricle to the aorta in midsystole is often reduced and the aortic valve may demonstrate midsystolic closure (33) (Fig. 27–3B). This occurs at a later time in systole as compared with discrete membranous subaortic stenosis and also is usually of a lesser amplitude (60). The abnormal systolic movement of the aortic valve in IHSS should also be distinguished from that which has been described in the presence of ruptured right coronary sinus of Valsalva aneurysm (53).

The diagnosis of idiopathic hypertrophic subaortic stenosis should be made with care, since either what may appear to be systolic anterior motion of the mitral valve or disproportionate thickening of the interventricular septum has been described in association with other conditions (42, 68, 77). Artifact due to beam width may result in superimposition of the mitral valve

annulus upon the mitral valve leaflets and produce so-called "pseudo-SAM." Additionally, exaggerated movement of the left ventricular posterior wall, chordae tendineae or mitral annulus can give a similar picture (33). Systolic anterior motion of the mitral valve has been described in the presence of hypovolemia (13), left ventricular aneurysm (44), pericardial effusion (76), atrial septal defect (87, 109), and in association with aortic valve disease and left ventricular hypertrophy (33). Mintz et al (74) reported the findings of dynamic left ventricular outflow tract obstruction (with a systolic pressure gradient within the left ventricle) and echocardiographic demonstration of SAM in the absence of echocardiographic evidence for asymmetric septal hypertrophy. The presence of SAM in patients with the physical findings suggestive of idiopathic hypertrophic subaortic stenosis but without asymmetric septal hypertrophy was reported by Come et al (17). Maron et al (67) collected echocardiographic and postmortem data in patients who had been found to have coronary artery disease and noted the presence of disproportionate interventricular septal thickening (interventricular septal thickness/posterior left ventricular wall thickness ≧1.3). Although in a few instances it appeared to be the result of genetic transmission, in others it was thought the interventricular septum might have become thickened to compensate for segments of myocardium that were not functioning appropriately. The possibility of interventricular septal thickening secondary to the combination of systemic hypertension and coronary artery disease was suggested by the authors. They also raised the question that in some select instances it might be conceivable that there may be sufficient thinning of the posterobasal myocardium (as a result of scarring from infarction) that the ratio of interventricular septal thickness to left ventricular posterior wall thickness may be increased—in the absence of thickening of the interventricular septum. This latter possibility has also been suggested by Henning et al (46). Additionally, asymmetric septal hypertrophy has been reported in some well-trained athletes (95).

To properly diagnose asymmetric septal hypertrophy, it is important to identify the endocardial surfaces of both sides of the interventricular septum and the endocardial and epicardial surface of the left ventricular posterior wall. Further, the measurements should be made according to parameters decribed by Henry et al (47). Often the right side of the interventricular septum cannot be identified (possibly because of adjacent echoes from the tricuspid valve apparatus, heavy trabeculations, and curvature), and accurate measurements cannot be made (2). On occasion contrast echocardiography (performed by rapid injection of either indocyanine green, normal saline or the patient's own blood—producing echoes as the injectate enters the heart) may be used to identify more clearly the right border of the interventricular septum.

AORTIC STENOSIS

In the presence of aortic valvular stenosis, the aortic valve leaflets may appear thickened and the usual fine fluttering that can occur normally may be absent (Fig. 27–8). Further, the maximal opening of the aortic valve may be reduced. The exact orientation of the ultrasound beam with respect to the aortic valve orifice is difficult to ascertain because of the irregular shape of that orifice in calcific aortic stenosis and the dome-like shape of the aortic valve (during systole) in congenital aortic stenosis (33). In general the size of the aortic valve cannot be accurately derived from the M-mode echocardiogram.

In the presence of decreased cardiac output the aortic valve opening also appears reduced, especially during late systole, even in the presence of a normal aortic valve. The homogeneous, thickened, dense echocardiographic appearance of calcification may be seen in conjunction with the aortic valve. In the presence of significant aortic valvular stenosis there may be thickening of the left ventricular posterior wall and the interventricular septum, usually to the same extent—the concentric form of left ventricular hypertrophy. There may be some widening (poststenotic dilatation) of the ascending aorta.

BICUSPID AORTIC VALVE

Recognition of the presence of a bicuspid aortic valve is important because it is one of the most common congenital heart abnormalities, presents an increased risk for bacterial endocarditis, and may progress to calcification and stenosis. The major diagnostic echocardiographic feature is the eccentric position of the aortic valve echo during diastole with respect to the center of the aortic lumen at the same time (78, 93) (Fig. 27–14). In such instances the diastolic aortic valve echo may be either anterior or posterior to the center of the aortic lumen. To determine the relative amount of eccentricity of the aortic valve echo, the aortic lumen diameter is measured, at the onset of diastole, between the inside echoes of the anterior and posterior walls—identified as the point of closure (coming together) of the aortic valve leaflets. The shortest distance between the echo of the aortic valve leaflets at the onset of diastole and the inner border of the closest aortic wall is also measured. The eccentricity index is calculated as:

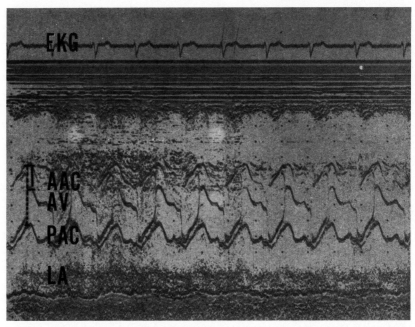

FIG. 27-14. Aortic valve (AV) with eccentric closure suggesting a bicuspid aortic valve. The solid line represents the distance between the diastolic position of the aortic leaflets and the closest aortic wall. The dashed line represents the internal aortic root dimension at the onset of diastole. See text for description of eccentricity index. AAC—anterior (right) aortic leaflet; PAC—posterior (noncoronary) aortic leaflet; LA—left atrium.

aortic root diameter at the onset of diastole × 1/2/shortest distance between aortic valve and aortic wall at onset of diastole.

If the diastolic aortic valve echo were centric, the eccentricity index would be 1.0. As the extent of eccentricity of the aortic valve echo increases, so does the numerical value for the calculated eccentricity index. Radford et al (93) found that an eccentricity index ≥ 1.3 was consistent with the presence of a bicuspid aortic valve. False-positive values for the eccentricity index, that is, ≥ 1.3, have been reported to occur in the presence of a tricuspid aortic valve in combination with a high membranous interventricular septal defect (93). Several of the patients in the latter group were found to have prolapse of an aortic cusp through the membranous ventricular septal defect. Variation in the degree of eccentricity of the diastolic aortic valve leaflet echo within the aortic root has been observed to occur within the same patient either during the same cycle (78) or

changing from cycle to cycle (78, 93). This has been thought to be due either to slight changes in the relationship of the transducer and sonic beam to the aorta and aortic valve or to a redundant aortic valve leaflet.

The aortic cusps may appear asymmetrical during systole, one having a greater systolic excursion than the other (78). Multiple echoes appearing in layers during diastole have been seen frequently in the presence of a bicuspid aortic valve, and these have been ascribed to the presence of either a redundant aortic valve leaflet or abnormal thickening of the aortic valve secondary to fibrosis or calcification (78).

Although the presence of an eccentric diastolic aortic valve echo appears to identify a bicuspid aortic valve, the absence of such eccentricity does not exclude this possibility, since it may not be present in as many as one-fourth of cases with bicuspid aortic valve. Multiple, layered diastolic echoes in proximity to the aortic valve appear more likely to suggest either a redundant aortic leaflet or an abnormally thickened (fibrosed or calcified) aortic valve rather than a bicuspid aortic valve.

SUBVALVULAR AORTIC STENOSIS

With discrete subvalvular aortic stenosis the aortic leaflets open promptly, only to be followed by early and then continued gradual closure of the leaflets (22). The initial closure occurs earlier than that seen in idiopathic hypertrophic subaortic stenosis. (60). The extent of partial closure of the aortic valve leaflets appears to be greater in degree than that usually seen in idiopathic hypertrophic subaortic stenosis. Further, there are 1) coarse fluttering of the aortic leaflets in systole (22), 2) narrowing of the left ventricular outflow tract, and 3) a band of echoes between the anterior mitral leaflet and the left side of the interventricular septum. In a report by Popp et al (89) a thin echo was seen between the interventricular septum and the anterior mitral leaflet, near the point of its insertion into the annulus. It remained within the left ventricular outflow tract throughout the cardiac cycle, appearing to make contact with the anterior mitral leaflet during diastole and separate from it in systole to move anteriorly toward the interventricular septum. This was felt to represent the subvalvular membrane. More recently Popp et al have shown that the ratio of left ventricular outflow tract size to aortic root at the aortic valve is a more sensitive measure of subvalvular versus valvular stenosis.

SUPRAVALVULAR AORTIC STENOSIS

In supravalvular aortic stenosis the echocardiogram demonstrates narrowing of the aorta above the level of the aortic valve. However, beyond this level (cephalad) the aorta widens again. Comparison of the percentage of narrowing of the aorta by echocardiography and by angiography was good in one study (81). By contrast, Bolen et al (8) described their experience in evaluating six patients with supravalvular aortic stenosis by using echocardiography. Although supravalvular narrowing was demonstrated, a

wider aortic lumen superior to the narrowed segment could not be visualized. Moreover, the percentage narrowing determined by echocardiography was less than by angiography, though the trend was similar.

AORTIC REGURGITATION

Aortic regurgitation is usually not appreciated by direct inspection of the aortic valve. If the latter is prolapsed, however, aortic regurgitation may be suspected. In the presence of aortic regurgitation fine fluttering of the anterior mitral leaflet may be seen during diastole (33) (Fig. 27–15); care must be taken not to confuse this with a similar appearance resulting from technical distortion produced by echocardiographic equipment. Fine fluttering is also dissimilar from the coarse, undulating movement of the mitral valve seen with atrial fibrillation.

If aortic regurgitation is severe, fluttering of the interventricular septum may be seen (20). Further, the pattern of left ventricular volume overload may be present. In cases with severe but recently acquired aortic regurgitation the mitral valve leaflets may close before the onset of ventricular systole (premature closing) (11, 91) (Fig. 27–16). Depending on left atrial pressure, left ventricular end-diastolic pressure, and the mechanical effectiveness of atrial systole, there may not be reopening of the mitral valve with atrial systole. Diastolic vibrations of the aortic leaflets were seen in a patient with a torn aortic cusp reported by Corrigall et al (21).

DISSECTING AORTIC ANEURYSM

Echocardiography may provide a means of suspecting aortic root dissection. But the diagnosis should be confirmed by using other currently accepted diagnostic techniques. One should be aware of the vast technical and pathologic pitfalls (see later) that may lead to an erroneous diagnosis; thus, extreme care should be taken to adhere to the following criteria suggested by Nanda (75): 1) the aortic root diameter should be ≥ 42 mm; 2) one or both aortic walls should be ≥ 16 mm in thickness; 3) the echo of the outer

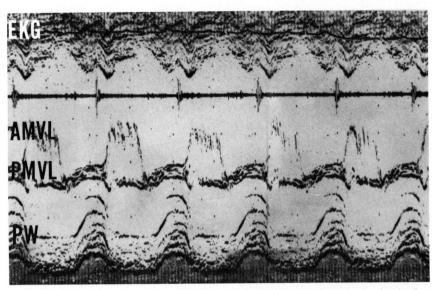

FIG. 27–15. Aortic regurgitation. There is fluttering of the anterior mitral valve leaflet (AMVL) during diastole suggesting aortic regurgitation. There is an increased left ventricular interval dimension in diastole and increased interventricular septal (IVS) excursion in systole, both findings suggesting left ventricular volume overload. PMVL—posterior mitral valve leaflet; PW—posterior wall of the left ventricle.

FIG. 27–16. Severe acute aortic regurgitation with premature closure (**open arrow**) of the mitral valve occurring before the onset of ventricular systole (**dashed line**); ivs—interventricular septum; aml—anterior mitral leaflet; pml—posterior mitral leaflet; pw—left ventricular posterior wall. The left ventricular internal dimension in diastole is increased and there is increased interventricular septal excursion, both features suggesting left ventricular volume overload.

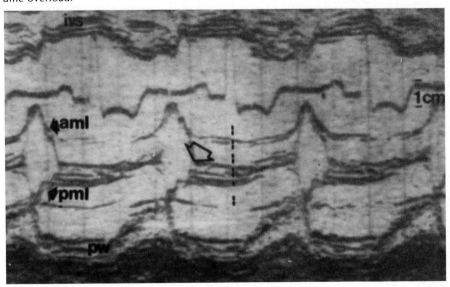

margin of the abnormal wall should be more dense than that of the inner component, or the echoes of the inner and outer components of the aortic walls should be parallel or almost parallel; 4) aortic valve cusps should be normal in appearance and remain within the true lumen.

Dissecting aortic root aneurysms may be accompanied by diastolic fluttering of the anterior mitral valve leaflet (secondary to aortic regurgitation) or pericardial effusion (if there has been a rupture of the aneurysm into the pericardial space) or both.

We have observed two instances in which the aortic valve cusps were not confined to the true lumen. In both instances the right aortic leaflet was seen to cross the thin inner margin of the anterior aortic wall. We postulated that this may represent movement of the right aortic leaflet into the false lumen through an intimal tear—in both cases this was supported by other examinations (angiographic, surgical, and postmortem). Despite such convincing evidence, the apparent movement of the aortic leaflet into the false lumen may result from superimposition of adjacent echoes attributed to the sonic beam band width. Other moving echoes within the false lumen have been described. For example, Nicholson noted a regularly oscillating flap in the false lumen posteriorly (83).

As previously mentioned, there are many pitfalls in the echocardiographic diagnosis of dissecting aortic room aneurysms: calcific disease of the aortic valve (multiple echoes may be seen in the aortic lumen); improper angulation of the sonic beam; the presence of a Swan–Ganz catheter in the pulmonary artery or displacement of a right ventricular pacing catheter (two echoes resulting from the catheter and anterior aortic wall simulate a false lumen) (80); simultaneous recording of the mitral annulus and the posterior aortic wall (simulate dissection of the posterior aortic wall); thick aortic plaques (61).

PERICARDIAL EFFUSION

Echocardiography is presently the procedure of choice for the diagnosis of pericardial effusion. Normally there is very little separation between the epicardial and pericardial echoes. In the presence of pericardial effusion there appears a separation, usually free of echoes, between the epicardial and pericardial echoes (52) (Figs. 27–17, 18). As the effusion becomes larger, the extent (distance between epicardium and pericardium) and duration (lasting throughout diastole) of this separation increases. Additionally, with the presence of increased fluid in the pericardial space, the motion of the pericardium decreases and its echo often resembles a flat line.

In the presence of pericardial effusion, as one does an M-mode scan from the apex to the base of the heart, the separation between the epicardium and pericardium appears to end at the level of the left atrium. (Fig. 27–19). This is because one of the pericardial reflections occurs where the pulmonary veins enter the left atrium, and the potential pericardial space disappears. This feature can be useful not only in helping to identify pericardial effusion but also in distinguishing between pericardial effusion and left-sided pleural effusion. In the latter entity an echo-free space is seen extending behind the left atrium. Nevertheless, in the presence of large pericardial effusion, fluid may appear posterior to the left atrium (43). In such instances the left atrial wall has a hyperdynamic movement with anterior excursion persisting into early ventricular systole (108).

With increasing quantity of pericardial effusion an echo-free space may appear anterior to the right ventricle. However, because such a space may normally exist, the diagnosis of pericardial effusion should not be made unless a posterior echo-free space is also present. With massive effusions (greater than 1000–1500 mm) mechanical alternation may appear (38) (i.e., the position of the heart shifts between an anterior and a posterior position with alternate cardiac cycles).

The amount of pericardial fluid can only be grossly approximated because 1) the pericardial space is not symmetrical; 2) the fluid around the heart is often unevenly distributed; and 3) the limited views of the cardiac circumference prevent accurate quantitation by M-mode echocardiography (24, 52).

The echocardiographer must be aware of some of the potential pitfalls of diagnosing pericardial effusion, as follows: loculated fluid,

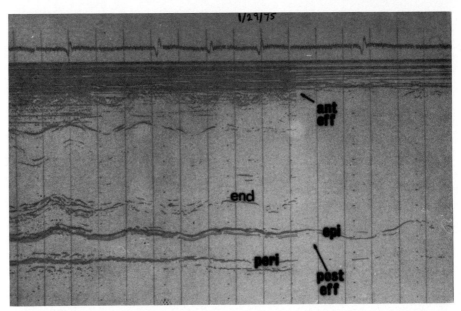

FIG. 27-17. Pericardial effusion manifested by a small echo-free (ant eff) located near the top of the picture anterior to the anterior wall of the right ventricle and a larger echo-free space (post eff) located between the epicardium (epi) and the pericardium (peri). Note the flattened movement of the pericardium. There is progressive dampening from left to right; end—endocardial surface of posterior wall of left ventricle.

FIG. 27-18. Echo-free space representing a pericardial effusion (PE) between the epicardium and the pericardium of the posterior wall (PW) of the left ventricle. Note that this space ends at the level of the left atrium (LA). The left ventricle appears dilated, as well as slight enlargement of the left atrium (LA). AAW—anterior aortic wall; PAW—posterior aortic wall; RV—right ventricle; IVS—interventricular septum.

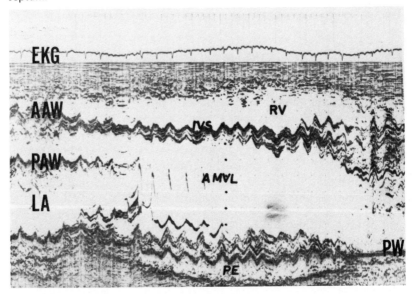

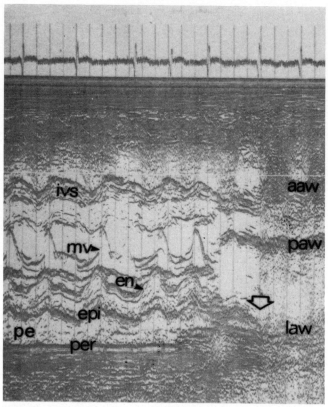

FIG. 27-19. Pericardial effusion (pe) is seen as the echo-free space between the epicardium (epi) and the pericardium (per). This space ends at the level of the left atrium (**open arrow**). Note the absence of movement of the pericardium; ivs—interventricular septum; mv—mitral valve; en—endocardium; law—left atrial wall; aaw—anterior aortic wall; paw—posterior aortic wall.

lesions mimicking the appearance of pericardial effusion, and a giant left atrium (94). Finally it is important to note that, if the transducer is medially angulated, the coronary sinus or pulmonary veins may appear as a clear space behind the posterior wall simulating a pericardial effusion (108).

Allen et al (1) using serial echocardiograms have shown that 1) as blood clots in the pericardial space or as fibrous material replaces serous fluid the intensity of reflected sound increases, and 2) as epicardial–pericardial adhesions develop, systolic anterior movement of the pericardial echo (previously flat) occurs.

In the presence of constrictive pericarditis Feigenbaum has described abnormal movement of the left ventricular posterior wall, as follows: 1) rapid anterior movement of the epicardium and pericardium in systole, 2) rapid posterior movement in early diastole, and 3) flattened movement during middiastole and late diastole (33). There findings are suggestive rather than pathognomonic of constrictive pericarditis.

Other changes seen in constrictive pericarditis are premature opening of the pulmonic valve (33) (thought to be due to an abrupt change and overshoot of right ventricular pressure) and abnormal interventricular septal motion (39).

Schnittger et al (103) have recently described echocardiographic patterns that appear to be consistent with pericardial disease. These echo patterns vary in appearance from two prominent parallel lines separated by a clear space to dense layers of parallel echoes. These authors did not find a specific echocardiographic pattern diagnostic of constrictive pericarditis. They noted, however, that other echocardiographic findings such as increased mitral E–F slope, abnormal interventricular septal motion, and flat diastolic motion of the left ventricular posterior wall are seen in patients with constrictive pericarditis.

In the presence of cardiac tamponade cyclic changes in respiration affect the mitral E–F slope, mitral valve excursion, and right ventricular dimension (with reciprocal changes in left ventricular dimension) (23). However, Schiller and Botvinick (102) find that these patterns are also seen in patients with pure pericardial effusion. In addition they emphasize that in the presence of clinical cardiac tamponade the echocardiographic appearance of right ventricular narrowing (measured at end-diastole during end-expiration) is seen.

In a small series of four patients with pericardial effusion and clinical evidence of pericardial tamponade Vignola et al (112) described the appearance of a notch on the epicardial surface of the right ventricle approximately 0.04 sec after the QRS. In some instances this notch was also seen superimposed on the interventricular septum and associated with coarse oscillations of the posterior wall of the left ventricle and a reduction of the E–F slope to less than 50 mm/sec.

CONGENITAL ABSENCE OF THE PERICARDIUM

The pattern of congenital absence of the left pericardium includes an increased right ventricular dimension and abnormal interventricular septal motion. Both features look similar, however, to that of right ventricular volume overload (84). Payvandi and Kerber also reported similar findings in patients with acquired absence of the pericardium (84). In addition to pointing out that the echocardiographic pattern of absence of the pericardium is similar to that of atrial septal defect, they also noted that, since the clinical findings may be similar in both entities, careful clinical evaluation is required.

ATRIAL MYXOMA

Atrial myxoma is commonly multilobulated and often accompanied by thrombus. As a result it produces a dense cloud of echoes (82). In rare instances, when the surface of the myxoma is calcified, a dense, well-defined echo may be seen (33). Optimal adjustment of the equipment is necessary to visualize echoes of small amplitude.

Most atrial myxomas are pedunculated masses attached to the interatrial septum by a stalk. During ventricular diastole left atrial myxomas prolapse from left atrium into the left ventricle, and the mass of echoes is seen to lie posterior to the anterior mitral leaflet (Fig. 27–20). During ventricular systole the mass of echoes is seen to return into the left atrium. Initially in early diastole the mitral leaflets move into the ventricle. Thus, an echo-free space posterior to the anterior mitral leaflet is seen. The tumor echoes appear later in diastole. If the tumor mass is sufficiently large, the diastolic closing velocity (E–F slope) of the anterior leaflet of the mitral valve may be reduced. This may be attributed either to interference with blood flow from the left atrium to left ventricle or simply to mechanical factors. It is the prolapsing feature of the atrial myxoma that permits visualization of the dense echoes behind the mitral valve leaflet (as it opens into the left ventricle). Occasionally, especially if the equipment is improperly adjusted, the reduced E–F slope of the anterior leaflet of the mitral valve and the dense band of echoes (parallel and slightly posterior to the anterior leaflet of the mitral valve) are mistaken for mitral stenosis. An M-mode scan from apex of the left ventricle to the left atrium should help clarify these findings. In the presence of a left atrial myxoma the quantity and density of the echo should increase as one approaches the left atrium, whereas commonly in the presence of a thickened stenotic mitral valve, the density of echoes is usually greatest within the left ventricle. Following surgical removal of the left atrial myxoma the mitral valve movement should return to normal and the left atrium should appear free of echoes.

RIGHT ATRIAL MYXOMA

In the instance of right atrial myxoma prolapsing across the tricuspid valve during diastole, the abnormal echoes appear within the right ventricular chamber posterior to the anterior leaflet of the tricuspid valve (73).

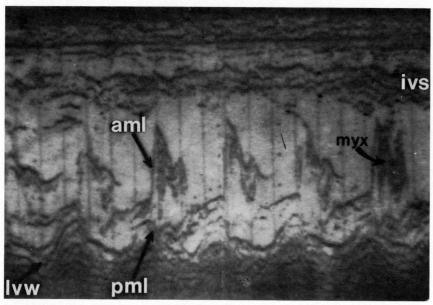

FIG. 27–20. Left atrial myxoma (myx) appears as a dense cloud of echoes posterior to the anterior mitral leaflet (aml) during diastole. Note that the anterior mitral leaflet first opens anteriorly (toward the transducer on the anterior chest wall) in diastole, and then slightly later the myxoma appears behind it. The movement of the posterior mitral leaflet (pml) appears normal; ivs—interventricular septum; lvw—posterior left ventricular wall.

ENDOCARDITIS AND VEGETATIONS

In the presence of infective endocarditis, vegetations may occasionally be demonstrable by echocardiography (30, 99, 115). These are represented by echoes showing a nonuniform distribution in close proximity to the valve structure (Figs. 27–21, 22). In the absence of other underlying valvular abnormalities (Figs. 27–21, 22) the valve motion seems to be unrestricted. In general, vegetations must be at least 2 mm in size to be recorded.

The abnormal echoes produced by mitral valve vegetations may occasionally be seen moving into the left atrium during ventricular systole. On the other hand aortic valvular vegetations may be seen moving into the left ventricular outflow tract during diastole and into the aorta during systole.

Yoshikawa et al (121) reported a case in which a long cordlike aortic valvular vegetation appeared by M-mode echocardiography during diastole as fine fluttering echoes extending from the left ventricular outflow tract into the aortic root. As the ultrasound beam was angulated more cephalad, coarse fluttering echoes appeared in the aortic root during systole and multiple linear echoes were recorded in the aortic root during diastole. Thus the cordlike structure appeared to completely enter the aorta in systole and the left ventricle in diastole. In the opinion of the authors these ultrasound findings were characteristic enough to differentiate this entity from a flail aortic valve leaflet.

FLAIL AORTIC VALVE

Wray (120) reported a case of a flail aortic valve leaflet secondary to bacterial endocarditis. The echocardiogram showed disorganized echoes between the interventricular septum and the anterior mitral leaflet. With more cephalad angulation of the ultrasonic beam (toward the aortic root) these echoes become more dense and continuous with disorganized echoes in the aortic root during diastole. This echocardiographic pattern should be distinguished from that obtained from a right sinus of Valsalva aneurysm (98). Rothbaum et al (98) described an echocar-

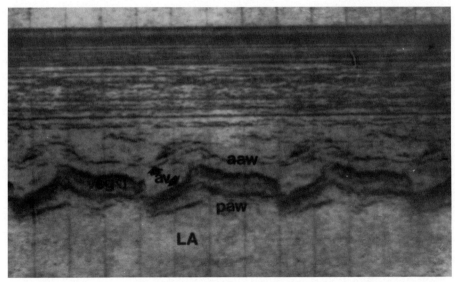

FIG. 27-21. Aortic valve with vegetations. The aortic valve leaflets (av—**solid arrow**) are thin and movement does not appear to be impaired by the vegetation. The vegetation (veg—**open arrow**) appears as a thick, fuzzy, echo; paw—posterior aortic wall; aaw—anterior aortic wall; LA—left atrium.

FIG. 27-22. Aortic valve (AO) with vegetation (VEG **arrow**). CW—chest wall; AAW—anterior aortic wall; PAW—posterior aortic wall; LA—left atrium; ECG—electrocardiogram.

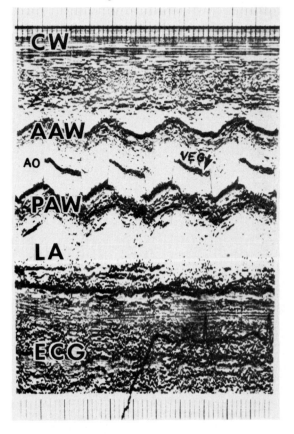

diogram showing an echo that appeared to be the right aortic cusp but that also continued into the left ventricle, where it was positioned between the anterior mitral leaflet and the interventricular septum. In the left ventricle, this echo moved away from the interventricular septum during diastole and toward the interventricular septum and into the aortic root during systole. This phenomenon was thought to be related to filling and emptying of the aneurysm. In addition, eccentricity of the aortic valve leaflets was noted. Johnson et al in their discussion of aortic valve lesions (53) include a description of the aortic valve in the setting of ruptured sinus of Valsalva aneurysms with left-to-right shunt. They found a "see-saw" pattern of movement of the right coronary cusp during systole (early systolic closure with late systolic reopening) and normal systolic movement of the noncoronary cusp.

CONGENITAL HEART DISEASE

ATRIAL SEPTAL DEFECT

Atrial septal defect of clinical significance may be suspected from the echocardiogram. The pattern of right ventricular volume overload (abnormal interventricular septal motion and increased right ventricular dimension) is seen in the presence of a significant left-to-right intracardiac shunt and normal left ventricular function (90). In normal hearts the interventricular septum moves posteriorly and thickens with the onset of systole. However, in the presence of right ventricular volume overload the interventricular septum moves anteriorly with the onset of systole and then returns posteriorly at the end of systole (Fig. 27–23). Using cross-sectional echocardiography to study septal motion, Weyman et al (119) have said that paradoxical movement of the interventricular septum in patients with right ventricular volume overload appears

to be related to an altered shape of the left ventricle during diastole. The interventricular septum thickens during systole, a finding that distinguishes this from the abnormal interventricular septal motion sometimes observed in the presence of interventricular septal aneurysms—the result of ischemic heart disease and scar formation in the septum.

In atrial septal defect the right ventricular diameter measured at end-diastole is increased because of excessive blood flow into the right ventricle. In the presence of a very large left-to-right intracardiac shunt the separation between the anterior and posterior tricuspid leaflets may be significantly greater than that seen between

FIG. 27–23. Atrial septal defect, secundum type with large left-to-right shunt. Increased right ventricular dimension (RVD). Note that at the beginning of systole the interventricular septum (ivs) moves anteriorly (**solid arrow**), thickens, and returns posteriorly at the end of systole (abnormal or paradoxical motion of the interventricular septum). The enlarged right ventricle and the paradoxical motion of the interventricular septum represents the pattern of right ventricular volume overload. Note also that the opening excursion (D–E) of the tricuspid valve (TV) is greater than the opening excursion of the mitral valve (MV), suggesting greater flow through the tricuspid valve. LVID$_d$—left ventricular internal dimension in diastole; en—endocardial surface left ventricular posterior wall; rss—right side of interventricular septum; lss—left side of interventricular septum.

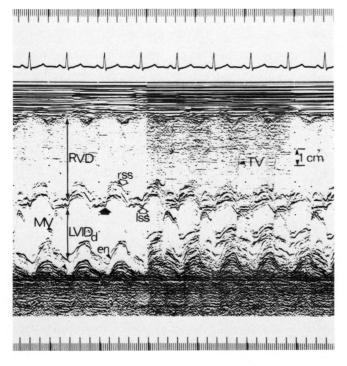

the anterior and posterior mitral leaflets in the same patient (33) (Fig. 27–23). This may be due to a relationship between the blood flow through the valve and the amount of separation between its leaflets. In atrial septal defect paradoxical motion of the interventricular septum is seen. This finding is, however, nonspecific and may be observed in the presence of other disease processes resulting in increased right ventricular volume overload. These are the following: tricuspid regurgitation (28, 42), pulmonic regurgitation (42), partial anomalous pulmonary venous drainage and total anomalous pulmonary venous drainage (if there is right ventricular volume overload but not right ventricular hypertension due to pulmonary venous obstruction) (3, 55, 64, 72) constrictive pericarditis (39) and anomalous origin of the left coronary artery (40). Sometimes this abnormal septal movement may appear following cardiovascular surgery (72).

The degree of abnormal movement of the interventricular septum may be quite variable, ranging from clearly paradoxical to flattened and may depend on what part of the interventricular septum is in view. It should be remembered that the motion of the basal portion of the interventricular septum (that portion close to the aorta) becomes similar to that of the aorta. Certainly, one should insist on the presence of an increased right ventricular dimension before one assumes that abnormal interventricular septal motion is related to right ventricular volume overload, as may be seen in atrial septal defect.

The paradoxical interventricular septal motion just described should not be confused with the altered interventricular septal motion seen with complete left bundle branch block (29). In this latter instance there is an initial abrupt posterior movement of the interventricular septum followed by an anterior motion. Changes in movement of the interventricular septum have also been reported to occur in the presence of preexcitation (i.e., Wolff–Parkinson–White syndrome) (27, 51).

The pattern just described above (abnormal interventricular septal motion) is more often seen with the ostium secundum type of atrial septal defect. Ostium primum septal defect has a right ventricle with increased diameter, but if the amount of mitral regurgitation is significant, its effect on left ventricular function may mask paradoxical interventricular septal motion. The echocardiogram may also show the anterior mitral leaflet to be abnormally close to the interventricular septum during systole and diastole, because of the abnormal insertion of the anterior mitral leaflet on the interventricular septum (58, 70). Multiple echoes of the mitral valve are also seen during systole (58, 70). Late systolic anterior motion of the mitral valve has been described (5). There is lack of continuity of the mitral and tricuspid valves—each valve can be seen separately (5). This is different from the pattern described for a complete atrioventricular canal wherein the mitral valve appears to cross the interventricular septum (5, 70). In the latter defect the interventricular septum may appear to be "fragmented" or absent near the aorta (70).

VENTRICULAR SEPTAL DEFECT

Isolated ventricular septal defects unless very large do not usually demonstrate discontinuity of the interventricular septum on the echocardiogram. Effects of the ventricular septal defect may, however, be seen, namely, 1) an increase in both left ventricular and left atrial dimensions resulting from increased blood volume in these chambers (33) 2) an increase in the ratio of the left atrial diameter to the aortic diameter, 3) a left ventricular volume overload pattern (if the left-to-right shunt is of sufficient size).

PATENT DUCTUS ARTERIOSUS

A large patent ductus arteriosus accompanied by a significant left-to-right shunt may demonstrate an increased left atrial dimension and the pattern of left ventricular volume overload.

In normal adults the LA/Ao ratio (left atrial dimension/aortic dimension) has been reported to be 0.87–1.11 (12). In normal premature and full-term infants Goldberg et al (41) reported the LA/Ao ratio of 0.74 ± 0.13. In premature infants Silverman et al (105) found an LA/Ao ratio of 0.86 ± 0.10.

By contrast, in infants with a large patent ductus arteriosus and significant left-to-right shunt the same investigators found the LA/Ao ratio to vary between 1.19(±0.18)–1.28(±0.23) (41, 105). Moreover, Silverman et al (105) stated that the LA/Ao ratio was greater than 1.15 in premature infants with significant cardiomegaly and a large left-to-right shunt. Serial measurements of LA/Ao ratio are more informative than an individual determination because the LA/Ao ratio increases with more left-to-right shunting of blood and decreases either with spontaneous or surgical closure (41). Baylen et al (6) found that in premature infants with large left-to-right shunts and left ventricular volume overload the percent shortening of the left ventricular internal diameter was increased, but they thought that when this value decreased it suggested decreased left ventricular contractility.

Echocardiography is especially useful in the evaluation of patent ductus arteriosus in the premature infant because the incidence of this anomaly is significantly increased (57). Thibeault et al (111) reported that a ductal murmur may not be heard even when a patent ductus arteriosus with left-to-right shunt was demonstrated by angiography. They also stated that massive cardiomegaly could in some instances

be observed before the ductal murmur was heard.

In some instances the communication between the aorta and the left pulmonary artery was visualized by cross-sectional echocardiography (Fig. 27–24).

Sahn et al (101) discussed the value in using the combination of Vcf, (mean velocity of shortening, an index of LV function) and LA/Ao ratio to differentiate between normal children and those with 1) myopathy, myocarditis, or metabolic heart disease and 2) a large left-to-right shunt (patent ductus arteriosus, ventricular septal defect). In the presence of a large left-to-right shunt there is an increase in value for both Vcf and LA/Ao ratio, while in the presence of myocardial disease the Vcf is decreased and the LA/Ao ratio is increased.

TETRALOGY OF FALLOT

Tetralogy of Fallot demonstrates a large aorta (16). The aorta straddles (overrides) the interventricular septum—the amount varies between individuals. In the longitudinal M-mode scan, with the transducer directed toward the base of

FIG. 27–24. A 30° sector scan from suprasternal notch of a patient with patent ductus arteriosus, where the left pulmonary artery (LPA) enters the transverse aorta (aorta) to takeoff of left subclavian artery (L. Subclavian).

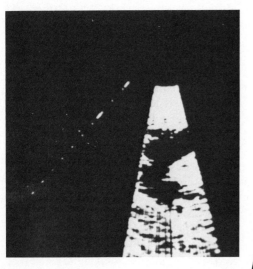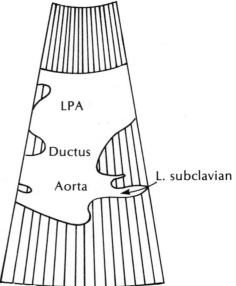

the heart, the normal interventricular septal–aortic continuity is lost. The anterior wall of the right ventricle may appear thickened. There may appear dilatation of the right ventricle and narrowing of the right ventricular outflow tract (16). In Tetralogy of Fallot the mitral valve–semilunar valve *continuity* is preserved (71). By contrast, in double-outlet right ventricle, with features similar to those of Tetralogy of Fallot, mitral valve–semilunar valve *discontinuity* occurs (71). If a pulmonic valve can be demonstrated, the possibility of truncus arteriosus can be excluded (15).

EBSTEIN'S ANOMALY

Ebstein's anomaly is a congenital lesion, its major pathologic features including deformity of the tricuspid valve and displacement of portions of the tricuspid valve into the right ventricle. Given this finding, the tricuspid valve is easily recorded leftward of the usual position. The amplitude of movement of the tricuspid valve may be increased. Tricuspid valve closure follows mitral valve closure by a greater than normal interval (greater than 55 msec) (32).

PROSTHETIC VALVE EVALUATION BY M-MODE

With the number of prosthetic valves available for cardiac valve replacement, a clinical challenge faces the physician who attempts to follow and assess the function of these valves. Each prosthetic valve has different opening and closing characteristics, ball, disc or leaflet excursions, and a variety of supporting struts or cage. To standardize evaluation of each individual valve the sonologist should 1) image the prosthetic valve from a common chest wall position to allow the disc to be perpendicular to the transducer, 2) image the cage or struts so that the transducer is aimed up the cone of the struts chamber or cage, 3) use a simultaneous phonocardiogram for timing and intensity of opening and closing sounds. By using these principles useful data can be derived and compared to the "standard ultrasound profile" of each valve type. As a result abnormal prosthetic valve function may be delineated. The commonly used types of prosthetic valves are listed here. In this chapter only the ball-cage mitral valve is described (Fig. 27–25).

FIG. 27–25. M-mode echocardiogram and phonocardiogram (**top line**) of a normal Starr-Edwards Ball-Cage Mitral Valve. The valve *ring*, the *ball*, and top of the cage are identified. The valve closing sound (phono) occurs in early systole at the end of downward excursion of the valve. Valve opening sound occurs as the ball impinges the cage (upward motion of the ball).

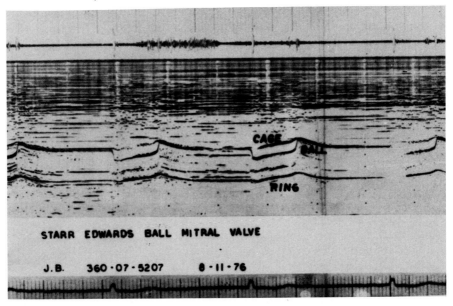

Common Prosthetic Valves
  Ball and cage valve
  Disc-strut valve
  Tilting disc valve
  Bioprosthetic valve (Porcine valve)

This valve is mounted on a sewing ring appearing as a persistent echo with decreased excursion (ring—bottom of Fig. 27–25). The ball echoes are seen as generally two parallel echoes moving toward the ring in systole (valve closure) and toward the cage in diastole (valve opening). The ball moves up to and touches the cage margins during diastole. The opening velocity (mm/sec) of the ball (early diastole) is generally one-half the closing velocity (systole). The ball excursion can be measured and is generally 8–11 mm. A phonocardiogram is taken to measure intensity and timing of the opening and closing sounds. The closing sound of the valve is loud, single, and crisp; the opening sound is generally less intense, single or narrowly split (<0.02 sec), and occurs 0.08 to 0.12 sec after aortic closure. In prosthetic valve malfunction with thrombus present on the valve ring, several features are present, as follows: the ring "echoes" lose their linear appearance and become multiple, the opening velocity decreases, the ball excursion diminishes, the closing sound decreases in intensity and may reduplicate, the opening sound is delayed greater than 0.12 sec, and the disc excursion diminishes. If thrombus is present on the cage, generally the ball excursion also diminishes and a separation is seen in diastole between the ball echo and cage. Whereas these findings are specific for the malfunctioning of the caged-ball mitral valve, they are applicable to other prosthetic valves with a known "ultrasound valve profile."

CROSS-SECTIONAL CROSS-SECTIONAL ECHOCARDIOGRAPHY

Cross section echocardiography or sector scanning examination of the heart has enhanced ultrasound examinations of the heart. There are many varieties of cross-sectional instruments and design concepts. However, the technique of real-time cross-sectional echocardiography is gaining acceptance among cardiologists. In this technique, an image of the heart is obtained in real-time similar to the cine-angiocardiography. The following two varieties of real-time scans are used: 1) the sector scan—where the point of the transducer is stationary on the chest wall and only the angle of the beam is changed, inscribing a sector image of the heart (45) and 2) the linear scan in which multiple transducers are positioned parallel to each other, providing a cross-sectional linear scan of the heart (10).

The most sophisticated and interesting device developed in sector scanning is probably the phased-array scanner (114). This technique employs multiple-element transducers in which there is a series of delays in firing of the elements. By controlling the time sequences of firing, the beam is swept electronically through a sector, providing a high-quality electronic scan of the heart.

In this chapter we describe a series of cardiac problems in which sector scanning has provided additional information (over M-mode) in the assessment of the cardiac status of the gravid pa-

FIG. 27-26. Long axis of 30° sector scan of aortic root and left ventricle. AR—aortic root; AV—aortic valve; RV—right ventricle; S—interventricular septum; PM—papillary muscle; LV—left ventricular cavity; P—pericardium; EP—epicardium; EN—endocardium; PML—posterior mitral leaflet; AML—anterior mitral leaflet; LA—left atrium.

Long axis 30° sector scan

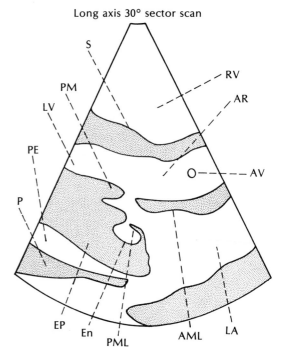

tient. Two views of the heart are considered, as follows: 1) a long-axis view with the arc inscribed to provide an image from the base of the aorta through the interventricular septum and mitral valve to the apex of the left ventricular cavity (Fig. 27–26) and 2) a short-axis (perpendicular to the long-axis) view providing a cross section in which the left ventricle appears circular and with the right ventricle seen above and toward the left as viewed from the apex (Fig. 27–27). Superior angulation in this view provides a cross section through anterior and poste-

rior mitral leaflets, whereas inferior angulation provides a cross section through the left ventricular cavity and papillary muscle.

AORTIC STENOSIS

Congenital aortic stenosis can complicate a pregnancy if the degree of stenosis is severe. Whereas M-mode provides useful information in calcified or deformed aortic valves in the older patient, a congenital stenotic valve in a child may have a normal appearance on M-mode.

FIG. 27–27. Long axis (**upper panel**) and short axis (**lower panel**) of 30° sector scanning. The short-axis view is perpendicular to long axis and images the heart as in 2 (**lower panel**).

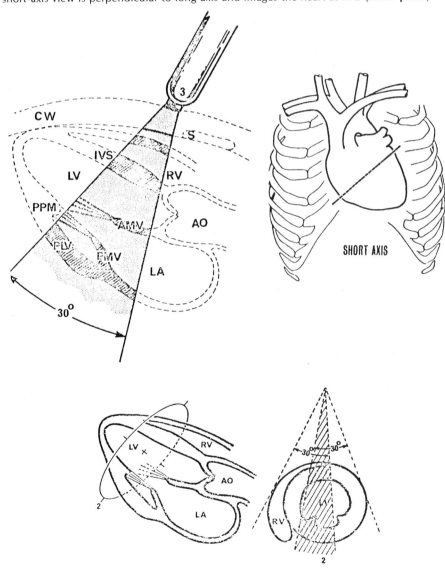

This occurs when the angle of the transducer is aimed at the tip of the leaflets. Also discrete subvalvular and supravalvular aortic stenosis may be difficult to image by M-mode owing to subtle change in the left ventricular outflow tract or aorta with minor changes in the aortic valve (see above). With cross-sectional echocardiography, the aortic valve is best imaged in the long axis, providing a view of the supravalvular chamber, aortic valve coaptation, and the subvalvular outflow tract. With regard to supravalvular aortic stenosis, the tubular narrowing in the ascending aorta can be imaged with scanning from aortic valve upward. In valvular aortic stenosis, the anterior and posterior aortic leaflets are seen as thickened leaflets with decreased separation during systole (usually less than 1.1 cm) (Fig. 27–28). In this figure the aortic leaflets appear thickened allowing discrete images to be seen during systole and diastole. Maximum separation of the leaflets during systole is normally greater than 1.5 cm. In this patient the systolic separation was less than 1.0 cm. In short-axis view of the aortic valve the superior and inferior margins of the aortic leaflets are seen. The lateral margins are not, however, readily imaged by mechanical scanning. Hence the

aortic leaflets can be seen in apposition during diastole distinguishing between a congenital bicuspid and a tricuspid aortic valve. Presently the aortic valve orifice cannot be readily or accurately measured. Nonetheless, cross-sectional echocardiography has improved the qualitative diagnosis of aortic stenosis. Preliminary data by Weyman et al do indicate that aortic leaflet separation during systole may correlate well with the severity of obstruction (118).

MITRAL STENOSIS

Although M-mode has provided a useful qualitative tool in the diagnosis of rheumatic valvular heart disease, none of the M-mode criteria have reproducibly held up in the quantitative diagnosis of the disease. With cross-sectional echocardiography the mitral leaflets can be readily imaged in long and short axis, and the relationship of the leaflets to the mitral annulus, left ventricular posterior wall, and chordae tendineae can be readily seen. Whereas the 30 scanner (Fig. 27–29) has provided useful information, the 90 scanner allows the entire mitral orifice to be viewed in one sector. Thickening of the leaflets, parallel motion of the anterior and posterior

FIG. 27–28. A 90° Sector aortic root and left ventricular outflow in patient with aortic stenosis. Note thickening of aortic leaflets (AVL) in midsystole. The aortic opening (AO) with separation of AVL is less than 1.0 cm, AAW—anterior aortic wall; PAW—posterior aortic wall; RVOT—right ventricular outflow tract; IVS—interventricular septum; PPM—posterior papillary muscle; LVPW—left ventricular posterior wall.

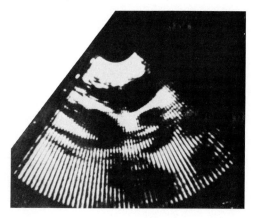
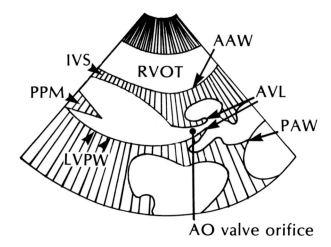

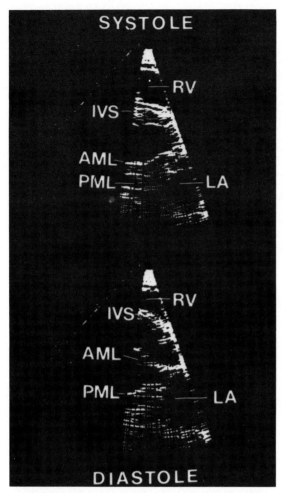

SYSTOLE

RV
IVS
AML
PML — LA

RV
IVS
AML
PML — LA

DIASTOLE

FIG. 27-29. A 30° sector in patient with mitral stenosis. Note thickening of anterior mitral leaflet during diastole, which is seen as the inferior extension of the posterior aortic wall, AML—anterior leaflet; PML—posterior leaflet; LA—left atrium.

ative technique in determining severity of mitral stenosis.

MITRAL VALVE PROLAPSE

Barlow described a syndrome encompassing thoracic–skeletal deformities, chest pain, systolic clicks, late systolic murmurs, dysrhythmia, and electrocardiographic ST–T changes (4). Myxomatous degeneration of the mitral valve is frequently associated with this syndrome. By use of M-mode the echocardiographic pattern of mitral valve prolapse correlates well with auscultatory and phonocardiographic findings (66). However, "false positives" and "false negatives" commonly occur. With cross-sectional echocardiography mitral coaptation can be categorized more accurately and the sensitivity of echocardiography enhanced (100). The redundant posterior leaflet with myxomatous degeneration on M-mode may appear as multiple echoes during the cardiac cycle, precluding proper imaging of the prolapsed mitral valve. In Figure 27–30 the anterior mitral leaflet (AML) and posterior mitral leaflet (PML) are seen to coapt in mid systole at the end of an imaginary line drawn from the AML hinge point of the aortic posterior wall (AR) to the posterior atrioventricular groove. In late systole both the anterior and posterior leaflets **(arrow)** prolapse into the left atrium. With this view precise measurements of degree of prolapse can be made, improving the specificity and sensitivity of echocardiography.

VALVULAR VEGETATIONS

When infective endocarditis involves the cardiac valves, the M-mode echo can provide information regarding torn leaflets, ruptured chordae tendineae, and flail cusps. When flail, the leaflets generally have an erratic, haphazard appearance. When vegetations accumulate on the leaflets beyond 2–3 mm, the M-mode can generally identify vegetations as echo-producing masses, provided the leaflets have not been previously deformed or calcified. Echocardiographic identification of vegetations generally indicates severe valvular destruction and the urgent need

mitral leaflets, thickened chordae tendineae, and left atrial dimension can be viewed in one 90 arc scan in long axis. In short axis, generally the entire mitral orifice can be imaged during diastole. With planimetry the mitral valve orifice can be measured and compared to hemodynamic measurements, as well as direct surgical measurements. When comparisons were made using a 30 mechanical scanner, measurements of mitral valve orifice were accurate when compared to direct measurements (50). Further studies in this area should establish cross-sectional echocardiography as the most accurate preoper-

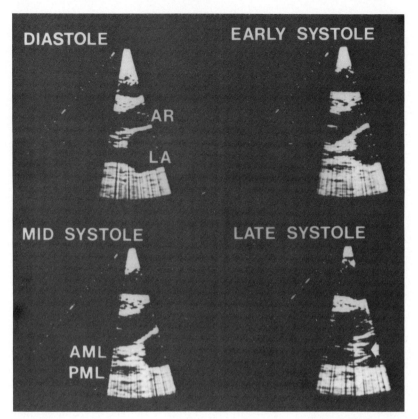

FIG. 27–30. Four 30° sector views taken during four phases of the cardiac cycle. AR—aortic root; LA—left atrium; AML—anterior mitral leaflet; PML—posterior mitral leaflet. Note prolapse of AML and PML into LA during late systole (**arrow**).

for surgical replacement of the valve (115). With M-mode, however, patients with myxomatous degeneration of the mitral valve may have echocardiograms indistinguishable from vegetations. With cross-sectional echocardiography there has been less of a problem in distinguishing these two states; in myxomatous degeneration the multiple echoes are uniformly distributed throughout the valve, whereas vegetation tends to clump on several loci of the leaflets. In Figure 27–31 a patient presented with streptococcus viridans endocarditis and a systolic murmur of mitral regurgitation; heavy, dense echoes from the anterior mitral leaflet are seen. They appear as "soft" echoes with attachment to the left atrial aspect of the leaflet. During real-time imaging these can be seen to oscillate at times independent of the valve leaflets, allowing for their recognition as vegetations.

With aortic valve vegetations M-mode studies generally reveal a mass just below the aortic valve. Careful scanning from left ventricular outflow tract to aortic root usually demonstrates an attachment of the aortic leaflets. But whether this echo-producing mass is a portion of flail aortic cusp or a vegetation is indistinguishable. Recently with cross-sectional echocardiography we have seen several patients with similar masses identified in the left ventricular outflow tract below the aortic valve. Their size and echocardiographic appearance have distinguished them correctly as vegetations. Whether sensitivity and specificity of echocardiography in identifying vegetation are improved by cross-sectional echocardiography is unknown. Initial impressions are, however, that cross-sectional echocardiography provides a more useful tool in the diagnosis of infective endocarditis.

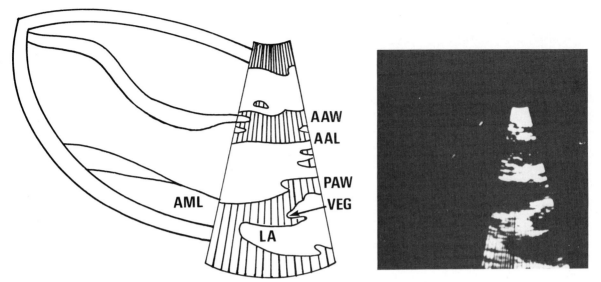

FIG. 27–31. A 30° sector long-axis scan of AML during early systole with vegetation (VEG) attached to AML in patient with infective endocarditis.

CONGENITAL HEART DISEASE

ATRIAL SEPTAL DEFECT

As previously cited, the M-mode diagnosis of atrial septal defect is an indirect diagnosis that examines the hemodynamic changes produced by right ventricular volume overload (findings not specific for this defect). By directly viewing the interatrial septum with cross-sectional echocardiography, a primary defect in the interatrial septum can be identified (69). Atrial septal defects are generally large enough that the entire ultrasonic beam can traverse the defect and produce an "echo dropout" area. More recent studies using contrast with cross-sectional echocardiography have been useful in identifying atrial septal defects. With peripheral injection of cardiogreen dye, or normal saline, some right to left streaming of "contrast" is seen across an echo dropout area in the interatrial septum, identifying most patients with atrial septal defect.

VENTRICULAR SEPTAL DEFECT

Ventricular septal defects are more difficult to identify by M-mode echocardiography. It might be anticipated that scanning of the interventricular septum from aorta to apex of the left ventricle would identify a dropout of echoes at the site of the ventricular septal defect. In actual practice, demonstration of this is very difficult, and the results are often inaccurate, for the following reasons: first, the M-mode records interventricular septal echoes best from the anterior upper third of the septum while most ventricular septal defects occur in the middle third. Secondly, because of wide beam angle of the transducer, a large defect must be present before recognition of the defect is possible. Thirdly, the ultrasonic beam must completely traverse the defect without reflection from the edge or margins before it can be recognized. In addition "false" dropout of interventricular septum echoes can be caused by faulty angulation of the transducer. Dropout of echoes has also been seen in ventricular septal defects by use of cross-sectional echocardiography (56).

In the A–V canal deformity (endocardial cushion defects) we can image the ventricular septal defect margin, but the recognition of the common A–V valve is generally most helpful in identifying this lesion as the leaflet is seen traversing the ventricular septum from left to right ventricle during diastole.

PATENT DUCTUS ARTERIOSUS

The M-mode diagnosis of patent ductus is based on the increased left atrial size that handles the large left-to-right shunt from the pulmonary circuit. The ratio of aortic root dimension to left atrial size has been previously cited as a useful adjunct in determining the size of the ductus. More recently with cross-sectional echocardiography the patent ductus can be identified and its size determined. With the transducer in the suprasternal notch the ductus can be visualized as the transducer images the left pulmonary artery over the ductus as it enters the aorta. In Figure 27–24 the left pulmonary artery (LPA), patent ductus (PDA), and aorta (Ar) are imaged from the suprasternal notch position. Closures of the defect resulted in separation of the left pulmonary artery and aorta structure.

REFERENCES

1. ALLEN JW, HARRISON EC, CAMP JC, BORSARI A, TURNIER E, LAU FYK: The role of serial echocardiography in evaluation and differential diagnosis of pericardial disease. Am Heart J 93:560–567, 1977

2. ALLEN JW, KIM SJ, EDMISTON WA, VENKATARAMAN K: Problems in ultrasonic estimates of septal thickness. Am J Cardiol 42:89–96, 1978

3. AZIZ KU, PAUL MH, BHARATI S, LEV M, SHANNON K: Echocardiographic features of total anomalous pulmonary venous drainage into the coronary sinus. Am J Cardiol 42:108–113, 1978

4. BARLOW JB, BOSMAN CK, POCOCK WA, MARCHAND P: Late systolic murmurs and non-ejection ("mid-late") systolic clicks: an analysis of 90 patients. Br Heart J 30:203–218, 1968

5. BASS JL, BESSINGER FB, LAWRENCE C: Echocardiographic differentiation of partial and complete atrioventricular canal. Circulation 57:1144–1150, 1978

6. BAYLEN B, MEYER RA, KORFHAGEN J, BENZING G III, BUBB ME, KAPLAN S: Left ventricular performance in the critically ill premature infant with patent ductus arteriosus and pulmonary disease. Circulation 55:182–188, 1977

7. BERMAN ND, GILBERT BW, MCLAUGHLIN PR, MARCH JE: Mitral stenosis with posterior diastolic movement of posterior leaflet. Cardiovasc Med Assoc J 112:976–979, 1975

8. BOLEN JL, POPP RL, FRENCH JW: Echocardiographic feature of supravalvular aortic stenosis. Circulation 52:817–822, 1975

9. BOLTON MR, KING JF, PLUMBO RA, MASON D, PUGH DM, REIS RL, DUNN MI: The effects of operation on the echocardiographic features of idiopathic hypertrophic subaortic stenosis. Circulation 50:897–900, 1974

10. BOM N, LANIER CT, VAN ZWEETEN G, KLOSTER FE: Multiscan echocardiography. I. Technical description. Circulation 48:1066, 1973

11. BOTVINICK EH, SCHILLER NB, WICKRAMASEKARAN R, KLAUSNER SC, GERTZ E: Echocardiographic demonstration of early mitral valve closure in severe aortic insufficiency. Its clinical implication. Circulation 51:836–847, 1975

12. BROWN OR, HARRISON DC, POPP RL: An improved method for echocardiographic detection of left atrial enlargement. Circulation 50:58–64, 1974

13. BULKLEY BH, FORTUIN NJ: Systolic anterior motion of the mitral valve without asymmetric septal hypertrophy. Chest 69:694, 1976

14. BURGESS J, CLARK R, KAMIGAKI M, COHN K: Echocardiographic findings in different types of mitral regurgitation. Circulation 48: 97–106, 1973

15. CHUNG KJ, ALEXSON CG, MANNING JA, GRAMIAK R: Echocardiography in truncus arteriosus. The value of pulmonic valve detection. Circulation 48:281–286, 1973

16. CHUNG KJ, NANDA NC, MANNING JA, GRAMIAK R: Echocardiographic findings in tetralogy of Fallot. Am J Cardiol 31:126, 1973

17. COME PC, BULKLEY BH, GOODMAN ZD, HUTCHINS GM, PITT B, FORTUIN NJ: Hypercontractile cardiac states simulating hypertrophic cardiomyopathy. Circulation 55:901–908, 1977

18. COOPER RH, O'ROURKE RA, KARLINER JS, PETERSON KL, LEOPOLD GR: Comparison of ultrasound and cineangiographic measurements of the mean rate of circumferential fiber shortening in man. Circulation 46:914–923, 1972

19. COPE GD, KISSLO JA, JOHNSON ML, BEHAR VS: A reassessment of the echocardiogram in mitral stenosis. Circulation 52:664–670, 1975

20. COPE GD, KISSLO JA, JOHNSON ML, MYERS S: Diastolic vibration of the interventricular septum in aortic insufficiency. Circulation 51:589, 1975

21. CORRIGALL DM, STRUNK BL, POPP RL: Phonocardiographic and echocardiographic features of ruptured aortic valvular cusp. Chest 69:669, 1976

22. DAVIS RH, FEIGENBAUM H, CHANG S, KONECKE LL, DILLON JC: Echocardiographic manifestations of discrete subaortic stenosis. Am J Cardiol 33:277–280, 1974

23. D'CRUZ IA, COHEN HC, PRABHU R, GLICK G: Diagnosis of cardiac tamponade by echocardiography. Changes in mitral valve motion and ventricular dimensions, with special reference to paradoxical pulse. Circulation 52:460–465, 1975

24. D'CRUZ IA, PRABHU R, COHEN HC, GLICK G: Potential

pitfalls in quantification of pericardial effusion by echocardiography. Br Heart J 39:529–535, 1977

25. DASHKOFF N, KARACUSCHANSKY M, COME PC, FORTUIN NJ: Echocardiographic features of mitral annulus calcification. Am Heart J 94:585–592, 1977

26. DEMARIA AN, KING JF, BOGREN HG, LIES JE, MASON DT: The variable spectrum of echocardiographic manifestation of the mitral valve prolapse syndrome. Circulation 50:33–41, 1974

27. DEMARIA AN, VERA Z, NEUMANN A, AWAN N, MASON D: Alterations in ventricular contraction pattern in the Wolff-Parkinson-White syndrome: detection by echocardiography. Circulation 53:249, 1976

28. DIAMOND MA, DILLON JC, HAINE CL, CHANG S, FEIGENBAUM H: Echocardiographic features of atrial septal defect. Circulation 43:129, 1971

29. DILLON JC, CHANG S, FEIGENBAUM H: Echocardiographic manifestation of left bundle branch block. Circulation 49:876–880, 1974

30. DILLON JC, FEIGENBAUM H, KONECKE LL, DAVIS RH, CHANG S: Echocardiographic manifestation of valvular vegetation. Am Heart J 86:698, 1973

31. DUCHAK JM, CHANG S, FEIGENBAUM H: The posterior mitral valve echo and echocardiographic diagnosis of mitral stenosis. Am J Cardiol 29:628, 1972

32. FAROOKI ZQ, HENRY JC, GREEN EW: Echocardiographic spectrum of Ebstein's anomaly of the tricuspid valve. Circulation 53:63–68, 1976

33. FEIGENBAUM H: Echocardiography, 2nd ed. Philadelphia, Lea & Febiger, 1976, p 87

34. FLAHERTY JT, LIVENGOOD S, FORTUIN NJ: Atypical posterior leaflet motion in echocardiogram in mitral stenosis. Am J Cardiol 35:675–678, 1975

35. FORTUIN NJ, HOOD WP, SHERMAN ME, CRAIGE E: Determination of left ventricular volumes by ultrasound. Circulation 44:575–584, 1971

36. FRAZIN L, TALANO JV, STEPHANIDES L, LOEB HS, KOPEL L, GUNNAR RM: Esophageal echocardiography. Circulation 54:102, 1976

37. GABOR GE, MOHR BD, GOEL PC, COHEN B: Echocardiographic and clinical spectrum of mitral annular calcification. Am J Cardiol 38:836–843, 1976

38. GABOR GE, WINSBERG F, BLOOM HS: Electrical and mechanical alternation in pericardial effusion. Chest 59:341–344, 1971

39. GIBSON TC, GROSSMAN W, MCLAURIN LP, MOOS S, CRAIGE E: An echocardiographic study of the interventricular septum in constrictive pericarditis. Br Heart J 38:738–743, 1976

40. GLASER J, BHARATI S, WHITMAN V, LIEBMAN J: Echocardiographic (EG) findings in patients (pts) with anomalous origin of the left coronary artery (ALCA). Circulation [Suppl] 48 (IV):63, 1973

41. GOLDBERG SJ, ALLEN HD, SAHN DJ: Pediatric and adolescent echocardiography. Chicago, Year Book Medical, 1975

42. GOODMAN DJ, HARRISON DC, POPP RL: Echocardiographic features of primary pulmonary hypertension. Am J Cardiol 39:438–443, 1974

43. GREENE DA, KLEID JJ, NAIDU S: Unusual echocardiographic manifestation of pericardial effusion. Am J Cardiol 39:112–115, 1977

44. GREENWALD J, YAP JF, FRANKLIN M, LICHTMAN AM: Echocardiographic mitral systolic motion in left ventricular aneurysm. Br Heart J 37:684, 1975

45. GRIFFITH JM, HENRY WL: A sector scanning for real-time two dimentional echocardiography. Circulation 49:1147, 1974

46. HENNING H, O'ROURKE RA, CRAWFORD MH, RIGLETTI A, KARLINER JS: Inferior myocardial infarction as a cause of asymmetric septal hypertrophy. An echocardiographic study. Am J Cardiol 41:817–822, 1978

47. HENRY WL, CLARK CE, EPSTEIN SE: Asymmetric septal hypertrophy: echocardiographic identification of the pathognomonic anatomic abnormality of IHSS. Circulation 47:225, 1973

48. HENRY WL, CLARK CE, GLANCY DL, EPSTEIN SE: Echocardiographic measurement of the left ventricular outflow gradient in idiopathic hypertrophic subaortic stenosis. N Engl J Med 288:989, 1973

49. HENRY WL, CLARK CE, ROBERTS WC, MORROW AG, EPSTEIN SE: Differences in distribution of myocardial abnormalities in patients with obstructive and non-obstructive asymmetric septal hypertrophy (ASH): echocardiographic and gross anatomic findings. Circulation 50:447, 1974

50. HENRY WL, GRIFFITH JM, MICHAELIS LL, MCINTOSH CL, MORROW AG, EPSTEIN S: Measurement of mitral valve orifice area in patients with mitral valve disease by real-time echocardiography. Circulation 51:827, 1975

51. HISHIDA H, SOTOBATA I, KOIKE Y, OKUMURA M, MIZUMO Y: Echocardiographic patterns of ventricular contraction in the Wolff-Parkinson-White syndrome. Circulation 54:567–570, 1976

52. HOROWITZ MS, SCHULTZ CS, STINSON EB, HARRISON DC, POPP RL: Sensitivity and specificity of echocardiographic diagnosis of pericardial effusion. Circulation 50:239–247, 1974

53. JOHNSON ML, WARREN SG, WAUGH RA, KISSLO JA, SABISTON DC, LESTER RG: Echocardiography of the aortic valve in non-rheumatic left ventricular outflow tract lesion. Radiology 112:677–684, 1974

54. KATZ R, KARLINER JS, RESNIK R: Effects of a natural volume overload state (pregnancy) on left ventricular performance in normal human subjects. Circulation 58:434, 1978

55. KERBER RE, DIPPEL WF, ABBUND FM: Abnormal motion of the interventricular septum in right ventricular volume overload. Experimental and clinical echocardiographic studies. Circulation 48:86–96, 1973

56. KING D, STEEG C, ELLIS K: Visualization of ventricular septal defect by cardiac ultrasonography. Circulation 48:1215–1220, 1973

57. KITTERMAN JA, EDMUNDS LH, GREGORY GA, HEYMANN MA, TOOLEY WH, RUDOLPH AM: Patent ductus arteriosus in premature infants. Incidence, relation to pulmonary disease and management. N Engl J Med 287:473–477, 1972

58. KOMATSU Y, NAGAI Y, SHIBUYA M, TAKAO A, HIROSAWA K: Echocardiographic analysis of intracardiac anatomy in endocardial cushion defect. Am Heart J 91:210–218, 1976

59. KONECKE LL, FEIGENBAUM H, CHANG S, CORYA BC, FISCHER JC: Abnormal mitral valve motion in patients with elevated left ventricular diastolic pressures. Circulation 47:989–996, 1973

60. KRAJCER Z, ORZAN F, PECHACEK LW, GARCIA E, LEACHMAN RD: Early systolic closure of the aortic valve in patients with hypertrophic subaortic stenosis and discrete subaortic stenosis. Correlation with preoperative and postoperative hemodynamics. Am J Cardiol 41:823–829, 1978

61. KRUEGER SK, STARKE H, FARKER AD, ELIOT RS: Echocardiographic mimics of aortic root dissection. Chest 67:441–444, 1975

62. LEVISMAN JA, ABASSI AS, PEARCE ML: Posterior mitral leaflet motion in mitral stenosis. Circulation 51:511–514, 1975

63. LEWIS JR, PARKER J, BURGGRAF GW: Mitral valve motion and changes in left ventricular end-diastolic pressure: a correlative study of the PR-AC interval. Am J Cardiol 42:383, 1978

64. MCCANN WD, HARBOLD NB JR, GIULIANI ER: The echocardiogram in right ventricular overload. JAMA 221:1243–1245, 1972

65. MCDONALD IG, FEIGENBAUM HA, CHANG S: Analysis of left ventricular wall motion by reflected ultrasound. Application to assessment of myocardial function. Circulation 46:14–25, 1972

66. MARKIEWICZ W, STONER J, LONDON E, HUNT SA, POPP RL: Mitral valve prolapse in one hundred presumably healthy young females. Circulation 53:464–473, 1975

67. MARON BJ, SAVAGE DD, CLARK CE, HENRY WL, VLODAVER Z, EDWARDS JE, EPSTEIN SE: Prevalence and characteristics of disproportionate ventricular septal thickening in patients with coronary artery disease. Circulation 57:250–256, 1978

68. MARON BJ, EDWARDS JE, FERRANS VJ, CLARK CE, LEBOWITZ EA, HENRY WL, EPSTEIN SE: Congenital heart malformation associated with disproportionate ventricular septal thickening. Circulation 52:926, 1975

69. MATSUMATO M: Ultrasonic features of inter-atrial septum: its motion analysis and detection of its defect. Jpn Circ J 37:1383, 1973

70. MEYER RA: Echocardiography in congenital heart disease. Am J Med 63:41–49, 1977

71. MEYER RA, KAPLAN S: Non-invasive techniques in pediatric cardiovascular disease. Prog Cardiovascular Dis 15:350, 1973

72. MEYER RA, SCHWARTZ DC, BENZING G, KAPLAN S: Ventricular septum in right ventricular volume overload. An echocardiographic study. Am J Cardiol 30:349, 1972

73. MEYERS SN, SHAPIRO JE, BARRESI V, DEBOER AA, PAVEL DI, GRACEY DR, SUHRE DE, BUEHLER JH: Right atrial myxoma with right to left shunting and mitral valve prolapse. Am J Med 62:308–314, 1977

74. MINTZ GS, KOTLER MN, SEGAL BL, PARRY WR: Systolic anterior motion of mitral valve in the absence of asymmetric septal hypertrophy. Circulation 57:256–263, 1978

75. NANDA NC: Echocardiography of the aortic root. Am J Med 62:836–842, 1977

76. NANDA NC, GRAMIAK R, GROSS CM: Echocardiography of cardiac valves in pericardial effusion. Circulation 54:500, 1976

77. NANDA NC, GRAMIAK R, MANNING JA, LIPCHIK EO: Echocardiographic features of subpulmonic obstruction in dextroposition of the great vessels. Circulation 51:515, 1975

78. NANDA NC, GRAMIAK R, MANNING J, MAHONEY EB, LIPCHIK EO, DEWEESE JA: Echocardiographic recognition of the congenital bicuspid aortic valve. Circulation 49:870, 1974

79. NANDA NC, GRAMIAK R, ROBINSON TI, SHAH PM: Echocardiographic evaluation of pulmonary hypertension. Circulation 50:575, 1974

80. NANDA NC, GRAMIAK R, SHAH PM: Diagnosis of aortic root dissection by echocardiography. Circulation 48:506–513, 1973

81. NASRALLAH AT, NIHILL M: Supravalvular aortic stenosis. Echocardiographic features. Br Heart J 37:662–667, 1975

82. NASSER WK, DAVIS RH, DILLON JC, TAVEL ME, HELMEN CH, FEIGENBAUM H, FISCH C: Atrial myxoma. II. Phonocardiographic, echocardiographic, hemodynamic and angiographic features in nine cases. Am Heart J 83:810–824, 1972

83. NICHOLSON WJ, COBBS BW JR: Echocardiographic oscillating flap in aortic root dissecting aneurysm. Chest 70:305–307, 1976

84. PAYVANDI MN, KERBER RE: Echocardiography in congenital and acquired absence of the pericardium. An echocardiographic mimic of right ventricular volume overload. Circulation 53:86–92, 1976

85. POMBO JF, TROY BL, RUSSELL RO: Left ventricular volume and ejection fraction by echocardiography. Circulation 43:480–490, 1971

86. POPP RL, BROWN OR, SILVERMAN JF, HARRISON DC: Echocardiographic abnormalities in the mitral valve prolapse syndrome. Circulation 49:428, 1974

87. POPP RL, HARRISON DC: Ultrasound in the diagnosis and evaluation of therapy of idiopathic hypertro-

phic subaortic stenosis. Circulation 40:905–914, 1969

88. POPP RL, HARRISON DC: Ultrasonic cardiac echocardiography for determining stroke volume and valvular regurgitation. Circulation 41:493–502, 1970

89. POPP RL, SILVERMAN JF, FRENCH JW, STINSON EB, HARRISON DC: Echocardiographic findings in discrete subvalvular aortic stenosis. Circulation 49:226–231, 1974

90. POPP RL, WOLFE SB, HIRATA T, FEIGENBAUM H: Extension of right and left ventricular size by ultrasound. A study of the echoes from the interventricular septum. Am J Cardiol 24:523, 1969

91. PRIDIE RB, BENHAM R, OAKLEY CM: Echocardiography of the mitral valve in aortic valve disease. Br Heart J 33:296–304, 1971

92. QUINONES MA, GAASH WH, WAISSER E, ALEXANDER JK: Reduction in the rate of diastolic descent of the mitral valve echocardiogram in patients with altered left ventricular diastolic pressure-valve relations. Circulation 49:246, 1974

93. RADFORD DJ, BLOOM KR, IZUKAWA T, MOES CAF, ROWE RD: Echocardiographic assessment of bicuspid aortic valves. Angiographic and pathological correlations. Circulation 53:80–85, 1976

94. RATSHIN RA, SMITH M, HOOD WP: Possible false-positive diagnosis of pericardial effusion by echocardiography in presence of large left atrium. Chest 65:112–114, 1974

95. ROESKE WR, O'ROURKE RA, KLEIN A, LEOPOLD G, KARLINER JS: Non-invasive evaluation of ventricular hypertrophy in professional athletes. Circulation 53:286–291, 1976

96. ROSENBLATT A, CLARK R, BURGESS J, COHN K: Echocardiographic assessment of the level of cardiac compensation in valvular heart disease. Circulation 54:509–518, 1976

97. ROSSEN RM, GOODMAN DJ, INGHAM RE, POPP RL: Ventricular systolic septal thickening and excursion in idiopathic hypertrophic subaortic stenosis. N Engl J Med 291:1317, 1974

98. ROTHBAUM DA, DILLON JC, CHANG S, FEIGENBAUM H: Echocardiographic manifestations of right sinus of valsalva aneurysm. Circulation 49:768–771, 1974

99. ROY P, TAJIK AJ, GIULIANI ER, SCHATTENBERG TT, GAU GT, FRYE RL: Spectrum of echocardiographic findings in bacterial endocarditis. Circulation 53:474–482, 1976

100. SAHN DJ, ALLEN HD, GOLDBERG SJ, FRIEDMAN WF: Cross-sectional echocardiographic evaluation of mitral prolapse in children. A problem defined by real-time cross-section echocardiography. Circulation 53:651, 1976

101. SAHN DJ, VANEHER Y, WILLIAMS DE, ALLEN HG, GOLDBERG SJ, FRIEDMAN WF: Echocardiographic detection of large left to right shunt and cardiomyopathies in infants and children.

102. SCHILLER NB, BOTVINICK EH: Right ventricular compression as a sign of cardiac tamponade. An analysis of echocardiographic ventricular dimensions and their clinical implication. Circulation 56:774–776, 1977

103. SCHNITTGER I, BOWDEN RE, ABRAMS J, POPP RL: Echocardiography: pericardial thickening and constrictive pericarditis. Am J Cardiol 42:388–395, 1978

104. SHAH PM, GRAMIAK R, ADELMAN AG, WIGLE ED: Echocardiographic assessment of the effects of surgery and propanolol on the diagnosis of outflow obstruction in hypertrophic subaortic stenosis. Circulation 45:516–521, 1972

105. SILVERMAN NH, LEWIS AB, HEYMANN MA, RUDOLPH AM: Echocardiographic assessment of ductus arteriosus shunt in premature infants. Circulation 50:821–825, 1974

106. STRUNK BL, LONDON EJ, FITZGERALD J, POPP RL, BARRY WH: The assessment of mitral stenosis and prosthetic mitral valve obstruction, using the posterior aortic wall echocardiogram. Circulation 55:885–891, 1977

107. SWEATMAN T, SELZER A, KAMAGAKI M, COHN L: Echocardiographic diagnosis of mitral regurgitation due to ruptured chordae tendineae. Circulation 46:580–586, 1972

108. TAJIK AJ: Echocardiography in pericardial effusion. Am J Med 63:29–40, 1977

109. TAJIK AJ, GAU GT, SCHATTENBERG TT: Echocardiographic "pseudo-IHSS" pattern in atrial septal defect. Chest 62:324, 1972

110. TEICHHOLZ LE, KRUELEN T, HERMAN MV, GORLIN R: Problems in echocardiographic volume determination: echocardiographic-angiographic correlation in the presence or absence of asynergy. Am J Cardiol 37:7–11, 1976

111. THIBEAULT DW, EMMANOUILIDES GC, NELSON RJ, LACHMAN RS, ROSENGART RM, OH W: Patent ductus arteriosus complicating the respiratory distress in preterm infants. J Pediatr 86:120–126, 1975

112. VIGNOLA PA, POHOST GM, CURFMAN GD, MYERS AS: Correlations of echocardiographic and clinical findings in patients with pericardial effusion. Am J Cardiol 37:701–707, 1976

113. VIGNOLA PA, WALKER HJ, GOLD HK, LEIMBACH RC: Alteration of the left ventricular pressure-volume relationship in man and the effect on the mitral echocardiographic early diastolic closure slope. Circulation 56:586–592, 1977

114. VON RAMM OT, THURSTINE FL: Cardiac imaging using a phased-array ultrasound system. Circulation 53:258, 1976

115. WANN LS, DILLON JC, WEYMAN AE, FEIGENBAUM H: Echocardiography in bacterial endocarditis. N Engl J Med 295:135, 1976

116. WEYMAN AE, DILLON JC, FEIGENBAUM H, CHANG S: Echocardiographic pattern of pulmonic valve mo-

tion with pulmonary hypertension. Circulation 50:905–910, 1974

117. WEYMAN AE, DILLON JC, FEIGENBAUM H, CHANG S: Echocardiographic differentiation of infundibular from valvular pulmonary stenosis. Am J Cardiol 36:21–26, 1975

118. WEYMAN AE, FEIGENBAUM H, DILLON JC, CHANG S: Cross-sectional echocardiography in assessing the severity of valvular aortic stenosis. Circulation 52:828, 1975

119. WEYMAN AE, WANN LS, FEIGENBAUM H, DILLON JC: Mechanism of abnormal septal motion in patients with right ventricular volume overload. A cross-sectional echocardiographic study. Circulation 54:179–186, 1976

120. WRAY TM: Echocardiographic manifestation of flail aortic valve leaflets in bacterial endocarditis. Circulation 51:832–835, 1975

121. YOSHIKAWA J, TANAKA K, OWAKI T, KATO H: Cord-like aortic valve vegetation in bacterial endocarditis. Demonstration by cardiac ultrasonography. Report of a case. Circulation 53:911–914, 1976

122. YOW MV, REICHEK N: Left ventricular end-diastolic pressure and echocardiographic mitral valve closure. Circulation [Suppl] (II):51, 1975

123. ZAKY A, NASSER WK, FEIGENBAUM H: Study of mitral valve action recorded by ultrasound and its application in the diagnosis of mitral stenosis. Circulation 37:789, 1968

28

A biophysical profile of the human fetus

LAWRENCE D. PLATT, FRANK A. MANNING

The wide spectrum of uses of ultrasound imaging has been exemplified by the variety of topics covered in this text. Most uses have assessed events that change over relatively long periods of time, such as biparietal diameter, fetal weight, other fetal measurements, and congenital anomalies. It has only recently been possible to assess accurately biophysical gauges of fetal condition based on short time constants, such as fetal breathing movements (FBM), fetal movements (FM), and fetal heart rate (FHR). The advent of dynamic ultrasound imaging, and in particular real-time B scanning, has allowed the perinatal physiologist and obstetrician to evaluate these functions more accurately. Chapter 18 in this text has given us an understanding of the physiology of fetal breathing movements and their clinical significance. It is apparent from Chapter 18 that we are at the beginning of an era of physical diagnosis of the human fetus. This chapter explores the information regarding evaluation of FBM, and incorporates the relationship of other biophysical variables in the overall assessment of fetal condition.

THE ASSESSMENT OF FETAL BREATHING MOVEMENTS

The assessment of FBM has become an integral part of the research in evaluating fetal condition.

Various methods have been used to evaluate FBM, and controversy exists at present regarding the best method. It is generally accepted that the A scan produces many artifactual "movements" and is thus an unreliable method of recording FBM (2). Limited studies have been done using M-mode ultrasound. Some centers (1, 8) are investigating the Doppler ultrasound method because of its ability to provide adequate signal recording which can later be used to analyze the results. We believe that real-time B-scan ultrasound (RTBS) is the most reliable method for direct observation of the fetal chest wall movements (10). Most centers have used the cathode ray tube (CRT) display to demonstrate FBM and indicate these movements by means of an event marker. These events are recorded on a tape recorder or strip chart for later analysis. A method described by Marsal et al, which utilizes a time–distance gating system to record FBM, has met with only limited success (9). We have explored a similar method (3) but it also has proved to be of limited value. In spite of the less than ideal recording method, we have utilized RTBS to assess FBM in our laboratory, using the event marker technique, and found it useful. Because of our earlier observations and because of limitations in the technique we merely assessed the presence or absence of FBM in 30-min periods. This approach differs from those used in previous studies which attempted to define the incidence of occurrence of FBM in a given observation period. This design has permitted a simpler approach in an attempt to evaluate the clinical significance of such observations.

THE DEVELOPMENT OF A CLINICAL TEST

The observed relationship between FBM and fetal condition in the animal model prompted us to evaluate this relationship in the human. Prior to the initiation of these studies, it became apparent that in order for a test to be used clinically certain criteria had to be met: the test must be simple to perform, must be easily reproducible, and must be performed in a short period of time. The first two criteria are met by utilizing the real-time method. The last criterion must be satisfied arbitrarily. We selected a 30-min maximum observation period, recognizing that this is likely not to be representative of every aspect of fetal-state cycles. In addition, factors which are known to affect FBM must be considered. For this reason we standardized the testing protocol, which 1) excluded patients' smoking prior to the test period, 2) required a rest period prior to the testing, and 3) required observing patients in the same physical position (semi-Fowler's).

FETAL BREATHING MOVEMENTS AND FETAL CONDITION

In our initial study of 134 pregnancies (136 fetuses) we evaluated the presence or absence of FBM during the last observation before delivery and their relationship to the outcome of pregnancy (10). Using the real-time method, FBM were present in 116 fetuses and absent in 20. The incidence of fetal distress during labor was significantly higher in fetuses with breathing movements absent, then in those with FBM. A similar relationship was found between a high and a low 5-min Apgar score (<7 or ≧7). Initial studies suggested that the mere presence or FBM reflects fetal health and that it was unnecessary to determine the time during which FBM occurred. The data also indicated that the presence of FBM was better as a predictor of fetal health than the absence of FBM was as a predictor of fetal compromise. Nevertheless, while the re-

sults were most encouraging, it became apparent that using FBM alone produced the same high rate of both false-positive and false-negative results as other antepartum tests did and thus, as a test alone, FBM would be unacceptable in clinical practice.

In our next series of studies we began looking at the association between FBM and the nonstress test (NST) (5), a standard test used to assess fetal condition. This test is based on the association of fetal heart rate acceleration with fetal movements (11). In 398 observations in 223 patients we found that the NST was reactive more often when FBM were present (80%) than when FBM were absent (49%). When these tests were looked at in combination, additional information was gained. We found that when both of the tests were normal, ie the NST was reactive and FBM were present, a low 5-min Apgar score was unlikely. Similarly, when both tests were abnormal, the incidence of low 5-min scores (45.5%) was significantly greater than when either test alone was abnormal (16.3% when NSTs were nonreactive; 25% when FBM were absent). These relationships also held for the incidence of fetal distress during labor.

From our review of these data, certain concepts developed. It is evident that a normal FBM test may be used as a screening test for the normal fetus. However, an abnormal test does not allow one to draw the opposite conclusion because of the high false-positive rate of single FBM tests. Therefore, it became clear that combining different tests gives one a more accurate identification of the fetus at risk. Thus, for example, the absence of FBM is associated with a low 5-min Apgar score in 25% of cases; when the NST is abnormal, ie, nonreactive, the low Apgar now occurs 45.5% of the time, and when a contraction stress test is also abnormal this incidence approaches 100%, within our limited experience (4).

With these encouraging results we began to consider the predictive value of other physiologic functions of the fetus.

FETAL MOVEMENTS AND FETAL BREATHING MOVEMENTS

Sadovsky and Yaffe first suggested that monitoring fetal movements (FM) during pregnancy may be a useful means of identifying fetuses at risk for antepartum demise (13). Since then, other reports have appeared supporting this work (12, 14). In an attempt to evaluate these observations we studied FM in the last week of 50 pregnancies, using RTBS (7). When at least one fetal movement was present in a 20-min observation period before delivery, 93% of the infants (43/46) had 5-min Apgar scores of 7 or greater. In three others the 5-min Apgar score was less than 7. FBM were present in two of these infants, both of whom died in utero, one following decompression of hydrocephaly and the other following an episode of diabetic ketoacidosis in the mother. FBM were absent in the third, also decompressed, infant (with a 5-min Apgar score of 4).

No FM were observed in four fetuses. Three of these four died in utero; FBM were also absent in each of these fetuses. In the remaining fetus with no FM, FBM were present. In this case the NST was nonreactive and the contraction stress test was positive. The patient delivered a nondepressed infant following induction of labor. This small study has confirmed the usefulness of monitoring fetal movements in late pregnancy.

ASSESSMENT OF OTHER BIOPHYSICAL VARIABLES

The interest in combining tests led us to evaluate two other biophysical variables as possible aids in assessing fetal condition: 1) fetal tone and 2) amniotic fluid volume (AFV). Tone, a component of the Apgar score, was judged to be either normal or decreased—normal if the fetus was in a position of full flexion in the upper and lower extremities, and the trunk was in a state of flexion, with the head flexed upon the chest. Also, during the observation period, at least one episode of extension of the extremities or spine had to be observed with a rapid recoil to the original position. If only a partial recoil was seen during this period or if fetal movement was not followed by a return to a flexed position, fetal tone was said to be decreased. AFV was assessed as a reflection of the fetal intrauterine environment. Oligohydramnios, a hallmark of the growth-retarded fetus and the fetus at risk, can be detected by using RTBS screening. Thus, AFV was

judged normal when fluid was evident throughout the uterine cavity and when greater than 1-cm fluid pockets were seen in all vertical axes. When these criteria were not met, and when fetal crowding was present, AFV was considered to be decreased. Results using these additional individual variables have proved to be useful.

EVOLUTION OF A SCORING SYSTEM

Much of what has been applied and accepted in the assessment of the adult patient or the newborn can now be applied to the fetus. If one were to use only a single abnormal test as the basis of management in the adult, an erroneous conclusion might be drawn. Thus, for example, if one applied a stimulus to an adult, such as a loud noise, and if no response was elicited, a number of conditions might exist: the patient might be deaf, asleep, comatose, or dead. To differentiate these states, and to make a valid diagnosis, one would necessarily have to evaluate other variables. It therefore seems reasonable to apply a similar conceptual approach in evaluating the human fetus. In this regard we have developed a method of simultaneously assessing multiple fetal variables (FBM, FM, FT, AFV, NST), utilizing dynamic ultrasound imaging.

In a pilot study (6) we have devised a scoring system (planning score), assigning scores to these five biophysical parameters. Observations were made in 216 high-risk patients in the third trimester of pregnancy (mean gestational age 38.7 ± 1 week). All observations were made within one week of delivery. An arbitrary value of 2 was given for each normal observation, with a 0 for each abnormal variable (lowest and highest possible scores, 0 and 10).

An inverse relationship between the planning score and the outcome of pregnancy was observed (Figs. 28–1 through 28–4). In fetuses with a score of 10 (ie, with five normal variables), the incidence of low 5-min Apgar scores was less than 2% (N = 119); the incidence of fetal distress during labor was less than 4% (N = 102) and the perinatal mortality rate was 0 (N = 119). Conversely, when the planning score was 0, the incidence of low 5-min Apgar scores was 80% (N = 5); the incidence of fetal distress during labor was 100% (N = 5) and the perinatal mortality rate was 600/1000 (N = 5). These differences are

(*Text continues on p. 420*)

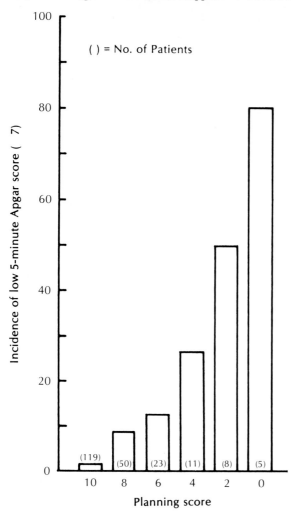

FIG. 28–1. The relationship of a fetal biophysical variable score (planning score) to the incidence of low 5-min Apgar scores. A 47-fold increase in the incidence of low Apgar scores is observed between a planning score of 10 (all normal) and a planning score of 0 (all abnormal). (Manning FA et al: Am J Obstet Gynecol, CV Mosby Company, in press.)

FIG. 28–2. The relationship of a fetal biophysical variable score (planning score) to the incidence of fetal distress in labor. A 37.5-fold increase in the incidence of fetal distress was observed between a planning score of 10 (all normal) and one of 0 (all abnormal). (Manning FA et al: Am J Obstet Gynecol, CV Mosby Company, in press)

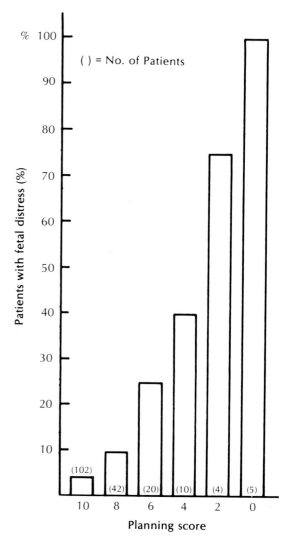

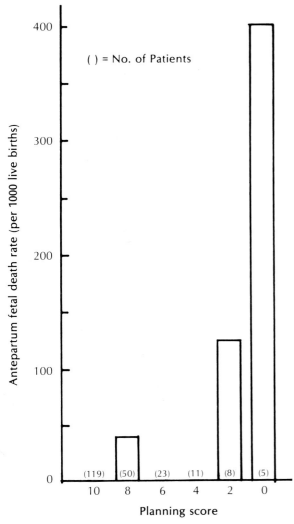

FIG. 28-3. The relationship between a fetal biophysical variable score (planning score) and the incidence of antepartum fetal death. (Manning FA et al: Am J Obstet Gynecol. CV Mosby Company, in press)

FIG. 28-4. The relationship of a fetal biophysical variable score (planning score) to perinatal mortality. (Manning FA et al: Am J Obstet Gynecol, CV Mosby Company, in press)

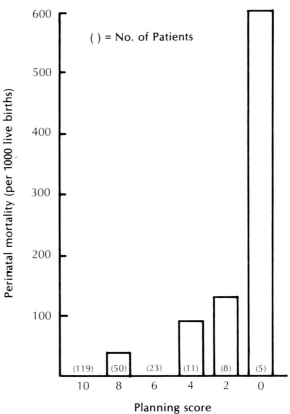

highly significant ($p < 0.001$). While these examples are at the extremes of the scoring system, significant relationships also hold for the intermediate scores as well.

CONCLUSIONS

Antepartum assessment of fetal risk based on these five biophysical variables has become an attractive method of evaluation for a variety of reasons. First, the results can be obtained both rapidly and without difficulty. Second, the assessments are independent of gestational age, and thus are related directly to the fetus being tested. Finally, these procedures are noninvasive and cause no known danger to the intrauterine environment. Combining the individual tests into a profile score has yielded the most discriminating method of identifying both the normal and the compromised fetus.

REFERENCES

1. BOYCE ES, DAWES GS, GOUGH JD, POOR ER: Doppler ultrasound method for detecting human fetal breathing in utero. Br Med J 2:17, 1976

2. FORMAN DJ, THOMAS G, BLACKWELL RJ: Errors and artifacts encountered in the monitoring of fetal respiratory movements using ultrasound. Ultrasound Med Biol 2:1, 1975

3. HON E, JILIK J, MANNING FA, PLATT LD: Unpublished data

4. MANNING FA, PLATT LD: Fetal breathing movements and the abnormal contraction stress test. Am J Obstet Gynecol 133:590, 1979

5. MANNING FA, PLATT LD, KEEGAN KA, SIPOS L: Fetal breathing movements and the non-stress test in high risk pregnancies. Am J Obstet Gynecol (in press)

6. MANNING FA, PLATT LD, SIPOS L: Antepartum fetal evaluation: development of a fetal biophysical profile. Am J Obstet Gynecol (in press)

7. MANNING FA, PLATT LD, SIPOS L: Fetal movements in human pregnancy in the third trimester. Obstet Gynecol (in press)

8. MANTELL C: The Auckland versus the Oxford Sound. Proc Sixth Annual Fetal Breathing Meeting, Paris, France, May 1979

9. MARSAL K, ULMSTEN V, LINDSTROM K: Device for measurement of fetal breathing movements. II. Accuracy of in vitro measurements, filtering of output signals and clinical application. Ultrasound Med Biol 4:1, 1979

10. PLATT LD, MANNING FA, LEMAY M, SIPOS L: Human fetal breathing—relationship to fetal condition. Am J Obstet Gynecol 132:906, 1978

11. ROCHARD F, SCHIFRIN BS, SUREAU C, et al: Non-stress cardiotachymetry for antepartum fetal evaluation. Obstet Gynecol 45:433, 1975

12. SADOVSKY E, POLISHOK WZ: Fetal movements in utero: nature, assessment, prognostic value, timing of delivery. Obstet Gynecol 50:49, 1977

13. SADOVSKY E, YAFFE M: Daily fetal movement recording and fetal diagnosis. Obstet Gynecol 41:845, 1973

14. SPELLACY WN, CRUZ AC, GELMAN SR, BUM WC: Fetal movements and placental lactogen levels for fetal-placental evaluation. A preliminary report. Obstet Gynecol 49:113, 1977

Index

Numerials in *italics* indicate a figure; "t" following a page number indicates a table.

421